COMMUNICATION ASSESSMENT AND INTERVENTION STRATEGIES

COMMUNICATION ASSESSMENT AND INTERVENTION STRATEGIES

Edited by

Lyle L. Lloyd, Ph.D.

Chairman and Professor
Special Education Section
Department of Education
and
Professor
Department of Audiology and Speech Sciences
Purdue University

University Park Press
Baltimore • London • Tokyo

UNIVERSITY PARK PRESS
International Publishers in Science and Medicine
Chamber of Commerce Building
Baltimore, Maryland 21202
Copyright © 1976 by University Park Press
Second printing, December 1977
Typeset by Service Composition Co.
Manufactured in the United States of America by
Universal Lithographers, Inc., and The Maple Press Co.

Library of Congress Cataloging in Publication Data

Main entry under title:

Communication assessment and intervention strategies.

Includes bibliographical references and indexes.
1. Communicative disorders in children. 2. Mentally
handicapped children—Language. 3. Hearing disorders
in children. I. Lloyd, Lyle L. [DNLM: 1. Hearing
disorders—Rehabilitation. 2. Speech disorders—
Rehabilitation. 3. Hearing disorders—In infancy
and childhood. 4. Speech disorders—In infancy and
childhood. 5. Communication—In infancy and childhood.
6. Mental retardation. [WV270 C734]
RJ496.C67C65   618.9'28'55   76-16141

ISBN 0-8391-0758-7

University Park Press would like to thank the following people for providing symbols

used on the jacket: Charlotte Clark: ʒ 𝄞 (manual sign for "communication"),

♫ (rebus symbol; American Guidance Service), and Ô (Bliss symbol for "talk" or "say");

Deberah Harris-Vanderheiden: ↓ₓ↑ (Bliss symbol representation for "exchange of

ideas"); and John Hollis: ⊓ , ⊏ , ♡ and ⌇ , 🐾 , ⇶

(Non-SLIP and Signing Exact English, respectively, for "the," "girl," and "on").

"Communication" is represented in T. O., fingerspelling, i. t. a. (cummʉenicæʃhon),
IPA (kəmjunəkeɪʃən), DMS (cummūnicătjon), UNIFON (KUMƱNƗKΔ8UN),

Fōnetic English (cumūnicāshun), Chinese (諮大), and Japanese kanji (伝達). The sound

spectrogram for "sauce" is taken from *Phonetics: Principles and Practices* (by S. Singh
and K. Singh,© 1976 by University Park Press).

CONTENTS

Contributors _____ vii

Preface _____ xi

1   A Model for Communication _____ 1
    Derek A. Sanders

2   Definitions and Prevalence _____ 33
    Gerard J. Bensberg and Carol K. Sigelman

3   Language Assessment _____ 73
    Gerald M. Siegel and Patricia A. Broen

4   Audiologic Considerations _____ 123
    B. Patrick Cox and Lyle L. Lloyd

5   Psychologic Evaluation of Hearing-Impaired Children ___ 195
    McCay Vernon

6   Behavior Analysis, Behavior Modification, and
    Developmental Disabilities _____ 225
    Joseph E. Spradlin, George R. Karlan,
    and Bruce Wetherby

7   An Approach to Remediation of Communication and
    Learning Deficiencies _____ 265
    John H. Hollis, Joseph K. Carrier, Jr.,
    and Joseph E. Spradlin

8   Amplification Systems _____ 295
    Mark Ross

9   Articulation _____ 325
    James E. McLean

10 Language Programming and Intervention _____ 371
    Louella W. Graham

11 The Linguistics of Manual Languages and
    Manual Systems _____ 423
    Ronnie Bring Wilbur

12 Total Communication for the Severely Language
    Impaired: A 24-Hour Approach _____ 501
    George A. Kopchick and Lyle L. Lloyd

**13 Application of a Nonspeech Language System with the
Severely Language Handicapped** _____ 523
Joseph K. Carrier

14 Graphic Systems of Communication _____ 549
Charlotte R. Clark and Richard W. Woodcock

**15 Communication Techniques and Aids for the
Nonvocal Severely Handicapped** _____ 607
Gregg C. Vanderheiden and
Deberah Harris-Vanderheiden

16 Supportive Personnel for the Developmentally Disabled _____ 653
Carol K. Sigelman and Gerard J. Bensberg

**17 Parent Involvement in Programming for
Developmentally Disabled Children** _____ 691
Bruce L. Baker

18 Audiovisual Media and Materials _____ 735
Sebastian Striefel, Richard Baer, and Vonda Douglass

Appendices _____ 775

Appendix A/**Language Assessment Procedures** _____ 777
Anthony Cicciarelli, Patricia A. Broen,
and Gerald M. Siegel

Appendix B/**International Phonetic Association (IPA)
Alphabet Pronunciation Key** _____ 801

Appendix C/**Standards for Speech Pathology
and Audiology Services** _____ 803

Appendix D/**Language Intervention Systems:
Programs Published in Kit Form** _____ 813
Macalyne Fristoe

Appendix E/**Rules of Talking** _____ 861

Appendix F/**A Functional or Basic Vocabulary** _____ 863

Appendix G/**Audiovisual Information Sources** _____ 867

Author Index _____ 873
Subject Index _____ 894

CONTRIBUTORS

Richard Baer, M.A., Psychologist, University Affiliated Exceptional Child Center, Utah State University, Logan, Utah 84322

Bruce L. Baker, Ph.D., Associate Professor, Department of Psychology, University of California, Los Angeles, California 90024

Gerard J. Bensberg, Ph.D., Director, Research and Training Center in Mental Retardation; Professor, Departments of Special Education and Psychology; and Clinical Professor, Department of Psychiatry, Texas Tech University, Lubbock, Texas 79409

Patricia A. Broen, Ph.D., Assistant Professor and Director of Clinical Training, Department of Communication Disorders, University of Minnesota, Minneapolis, Minnesota 55455

Joseph K. Carrier, Jr., Ph.D., Language Consultant, 208 East Oak, Fort Collins, Colorado 80521

Anthony Cicciarelli, M.A., Doctoral Student, Department of Communication Disorders, University of Minnesota, Minneapolis, Minnesota 55455

Charlotte R. Clark, M.A., Research Associate, Research, Development, and Demonstration Center in Education of Handicapped Children, University of Minnesota, Minneapolis, Minnesota 55455

B. Patrick Cox, Ph.D., Assistant Professor in Pediatrics, and Director, Division of Communication Disorders, University Affiliated Program for Child Development, Georgetown University Hospital, Washington, D.C. 20007

Vonda Douglass, M.S., Coordinator of Speech and Hearing Services, University Affiliated Exceptional Child Center, Utah State University, Logan, Utah 84322

Macalyne Fristoe, Ph.D., Director, Speech Clinic, and Associate Professor, Department of Audiology and Speech Sciences, Purdue University, West Lafayette, Indiana 47907

Louella W. Graham, Ph.D., Program Unit Director, Georgia Retardation Center, 4770 North Peachtree Road, Atlanta, Georgia 30341; Assistant Professor, Communicative Disorders, Emory University, Atlanta, Georgia 30322

Deberah Harris-Vanderheiden, M.S., Area Coordinator, Communication Research and Clinical Services, Trace Research and Development Center for the Severely Communicatively Handicapped, University of Wisconsin, Madison, Wisconsin 53706

John H. Hollis, Ed.D., Research Associate, Bureau of Child Research and Department of Human Development, University of Kansas, Lawrence, Kansas 66045; Research Psychologist, Kansas Neurological Institute, Topeka, Kansas 66604

George R. Karlan, M.A., Bureau of Child Research and Department of Human Development, University of Kansas, Lawrence, Kansas 66045

George A. Kopchick, Jr., M.A., Program Director, Rosewood Center, Owings Mills, Maryland 21117

Lyle L. Lloyd, Ph.D., Chairman and Professor, Special Education Section, and Professor, Department of Audiology and Speech Sciences, Purdue University, West Lafayette, Indiana 47907

James E. McLean, Ph.D., Research Associate, Bureau of Child Research, University of Kansas, Parsons State Hospital and Training Center, Parsons, Kansas 67357

Mark Ross, Ph.D., Professor of Audiology, Department of Speech, University of Connecticut, Storrs, Connecticut 06268

Derek A. Sanders, Ph.D., Professor, Director of Audiology Studies, Division of Communicative Disorders and Sciences, Department of Speech Communication, State University of New York, Buffalo, New York 14226

Gerald M. Siegel, Ph.D., Professor, Department of Communication Disorders, and Member, Center for Research in Human Learning, University of Minnesota, Minneapolis, Minnesota 55455

Carol K. Sigelman, Ph.D., Director of Research, Research and Training Center in Mental Retardation, and Adjunct Assistant Professor, Department of Psychology, Texas Tech University, Lubbock, Texas 79409

Joseph E. Spradlin, Ph.D., Bureau of Child Research and Department of Human Development, University of Kansas, Lawrence, Kansas 66045

Sebastian Striefel, Ph.D., Director, Division of Services, University Affiliated Exceptional Child Center, and Psychology Department, Utah State University, Logan, Utah 84322

Gregg C. Vanderheiden, M.S., Director, Trace Research and Development Center for the Severely Communicatively Handicapped, University of Wisconsin, Madison, Wisconsin 53706

McCay Vernon, Ph.D., Professor, Department of Psychology, Western Maryland College, Westminster, Maryland 21157

Bruce Wetherby, M.A., Bureau of Child Research and Department of Human Development, University of Kansas, Lawrence, Kansas 66045

Ronnie Bring Wilbur, Ph.D., Assistant Professor, School of Education, Boston University, Boston, Massachusetts 02215

Richard W. Woodcock, Ed.D., Measurement Learning Consultants, 920 North Lexington Avenue, Circle Pines, Minnesota 55014

PREFACE

The most pervasive problems resulting from hearing impairment, mental retardation, and other developmental disabilities lie in the area of communication. The exact nature of these problems varies considerably according to the disability and the individual. The problems have no single solution. This book therefore has been developed to provide clinicians, teachers, and professionals-in-training with basic information covering a wide variety of assessment and intervention strategies necessary to modify and alleviate the communication problems of children with developmental disabilities.

The book is basically noncategorical. Many chapters use the communication problems of the hearing impaired and mentally retarded as exemplars because sensory input and cognitive limitations are the primary cause of communication disorders. However, in most cases these approaches can be generalized for use with persons whose communication problems originate from other causes.

The book is designed around a reciprocal and multichanneled approach to communication. By using this approach, the book capitalizes on the best of linguistic theory and operant technology rather than simply representing a single polar position. Such an approach also provides a framework for using all communication modes. Whereas other books tend to stress the speech aspects of language and communication, this volume provides a balance by including several nonspeech approaches. Human communication, both in its development and in its everyday use, is primarily based on the aural input and oral output channels. With most communication-disordered children, the aural-oral channels may be used for remedial purposes, exclusively or at least primarily. However, the normal development of language and communication skills also is based on other input and output channels. These other channels play a critical, and in some cases, primary, role in remedial programming for some communication-disordered children. The more severely impaired the individual, the more likely the need for the clinician to supplement the aural-oral channel.

The role of various communication channels is discussed by Sanders in the first chapter. Sanders presents a reciprocal and multichanneled model of communication that provides a broad framework for the assessment and intervention strategies presented in subsequent chapters.

The second chapter (Bensberg and Sigelman) presents information on the etiology, definition, incidence, and prevalence of communication disorders relative to the broad area of developmental disabilities. These topics have engendered much confusion, which the chapter clarifies. Three other chapters (Cox and Lloyd; Ross; and Vernon) also focus on hearing impairment. However, the book does not emphasize etiologic categorization but primarily provides noncategorical assessment and intervention strategies.

The three chapters focusing on hearing impairment are included in a generic text on communication disorders for several reasons. Although hearing impairment usually results in a communication problem of some type, and a high prevalence of hearing impairment exists among the developmentally disabled regardless of etiology, most books on language, speech pathology, and communication disorders provide little or no information on the topic. Therefore, the three chapters are included to provide a broader coverage of assessment and intervention strategies.

All communicatively impaired persons should have the benefit of at least an audiometric screening if not a comprehensive audiologic assessment. The Cox and Lloyd chapter provides an overview of such procedures for clinicians and teachers who may lack extensive training in audiology. Similarly, the Vernon chapter considers special problems encountered in psychologic evaluation and test interpretation in instances where the client has a language or other communication problem, specifically one caused by hearing impairment. The basic considerations of this chapter, however, can be generalized to other communicatively impaired individuals.

Because clinical and classroom services for the majority of hearing-impaired children are provided by individuals who lack extensive training in audiology and/or education of the hearing impaired, information on aural habilitation (Cox and Lloyd) and amplification systems (Ross) is presented. Ross avoids relying on technical jargon and explains hearing aids and auditory training equipment in practical terms. He also provides information to facilitate the maximum use of aural input.

Siegel and Broen present a major chapter on the theoretical and applied considerations in language assessment without being limited to commercially available tests. This chapter is supplemented by an extensive appendix (by Cicciarelli, Broen, and Siegel) that provides abstracts of available language assessment procedures.

Although a considerable amount of literature on behavior analysis and modification is already available, the chapter by Spradlin, Karlan, and Wetherby provides clinicians and teachers with the most current thinking on this topic, with specific reference to the assessment and remediation of communication disorders. This is followed by a bridging chapter by Hollis, Carrier, and Spradlin which presents a noncategorical approach to remediation based on the integration of the functional analysis of behavior (involving four basic components: stimulus, response, contingency, and reinforcement) and Osgood's input-integration-output model (which also can be related to Sanders' communication model).

The chapter on articulation (McLean) focuses on the more severely impaired, in part because previous writers on articulation have paid little attention to this end of the continuum. However, the basic considerations and approaches presented can be generalized to the less severely impaired.

Graham provides an integrative chapter on a variety of language intervention strategies. This chapter is supplemented by an appendix containing Fristoe's report of her national survey and the summary of 39 language intervention systems published in kit form.

The following five chapters emphasizing nonspeech systems are unique in a broad book on communication disorders. Wilbur's chapter provides a comprehensive discussion of the linguistics of manual languages (e.g., Ameslan) and the pedagogical manual systems (e.g., Signed English). In recent years these communication systems used by and/or developed for use with the hearing impaired also have become the basis of an important new intervention strategy for the severely language impaired without significant hearing impairment. The chapter by Kopchick and Lloyd presents a practical application of this strategy.

Additional nonspeech communication systems that may be used as augmentative and/or complementary modes of communication are discussed in the next three chapters. Carrier presents the practical application of the Non-Speech Language Initiation Program (Non-SLIP), based on the plastic symbol system developed by Premack in his work with the chimpanzee Sarah. Vanderheiden and Harris-Vanderheiden provide a comprehensive overview of communication techniques and aids for the nonvocal severely physically handicapped.

To round out the consideration of nonspeech communication, the chapter by Clark and Woodcock acquaints clinicians and teachers with the wide variety of graphic systems used in reading that may be employed in developing communication intervention strategies.

Another special feature of this volume is the inclusion of chapters on the uses of supportive personnel (Sigelman and Bensberg), parent involvement (Baker), and audiovisual aids (Striefel, Baer, and Douglass). These often overlooked resources seem critical to optimal intervention programming.

Because no single volume can provide an exhaustive coverage of the many facets of intervention programming, each chapter is extensively referenced to guide clinicians and teachers to additional information. Because of the large number of citations and references, this book has an author index in addition to the usual subject index to increase its use as an authoritative reference volume. In addition, appendices are included as practical resources. Besides the two previously mentioned appendices, the IPA pronunciation key is provided to assist persons not familiar with the International Phonetic Association alphabet, which is used occasionally in this book as a useful notation system for describing spoken communication. This appendix also functions as a convenient reference for those trained in IPA transcription but who do not use it every day.

Since many readers have as their major goal improvement of services, the Accreditation Council for Facilities for the Mentally Retarded (AC/

FMR) Standards for Speech Pathology and Audiology Services are included in an appendix as a handy reference. The "Rules of Talking," from the Bill Wilkerson Hearing and Speech Center, are reprinted as an outstanding example of specific suggestions to improve language development. An example of a functional or basic vocabulary, an important consideration in many intervention programs, is provided in another appendix. Because many clinicians are just beginning to use audiovisual materials, sources of audiovisual information are provided in the concluding appendix.

The wide range of contributors to this volume—audiologists, linguists, psychologists, special educators, and speech pathologists—provides a broad and integrative approach to the remediation of communication disorders. However, technical terms and jargon may vary considerably when used by professionals from different fields. This volume therefore is edited to make the usage of technical language as consistent as possible without sacrificing meaning or creativity. For example, although the jargon in some fields continues to use the redundant suffix in terms such as *audiological, morphological, phonological,* and *psychological,* this volume consistently uses the shorter suffix, as in *audiologic,* which is emerging more often in the literature. Other examples of editing to make the language more consistent from chapter to chapter include the use of *caregiver* instead of *caretaker, multiply handicapped* rather than *multihandicapped,* and *hearing impaired* in place of *hard of hearing.*

The remediation of severe communication problems is never a simple task. It is hoped that the thoughts and information presented in this volume will prove a significant aid to clinicians and teachers who seek to alleviate these problems.

Lyle L. Lloyd

to M

COMMUNICATION ASSESSMENT AND INTERVENTION STRATEGIES

1

A MODEL FOR COMMUNICATION

Derek A. Sanders

CONTENTS

Communication as Adaptive Behavior _____ 3

Origin of Communication Needs _____ 4
  Maturational influences/5
  Development adaptation/6
  Environmental influences/8

Nature and Role of Stimulus in Communication _____ 10

Equivalence of Stimulus Patterns _____ 11

Channels of Interaction between the Individual
  and the Environment _____ 14
  Encoding and transmitting patterned information/15
  Monitoring the transmission process/19

Environment _____ 22

Receiving and Decoding Patterned Information _____ 23

Summary _____ 28

References _____ 29

This book is primarily concerned with preventing or ameliorating a disruption of the process of communication that arises from any one of several causes. Each writer focuses expertise on a particular aspect of the problem. Together, these specialists represent the various facets of the task of offering professional advice and of providing for intervention in the communicative behavior of a person experiencing speech and language problems.

While the task at times may seem awesome, it is encouraging to realize how rapidly our capacity to help these individuals has grown. There is cause for optimism, for, although human communication is an enormously complex process and its disturbances are confounding, much progress has been made toward unraveling the critical elements of its operation. It would be foolish to suggest that all the intricacies of the process are known; indeed, a detailed understanding of these may never be achieved. However, enough is known to permit the construction of theoretical models based upon research findings, empirical data, and reasoning. Theoretical models, if well conceived, can be very helpful. They provide a perspective from which to examine the problem; they facilitate the integration of the increasing knowledge of the various aspects of the process; and they provide a basis for the planning of intervention strategies.

This chapter presents one way of looking at communication. It is hoped that this approach will contribute to the understanding and integration of the information in subsequent chapters.

COMMUNICATION AS ADAPTIVE BEHAVIOR

This text is intended to provide a resource to assist in planning an intervention program aimed at improving the communicative effectiveness of persons whose communication ability is impaired. The assumption is made that the role of positive intervention in the management of the communicatively handicapped person is to seek improvement in adaptive behavior. The need for adaptive behavior arises because of the constant change in the patterns of relationship between the individual and the individual's environment. These changes motivate the human organism to enter into a transactional relationship with its environment. In order to survive, living organisms must adapt to changes in demands originating from their physical environment. Because humans have evolved to a very high level of socialization, their progress, if not their existence, has also become dependent upon the ability to adapt to demands generated by society. It is communication that makes societal adaptation possible. Through the function of the language system, it not only permits humans to adapt to their environment, but also to exert control over it.

Human communication, therefore, first must be viewed within its broadest sense, as an outgrowth of all forms of controlled interrelationships with the environment. Its function is to provide greater behavioral alternatives for the successful gratification of needs. This is an important point to remember when planning intervention strategies. Unless activities are associated with naturally arising needs, or are designed to create need for adaptation, their chance of success will be seriously limited.

ORIGIN OF COMMUNICATION NEEDS

It is appropriate to consider the ways in which needs arise because intervention strategies should be planned to provide for more effective need gratification.

In the generation of needs in the growing child, two elements operate. The first is *maturation,* and the second is the *changing environment.* The environment consists of things and people. These interact among and between themselves to give rise to events that impinge upon the child's world. It is convenient, for the purpose of discussion, to separate maturational and environmental factors, However, it is very important to realize that these two influences are not independent parallel factors. Maturation and environment are totally interdependent factors in the development of communicative behavior in the child. Church (1961) called these two factors "biological" and "experiential" factors. He stressed that they stand in a symbiotic feedback relationship. He asserted that:

> . . . theories which assume that ontogenetic changes in behavior are produced by maturational changes must take account of the possibility that many maturational changes are in turn induced by perceptual stimulation (p. 30).

> . . . while some part of the change that occurs in infancy can be accounted for in terms of physical maturation, we know that maturation stands in a circular feedback relationship to experience—the things the organism does, feels, and has done to it (p. 36).

Effective intervention to a large part will depend upon how the clinician or teacher manipulates the environment to stimulate desired maturational patterns.

Maturational Influences

The processes of human communication are complex. This is true even when the communication code is kept relatively simple, as, for example, when a picture board is used to identify selected people, objects, or events. When communication involves the use of spoken language, the complexity is at its highest. At birth the infant already has fully developed peripheral sensory systems. However, the infant is protected from being overwhelmed by the multitude of sensory stimuli that impinge upon these sensory systems by what Spitz (1965) and Broadbent (1958) have referred to as the "sensory barrier." This barrier primarily arises from the fact that mental processing capabilities grow gradually over the early months as a function of the growing child's maturing capacity for voluntary action. Spitz (1965) strongly emphasized that perception in the infant can be said to have taken place only when the stimuli reaching the sensorium have been processed and made meaningful through the infant's experience.

Maturation, both of the physical system and the nervous system, therefore, is extremely important to the development of communication in the child. The capacity of the nervous system to receive and process the incoming signal will be the overriding factor in determing the ultimate potential for the development of communicative abilities.

Because this text specifically refers to the effects of hearing impairment and mental retardation on communication, it is particularly important to differentiate between the two aspects of perception that Watson (1973, 1974) has referred to as *sensory capability* and *response proclivity*. The former refers to the measure of the limits or capacity of the sensory system's function, while the latter refers to the way in which we use our senses. Sensory capability is concerned with measures such as sensitivity, capacity for information transmission, and the resolving power of the system. It is determined by the genetic endowment of the organism and other physical influences. Response proclivity, concerned with the special way in which our auditory system adapts itself to the processing of spoken language, represents:

> . . . a systematic tendency to respond to a particular sensory stimulus or sequence of stimuli in a particular way, even though a variety of

other responses are clearly within the capability of the organism (Watson, 1974, p. 103).

Speech perception may depend upon the evolution of specialized neural detectors and systems within the auditory system (Desmedt, 1960; Neff, 1961; Abbs and Sussman, 1971). Nevertheless, continuous exposure to speech from an early age plays a major role in triggering the maturational processes necessary for the organization of these specialized circuits (Stark, 1974, p. 263). Response proclivity, as Watson (1974) used the term, specifically refers to psychoacoustic functions assessed in experimental situations. The term is very useful. In this chapter the liberty is taken of extending its use to cover the tendency of the individual to respond to a particular communicative stimulus in a given manner despite the capability, or at least the assumed potential, to respond in other ways. Such a distinction between these two aspects of perceptual processing is important to the topic of this text. It emphasizes the need to differentiate between components of communication disabilities that are attributable to limitations in the neurophysiologic capacities of the system from those that arise from habituated patterns of response. The latter type of response may be amenable to positive intervention programs. It is reasonable to hope that greater understanding of the factors involved will lead to specialized early intervention strategies. These must be designed to ensure that the response proclivity will be directed toward productive patterns of communicative processing.

Developmental Adaptation

As the infant matures, sensory capability grows. The infant begins to have available an increasing amount of information about how the world around him is affecting his sensory perceptual system. Greater demands are placed upon this system to evolve in a manner that facilitates the more complex processing necessitated by adaptive behavior. This results in further neurologic maturation which, in concert with the motor system, occurs in a manner concurrent with the demands placed upon it.

Thus the child, by virtue of his own growth and development, is instrumental in increasing the demands he experiences for increasingly complex adaptive procedures (Lenneberg, 1967, p. 178). The growing sophistication of his sensory perceptual system, together with the growing mobility that physical growth makes possible, forces the child into closer contact with his environment.

A further aspect of maturational influences that must be considered is the role of optimal learning periods. Lenneberg (1967) has referred to the critical period for language acquisition. He maintained that this is bounded by lack of maturation at the lower limit and loss of adaptability and inability for reorganization in the brain at the upper limit. On the basis of findings derived from the study of the effects of traumatic cerebral lesions on language learning, Lenneberg (1967, p. 153) has inferred that "language learning can take place, at least in the right hemisphere, only between the ages of two to about thirteen."

Fry (1966), McConnell (1970), Horton (1974), Schiefelbusch and Lloyd (1974), and Lloyd (1976) have all stressed the critical role of the first 2 years of life in determining the ultimate potential for the development of speech communication skills in hearing-impaired children. Early exposure to sound patterns of spoken language is critically important for maximal language development in these children. It is equally important that, whenever possible, intervention strategies for the mentally retarded child be directed at the child's maturational readiness level for acquisition of a communication skill at the time he reaches it. This is not to imply that intervention at a later age will be unproductive. For example, the work of Carrier (this volume; Carrier and Peak, 1975) in teaching symbolic communication by a system other than speech indicates that even mentally retarded persons in their midteens are not beyond the reach of appropriate intervention procedures. However, it is apparent that the rate and level of achievement in the acquisition of spoken language is inversely related to the age at which intervention first occurs.

In considering intervention strategies, it must be borne in mind that speech is only a symptom of language. It is language that constitutes the underlying symbolic system. In turn, the language system has its roots in the child's knowledge of the world around him, a knowledge defined in terms of his own experience of it. Any system of symbolic communication, verbal or nonverbal, must be preceded by a representational stage of cognitive development. Piaget (1951; Piaget and Inhelder, 1966) has argued that the child first constructs a *reality-as-known*. He then subjects that knowledge to a process that reduces, refines, and re-presents the real event. Initially, the child "knows" his world only in a very concrete sensorimotor sense. Through the interaction of the organism with person, object, or event, the perceptual organism is itself modified. Its relationship to the physical event is expanded. A representational function develops. This function can operate independently of sensorimotor involvement of the physical world; that is, it does not depend upon the child sensing or doing. The child at this stage can now re-create, re-presenting his experience of people, objects, and events in the absence of their physical realities. Only at this stage of development can a child learn to use a system of referential symbols for the purpose of evoking, in himself and in others, the memory image that is now the substitute for the sensorimotor experience.

If Piaget's view is accepted, then language intervention can be successful only if it is accepted that a sensorimotor knowledge of what is to be learned is a prerequisite to knowing the world at a representational level.

Environmental Influences

Maturational influences bring about certain changes in the behavior of a growing child regardless of the effects of the environment. By virtue of growth, the child is automatically placed in a situation of change. Certain genetically encoded processes then operate to effect maturation. This in turn creates further demands for adaptation. If the system is endowed with adequate capacity, it adjusts to satisfy these internal needs. Most forms of adaptive behavior, however, even when they are genetically encoded, require triggering by environmental stimulation. Furthermore, many behavioral patterns not genetically encoded result from the organism adjusting to environmental demands. The environment, therefore, plays a critical role in stimulating maturational growth and in originating certain forms of adaptation that have their origins purely in environmentally generated demand.

It has been pointed out that the child's physical maturation expands his contact with the environment at the same time that his sensory perceptual system develops the capacity to process more sophisticated patterns of information. The environment, by the nature of the demands it places on the organism, exerts a strong influence on the way in which the individual's system evolves. It constrains the pattern of development, molding the behavior of the growing child. Among the extrinsic demands placed upon the child are pressures for social behavior. These pressures are age related, because expectancies for social behavior become increasingly more demanding, both in intensity and complexity, as the child grows older. Even during the first 2 years of the child's life, his parents expect to be able to modify his behavior through the use of speech and nonverbal behavior. Research on infant speech perception (Eimas et al., 1971; Eimas, 1974; Butterfield and Cairns, 1974; Morse, 1974, 1976) confirms that even very young infants have the capacity to discriminate between speech sounds. Furthermore, they discriminate in terms of the linguistic categories of the adult. This suggests that the child may be genetically endowed with the capacity to be influenced by speech communication from his earliest days of life. Certainly from her earliest contacts with the child, the mother exposes him to nonverbal and verbal communicative behavior.

Through what is probably a combination of genetic coding abilities and exposure to the communication model, the child begins to acquire the ability to modify his behavior in a manner compatible with the intent of the communication. In other words, it begins to be possible to effect certain types of desired adaptive behavior in the child by using the communication system as the medium for initiating the change. Somewhat later, the child likewise begins to make purposeful use of speech and gesture to constrain others in his environment. It is of interest to note that several authors (e.g., Schlesinger and Meadow, 1972; Boyes-Braem, 1973; McIntire, 1974; Wilbur and Jones, 1974) have reported that the time at which signing occurs among deaf children of deaf parents and among normal hearing children of deaf parents is earlier than the occurrence of speech in hearing children of hearing parents. The sign vocabulary and the use of two- and three-word sign utterances of deaf children also occur significantly earlier than the norms for spoken utterances of equivalent length. These findings may be explained by the difference in the neuromotor sophistication required for encoding the larger manual signs compared with the finer motor control required for speech production. A similar explanation may clarify the difference in the receptive vocabularies for signed and spoken English between deaf children of deaf parents and hearing children of hearing parents. The processing of spoken language requires several transformations through several levels of language complexity (Liberman, 1970; Liberman, Mattingly, and Turvey, 1972). It is likely that the ability to achieve this processing depends upon a level of maturation of the auditory system which exceeds that necessary to decode signs through the visual system. At this point, the use of the communication system has been established as an effective mediator between the child and his environment and between the environment and the child. The potential of the communication system for exerting control over the dynamic relationship between the child and his environment for the first time has been demonstrated. The system has the potential for greatly facilitating the organism's search for homeostasis and for providing the plasticity of behavior so essential to successful adaptive behavior. Communication thus serves as a mediative device. Through the mechanism of feedback, the system is progressively developed and modified. The result of the refinement is to enhance the effectiveness of the adaptation necessary for the satisfaction of externally and internally generated needs.

NATURE AND ROLE OF STIMULUS IN COMMUNICATION

A *stimulus* is a complex entity that constitutes an integral component of a whole. It arises from the changing status of a source. This in turn changes the status of one or more of the environmental media to which the person is sensitive. The behavior of the source occurs in space over time, giving rise to an event. As a result the stimulus event will have temporospatial characteristics equivalent to the particular pattern of behavior of the source. The stimulus event, therefore, has the potential to serve in a referential capacity once the relationship of the stimulus to its source has been learned.

Because a stimulus is part of a temporospatial event, its components are related. Thus, any section of the total event stands in a regular relationship to the components that precede it, to those that coexist with it, and to those that succeed it. The product of these relationships is a pattern that builds over time. The importance of the ordering of the components of a pattern is that, once a person is familiar with the whole, it is no longer necessary to receive all the components in order to identify it. It becomes possible to complete the pattern from less than all the parts. Even more important, prediction of the probable evolution of the pattern is made possible, often on the basis of only a very few of its components.

This capacity of the sensory perceptual system to process informational components makes human communication possible. Communication systems, regardless of their nature or complexity, are all based upon predicting intended meanings through the identification of stimulus patterns. This necessitates that a person:

1.   Be familiar with the rules used for the generation of the pattern
2.   Have appropriate semantic and conceptual values for the patterns received

3. Have established the relationship between pattern and value (meaning)

It has already been explained that the individual components of a stimulus event are informational. The term *information,* in this context, refers to the structure or organization of a medium that reduces the degrees of freedom within which choices may be made. In other words, information is generated by any constraining influence that reduces the number of alternative categories within which an item to be identified (object, person, word, idea, etc.) might be located.

Communication essentially involves a process in which two or more people, operating under a common set of rules, attempt to constrain the thoughts of each other. They do this by imposing a structure, or pattern, on one or more of the environmental media to which the human sensory perceptual system is sensitive. By controlling the patterning, they are able to transmit to each other information concerning which combination of rules is being used. Once the rule system is known by each participant, it can be used by the person receiving the information pattern to regenerate or reconstruct an equivalent of the original idea. An attempt is made, therefore, to predict with an acceptable degree of accuracy what another person is thinking. When a match occurs, communication is said to be effective. It is important to realize that what is transmitted between individuals is not the idea or message, but information about how to restructure an idea of equivalent value.

It should be clear, then, that the aim in communication is to evoke in others thoughts or ideas that match those we ourselves have selected. The semantic and conceptual values, therefore, lie, within the listener, not within the pattern of information received. Information serves only to identify those values. It provides the listener with the constraints necessary to reconstruct a pattern or message similar to the one that the speaker constructed.

EQUIVALENCE OF STIMULUS PATTERNS

Because the concern is with the evoking of an idea, rather than with the actual sending of a message, communication is not limited to a single medium. Information, existing as pattern or structure, can be encoded and transmitted through any of the media to which our sensory systems are sensitive. It is most important to realize that, although spoken language constitutes the most efficient and acceptable form for social interaction, it is by no means the only form used. Information is communicated in a wide range of codes, each with a particular degree of specificity dependent upon the strictness of the constraints operating. Mathematics and logic are subject to very stringent rules, while dance and Japanese flower arrangements are subject to far fewer constraints.

The establishment of a communication system requires that the communicating partners each:

1.   Possess a set of referents or values
2.   Share a common set of tokens (symbols) with which to identify those values
3.   Be familiar with generative rules governing the manner in which tokens may be used to construct patterns

Through experience the partners learn to ascribe values to the different patterns.

The tokens used may vary in size; however, each consists of a unit that has been ascribed to a particular referent and is, therefore, meaningful to each partner. By patterning units into different combinations, complex meanings can be conveyed. It is essential, however, that there be compatibility between the communicating partners —that is, that they share the same tokens and are both well familiar with the rules for using the system. Without this compatibility, communication will not take place.

The work of Premack and Premack (1974), both with mentally retarded children and with apes, and of Carrier (this volume; Carrier and Peak, 1975) with mentally retarded children illustrates how equivalency permits communication systems to be established. Pieces of plastic, varied by color and shape, were used as tokens. The subject was taught to relate a plastic shape to a particular object or object relationship. Later the subject was trained to relate arrangements or patterns of tokens to different relationships between objects, and to generate questions. Working with an ape named Sarah, Premack and Premack were able to teach a visual language vocabulary of 130 words representing eight functional categories. Sarah was capable of producing and comprehending a variety of simple sentences and several types of questions. She was even able to generate a compound and a complex sentence, although these were limited to only one example.

Premack and Premack also demonstrated that language acquired in this manner by a severely autistic child showed a degree of transferability to natural language. They were able to demonstrate equivalence between the systems and suggest that the system of using concrete tokens not only provides a means of communication that is relatively easily taught but also may enhance the acquisition of natural language.

Carrier modeled his work on that of Premack and Premack. Working with mentally retarded children, he developed a program that he called Non-Speech Language Initiation Program (Non-SLIP). This involved a core vocabulary of approximately 30 concrete words together with a simplified set of grammatical rules. A sentence pattern was first taught through establishing color equivalency for the various classes of words—noun symbols had an orange tape strip on them; verbs, a blue strip; articles, a red strip; and prepositions, a black strip. He then used the colors to drill the rote learning of the sentence pattern: red, orange, blue, black, red, orange. This represents the grammatical structure of a simple sentence. Coding of pictures according to word class then permitted the child to communicate an idea or experience within the limits of the patterns he could produce using the words and the single generative rule he learned.

Equivalence also exists in communication when information about a person, object, or event is broadcast simultaneously into more than a single medium. Although the nature of the patterning of the media differs, it is effected by the same source. Thus, the information in each medium has equivalency and is referential to the source. This occurs, for example, when speech and fingerspelling occur simultaneously. An observer receives both an auditory and a visual pattern imposed by the speaker on his environment. If the observer is familiar with the cultural constraints governing the use of speech and fingerspelling by the speaker, the amount of information potentially available to him is greatly enhanced by the bimodal transmission.

Even the very act of speaking generates both auditory and visual patterns of information that have equivalency. The availability of visual cues to speech provides the hearing-impaired person, whose access to auditory cues is reduced by hearing deficiency, with additional constraint information. Often this may play an important role in learning to understand speech communication.

It is the complex of information with patterning within and between sensory channels that permits a person to predict preconsciously how the pattern will evolve. This process applies at all levels of pattern processing involving both small and large units. In verbal language it occurs in the processing of phonemes and morphemes, and in restructuring the syntactic and semantic information. The ability to preguess the incoming signal by virtue of a knowledge of the communication rules permits information to be processed rapidly (Carroll, 1964; Sanders, 1971, p. 30). Intervention procedures, therefore, concentrate on stimulating the learning of the rules of the communication game regardless of the type of communication system being used. For this reason every system places demands upon cognitive function. The extent of the demand varies with the sophistication of the system. Verbal language requires a sophisticated use of linguistic rules in addition to the cognitive function.

For comprehension to occur it is necessary that a minimal amount of information be available. This minimal level constitutes the least amount of the information pattern necessary for its correct identification. It is usually met by the interaction of information derived from the external signal with information generated by the individual in the form of constraints or expectancies. The relative dependency on the external signal varies inversely with the person's ability to preguess its content.

Thus, the very aspect of information processing that facilitates communication in normal subjects is the one that is weak or absent in communicatively impaired children. Internal redundancy depends upon normal language function; therefore, any impairment in cognitive or linguistic processes maximizes the subject's dependency upon the external stimulus constraints. If the subject, in addition to impairment in cognitive development, has a peripheral hearing defect, he will be placed in double jeopardy. He not only brings a reduced internal redundancy to the communication task, but he is faced with a reduction in extrinsic information resulting from the distortion of the speech signal caused by the hearing impairment.

CHANNELS OF INTERACTION
BETWEEN THE INDIVIDUAL AND THE ENVIRONMENT

As explained earlier, an individual transacts with his environment through the modification of the media to which he is sensitive. Figure 1 indicates the channels involved in the transmission of information into the environmental media.

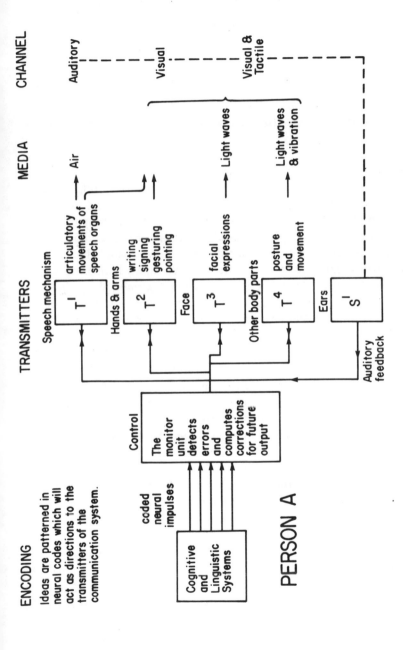

Figure 1. The encoding and transmitting of patterned information. (Modified from Sanders, 1971.)

Encoding and Transmitting Patterned Information

The primary effectors for the output of encoded information are the articulatory organs of speech, the hands and arms, and the facial muscles. However, other body parts also may be involved. For example, shoulders may be shrugged, the head may be nodded affirmatively or shaken negatively, or the foot stamped defiantly. Adaptive communicative behavior is, therefore, motoric.

Vocal Patterning   In normal social communication the vocal/articulatory system plays the primary role. One of the earliest and simplest means of communication used by a baby is purposeful crying, through which the child controls the mother's behavior. Although this is a very primal form of adaptation, if it is successful, it will be reinforced as an effective adaptive procedure. Purposeful crying has been identified by Kaplan and Kaplan (1971) as occurring in the age range 3 weeks to 5 months. The infant begins to use modification of his crying pattern to communicate different states of maladaptation. A parent soon learns to differentiate between the whimpering cry of mild discomfort and the intense cry of anger exhibited by the child when put down. In the latter instance, the child, when picked up again, may cease screaming, thus communicating the end of his state of distress.

This crude use of vocalization is not clearly differentiated from physiologically induced crying. It does, however, provide the earliest form of primitive communicative interaction between mother and child. It is augmented by the emergence of the cooing vocalizations most frequently associated with pleasure states.

During a subsequent stage, identified by Kaplan and Kaplan (1971) as occurring around 6 months, the purposeful use of vocalization becomes more sophisticated as intonational variations begin to expand in pitch variation and in complexity of patterning. Babbling also occurs during this stage. It is not used purposely as a communication-controlling behavior, although it does seem to be important to subsequent speech development.

Phonemic Patterning   The next stage of development of speech communication, occurring between 9 and 12 months, involves the sequential patterning of phonemes according to the rules of the language culture. It is a gradual process that involves identifying the sound patterns that are the tokens of specific experiences and perfecting their production. At the same time, these phonemic (segmental) patterns are combined with the melodic (suprasegmental) patterns of vocalization to communicate needs in a far more specific manner than is possible through the use of inarticulated vocalizations.

It must be stressed that this is not simply a process of a child learning to speak. This is a process of learning to adapt to more sophisticated environmental demands through the use of a more sophisticated tool of communication. It involves learning how the system operates and experimenting in its use. The success that the child experiences in these early attempts depends heavily upon the ability of the listener to compensate for the child's crude use of the system— that is, the familiarity of the receiver with the rules of the language game. The mother generally can compensate in this manner with some success, because she is able to predict need, intent, or meaning on the basis of probabilities generated by situational constraints. Bear in mind that she is also a component of this communication transaction. From the start she makes every attempt to adapt to the communicative strategies used by her child.

Ingram (1974) has identified some of these strategies used by young children. A similar adjustment or "normalization" of our processes of speech perception seems to take place when we listen to speakers whose speech differs from our own (Broadbent, 1958).

The language interventionist similarly adapts to the child's communication patterns. He does so with the conscious intent of analyzing the strategies being used by the child. His purpose is to utilize procedures to reinforce and shape those patterns toward a closer approximation of normal structures (Winitz, 1975).

Syntactic Patterning   The final stage of constraints imposed by speech structure lies within the syntax and grammar of the language. Syntax permits highly sophisticated patterns to be generated to serve as tokens for complex ideas. The child first begins to use this form of refined communication behavior when he begins to combine the word units he knows. Concatenation is the capacity to combine and recombine words to form different patterns, just as phonemes are combined and recombined. Each pattern becomes a new token that increases the child's ability to transact with his environment, to further his level of adaptation.

Speech, therefore, must, be seen as a sophisticated form of adaptive behavior. It is rule based, involving the use of the articulators and resonators of the speech production mechanism to pattern or constrain the air medium. The rules are an integral part of the rules of language processing and relate to semantic values. Speech information is encoded into melodic patterns, or suprasegmental cues, and into articulatory resonant patterns, or segmental cues, both of which stand in a symbiotic relationship (Martin, 1972). The complexity of the patterns that can be generated makes speech the most effective means of adaptation in a hearing society, where speech constitutes the dominant form of interpersonal communication. Speech provides the user with what is potentially a highly sophisticated means of influencing and being influenced by other people.

Fingerspelling and Signing   Fingerspelling and signing are forms of adaptive motor behavior that involve the use of structured systems of information processing. Fingerspelling is directly tied to the spoken language system. It involves the use of a manual alphabet with a hand-finger pattern, or token, for each letter. Its use is tied to the traditional orthography and limited by the language and spelling ability of the communicants.

Signing involves the use of a repertoire of patterned movements of the hand (and face). The patterning arises from the constraints of hand configurations, the placement of the hands with regard to the body, and the movement of the hands (Moores, 1974). These three variables combine in different patterns to produce different signs (words and/or concepts). Signs can be combined in different syntactic patterns to produce sentences. The syntactic patterns of American Sign Language (ASL or Ameslan) are different from those of Signed English and other manual systems that are intended to parallel spoken English. Wilbur (this volume) provides an extensive review of the linguistics of manual language and manual systems.

Writing   The written form of communication, existing between a writer and a reader, provides another vitally important channel of interaction. Reading and writing are both derived from the verbal language system and are therefore limited to the level of language competence. For persons with a poor ability to produce and understand speech, writing can become the major channel of communication. The role of this channel is discussed by Clark and Woodcock (this volume).

Pointing   Pointing is a simple motor means of communication and is very evident in the prelingual child. It serves as a constraint placed upon the possible alternative points of visual focus of the observer. Adults use pointing to help to identify a referent: "That one, over there" (pointing). Pointing serves as a very helpful communication device for children or adults who have not yet learned to use speech or sign language. It is limited to the physical presence of the referent and depends upon the observer's ability to narrow down the probabilities of the desired object through the use of situational cues. In establishing a communication system dependent upon this limited constraint behavior, the observer can establish categories of referents representing common needs of the communicatively handicapped person, for example, basic needs (toilet needs, food, drink, pillows, toys, etc.). The word or pictures used to represent the person, object, or event comprise the tokens that are identified by pointing.

Facial Expressions and Natural Gestures   The emotive content of the idea to be communicated is embodied in linguistic form both in segmental and suprasegmental information. It is also frequently encoded into potentially informative patterns transmitted to the facial muscles and the hands and arms. Expressions of surprise, puzzlement, joy, anxiety, anger, and so on, serve to place further constraints on the manner in which the person receiving the verbal and nonverbal information decodes it. Facial expressions and gestures that arise naturally as part of the act of communication serve to reduce the listener's dependency upon the speech pattern. They provide very valuable additional speech-related cues to facilitate communication because they are broader and more easily categorized than verbal patterns.

Movement or Posture   Information is given either intentionally or unintentionally by the behavior of a person. When such behavior is interpreted by an observer, it has been attributed token value. Communicative behavior is part of a larger pattern of adaptive behavior. It is, therefore, frequently associated with pattern of movement (pacing up and down, turning toward a figure or a diagram being discussed, and so on) or with certain body postures reflective of a mood that is in keeping with the verbal message. Nonverbal behavior of this type serves to provide a broader frame of reference into which the verbal messages are fitted. It helps to generate the expectancies that constitute such an important part of easy comprehension of spoken or signed language.

Monitoring the Transmission Process

We have seen that the message is transmitted in the form of an energy pattern impressed upon an environmental medium. It changes the existing status of the medium in accordance with rules. We have examined the various channels into which the information pattern may be encoded. However, it is necessary to ensure that the signal generated conforms to the desired pattern and produces the desired effect. This is provided by a monitoring process known as auditory *feedback*. As shown in Figure 2, the feedback occurs in two forms, internal and external. Internal feedback originates from sensory information arising from the monitoring of the activities of the motor system. It involves feeding back into the system a part of the output for

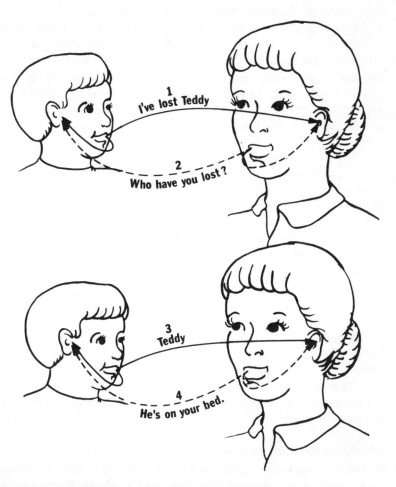

Figure 2. Communication involves the use of internal and external auditory feedback to ensure correctness. (Modified from Sanders, 1971.)

purposes of comparison of the signal produced with the signal intended (Sanders, 1971, pp. 16–22). This is a process of quality control. External feedback arises from objects or people in our environment. It involves a monitoring of the effectiveness of our communicative actions and our adaptive behavior in terms of what we sought to achieve. In both cases feedback consists of the checking of performance against expectancies. The information thus obtained provides the speaker with a measure of the discrepancy between these two stages of information processing. The data are then used to compute a correction factor. It is predicted that when this anticipated error-correction factor is applied to the subsequent stages of the unit production, future error will be reduced.

Feedback, then, is a continuous self-adjusting monitoring system. It involves the use of output to compute ahead the anticipated adjustments that must be made to future output if the desired pattern is to be achieved.

In communication the sensory feedback channels that provide feedback information are: 1) the eyes for information encoded into the visual medium—for writing or drawing; 2) the ears, for acoustically encoded information—for vocalization and speech; 3) muscle and joint receptors and touch receptors—for speech, gesture, signing, writing, and the like.

The influence of the feedback system depends upon:

1. The quality or definition of the internal model of what the output should be
2. The sensitivity and fidelity of the sensory perceptual system, which processes both the output and the input of the external feedback

Among the population with which this text is concerned, problems may be expected to exist both in establishing a clearly defined internal model and in comparing the output to the model.

The mentally retarded child has difficulty in recording accurate images of external models because of reduced capacity for analysis and storage of complex patterns. A probable reduction in the capacity to record the details of motor output further reduces the effectiveness of the feedback system intended to monitor and correct production.

The hearing-impaired child's difficulty in achieving adequate feedback likewise involves difficulty in establishing adequate internal language and speech models, a difficulty attributable to a deficiency in the major channel (hearing) through which spoken language is processed. The child's problem is further complicated by the fact that the monitoring of speech production is primarily based on acoustic feedback. Part of intervention procedures is aimed at increasing the child's awareness of information pertaining to his own productive communication. For a hearing-impaired child, amplification is a prerequisite to increasing available auditory cues. Visual and tactile feedback play an important role in improving the speech production of all communicatively handicapped children. The child is presented with informal or formal models of the desired patterns with the aim of providing new models for internalization or modification of unsatisfactory models.

ENVIRONMENT

Because the only way in which information can travel from sender to receiver is through the patterning of environmental media, the status of the medium either facilitates or impedes the transmission of information. Any activity within a medium that has the effect of impeding the flow of the energy pattern generated by the sender is known as *noise*. Noise constitutes an interference factor that may exist in any medium. It results in a distortion of the true pattern by adding or subtracting energy from the wave pattern originated by the source. In most situations our familiarity with the language structure and rules, together with the effects of contextual and situational constraints, results in high levels of predictability. Our dependency upon the acoustic signal, therefore, is relatively low. In other words, a high internal redundancy compensates for the effects of noise. Under normal conditions, therefore, the visual or auditory noise in the communication system is not sufficiently high as to interfere with a person's ability to understand. However, from time to time, the acoustics of a room are so poor that comprehension becomes difficult (Ross, 1972). Competing auditory stimuli may mask out the speech message, or the medium may badly distort the signal pattern, as occurs when room reverberation levels are high. Transmission of the signal through a telephone, radio, or, most importantly, a hearing aid, may result in substantial distortion.

The problems of acoustic distortion and acoustic noise only occasionally become of real significance to the normal hearing person. The child or adult with a receptive communication problem, on the other hand, is disproportionally affected. Not only does this individual experience a reduction and/or distortion of the input information, but he is also affected by his reduced ability to predict the message because of low internal redundancy.

Acoustic noise arises from the adding or subtracting from components of the message signal. This may have the effect of overwhelming the pattern, a phenomenon called *masking,* or it may distort the pattern by interfering with the particular relationship of the components, which is called frequency or *intensity distortion.* Reverberation and poor quality audiotransmission systems, which include hearing aids, are frequent contributors to distortion. The management implications of these factors along with the effect of visual noise are discussed more fully in subsequent chapters (Cox and Lloyd, this volume; Ross, this volume).

Visual noise also results in the addition of unwanted stimuli or the deletion of important stimulus information. Many mentally retarded children have a limited capacity to control the effects of environmental change on their system. They have low channel capacity and may rapidly experience an overload. This factor makes them very prone to visual distractibility or to the opposite phenomenon of *perseveration,* that is, difficulty in shifting attention once focused. Controlling the nature, amount, and relevance of the visual information present in a learning situation becomes an important consideration in planning intervention strategies.

The child with reduced auditory information caused by a hearing impairment needs to be trained to make greater use of relevant visual cues. The most important of these are those arising from the visible components of speech articulation, from manually encoded information, or from a combination of both. The child must be able to see the signals as clearly as possible. The vision of the child must be carefully assessed and corrective lenses fitted if necessary. It is additionally important to ensure good lighting of the person communicating the information and an optimal distance of 4 to 9 feet from speaker to listener. Therefore, one should avoid situations where the lighting originates from behind the speaker, placing his face and hands in shadow. These conditions are particularly important when trying to help the hearing-impaired child to increase the information he processes by use of speechreading and interpretation of facial cues.

The environment constitutes an important component of the communication system; its role must not be overlooked.

RECEIVING AND DECODING PATTERNED INFORMATION

To effect communication it is necessary to change the environment in some way, to pattern the environmental media. Information about such structured change is available to an individual through the afferent or sensory systems. It is the primitive "near" senses of the haptic (touch), olfactory (smell), and gustatory (taste) systems and the more sophisticated "distance" senses of vision and audition that define the breadth of the organism's experience of the sensory world. These receptive aspects are schematically represented in Figure 3.

In man, the auditory, visual, and haptic systems constitute the input channels that are most useful in communication. Information may be encoded into any sensory modality; thus, all sensory systems are potentially open for use in communication. The possible communicative value of the senses of smell and taste as avenues of reaching children with severe communication disorders (Hollis, Carrier, and Spradlin, this volume; Wood, 1975), however, remains to be fully explored.

Various codes have been developed for transmitting information to the three major pathways. These codes may involve the reception of information through a single sensory system, as occurs in listening to a speaker who cannot be seen, in reading, or in the use of braille by the blind. More often, information is received simultaneously by two sensory modalities, as in listening and watching a speaker (auditory-visual speech reception), in simultaneous presentation of speech and fingerspelling, or of speech and speech-vibration patterns presented to the fingers. Regardless of the medium into which the message is transmitted, the patterned information is initially detected in terms of changes induced in the relationship between the sensory end organs and the physical environment. The peripheral sense organs respond to these changes in a manner commensurate with them. In this way the patterned signal is internalized. The process of analysis involves the identification of the manner in which the acoustic signal was originally patterned. Two schools of thought exist concerning how this identification in fact occurs. One view suggests that specialized neural detector cells sense the presence or absence of various components of the incoming stimulus complex. The firing of various combinations of cells, on the basis of the particular combination of components present in the incoming signal, permits the internal restructuring of the pattern (Abbs and Sussman, 1971).

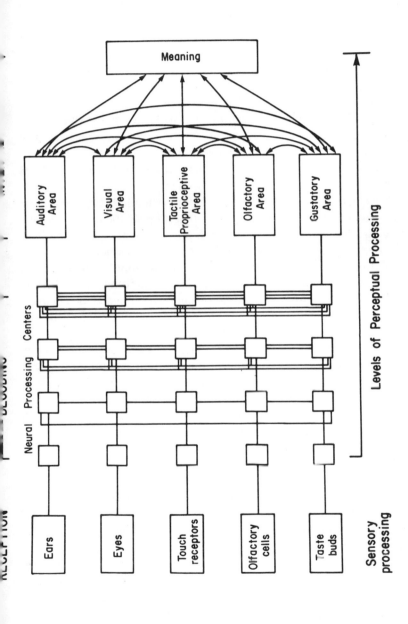

Figure 3. The receptive aspect of the communication system.

A more widely held view, although not disputing the existence of such a detector system, holds that the pattern is identified only after it has been compared to the internal model based on the expectancy computations (Stevens, 1960, 1972; Liberman et al., 1967; Stevens and Halle, 1967; Liberman, Mattingly, and Turvey, 1972). The nature of the internal model is believed to vary in detail from the articulatory features of phonemes to much larger linguistic segments.

It is possible to conceive of a quite viable compromise between the direct passive feature-detection theory and the active motor theory (Sanders, 1976). Whichever rationale proves most effective, some type of internal modeling must occur. This is necessary because perception depends upon the individual's ability to identify the value (meaning), which is within the system, from its token, which is received from without.

Thus, effective communication between individuals, regardless of the channel(s) used, involves the integration of the complete systems of two individuals. The relationship is therefore symbiotic. It is not correct to speak of a sender and a receiver, since both parties are transmitting and receiving information all the time in a feedback relationship. Only the relative emphasis on transmitting and receiving shifts between the parties. This relationship can be depicted schematically by combining Figures 1 and 3 for two people. The resultant, Figure 4, shows two persons in a communicative interaction. Information flows continuously and simultaneously from person A to person B, and from person B to person A. The amount flowing in a given direction varies, as does its distribution among channels. The result is an orchestrated interpersonal interaction. This is only at its best when each party makes maximal use of feedback to monitor and adjust both production and reception processes in a search for maximal compatibility between the two systems.

It is important to keep in mind that communication does not simply involve an ability to receive and analyze the incoming stimulus pattern. It equally involves the possession by the receiver of a conceptual library of experience. The receiver of the information must be able to encode the experiential value into a symbolic system shared with his communicant and must be able to recognize a similar pattern transmitted to him by the sender. Communication, therefore, involves the utilization of a mutual code used by one individual to direct the thoughts of another in a manner intended to establish equivalent value identification. This is done in a kind of linguistic guessing game. The

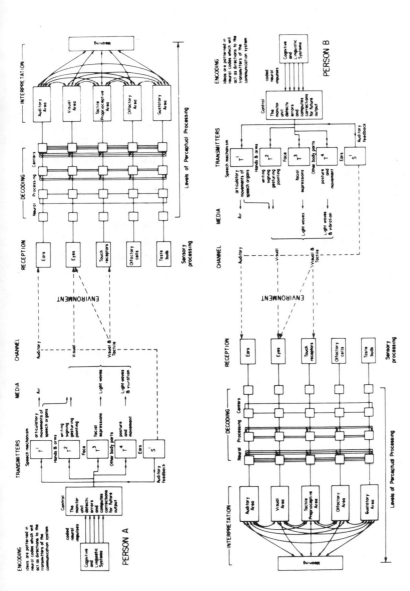

Figure 4. The continuous and stimultaneous flow of information between two people. (From Sanders, 1971; reprinted by permission.)

process is based upon the possession by each participant of a store of similar experiences. These experiences are then tapped by means of a symbolic language code. The process embodies the use of a variety of shared language-coding strategies.

With the use of any one of the several encoding channels, patterned changes are impressed upon the associated environmental medium shared by both communicants. Information in the form of constraints thus flows from one person to the other.

The physical patterning of the environment induces equivalent patterned changes in the sensory end organ sensitive to that medium. In this manner the patterned information is internalized. Because the pattern stands in a referential relationship to the particular combination of rules used to generate it, the identification of those rules by the receiver permits the re-creation of a reasonable facsimile of the original. The values intended are thus identified.

Communication is greatly facilitated by the fact that familiarity with the rules of the game permits the listener, well versed in the symbol system, to predict ahead of the speaker. The resultant redundancy decreases dependency on the message signal, permitting high rates of information processing.

Children with communication difficulties that involve language encoding and decoding are in a position of double jeopardy. Not only do they experience a distortion of the message signal received, but they also experience difficulty in predicting its evolution. They are thus more than usually dependent upon the very signal that they have so much difficulty in faithfully receiving and decoding. Communication intervention strategies are directed at reducing this impedance between the child and his society.

SUMMARY

The points stressed in this chapter arise from the fundamental concept that communication is adaptive behavior. Maturation of the organism and changing environmental demands interact to necessitate the development of increasingly complex adaptive strategies. Among the most sophisticated of these is communicative behavior.

It is necessary to bear in mind that, although verbal language represents the most socially useful and one of the most advanced methods of human interaction, it is only one of a number of methods of human communication. The critical factors common to all methods are that: 1) the tokens used have referential value, 2) both communicants are familiar with them, and 3) there is a shared understanding of the rules that are to be used form the communication.

The potential exists for interaction between the communicating individuals through any medium to which both partners are sensitive. This is an important factor because it does not confine us to the utilization of a single modality, such as hearing, in our attempts to teach communication skills to the handicapped. We have available a variety of input channels through which information can be transmitted with varying degrees of complexity.

Intervention procedures seek to determine the most appropriate channel for developing communicative behavior in a particular child at a given stage of development. A more complex system using a different channel may offer more potential after a period of training. In addition, communication involves the processing of constraint information, which is not sense specific. Equivalency exists across modalities. Through training, channels can serve in a symbiotic relationship. This greatly enhances the potential for language learning.

Intervention strategies arise from a clear concept of the nature of the communication process. The effectiveness of new approaches in turn adds to our understanding of communication. It is important, therefore, that in approaching the task of planning for the needs of communicatively handicapped children, we remain open minded and creative. It is these attitudes that are reflected in subsequent chapters.

REFERENCES

Abbs, J. H., and H. M. Sussman. 1971. Neurophysiological feature detectors and speech perception: A discussion of theoretical implications. J. Speech Hear. Res. 14:23–26.

Boyes-Braem, P. 1973. A study of the acquisition of the dez in American Sign Language. Working paper, Salk Institute for Biological Studies, La Jolla, Cal.

Broadbent, D. E. 1958. Perception and Communication. Pergamon Press, New York.

Butterfield, E. C., and G. F. Cairns. 1974. Discussion summary—Infant research. *In* R. L. Schiefelbusch and L. L. Lloyd (eds.), Language Perspectives—Acquisition, Retardation, and Intervention, pp. 75–102. University Park Press, Baltimore.

Carrier, J. K., Jr., and T. Peak. 1975. Nonspeech Language Initiation Program. H & H Enterprises, Lawrence, Kan.

Carroll, J. B. 1964. Language and Thought. Prentice-Hall, Englewood Cliffs, N.J.

Church, J. 1961. Language and the Discovery of Reality. Random House, New York.

Desmedt, J. E. 1960. Neurophysiological mechanisms controlling acoustic input. *In* G. L. Rasmussen and W. Windle (eds.), Neural Mechanisms of the Auditory and Vestibular System. Ch. 8. Charles C Thomas, Springfield, Ill.

Eimas, P. D. 1974. Linguistic processing of speech by young infants. *In* R. L. Schiefelbusch and L. L. Lloyd (eds.), Language Perspectives— Acquisition, Retardation, and Intervention, pp. 55–73. University Park Press, Baltimore.

Eimas, P. D., E. R. Siqueland, P. Jusczyk, and J. Vigorito. 1971. Speech perception in infants. Science 171:303–306.

Fry, D. B. 1966. The development of the phonological system in the normal and deaf child. *In* F. Smith and G. A. Miller (eds.), The Genesis of Language: A Psycholinguistic Approach. MIT Press, Cambridge, Mass.

Horton, K. B. 1974. Infant intervention and language learning. *In* R. L. Schiefelbusch and L. L. Lloyd (eds.), Language Perspectives—Acquisition, Retardation, and Intervention, pp. 469–491. University Park Press, Baltimore.

Ingram, D. 1974. Phonological rules in young children. J. Child. Lang. 1:49–64.

Kaplan, E., and G. Kaplan. 1971. The prelinguistic child. *In* J. Eliot (ed.), Human Development and Cognitive Processes. Holt, Rinehart and Winston, New York.

Lenneberg, E. H. 1967. Biological Foundations of Language. John Wiley & Sons, New York.

Liberman, A. M. 1970. The grammars of speech and language. Cog. Psychol. 1:301–323.

Liberman, A. M., F. S. Cooper, D. P. Shankweiler, and M. G. Studdert-Kennedy. 1967. Perception of the speech code. Psychol. Rev. 74 (6):431–461.

Liberman, A. M., I. G. Mattingly, and M. T. Turvey. 1972. Language Codes and Memory Codes, *In* A. W. Melton and E. Martin (eds.), Coding Processes in Human Memory, pp. 307–334. V. H. Winston & Sons, Washington, D.C.

Lloyd, L. L. 1976. Discussant's comment: Language and Communication Aspects. *In* T. D. Tjossem (ed.), Intervention Strategies for High Risk Infants and Young Children. University Park Press, Baltimore.

Martin, J. G. 1972. Rythmic hierarchical versus serial structure in speech and other behavior. Psychol. Rev. 79:487–509.

McConnell, F. 1970. A New Approach to the Management of Deafness. Ped. Clin. N. Amer. 17 (2):347–362.

McIntire, M. L. 1974. A modified model for the description of language acquisition in a deaf child. Unpublished masters thesis, California State College at Northridge, Cal.

Moores, D. L. 1974. Nonvocal systems of verbal behavior. *In* R. L. Schiefelbusch and L. L. Lloyd (eds.), Language Perspectives—Acquisition, Retardation, and Intervention, pp. 377–417. University Park Press, Baltimore.

Morse, P. A. 1974. Infant speech perception: A preliminary model and review of the literature. *In* R. L. Schiefelbusch and L. L. Lloyd (eds.), Language Perspectives—Acquisition, Retardation, and Intervention, pp. 19–53. University Park Press, Baltimore.

Morse, P. A. 1976. Auditory-perceptual development in infants. *In* D. A. Sanders, Auditory Perception of Speech—An Introduction to Principles and Problems. Prentice-Hall, Englewood Cliffs, N.J.

Neff, W. D. 1961. Neural mechanisms of auditory discrimination. *In* W. A. Rosenblith (ed.), Sensory Communications, pp. 259–278. MIT Press, Cambridge, Mass.

Premack, D., and A. J. Premack. 1974. Teaching visual language to apes and language-deficient persons. *In* R. L. Schiefelbusch and L. L. Lloyd (eds.), Language Perspectives—Acquisition, Retardation, and Intervention, pp. 347–376. University Park Press, Baltimore.

Piaget, J. 1951. Play Dreams and Imitation in Childhood. Norton, New York.

Piaget, J., and B. Inhelder. 1966. La psychologie de l'enfant. Collection "Que suis-je." No. 369. Presses Universitaires de France, Paris.

Ross, M. 1972. Hearing aid evaluation. *In* J. Katz (ed.), Handbook of Clinical Audiology, pp. 624–655. Williams & Wilkins, Baltimore.

Sanders, D. A. 1971. Aural Rehabilitation. Prentice-Hall, Englewood Cliffs, N.J.

Sanders, D. A. 1976. Auditory Perception of Speech: An Introduction to Principles and Problems. Prentice-Hall, Englewood Cliffs, N.J.

Schiefelbusch, R. L., and L. L. Lloyd. 1974. Introduction. *In* R. L. Schiefelbusch and L. L. Lloyd (eds.), Language Perspectives—Acquisition, Retardation, and Intervention pp. 1–15. University Park Press, Baltimore.

Schlesinger, H. S., and K. Meadow. 1972. Sound and Sign: Childhood Deafness and Mental Health. University of California Press, Berkeley.

Spitz, R. 1965. The First Year of Life. International Universities Press, New York.

Stark, R. 1974. Looking to the future: Overview and preview. *In* R. Stark (ed.), Sensory Capabilities of Hearing-Impaired Children, pp. 209–225. University Park Press, Baltimore.

Stevens, K. N. 1960. Toward a model for speech recognition. J. Acous. Soc. Amer. 32:45–55.

Stevens, K. N. 1972. Segments, features, and analysis-by-synthesis. *In* J. F. Kavanagh and I. G. Mattingly (eds.), Language by Eye and Ear. MIT Press, Cambridge, Mass.

Stevens, K. N., and M. Halle. 1967. Remarks on analysis-by-synthesis and distinctive features. *In* W. Wathen-Dunn (ed.), Models for the Perception of Speech and Visual Form, pp. 88–102. MIT Press, Cambridge, Mass.

Watson, C. S. 1973. Psychophysics. *In* B. Wolman (ed.), Handbook of General Psychology. Prentice-Hall, Englewood Cliffs, N.J.

Watson, C. S. 1974. Perceptual and cognitive strategies—Discussion: Perception of speech and nonspeech stimuli. *In* R. Stark (ed.), Sensory Capabilities of Hearing-Impaired Children, pp. 91–95. University Park Press, Baltimore.

Wilbur, R. B., and M. L. Jones. 1974. Some aspects of the bilingual/bimodal acquisition of sign and English by three hearing children of deaf parents. *In* M. LaGaly, R. Fox, and A. Bruck (eds.), Proceedings of the Tenth Regional Meeting, Chicago Linguistic Society. Chicago Linguistic Society, Chicago.

Winitz, H. 1975. From Syllable to Conversation. University Park Press, Baltimore.

Wood, M. M. 1975. Developmental Therapy: A Textbook for Teachers as Therapists for Emotionally Disturbed Young Children. University Park Press, Baltimore.

2

DEFINITIONS AND PREVALENCE

Gerard J. Bensberg and
Carol K. Sigelman

CONTENTS

Developmental Disabilities _____ 36

    Specific learning disabilities/38
    Autism/38
    Cerebral palsy/39
    Epilepsy/41
    Mental retardation/42

Hearing Impairment _____ 47

    Heredity and hearing impairment/52
    Cleft palate and hearing impairment/54
    Maternal rubella and hearing impairment/54
    Rh factor and hearing impairment/56
    Prematurity and hearing impairment/56
    Postnatal infections and hearing impairment/57

Multiple Handicaps _____ 58

    Communication disorders and mental retardation/59
    Hearing impairment and mental retardation/60

Summary and Recommendations _____ 61

References _____ 66

Adequate treatment of the prevalence of developmental disabilities, hearing impairment, and communicative disorders represents a challenge of considerable magnitude. Problems of definition of various handicapping conditions, biased samples used in studies and surveys, and the lack of uniform criteria for categorizing these conditions produce widely divergent statistics. However, information gained in recent years has resulted in a growing awareness of some of the commonly made errors and a movement toward a greater uniformity of definitions.

Within the past decade, there also have been increasing awareness and appreciation of the prevalence of multiple handicaps. Paralleling this change has been the realization that persons with multiple handicaps often require the coordinated services of many disciplines if proper diagnosis, education, and treatment are to be provided. The early 1960's were marked by attention given to categorical conditions such as mental retardation. This resulted in federal legislation that provided funds for the development of professional manpower to meet the needs of various handicapped groups, research funds to seek improved methods of prevention and treatment, and direct service monies to upgrade habilitation. The early 1970's have been marked by a blurring of crisp distinctions between disabilities and by attempts to merge training and service programs that have similar qualities or serve similar disabilities.

Because the methodology of prevalence studies has improved and because services for distinct handicapped groups are being integrated, a review of the more current literature is particularly instructive. This chapter examines the major developmental disabilities one by one, highlighting the nature of each, its prevalence, and the communication disorders that accompany it. Second, hearing impairment is described and related to a variety of causal factors ranging from heredity to early childhood diseases. Finally, multiple disabilities are considered, with emphasis placed on the combination of mental retardation with hearing impairment and communication disorders.

A few key terms facilitate understanding of the prevalence literature. *Epidemiology* is the study of the distribution and determinants of disease prevalence (MacMahon, Pugh, and Ipsen, 1960). *Descriptive epidemiology* is the study of the distribution of a disease. It represents an extension of the discipline of demography to health and disease by noting the relationships of factors such as age, sex, race, and geography to the prevalence of the condition. *Analytic epidemiology* seeks to determine the causes of the condition under study. Many feel that the major concern of epidemiology should be the discovery of factors essential or contributory to the occurrence of disease (Fox, Hall, and Elveback, 1970). Traditionally, emphasis was given to acute outbreaks of infectious diseases, called epidemics. More recently, however, this concern with epidemics (the unusual) has been supplemented by a growing appreciation for the study of disease frequency during endemic times (nonepidemic or usual times).

Common usage frequently confuses the terms *incidence* and *prevalence*. Incidence refers to the frequency with which a specific event occurs within a defined population during a stated period of time (Paul, 1966). Thus, the annual incidence of new cases of a given disease such as rheumatic fever is defined as the proportion of persons within a population who develop the disease for the first time during a 1-year period. It represents the frequency of the event.

Prevalence, by contrast, is the proportion of persons in a defined population who, at a specified time, are affected *or have been affected* by a particular disease. Hence, the prevalence of a condition such as coronary occlusion is given as the ratio of the number of affected persons to the total population. An affected person is defined as one who now has or has had one or more coronary attacks before the time of observation. Prevalence represents the accumulated incidence of new cases during previous years from which deaths from all causes have been subtracted. Prevalence, then, refers to the amount on hand, much like one's current bank balance (MacMahon, Pugh, and Ipsen, 1960).

DEVELOPMENTAL DISABILITIES

Because of the frequent occurrence of several handicapping conditions in the same individual and the resultant need for coordinated services from a variety of disciplines to assist that individual, the Developmental Disabilities Services and Facilities Construction Act (Public Law 91-517) was signed into law in 1970. The Act defines developmental disability to mean:

> . . . a disability attributable to mental retardation, cerebral palsy, epilepsy, or other neurological handicapping-condition of an individual, found to be closely related to mental retardation or to require treatment similar to that required by mentally retarded individuals,

and the disability originates before such individual attains 18 and has continued, or can be expected to continue, indefinitely, and constitutes a substantial handicap of such individuals.

The Act provides federal support for a wide range of diversified services in terms of life-time human needs of the developmentally disabled. It permits the co-mingling of federal funds with state funds to facilitate the development of comprehensive services by several state agencies representing diverse areas such as health, welfare, education, and rehabilitation, without imposing a set pattern of services on any one state. Its intent is to simulate the development of innovative programs to fill gaps in existing services and to integrate the services and resources of all state, regional, and local agencies assisting the developmentally disabled.

On October 7, 1975, President Ford signed into law The Developmentally Disabled Assistance and Bill of Rights Act (Public Law 94-103). This Act replaces Public Law 91-517. For the first time, autism is included in the definition of developmental disabilities. Dyslexia, a type of reading impairment, is also mentioned as a grounds for eligibility for services under this law if it represents a severe impairment of general intellectual functioning. Support for university-affiliated interdisciplinary training programs is continued. It is now possible to develop satellite programs in other universities that are associated with a recognized university-affiliated training program.

Perhaps the greatest change in the new law is the section dealing with provisions for the establishment and protection of rights of persons with developmental disabilities. This section specifies that the developmentally disabled have a right to appropriate treatment and services and that these services should be designed to maximize developmental potential and should be provided in a setting that is least restrictive to the person's personal liberty. Minimum standards for assuring the provision of these basic rights are included. If a state does not provide adequate assurance that it has met the requirements set forth in this Act by October 1, 1977, it is subject to a witholding of funds as provided under part C of the Act.

Two surveys that have attempted to identify children (under age 21) with developmental disabilities are those of Wishik (1956) and Richardson and Higgins (1964). Although there are many problems of methodology and definition in such surveys, it is helpful to review their findings. Table 1 presents a summary of those conditions

Table 1. Percentage of children (birth to age 21) with disabilities

Handicap	Wishik (1956)	Richardson and Higgins (1964)
Mental retardation	4.0	7.7
Speech	2.9	4.6
Emotional	2.9	10.6
Vision	2.4	12.3
Hearing	1.9	4.9
Orthopedic	1.7	6.0
Orthodontic	1.6	8.9
Heart	1.0	6.3
Cerebral palsy	0.5	0.8
Epilepsy	0.4	1.2[a]
Cleft lip and palate	0.1	0.3

[a]An adjusted percentage.

considered to occur during the developmental period and which therefore might be considered broadly as developmental disabilities.

Specific Learning Disabilities

Perhaps the most controversial class of handicaps that was considered by Congress for inclusion in the new developmental disabilities legislation is "specific learning disabilities." Whether or not they fit the current definition of developmental disability is unclear, particularly because dyslexia is considered by many to be a specific type of learning disability. Several professional groups and many professionals argue that there is little agreement as to the cause and treatment of specific learning disabilities. One of the biggest concerns is that provision of services to the many people with learning disabilities will so dilute existing federal monies that programs will have to be cut back for the more severely disabled. In testimony before the Senate committee (Senate Report 93-1169), the estimated prevalence of specific learning disabilities was 10% of all public school children or a half-million between the ages of 6 and 18.

Autism

As pointed out earlier, autism is mentioned as one of the conditions included in the new legislation. This condition frequently has been referred to as "infantile autism" because it seems to begin in the first 2 or 3 years of life. A dictionary definition is, "the condition of being dominated by subjective, self-centered trends of thought or behavior" (Dorland's Illustrated Medical Dictionary, 1965). Typically, autism is defined by the characteristic behavior exhibited. Four characteristics are most frequently observed in autistic children: 1) lack of social responsiveness to others; 2) ritualistic behavior, such as rocking back and forth or staring at one's hand; 3) obsessive-compulsive behavior, such as repeating an act over and over again; and 4) bizarre verbal behavior, such as repeating the last part of a sentence said to the child (echolalia) or perhaps being mute.

The estimates of the number of people with autism vary widely. Gallagher and Wiegerink (1973) reported that four out of every 10,000 births are later labeled autistic and estimate that there are 4000 preschool-age autistic children. In testimony before the Senate Committee, an estimated prevalence of 80,000 was given (Senate Report 93-1169). There is considerable disagreement on the cause of autism, but most theories place major emphasis on one of two possibilities: the child is the product of an emotionally starved environment, or else there is a biologic or even a genetic basis for the condition. Gallagher and Wiegerink (1973), after reviewing the treatment approaches that have been used, concluded that those methods which have achieved some success have been those which used an operant methodology (e.g., Ferster, 1961; Wolf, Risley, and Mees, 1964; Lovaas et al., 1973). By following a structured program that relies upon the use of appropriate reinforcement, considerable progress can be made in developing speech and language in these children.

Balthazar and Stevens (1975), in reviewing the literature, suggested that the root of professional disagreement regarding the etiology of autism, and how it differs from other conditions such as childhood schizophrenia, is probably the subjective judgments utilized in labeling. They recommended standardization of observational data in order to improve objectivity. Also, classification and diagnosis perhaps should place more emphasis upon strategies for treatment rather than for categorization.

Cerebral Palsy

Cerebral palsy is a term that has been applied to many different conditions whose primary characteristic is a motor disorder or difficulty in body movement or control. It is a descriptive term rather than an etiologic diagnosis and refers to motor dysfunction resulting from an injury to the brain during the developmental period (before age 18). The American Academy of Cerebral Palsy proposes seven different types of manifestations of the motor disorder: 1) rigidity, which is characterized by a stiffness of the body and limbs; 2) spasticity, which results in the muscle becoming stiff with increased movement; 3) tremor, in which the limb quivers when a voluntary and coordinated movement is attempted; 4) ataxia, which is usually shown by a staggering gait or jerky arm movements; 5) athetosis, which is characterized by a "writhing" or overflow of muscle movement that makes the whole body move when the person attempts to move only one part; 6) atonia, which is demonstrated by lack of sufficient muscle tone; and 7) mixed, a term used when an individual displays more than one of the above characteristics.

The causes of such a diverse symptomatology are also many and diverse. They include genetic conditions that produce inborn errors of metabolism that in turn cause brain damage and motor dysfunction; prenatal viral and bacterial infections; trauma at the time of birth that may produce anoxia (insufficient oxygen reaching the brain); and postnatal infections such as pneumococcus meningitis or measles encephalitis.

The United Cerebral Palsy Association, the national organization concerned with the problems of this disability group, reported a prevalence rate of about three cerebral palsied children per 1000 population (Taylor, 1961). The prevalence in the United States has been given as 750,000 (Senate Report 93-1169). Wishik (1956), in a 10% sampling of two counties in Georgia, found a prevalence rate of five per 1000 children under age 21. A similar finding was obtained in a 5% sample of Alamance County in North Carolina (Richardson and Higgins, 1964).

The same insult to the central nervous system that causes motor dysfunction also causes other handicaps. Taylor (1961) analyzed the records of 187 cerebral palsied children seen at the Boston Children's Hospital and found that the incidence of mental retardation in this group was approximately 50%. Hearing losses are also frequent, with an overall average of 25% (Cardwell, 1956). Some 50% of the cerebral palsied have vision defects, 60% have speech disorders, and at least one-third have had seizures at one time in their lives (Illingworth, 1958). R. O. Robinson (1973) found similar additional handicaps in a group of 80 cerebral palsied children. A total of 13% had hearing impairments and 31% visual handicaps.

Epilepsy

Epilepsy is, ". . . a clinical disorder involving impairment of consciousness, characterized by single or recurring attacks of loss of consciousness, convulsive movements, or disturbances of feeling or behavior. These transient episodes are associated with excessive neuronal discharge occurring diffusely or focally in the brain. The sites of neuronal discharges determine the clinical manifestations of the seizures" (testimony on Developmentally Disabled Assistance and Bill of Rights Act, 1974). Basically, epilepsy is a symptom of a central nervous system disorder in which there is a recurrent loss or impairment of consciousness. There may be associated muscular movements that range from a simple twitching of the eyelids to a convulsive shaking of the entire body (Arangio, 1974).

Estimates of the prevalence rate for epilepsy vary widely. Different surveys have used different criteria—for instance, either including or excluding individuals who have had febrile convulsions (seizures that occur during high fever). Because of the stigma attached to epilepsy, many physicians are hesitant to report patients who have it. Certainly, an epileptic is not likely to freely admit that he is an epileptic because he may be unable to obtain a driver's license or gain employment.

The National Institute of Neurological Diseases and Stroke has given the highest estimate of the number of epilepsy-affected persons in the United States, indicating that it is between 1 and 2% (Coatsworth and Penry, 1972). This estimate was based on a number of clinical studies and included persons with a history of convulsions in infancy. Folsom (1968) reported that epilepsy affects only four to seven of every 1000 individuals. She indicated that the best figures come from the World War II draft. Five to six draftees per 1000 were rejected from service because of reported epilepsy. As Table 1 reveals, there is a considerable difference in prevalence estimates obtained by Wishik (1956), who reported four in 1000, and Richardson and Higgins (1964), who reported 31 in 1000 among children under age 21. However, in a follow-up clinic examination of approximately one-half of the children in the Richardson and Higgins study, an adjusted, and lower, prevalence of 12 per 1000 was obtained.

The age of onset of febrile seizures is between 6 months and 3 years. One child in 50 under 5 years of age will have one or more seizures. About 50% of these children will have more than one seizure, and about 10% will have more than four seizures (Millichap, 1974). Lennox (1960) reported that 30.1% of epileptics begin having some seizures before age 5, 46.7% between ages 5 and 19, and 23.2% after age 19.

Mental Retardation

The definition of mental retardation is understandably complex—very simply, because of the difficulties in understanding and defining intelligence. Robinson and Robinson (1965) pointed out that there have been many diverse ideas about the nature of intelligence. However, most definitions have emphasized one of three themes: 1) capacity to learn; 2) knowledge acquired; or 3) ability to adjust or adapt to the total environment, particularly to novel situations.

Prehm (1974) indicated that definitions of mental retardation have stressed one or more of five concepts. Three of these are almost always used and two are used less frequently. The first of these is the notion that mental retardation arises during the developmental period. This is usually taken as being before 16 or 18 years of age and excludes conditions caused by trauma and disease that may produce intellectual impairments in adults. A second condition stipulated in all definitions is mental subnormality or subaverage intellectual functioning. The third condition relates to an inability to adjust socially. Fourth, some professionals have stipulated that an organic cause must be identifiable because they feel that mental retardation is basically a defect of the central nervous system. This leads to the fifth concept used in some definitions, that mental retardation is essentially incurable. If mental retardation arises only from central nervous system defect, then it would naturally follow that the condition is incurable because central nervous tissue cannot be regenerated.

Edgar A. Doll (1941) developed a widely accepted definition that attempted to include all of the essential elements thought to be present in menal retardation. His definition included six elements: 1) socially incompetent, that is, showing ". . . inherent incapacity for managing themselves independently beyond the marginal level of subsistence;" 2) mentally subnormal; 3) retarded intellectually from birth or early age; 4) caused by heredity or disease; 5) continuing to exist at maturity; and 6) essentially incurable. Doll (1953) was the first to attempt to standardize a measure of social competence with the development of the Vineland Social Maturity Scale.

Brison (1967) summarized the criticism that has been leveled at the use of intelligence tests as the sole criterion for labeling an individual as mentally retarded. For example, the intelligence test may not measure some aspects of behavior necessary for social adjustment. Intelligence test scores are subject to errors of measurement, resulting in fluctuations in IQ. Moreover, performance on an intelligence test is greatly influenced by cultural differences, sensory defects, and defects of the central nervous system. The early hope was that, with the development of standardized intelligence tests, much of the difficulty in comparing and classifying individuals, as well as establishing appropriate education programs, would be diminished. The intelligence test sought to measure the intellectual *potential* of the individual rather than his performance. Unfortunately, even tests specifically developed to reduce the influence of cultural factors upon test performance—such as the Arthur Adaptation of the Leiter and the Cattell Culture Free Test— have not proved effective in this regard (Bensberg and Sloan, 1954, 1955).

Because of the inadequacies of existing definitions and classification systems, the American Association on Mental Deficiency (AAMD) undertook a research project to develop and test a classification system that would be compatible with the International Classification of Diseases and that could be reliably used by professional persons working in this field. The system was developed in 1957, with subsequent revisions in 1959 and 1973 (Grossman, 1973). The major change between the earlier classification system and that currently in use is the deletion of the borderline category (70 to 79 IQ range). The AAMD definition currently is, "Mental retardation refers to significantly subaverage general intellect functioning existing concurrently with deficits in adaptive behavior and manifested during the developmental period."

The AAMD definition of mental retardation denotes a level of behavioral performance without reference to etiology. Hence, it makes no attempt to distinguish between retardation associated with psychosocial influences and that associated with biologic defects. In addition, an attempt is made to describe current behavior with no intention of implying prognosis. In spite of the shortcomings of psychologic tests, the AAMD has taken the position that these tests are still the most reliable and valid instruments available in diagnosing and classifying the retarded. For that reason, the evaluation of intellectual functioning, as well as adaptive behavior, is based upon test results.

Significantly subaverage intellectual functioning may be assessed by one or more of the standardized tests. It refers to performance that is two or more standard deviations below the mean of the test. In the case of the Stanford-Binet, this would mean an upper IQ limit of 68, and in the case of the Wechsler Intelligence Scale, an upper IQ limit of 70. Table 2 presents the IQ ranges for each level of retardation.

If the number within each level of retardation fits the normal curve expectancy, one would project only a total of 60 profoundly retarded in the United States (based on a population of 210 million). However, as Penrose (1954) and Dingman and Tarjan (1960) have pointed out, there are many more than this number within existing institutions. If one included those suspected of residing within the community, the excess number of retarded within the lower levels of intelligence would be sizable. Penrose, and Dingman and Tarjan argued that, although the "physiologically" retarded may fit the normal curve, people who are retarded as a result of disease or trauma create a larger than expected number. These researchers projected, for example, that, although one would predict only 60 individuals in the profound level of retardation, there are probably some 105,000. They projected some excess in the severe and moderate levels, with the mild level being approximately in keeping with the normal curve expectancy. This would lead to the expectation that nearly 5.5 million persons in the United States are mildly retarded.

Table 2. Levels and IQ ranges for Wechsler, Cattell, and Stanford-Binet

Levels	Intelligence quotient		
	Stanford-Binet, Cattell	Wechsler scales[a]	S.D. below mean
Mild	68–52	69–55	−2.00 to −3.00
Moderate	51–36	54–40	−3.00 to −4.00
Severe	35–20	39–25 (ext.)	−4.00 to −5.00
Profound	19 and below	24 and below (ext.)	Below −5.00

Adapted from Robinson and Robinson (1965).
[a]ext., extrapolated.

Adaptive behavior is defined as, "the effectiveness or degree with which the individual meets the standards of personal independence and social responsibility expected of his age and cultural group" (Grossman, 1973). Because these expectations vary for different ages and societal groups, deficits in adaptive behavior would be expected to vary as well. During early childhood, critical areas of adaptive behavior would be sensorimotor skills, communication skills, self-help skills, and social skills. During childhood, academic skills, appropriate reasoning and judgment, and interpersonal skills become important. In adults, vocationally related skills are expected to emerge. The AAMD Adaptive Behavior Scale (AAMD, 1969) was developed specifically for the purpose of assessing level of adaptive behavior. There is a positive relationship between measured intelligence and adaptive behavior. As the level of intelligence becomes lower, the level of adaptive behavior is also lower (Heber, 1965).

The most accepted prevalence rate of mental retardation is 3% of the population. However, this is based on expert opinion and the concept of the normal distribution of intelligence rather than on established fact because various epidemiologic studies have reported prevalence rates of 0.4% to 18.4%. Generally, epidemiologic studies are of three types: voluntary reporting, agency surveys, and household surveys. As Conley (1973) pointed out, the agency surveys generally produce relatively low prevalence figures because not all individuals possessing a particular trait are known to agencies. In addition, epidemiologic surveys have used widely differing definitions of retardation that greatly influence the prevalence figures. Surveys defining retardation on the basis of IQ tests alone usually produce the highest prevalences.

Wishik (1956) found a prevalence rate of 40 mentally retarded per 1000 population under age 21 in two counties in Georgia. This was based on a follow-up examination of children identified by a 10% sampling in a house-to-house canvas. This estimate was reduced to 36 per 1000 when those not showing "functional" retardation, or deficits in adaptive behavior, were excluded. This is half the rate found by Richardson and Higgins (1964) in their survey of 5% of the homes in Alamance County, North Carolina. An adjusted rate of 77 per 1000 (or 7.7%) was found in their survey. The researchers, recognizing that their rates were far higher than any reported by other researchers, suggested that their findings may be the result of the more inclusive definitions that they used. However, they felt that the major difference in their study was the whole-hearted support that they received from the agencies, volunteers collecting data, and participating public. A survey by the New York Department of Mental Hygiene (1955) reported a prevalence rate of 35.2 per 1000 population under age 18. Kirk and Weiner (1969) were critical of this finding because of the study's failure to differentiate mental retardation from educational retardation. The New York study found a very low prevalence rate below age 5 (0.5%) as compared to during the early teen years (8%). Kirk and Weiner felt that their definition included individuals who may have shown poor social and academic adaptation but who were otherwise intellectually normal.

Robinson and Robinson (1965) pointed out that most studies in the United States have found that black children, as well as children from several other minority groups, tend to obtain lower scores on intelligence tests than do white children. Kennedy, Van de Riet, and White (1963) confirmed this in their study of black children in the southeastern United States. Ginzberg and Bray (1953) found that the rejection of black men during World War II was 15.2% as compared with 2.5% for white men, with the rejection rate for the South generally greater than that for other parts of the country.

Socioeconomic conditions also influence the prevalence rates of mental retardation. Kirk (1963) suggested that mild retardation occurs about twice as frequently in low-income families as in middle-income families. Dr. Don Stedman of the University of North Carolina (personal communication) feels that there is sufficient evidence to predict the number of retarded people who would need services in various socioeconomic groups. He believes that the prevalence of retardation in middle- and upper-class suburbs is 2%, whereas in rural areas it is 5%, and in the inner city it is 7%.

In evaluating these findings, one must remember that the relationship between ethnic group and mental retardation is complicated and controversial, although prenatal and postnatal health problems may continue to lower intellectual functioning among lower-income groups of all ethnicities. Intelligence tests are not always fair to members of minority groups because their items are often based on information that is part of the mainstream white culture and because communication and cultural factors influence motivation and performance in testing situations. It is essential to note that rates of retardation in minority groups have been demonstrated to drop markedly when adaptive behavior is considered along with intelligence test score (Mercer, 1973).

HEARING IMPAIRMENT

Hearing impairment is not generally considered a developmental disability because it may occur at any age. However, because the onset of hearing loss often occurs at a very early age, one can argue convincingly that it should be considered a developmental disability. For example, the Office of Demographic Studies (1973b) reported that, of the 34,218 individuals being served by special education programs for the hearing impaired, 65.4% were congenitally deaf and an additional 12.1% became deaf before 3 years of age. Of course, these figures are exaggerated because adults were not included in the survey. When adults are appropriately represented in the sample, some 12% of the population of deaf have this handicap before the age of 3 (Schein and Delk, 1974).

Although one might presume that the identification and statistical reporting of individuals with hearing impairment would be much easier than that for a handicap such as mental retardation, this is not the case. The surveys that have been conducted are not only plagued by problems of biased samples and inadequate assessment techniques, but they have not used a standard criterion for degree of hearing loss. The standard definitions fall into two categories: 1) functional criteria in which the degree of hearing loss is expressed in terms of its influence on receiving and understanding spoken language; and 2) definitions expressed in terms of decibel loss on the basis of audiometric examinations.

There are many terms that refer to the hearing impaired. Lloyd's (1973, p. 47) operational or functional definition is as follows:

> "Hearing Impairment"—refers to a deviation in hearing sufficient to impair normal aural-oral communication. The degree of hearing impairment is the result of the degree of deviation in hearing (sensitivity and/or other auditory abilities) interacting with a number of other factors, e.g., age of onset, age of detection and intervention, duration, type of pathology and related factors, use of amplification, habilitative programming, family factors, and resilience or compensatory (or adaptive) abilities.

Lloyd reserves use of the term *deafness* for the extreme end of the continuum where the normal acquisition of oral language is precluded. The above definition is similar to that developed in 1938 by the Conference of Executives of American Schools for the Deaf (CEASD), who used the term *deaf* to apply to those in whom the sense of hearing is nonfunctional for ordinary purposes of life. The CEASD distinguishes between the congenitally deaf (those born deaf) and the adventitiously deaf (those who are born with hearing but later become deaf). Vernon (1969) felt that the age at which deafness occurs is most critical in determining the development of speech and language, and that those persons with the greatest handicap are those whose deafness is congenital or developed within the first 2 or 3 years of life.

Most authorities divide hearing impairments into three types (Lloyd, 1968; National Institute of Neurological Diseases and Stroke, 1970; Goodhill and Guggenheim, 1971). A *conductive loss* is one in which there is a defect in the conductive pathway of the hearing organ—that is, anything peripheral to the round or oval window. The term *sensorineural* has replaced the terms *nerve deafness* and *perceptive deafness* and refers to a second type of hearing impairment, involving the cochlear and neural auditory pathway. A *mixed* hearing impairment is one in which there are defects in both areas. For a fuller discussion of types of hearing impairment and audiometric findings, the reader is referred to Cox and Lloyd (this volume).

Most surveys have used the pure tone audiometer to determine degree of hearing loss. The pure tone frequencies that provide the best estimate of speech reception are 500, 1000, and 2000 Hz. Hz, the abbreviation for Hertz, stands for a unit of vibration frequency that has been adopted internationally to replace the term *cycles per second,* or cps. It was named after Heinrich Rudolph Hertz, the German physicist. Sensitivity to sound is expressed in decibels (or dB), a logarithmic ratio unit indicating by what proportion one intensity level differs from another. Studies before 1964 generally used the 1951 reference threshold developed by the American Standards Association (ASA). In 1964, the International Organization for Standardization (ISO) adopted a revised reference threshold. The American Standards Association, renamed the American National Standards Institute (ANSI) in 1969, adopted reference thresholds that approximate the 1964 ISO references (Lloyd, 1970; Melnick, 1971). Hence, in some recent studies, a reference to ANSI is given when referring to the newer threshold levels of the ISO. Table 3 shows the relationship of the ASA standards to the ISO and ANSI standards. The ISO and ANSI thresholds are approximately 10 dB lower at each frequency than the older ASA thresholds. This shift—attributable to improved subject selection, sound-treated rooms, equipment, and techniques—means that the person with average hearing can perceive a tone 10 dB lower than was indicated under the previous standard.

Eleven states now have some type of screening program for children entering into kindergarten or first grade. Although the states vary in the criteria used when deciding whether further testing is required, the usual criterion is a hearing loss of greater than 20 dB (ISO) in either or both ears for one or more frequency within the speech range.

There have been numerous classification systems developed in order to better categorize individuals with varying degrees of hearing loss. One of these was developed by Huizing (1953):

Grade I: 0–30 dB = slight loss
Grade II: 30–60 dB = moderate loss
Grade III: 60–90 dB = severe loss
Grade IV: more than 90 dB = deaf (no speech-understanding ability)

Early surveys of the general population used such biased samples that they have little value for estimating prevalence. However, within the past decade several studies have attempted to obtain a stratified sample. One recent survey is the 1960–1962 Health Examination Survey (Glorig and Roberts, 1965). Hearing tests were administered to 6672 persons selected to represent the 111 million adults aged 18 to 79 in the United States. Military and institutionalized individuals were excluded. A total of 1.6% had hearing losses

Table 3. Comparison between ASA, ISO, and ANSI reference thresholds in dB

	Frequency (Hz, or cycles/sec)					
	125	250	500	1000	2000	4000
1951 ASA	54.5	39.5	25.0	16.5	17.0	15.0
1964 ISO and 1970 ANSI	45.5	24.5	11.0	6.5	8.5	9.0
dB difference	10.0	15.0	14.0	10.0	8.5	6.0

in the 41- to 55-dB range (frequent difficulty with normal speech), and 1.1% had losses in the 56- to 70-dB range (frequent difficulty with loud speech). A second study derived its estimates from interviews obtained during a continuous probability sampling of the civilian, noninstitutional population of the United States (Gentile, Schein, and Hasse, 1967). All together, 134,000 persons representing the entire age span were included. The criteria of hearing impairment were qualitative, being expressed in terms of the kinds of trouble in everyday hearing that the respondents to the interviews observed in themselves and their relatives. In this survey, 1.7% reported impaired hearing but said they could hear and understand most normally spoken words, and 1.0% indicated that they could hear and understand only a few loudly spoken words.

A more recent study of the deaf population in the United States was sponsored by the National Association of the Deaf in cooperation with the Deafness Research and Training Center at New York University (Schein and Delk, 1974). Their study population was defined as those persons who could not hear and understand speech and who lost (or never had) that ability before they were 19 years old. This group was labeled *prevocationally deaf*. A national list of deaf persons was compiled, and then contacts were made to make sure that each nominee on the list met the project criteria. Next, a probability sample of 42,000 households in the United States was drawn, and interviews were conducted to locate all prevocationally deaf persons was compiled, and then contacts were made to make the deaf persons found in the household interviews, the completeness of the list then could be estimated. The verified list was then corrected to include those who had been identified in the household survey but had not been included in the original list. The hearing-impaired individuals identified by the Hearing Interview Survey (Gentile, Schein, and Hasse, 1967) who were not identified by the household survey were also added to the data. Military and institutionalized individuals were not included in the sample.

Degree of hearing loss was determined by the subject's responses to a series of questions that were ranked to indicate an increasing severity of hearing loss. This procedure resulted in a prevalence rate for prevocational deafness of 203 per 100,000 (0.2%), as compared with the generally accepted prevalence for the deaf of 100 per 100,000 (0.1%). Based upon those who indicated a hearing impairment ("I have trouble hearing in one or both ears"), a higher prevalence rate of 660 per 100,000 was obtained.

Schein and Delk (1974) found that prevocational deafness is not uniformly distributed across all ages. A greater prevalence rate appears in the 6 to 24 age range than in the 25 to 44 range. A higher percentage of men than women are prevocationally deaf, although women are affected vocationally and socially more than men. The black population shows a lower prevalence than the white, a finding that Schein and Delk interpreted as reflecting an inadequate sampling of the black population, making figures for blacks less reliable.

One of the best estimates of the prevalence of hearing impairment among public school children was derived from a study of Pittsburgh school children (Eagles et al., 1963). They found that 1.7% of children 5 to 10 years of age had losses greater than 26 dB.

The city schools of Stockholm, Sweden, have been screening all children over 7 years of age since 1951. In recent years, 2135 four-year-olds have been screened by well-baby clinics (Barr, Anderson, and Wedenberg, 1973). A total of over 500,000 children have been seen in all. An analysis of the audiograms indicated that prevalence had not changed greatly in the 13 years of the program. The incidence of temporary or conductive loss decreased with age, while permanent defects, particularly sensorineural, high frequency loss, increased with age. There was no sex difference for conductive loss, but boys showed a higher incidence of sensorineural loss. Bilateral severe to total deafness was found in 0.2% of the population. This no doubt underestimates the prevalence since children in schools for the deaf were excluded. Approximately 4% were found to have a loss greater than 20 dB.

Weber, McGovern, and Zink (1967) analyzed the records of 1000 school children who had been screened during a 5-year-period. All children who failed at 20 dB ISO in the speech range were referred for additional study. After further testing, the prevalence of hearing loss remained at approximately 3%. This finding is similar to that of Feinmesser, Baubergertell, and Bilski-Hirsch (1959), who found an overall rate of 3.08% hearing loss among school children in Jerusalem, Israel. The prevalence was greater among children from a lower socioeconomic group (3.5%) than among the middle class (2.1%). Using a definition of 40 dB ASA or greater in either ear, the National Society for the Study of Education (1950) found that, on the average, 5% of the general school population possessed a hearing loss.

Lipscomb (1973) reported the hearing examinations of 7119 school children considered to be representative of the 6 to 11 age group. He found that about 20% had at least one change or abnormality in an ear or in hearing acuity. About 14% had occluded auditory canals that prevented an examination. Some 9.7% had abnormal tympanic membranes on both sides. Some 4.2% of the parents reported that their child had a problem in hearing.

Although it is clearly difficult to arrive at generalizations given the diversity of samples studied and criteria used, it seems that approximately 0.2% of the school-age population (and the general population as well) are severely and bilaterally impaired or deaf. Approximately 3 to 5% of school children manifest some degree of hearing loss, and some types of hearing impairment increase as a function of age.

Heredity and Hearing Impairment

Kennedy (1967), after reviewing the literature, concluded that the incidence of congenital malformations of all types ranges from 0.15% (when the data used in arriving at the estimates are birth certificates and "official records") through a mean of 1.25% (when the data are derived from hospital records) to 4.5% (when the data are derived from special examinations). He inferred that the actual incidence of congenital defects must be at least 2%, even when minor defects are excluded.

There are about 70 types of hereditary defects in man (Konigswork, 1971). Fortunately, most of these are relatively rare causes of congenital deafness. As Fisch (1973) pointed out, it is not always easy to determine whether a hearing loss is congenital or acquired. During assessment, when no congenital etiologic causes can be discerned, one always must consider that the loss might have been acquired before the time of examination. Unilateral loss of congenital origin is typically discovered late and is rarely included in population statistics.

Table 4 summarizes the major surveys that have been conducted to determine the etiology of hearing impairment. There is wide variability depending upon the source and characteristics of the sample, the comprehensiveness of the evaluation, and, probably, the bias of the clinicians involved. If one were trying to average the findings of

Table 4. Etiology of hearing loss

Study	Population	N	Unknown (%)	Genetic (%)	Prenatal (%)	Perinatal (%)	Postnatal (%)
Vernon (1969)	Applicants to school for deaf	1468		5.4 (both parents deaf)	8.8 rubella	11.9 premature 3.1 Rh	40.4 total 8.1 meningitis 7.3 other infections 25.0 other
Fraser (1970)	Referred children	2355	36.2	30.4	5.9	5.4	19.7
Ruben and Rozycki (1971)	Referred children	348	20.0	60.0	20.0 acquired	20.0	
Fisch (1973)	Referred children	600	25.0	26.0	24.0 rubella	14.0	—
Lindsay (1973)	Referred children			51.5	6.0	10.0	30.0
Surjan, Dvald and Palvadi (1973)	Referred adult	32,397		1.5			71.8 approximate total 19.5 presbyacusis 19.0 noise induced 11.0 tympanosclerosis 12.0 chronic otitis
Wright (1973)	Referred young children	302	25.9	12.3	14.4 rubella 1.6 toxemia	10.2 anoxia 4.8 premature 6.4 kernicterus	17.5
Budden et al. (1974)	Referred preschool	500	48.4	18.2	15.2 rubella 1.2 other	6.4 total 5.25 kernicterus	10.6 total 7.8 meningitis
Schein and Delk (1974)	Adult deaf self-supporting	410,522	17.1	7.6	24.2 total 5.2 rubella	2.5	42.5 total 9.7 meningitis 6.2 scarlet fever

all of the studies, it would appear that approximately one-third seem to have a genetic component, one-third a posttraumatic or post-infectual etiology, and one-third an unknown etiology.

Cleft Palate and Hearing Impairment

Ingalls and Klingberg (1969), after reviewing the literature, concluded that the frequency of occurrence of palatolabial defects is between one and two cases per 1000 live births, whereas the frequency among relatives of affected babies is almost 10 times higher. They also noted that the incidence among Caucasians is almost twice that found among blacks. Spriestersbach et al. (1973) indicated that middle-ear disease only recently has been a universal and persistent problem in infants with unrepaired cleft palates. Those with otitis media (inflammation of the middle ear) experience conductive hearing losses of variable degree. There does seem to be a sharp reduction in middle-ear disease after palatal repair, but nonetheless the evidence suggests that cleft palate is often associated with hearing impairment.

Maternal Rubella and Hearing Impairment

Rubella is a cyclical viral disease that is very mild and usually causes a rash and sore throat. Unfortunately, when contracted by pregnant women, it frequently passes through the placental barrier and infects the unborn fetus. Although it is one of the mildest viruses, it is the only one that regularly causes birth defects (Cooper, 1969). Hardy et al. (1973) found that 37% of the rubella mothers studied did not know they had had the disease until it was confirmed by laboratory tests. Cooper found that the fetus, once infected in the uterus, usually remains infected, and approximately 85% are still shedding rubella virus in pharyngeal secretions at birth. By age 6 months, less than 50% of the infants infected in utero are still infected, and by 1 year, less than 10%.

During the rubella epidemic of 1964, 1% of the pregnancies in the United States became casualties and an estimated 30,000 infants were affected (Siegel, Fuerst, and Peress, 1966). The time at which the pregnant woman contracts rubella is most important in determining its influence on the developing fetus (Cooper and Krugman, 1967). From the 2nd to the 6th week after conception, the maximal hazard is to the heart and eyes. Deafness may be the only clinical manifestation of congenital rubella, especially if maternal infection occurs after the 8th week of pregnancy (Friedman and Wright, 1966). By the 5th month, the influence of maternal infection does not appear to be significant. For affected infants, low birth weight is the rule. Hepatitis, anemia, and disturbed bone growth are also frequently found. Hardy and Bordley (1973), in a study of 300 confirmed rubella cases, reported that 40% had impaired hearing, 25% had heart defects, 20% had visual problems, 60% showed slow motor development, and 50% had poor physical development. Vernon (1967a), in a study of rubella-induced deafness in children at the Riverside School for the Deaf, found that 43% were born prematurely and that males exceeded females, 59 to 41%. He reported that 53.8% had multiple handicaps.

Hearing loss attributable to rubella is generally considered to be sensorineural in character (Brookhauser and Bordley, 1973; Ojala, Timo, and Elo, 1973). Although defects in middle-ear structures have been reported, rubella deafness is generally the result of damage to the organ of Corti (Friedman and Wright, 1966).

Ojala, Timo, and Elo (1973) reported that, of all deafness among children, some 12% was caused by rubella. In a study of 128 rubella infants, they found that 20% had moderate to severe hearing loss, 34% had profound loss, 21% were mixed, and 14% were difficult to test. Similar findings were obtained by Hodgson (1969) for 43 postrubella children. Hardy et al. (1973), in a study of 129 cases, found that 17% had mild to severe losses and 24% had profound losses. Brookhauser and Bordley (1973) reported that, in about 25% of the cases, a progressive loss of hearing occurs as the child grows older.

Rubella seems to be associated with lower intelligence as well as with hearing impairment. Vernon (1967a), in his study of students from the Riverside School for the Deaf, found that the average IQ of the rubella group was significantly below that of other students. Some one-third of these students were below 90 IQ and 8% were below 70 IQ. Hardy (1973) reported that an intelligence evaluation of 171 rubella children up to age 5 indicated that 40.3% were average or above in intelligence, 31.1% borderline to dull normal, and 28.6% mentally retarded. A higher percentage of the retarded children possessed hearing impairments, visual impairments, and small head size.

Rh Factor and Hearing Impairment

A pregnant woman whose blood type is Rh negative and whose husband is heterozygous for Rh can expect half of her children to be Rh positive. In some instances, it is believed that blood may escape through the placental barrier into the mother's bloodstream. Because of the incompatibility of the Rh-positive blood with the mother's Rh-negative blood, the mother builds up antibodies against these cells. These antibodies then pass into the fetal circulation and destroy the Rh-positive cells by combining with them. The result is erythroblastosis fetalis (hemolytic anemia), which results in kernicterus or jaundiced areas of the brain (Goodhill, 1956).

Generally, the likelihood of the fetal blood passing through the placental barrier increases with successive pregnancies. Although approximately one out of 12 pregnancies represents the blood combinations that can produce erythroblastosis fetalis, it happens in only one out of 200 births (Ford, 1960). Fortunately, complete blood transfusions carried out during the first day or two following birth seem to prevent major damage from occurring. Goldstein, McRandle, and Rodman (1972) argued that the cause of deafness that may result from kernicterus may be damage to the hearing mechanism rather than damage to auditory areas of the brain. They cite findings indicating a defect in the cochlea. Vernon (1967c) felt that there is strong evidence of brain damage in these individuals. It seems logical to assume that the deficit may be a disorder of perceptual integration rather than an elevated threshold.

Vernon (1967c), in a survey of 1468 applicants to the California School for the Deaf from 1953 to 1964, found 45 educationally deaf (at 65 dB or higher) with a definitely established erythroblastosis fetalis condition. None of these was Oriental, black, or Mexican-American, and 71.1% were multiply handicapped. One out of four of these individuals could not maintain the minimal standards required by the schools for the deaf. Robinson (1964) considered complications of Rh incompatibility as the leading perinatal cause of deafness, accounting for about 3.1% of all profound hearing loss among school-age deaf children.

Prematurity and Hearing Impairment

There seems to be very little agreement among professionals in the field as to whether prematurity itself carries any particular risk to the child (Robinson and Robinson, 1965). Increasing knowledge is accumulating that prematurity tends to be associated with many factors such as socioeconomic status, prenatal health care, and whether the mother is a heavy smoker or drinker. Prematurity is also associated with factors related to the health of the mother such as maternal rubella and complications of the Rh factor. Research has been hampered by lack of agreement on the definition of prematurity, resulting from the problems in accurately determining gestational age. Consequently, most research has used birth weight as the criterion, usually defining prematurity as a birth weight under 5 pounds (or 2268 g).

It is generally accepted that the immature development of the prematurely born infant does make him more susceptible to injury. Desmond and Rudolph (1970) studied 6211 live births. Some 5300 of these were term infants, and 911 were low birth weight infants. Major malformations were present in 2.6% of the term births and 3.7% of the low birth weight infants. Neonatal deaths occurred in 0.5% of the term births and 12.3% of the low weight births. The incidence of other symptoms of central nervous system problems was much higher among the low birth weight group.

Vernon (1967d) found 257 premature births among 1468 applicants to the California School for the Deaf. This represents a prevalence rate of 17.4%, which is much higher than the 7.6% prevalence in the general population. He found that all but 11.9% of the premature children had other problems associated with prematurity, such as rubella or Rh complications. Thus, for a variety of reasons, there is a linkage between prematurity and hearing impairment.

Postnatal Infections and Hearing Impairment

Meningitis is the leading postnatal cause of hearing loss among school-age deaf children (Robinson, 1964). Unfortunately, as Vernon (1969) and Schein and Delk (1974) pointed out, it is difficult to pinpoint its exact incidence as an etiologic factor because there have not been any recent studies that have relied upon laboratory diagnoses. For example, the Schein and Delk study relied upon interview data that, in many instances, reflected what the parents of the deaf person told him caused his deafness. Also, medical advances over the past two decades have probably obscured the role of meningitis as a causative factor in deafness.

Meningitis is a disease that begins as an infection of the membranes surrounding the brain. It can be caused by a wide range of infectious organisms including bacteria, viruses, fungi, and spirochetes (Kelly, 1964). Meningitis occurs most frequently in young children, with some 50% of the cases being children under 5 years of age (Ford, 1960). Vernon (1967b), in a study of 1468 school-age deaf children, found 8% to be postmeningitic. Additional handicaps were detected in 38% of this group, with mental retardation, aphasia, and cerebral palsy being common.

Lindsay (1973a) indicated that the incidence of deafness attributable to measles accounts for 3 to 4% of the deaf. Mumps is another childhood disease that may infect the central nervous system and produce sensorineural deafness. Lindsay estimated that bilateral deafness caused by mumps affects from 0.5 to 5% of all deafness that occurs in childhood. In the Schein and Delk (1974) survey of adult deaf persons, three out of 10 cases were attributable to illnesses. Spinal meningitis was the most frequent cause and accounted for 9.7% of the cases. Scarlet fever was the attributed cause of deafness for 6.2%, measles for 4.3%, and whooping cough for 2.6%.

The bacterium of congenital syphilis has been long known to cause deafness as well as other mental and physical handicaps. With the discovery of penicillin, it was hoped that syphilis might be eradicated. However, it is apparently on the increase because of increased sexual activity among young people and reduced reliance upon the condom for birth control. Kerr, Smyth, and Cinnamond (1973) reported seeing 25 cases of congenital syphilis in an English clinic. They pointed out that inner-ear symptoms can develop years after the congenital condition seems to be cured.

MULTIPLE HANDICAPS

There is increasing evidence that many individuals possess more than one handicapping condition. This seems to be particularly true of conditions that arise during the developmental period. Wolf and Anderson (1969) and Doctor (1959) independently concluded that there is considerable evidence in the literature to support the hypothesis that the number of individuals with multiple handicaps has increased. They suggested that this may be partially explained by improved treatment of communicable and infectious disease, improved public health services, advances in prenatal care, and the prevention of infant mortality, increased education, and better housing—all of which have contributed to the survival of handicapped children who formerly would have died. (Of course, greater awareness and improved diagnostic and treatment procedures also may inflate incidence figures.)

In a study of 145 hearing-impaired individuals, Bolton (1972) found that 34% had a secondary disability and 12% had three handicapping conditions. Wishik's (1956) 10% sampling of two counties in Georgia revealed that 10% of all children under age 21 had one or more handicapping conditions. There was an average of 2.2 pathologic conditions per child. In a similar survey followed by clinical examination in a North Carolina county, Richardson and Higgins (1964) found an average of 1.6 handicapping conditions per child.

A New York public school, Junior High School #47, provides instruction for 45 deaf and 630 hearing-impaired mentally retarded students. A total of 85% have a hearing loss greater than 85 dB. Approximately 70% of these students have more than the dual handicaps of hearing impairment and mental retardation (Page and LaPlace, 1972).

Communication Disorders and Mental Retardation

The prevalence of speech disorders within the general population is difficult to determine. As with many other handicapping disorders, there is no universally accepted definition with criteria that permit reliable surveys. Milisen (1971) stated that a median figure might be as meaningful as any. He reported that, from kindergarten through the fourth-grade level, approximately 12 to 15% of the children have seriously deviant speech. Perhaps this reflects the high incidence of articulation problems in early childhood that do not require therapeutic intervention. Above the fourth grade, the prevalence would be approximately 4 to 5%.

Delayed speech is one of the common characteristics of the mentally retarded. The literature is also in general agreement that, when speech does emerge in mentally retarded children, it is more often defective than it is in the general population. Matthews (1971) reviewed 18 studies that surveyed the prevalence of speech defects among the retarded. A range of 18 to 94% was reported, with an approximate median of 56%. This is in general agreement with an estimate by Spradlin (1963), who set the prevalence at 52 to 57%.

Keane (1972) summarized the literature in this area and, among other things, concluded the following:

1. There is a higher than normal prevalence of communication disorders in the retarded
2. Those institutionalized have a higher prevalence than the non-institutionalized
3. Although the data are inconclusive, it seems that the lower the IQ, the more frequent the communication problems
4. The data are inconclusive regarding the prevalence of stuttering among the retarded

Hearing Impairment and Mental Retardation

The Task Force on the Mentally Retarded and the Deaf (1973) pointed out that mental retardation alone and an auditory deficit alone are significant handicapping conditions. When both intellectual and hearing impairment are present in the same individual, the combination of the two handicaps is frequently disastrous for the individual and his family.

The literature is in general agreement in indicating higher prevalences of mental retardation among the hearing impaired and higher prevalences of hearing impairment among the mentally retarded. In a survey of school children in California, Leenhouts (1969) found that about 15% of the deaf children of school age were retarded. In the 1971 to 1972 annual survey of the deaf (Office of Demographic Studies, 1973a), 19.3% of children enrolled in day classes for the hearing impaired were retarded. This is only slightly lower than the 23.4% rate of retardation found in residential schools for the deaf. Anderson and Stevens (1969) reported that a median of 19% of the deaf school population fell below 83 IQ. Powers and Quigley (1970), after a review of the literature, concluded that 11% of all deaf children may be classified as being educable mentally retarded (in the mild to moderate range of retardation). Conley (1973) estimated that if 0.1% of the population is deaf and 15% of these are retarded, then some 9000 school-age children have these dual handicaps.

Most of the hearing surveys of retarded populations have been carried out in state residential facilities for the mentally retarded. These surveys have produced widely differing results. Lloyd (1971, 1973; Lloyd and Moore, 1972) pointed out that these differences can be attributed to the criteria of hearing impairment used, characteristics of the retarded population, hearing assessments used, and expertise of the audiologist. Hogan (1973) pointed out that two different formulas have been used in deriving the percentage of the retarded who are hearing impaired. This same point was made by Lloyd and Reid (1967) in a survey of the complete population of the state school at Parsons, Kansas. In one case, the difficult-to-test retarded were added to the denominator of the total subjects, and in the other case, only those subjects who had valid audiograms were included in the denominator. Hogan argued that the latter formula is more accurate. However, in examining his data, a higher percentage of the more severely retarded fall in the difficult-to-test group, and this group would be expected to have a higher incidence of hearing impairment. Much of the difficulty in determining the relationship between mental retardation and hearing impairment stems from the difficulty of testing retarded persons.

Table 5 summarizes 12 studies that have surveyed hearing impairment among the retarded in state residential facilities for the mentally retarded. Although one can see the wide variability in prevalence among the different studies, it is clear that the prevalence of hearing impairment is much higher among the mentally retarded than among the general population. It would appear that the figure suggested by Lloyd (1971, 1973; Lloyd and Moore, 1972)—10 to 15%—probably approximates the actual prevalence.

SUMMARY AND RECOMMENDATIONS

Estimates of the prevalence of disorders of communication associated with developmental disabilities and hearing impairment are indeed only estimates. Problems of definition, lack of consensus on criteria or standards that can be communicated from one researcher to another and utilized in replicated studies, biased samples, and varying degrees of competency in diagnosis and assessment all present problems in arriving at precise figures. However, our technology has greatly improved in recent years, and appreciation for the interrelationships of many handicapping conditions is gradually filling gaps in our knowledge. A relatively recent concept, that of developmental disabilities, has helped to focus attention on the multiply handicapped and the need for coordinated services. The concept always includes mental retardation, cerebral palsy, and epilepsy, and recently has

Table 5. Selected studies of hearing impairment among institutionalized retarded[a]

Study	N	Sample characteristics[a]	Percent	Methods and criteria
Birch and Matthews (1951)	247	CA: 10–19, IQ: 49	55.5 44.5	Screening 15 dB (ASA), 512–8192 Hz 20 dB
Johnson and Farrell (1954)	270		24.0	Screening 20 dB (ASA), two or more frequencies
Schlanger and Gottsleben (1956)	498	Younger Older	25.7 41.4	Screening 30 dB either ear, 125–12,000 Hz
Kodman et al. (1959)	84 105	CA: 15.4, MA: 6.8 CA: 38.7, MA: 6.4	19.0 23.8	Screening 20 dB (ASA), two or more frequencies
Rittmanic (1959)	1220[b]	CA: 10–14 CA: over 59	19.8 84.0	Screening 15 dB (ASA) either ear, 250–8000 Hz, two or more frequencies
Sigenthaler and Krzywicki (1959)	638	Female adults	17.9	Screening 15 dB (ASA) either ear
Webb, Weber, and Biddle (1964)	369		25.0	Screening 20 dB (ASA) 500–2000 Hz

Continued

Table 5—*continued*

Study	N	Sample characteristics[a]	Percent	Methods and criteria
Lloyd and Reid (1967)	638[c]	CA: 6–22, all levels MR	22.0	Screening Poorer than 15 dB in either ear at one or more frequency octaves 250–8000 Hz plus 600 (excluding the difficult to test, there were 29%)
			19.0	Poorer than 25 dB as above
Mitra (1970)		Survey of MR facilities	4.3 median %; range 1–21%	Rating scale, questionnaire
				Questionnaire, criteria
Colpoys (1972)	2600	Survey of MR facilities	1.7 deaf	Not given
			6.3 hearing impaired	
Hogan (1973)	815[d]	51% severe and profound	42.0	Questionnaire, criteria Not given
Brannan, Sigelman, and Bensberg (1975)	98,034	Survey of state MR facilities	2.3 deaf	Questionnaire
			7.2 hearing impaired	Functional criteria

Adapted from: Lloyd, 1970. See his table (pp. 314–329) for a more complete summary of studies.
[a]Chronologic age (CA) and mental age (MA) in years; MR, mental retardation.
[b]30–129 excluded as untestable.
[c]24% classified as difficult to test.
[d]303 untestable.

been used to refer to autism, specific learning disabilities, and other handicaps arising in the developmental period. Although definitive studies have not been made to determine the prevalence of developmental disabilities, it is estimated that approximately 10% of the population has one or more of these handicapping conditions. The evidence is fairly clear that the number of individuals with multiple handicaps is increasing.

The prevalence of most handicapping conditions seems to be correlated with socioeconomic status. Most studies have indicated that the lower the socioeconomic level, the greater the incidence of prematurity, prenatal infection, congenital defects such as deafness, and mental retardation.

Special emphasis is placed in this chapter on the prevalence of hearing impairment, mental retardation, and the combination of both of these handicaps in an individual. Various surveys of public school children suggest that some 5% will show a hearing loss in one or both ears. Many of these are apparently temporary impairments attributable to ear infections. However, it seems that 1.7% of school children show a loss greater than 25 dB and that 0.2% suffer a bilateral loss of severe degree. The most recent study that sampled the general population used the functional definition of an "inability to understand and use speech." This study found 0.2% of the population deaf according to this definition. However, this increases to approximately 0.6% in the 45 to 64 age group and to 2.8% among those over age 64.

Estimates of prevalence of mental retardation are usually set at 3% of the general population. Several studies have suggested that the figures may run as low as 2% in middle- and upper-class neighborhoods, 5% in rural areas, and 7% in lower-income neighborhoods.

The prevalence of hearing impairment among the retarded has been found to be much greater than in the general population. As pointed out by Lloyd (1973), the deviation in functioning level of hearing-impaired, mentally retarded persons is greater than the sum of the deviations attributable to each handicap separately. The problems of hearing impairment and mental retardation do not add arithmetically; rather, they compound geometrically. Most studies conducted in schools for the deaf have indicated that 10 to 15% of the students are mentally retarded. Surveys in residential facilities for the mentally retarded have indicated a similar prevalence of hearing impairment.

Based on a review of the literature regarding the prevalence of various developmental disabilities, several clear recommendations can be made. Tremendous technical progress has been made within the past 10 years in the fields of audiology, medicine, psychology, and other disciplines concerned with the developmentally disabled. With the development of techniques and instruments such as the evoked response audiometer, impedance bridge, and improved operant audiometry, there should be very few individuals whose hearing level cannot be accurately assessed. An immediate need is for strengthening hearing screening services, particularly during the early preschool years. Well-baby clinics, public health nursing programs, and primary care physicians all represent resources that can implement hearing screening as a routine procedure. Those individuals identified as having suspected hearing impairment would be then referred to training audiologists, otolaryngologists, and other medical specialists. Currently, these more sophisticated services are in short supply and need to be expanded. Expanded speech and hearing clinics could provide continuing education for the frontline screening personnel to improve their skills and knowledge in this area.

Powers and Quigley (1971) recommended that centralized centers be established to assume responsibility for the upkeep of a register of multiply disabled children, the diagnosis and ascertainment of multiple handicaps, and the coordination of program and facilities for such children. It would seem that such services might be fostered and supported by the state developmental disabilities councils because they have this responsibility and also have some financial support at their disposal. This position was taken by the Task Force on the Mentally Retarded and the Deaf (1973).

Based upon information gained from several surveys in schools for the deaf and residential facilities for the retarded, it seems that persons with mental retardation and deafness are not being adequately served in either type of facility. With a few notable exceptions, audiologic assessment services seem to be particularly weak in facilities for the retarded. There are no college and university programs available that provide training in both deafness and mental retardation. Because some 15% of the population in schools for the deaf and facilities for the retarded possess both handicaps, there are obvious needs for the development and implementation of such training programs at the graduate level. No less important is the need for expertise and sophisticated services in school and community programs as "right to education" and "zero rejection" laws take hold.

In view of the current lack of comprehensive data on the prevalence of various handicapping conditions at a time when improved technology exists, it would seem appropriate to mount a large-scale, interdisciplinary prevalence survey to determine the number and characteristics of our handicapped population. Such a survey should include not only interview data but also clinical examinations of at least subsamples of the sample population. Perhaps an organization such as the Office of Demographic Studies of Gallaudet College, the National Association of the Deaf, or the Office of Child Development might be appropriate agencies to sponsor such a study. Accurate identification of the scope of the problem is the bedrock upon which sound programming must be based.

REFERENCES

AAMD. 1969. Adaptive Scale of Behavior. American Association on Mental Deficiency, Washington, D. C.

ANSI. 1969. American National Standard Specifications for Audiometers, S3.6-1969. American National Standards Institute, New York.

ASA. 1951. American Standard Specifications for Audiometers for General Diagnostic Purposes, A24.5-1951. American Standards Association, New York.

Anderson, R. M., and G. D. Stevens. 1969. Practices and problems in educating deaf retarded children in residential schools. Except. Child. 35:687–694.

Arangio, A. J. 1974. Behind the Stigma of Epilepsy. Epilepsy Foundation of America, Washington, D.C.

Balthazar, E. E., and H. A. Stevens. 1975. The Emotionally Disturbed Mentally Retarded: A Historical and Contemporary Perspective. Prentice-Hall, Englewood Cliffs, N.J.

Barr, B., J. Anderson, and E. Wedenberg. 1973. Epidemiology of hearing loss in childhood. Audiology 12:426–437.

Bensberg, G. J., and W. Sloan. 1954. Performance of brain injured defectives on the Arthur Adaption of the Leiter. Psychological Service Center, Syracuse University.

Bensberg, G. J., and W. Sloan. 1955. The use of the Cattell Culture Free Test with mental defectives. Amer. J. Ment. Defic. 23:134–144.

Birch, J. W., and J. Matthews, 1951. The hearing of mental defectives: Its measurement and characteristics. Amer. J. Ment. Defic. 55:384–393.

Bolton, B. 1972. A profile of the multiply handicapped deaf young adult. J. Rehab. Deaf, 5(4):7–11.

Brannan, C., C. Sigelman, and G. Bensberg. 1975. The Hearing Impaired/ Mentally Retarded: A Summary of State Institutions for the Retarded. Research and Training Center in Mental Retardation, Texas Tech University, Lubbock.

Brison, D. W. 1967. Definition, diagnosis and classification. In A. A. Baumeister (ed.), Mental Retardation: Appraisal, Education, and Rehabilitation. Aldine, Chicago.

Brookhauser, P. E., and J. E. Bordley. 1973. Congenital rubella deafness: Pathology and pathogenesis. Arch. Otolaryngol. 98: 252–257.

Budden, S. S., G. C. Robinson, C. D. MacLean, and K. G. Cambon. 1974. Deafness in infants and preschool children. Amer. Ann. Deaf 119(4): 387–395.

Cardwell, V. E. 1956. Cerebral Palsy: Advances in Understanding and Care. Association for the Aid of Crippled Children, New York.

Coatsworth, J. J., and J. K. Penry. 1972. Clinical efficiency and use. In M. Woodbury et al. (eds.), Pharmacology of Antiepileptic Drugs. Raven Press, New York.

Colpoys, B. P. 1972. The mentally retarded deaf in New York: Size and scope. In L. B. Stewart (ed.), Deafness and Mental Retardation. Deafness Research and Training Center, New York University, New York.

Conley, R. W. 1973. The Economics of Mental Retardation. Johns Hopkins University Press, Baltimore.

Cooper, L. 1969. The child with rubella syndrome. New Outlook Blind 63(10):290–298.

Cooper, L. Z., and S. C. Krugman. 1967. Clinical manifestations of postnatal and congenital rubella. Arch. Ophthalmol. 77:434–439.

Desmond, M. M., and A. Rudolph. 1970. The clinical evaluation of low-birth-weight infants with regard to head trauma. In C. R. Angle and E. A. Bering (eds.), Physical Trauma as an Etiological Agent in Mental Retardation. National Institute of Neurological Diseases and Stroke, Bethesda, Md.

Dingman, J. R., and G. Tarjan. 1960. Mental retardation and the normal distribution curve. Amer. J. Ment. Defic. 64:991–994.

Doctor, P. V. 1959. Multiple handicaps in the field of deafness. Except. Child. 46:214–219.

Doll, E. A. 1941. The essentials of an inclusive concept of mental deficiency. Amer. J. Ment. Defic. 46:214–219.

Doll, E. A. 1953. The Measurement of Social Competence: A Manual for the Vineland Social Maturity Scale. Educational Testing Bureau, Minneapolis.

Dorland's Illustrated Medical Dictionary. 1965. 24th Ed. W. B. Saunders, Philadelphia.

Eagles, E., S. Wishik, L. Doerfler, W. Melnick, and H. Levine. 1963. Hearing sensitivity and related factors in children. Laryngoscope (Special monograph, no number).

Feinmesser, M., L. Baubergertell, and R. Bilski-Hirsch. 1959. A hearing survey in the public schools of Jerusalem. Isr. Med. J. 18:59–63.

Ferster. C. B. 1961. Positive reinforcement and behavioral deficits of autistic children. Child Dev. 32:437–456.

Fisch, L. 1973. Epidemiology of congenital hearing loss. Audiology 12:411–425.

Folsom, A. T. 1968. The epilepsies. In H. C. Haywood (ed.), Brain Damage in School Age Children. The Council for Exceptional Children, Washington, D.C.

Ford, R. R. 1960. Diseases of the Nervous System in Infancy, Childhood and Adolescence. 4th Ed. Charles C Thomas, Springfield, Ill.

Fox, J. P., E. E. Hall, and L. R. Elveback. 1970. Epidemiology: man and Disease. Macmillan, New York.

Fraser, G. R. 1970. The causes of profound deafness in childhood. In G. E. W. Wolsterhome and J. Knight (eds.), Ciba Foundation Symposium on Sensorineural Hearing Loss. J. & A. Churchill, London.

Friedman, I., and M. I. Wright. 1966. Histopathological changes in the foetal and infantile inner ear caused by maternal rubella. Brit. Med. J. 2:20–23.

Gallagher, J. J., and R. Wiegerink. 1973. Educational strategies for the autistic child. Unpublished manuscript, Frank Porter Graham Center, University of North Carolina, Chapel Hill.

Gentile, A., J. D. Schein, and K. Hasse. 1967. Characteristics of persons with impaired hearing. Series 10, no. 35, U.S. Vital and Health Statistics. National Center for Health Statistics, Bethesda, Md.

Ginzberg, E., and D. W. Bray. 1953. The Uneducated. Columbia University Press, New York.

Glorig, A., and J. Roberts. 1965. Hearing levels of adults by age and sex. Series 11, no. 11, U.S. Vital and Health Statistics. National Center for Health Statistics, Bethesda, Md.

Goldstein, R., C. C. McRandle, and L. B. Rodman. 1972. Site of lesion in cases of hearing loss associated with Rh incompatibility: An argument for peripheral impairment. J. Speech Hear. Disord. 37:447–450.

Goodhill, V. 1956. Rh child: Deaf or aphasic? J. Speech Hear. Disord. 2:407–410.

Goodhill, V., and P. Guggenheim. 1971. Pathology, diagnosis and therapy of deafness. In L. E. Travis (ed.), Handbook of Speech Pathology and Audiology. Appleton-Century-Crofts, New York.

Grossman, H. J. (ed.). 1973. Manual on Terminology and Classification in Mental Retardation. Special Publication Series no. 2. American Association on Mental Deficiency, Washington, D.C. p. 180.

Hardy, J. B. 1973. Clinical and developmental aspects of rubella. Arch. Otolaryngol. 98:230–245.

Hardy, M. P., H. L. Haskins, W. G. Hardy, and H. Shimiz. 1973. Rubella: Audiologic evaluation and follow-up. Arch. Otolaryngol. 98:237–245.

Hardy, W. G., and J. E. Bordley. 1973. Problems in diagnosis and management of the multiply handicapped deaf child. Arch. Otolaryngol. 98:269–274.

Heber, R. G. (ed.) 1965. Special Problems in the Vocational Rehabilitation of the Mentally Retarded. Rehabilitation Services Series No.
65-16, U.S. Department of Health, Education, and Welfare, Bethesda,
Md.

Hodgson, W. R. 1969. Auditory characteristics of post-rubella impairment. Volta Rev. 71(2):97–103.

Hogan, D. D. 1973. Errors in computation of incidence of hearing loss
in studies of large populations. Ment. Retard. 11:15–17.

Huizing, J. 1953. Assessment and evaluation of hearing anomalies in
young children. *In* Proceedings of the International Course in Paedo-
Audiology. Vernigde Brukkerjen Hoitsema N. V., Groningen.

Illingworth, R. 1958. Recent Advances in Cerebral Palsy. Little, Brown,
Boston.

Ingalls, T. H., and M. A. Klingberg. 1969. Congenital malformations:
Clinical and community considerations. *In* J. M. Wolf and R. M.
Anderson (eds.), The Multiple Handicapped Child. Charles C Thomas,
Springfield, Ill.

ISO. 1964. ISO Recommendation, R 389, Standard Reference Zero for
Calibration of Pure-Tone Audiometers. International Organization for
Standardization, Switzerland.

Johnson, P. W., and M. J. Farrell. 1954. Auditory impairments among
resident school children at the Walter E. Fernald State School. Amer.
J. Ment. Defic. 58:640–643.

Keane, V. E. 1972. The incidence of speech and language problems in
the mentally retarded. Ment. Retard. 10:3–8.

Kelly, V. C. (ed.) 1964. Practices of Pediatrics. W. F. Prior, Hagers-
town, Md.

Kennedy, W. A., V. Van de Riet, and J. C. White, Jr. 1963. A normative
sample of intelligence and achievement of Negro elementary school
children in the southeastern United States. *In* Monographs of the
Society for Research in Child Development. Vol. 28(6). University
of Chicago Press, Chicago.

Kennedy, W. P. 1967. Epidemiologic aspects of the problem of congenital
malformations. *In* Birth Defects: Original Article Series. Vol. 3(2).
National Foundation–March of Dimes, New York.

Kerr, A. G., G. D. L. Smyth, and M. J. Cinnamond. 1973. Congenital
syphilitic deafness. J. Laryngol. Otol. 87:1–12.

Kirk, S. A. 1963. Educating Exceptional Children. Houghton-Mifflin,
Boston.

Kirk, S. A., and B. B. Weiner. 1969. The Onondaga Census—Fact or
artifact. *In* J. M. Wolf and R. M. Anderson (eds.), The Multiple
Handicapped Child. Charles C Thomas, Springfield, Ill.

Kodman, R., T. R. Powers, P. P. Philip, and G. M. Weller. 1959. An
investigation of hearing loss in mentally retarded children and adults.
Amer. J. Ment. Defic. 63:460–463.

Konigswork, B. W. 1971. Syndrome approaches to the nosology of
hereditary deafness. *In* Birth Defects: Original Article Series, pp.
2–20. Vol. 6(4). National Foundation–March of Dimes, New York.

Leenhouts, M. 1969. The mentally retarded deaf child. Proceedings of the Thirty-Ninth Meeting of the American Instructors of the Deaf. U.S. Government Printing Office, Washington, D.C. p. 56.

Lennox, W. 1960. Epilepsy and Related Disorders. Little, Brown, Boston.

Lindsay, J. R. 1973a. Histopathology of deafness due to postnatal viral disease. Arch. Otolaryngol. 98:258–264.

Lindsay, J. R. 1973b. Profound childhood deafness. Ann. Otol. Rhinol. Laryngol. 83(suppl. 5).

Lipscomb, D. M. 1973. How frequent are ear lesions and hearing defects among United States children? Clin. Ped. 12:125–126.

Lloyd, L. L. 1968. Operant conditioning with retarded children. In E. F. Walden (ed.), Differential Diagnosis of Speech and Hearing Problems of Mental Retardates. Catholic University of America Press, Washington, D.C.

Lloyd, L. L. 1970. Audiologic aspects of mental retardation. In N. R. Ellis (ed.), International Review of Research in Mental Retardation. Vol. 4. Academic Press, New York.

Lloyd, L. L. 1971. The establishment of standards for speech pathology and audiology in facilities for the retarded. Asha 13:607–610.

Lloyd, L. L. 1973. Mental retardation and hearing impairment. In A. G. Norris (ed.), PRWAD Deafness Annual. Vol. 3. Professional Rehabilitation Workers with the Adult Deaf, Washington, D.C.

Lloyd, L. L., and E. G. Moore. 1972. Audiology. In J. Wortis (ed.), Mental Retardation: An Annual Review. Vol. 4. Grune & Stratton, New York.

Lloyd, L. L., and M. J. Reid. 1967. The incidence of hearing impairment in an institutionalized mentally retarded population. Amer. J. Ment. Defic. 71:746–763.

Lovaas, O. I., R. Koegel, J. Q. Simmons, and J. Stevens. 1973. Some generalization and follow-up measures on autistic children in behavior therapy. J. Appl. Behav. Anal. 6:131–166.

MacMahon, B., T. F. Pugh, and J. Ipsen. 1960. Epidemiologic Methods. Little, Brown, Boston.

Matthews, J. 1971. Communication disorders in the mentally retarded. In L. E. Travis (ed.), Handbook of Speech Pathology and Audiology. Appleton-Century-Crofts, New York.

Melnick, W. 1971. American National Standard specifications for audiometers. Asha 13:203–206.

Mercer, J. R. 1973. Labeling the Mentally Retarded. University of California Press, Berkeley.

Milisen, R. 1971. The incidence of speech disorders. In L. E. Travis (ed.), Handbook of Speech Pathology and Audiology. Appleton-Century-Crofts, New York.

Millichap, J. G. 1974. Treatment needs of the epileptic: The child. In P. Hamilton (ed.), Modern Dimensions of Epilepsy: Proceedings of an Inter-regional Training Conference. Rehabilitation Institute of Chicago, Chicago.

Mitra, S. B. 1970. Educational provisions for mentally retarded deaf students in residential institutions for the retarded. Volta Rev. 72: 225–236.

National Institute of Neurological Diseases and Stroke. 1970. Human communication and its disorders: An overview. Department of Health, Education, and Welfare, Bethesda, Md.

National Society for the Study of Education. 1950. The Education of Exceptional Children. 49th Yrbk. Part 2. University of Chicago Press, Chicago.

New York State Department of Mental Hygiene. 1955. Technical Report of the Mental Health Research Unit. New York State Department of Mental Hygiene, Syracuse, N.Y.

Office of Demographic Studies. 1973a. Characteristics of Hearing Impaired Students by Hearing Status: United States, 1970–71. Gallaudet College, Washington, D.C.

Office of Demographic Studies. 1973b. Annual Survey of Hearing Impaired Children and Youth: Additional Handicapping Conditions Among Hearing Impaired Students—1971–72. Gallaudet College, Washington, D.C.

Ojala, P., V. Timo, and O. Elo. 1973. Rubella during pregnancy as a cause of hearing loss. Amer. J. Epidemiol. 98:395–401.

Page, H. A., and V. LaPlace. 1972. The mentally retarded deaf in New York: Size and scope of the problem. In L. G. Stewart (ed.), Deafness and Mental Retardation. Deafness Research and Training Center, New York University, New York.

Paul, J. R. (ed.) 1966. Clinical Epidemiology. 2nd Ed. University of Chicago Press, Chicago.

Penrose, L. S. 1954. The Biology of Mental Defect. Sidgwick & Jackson, London.

Powers, D. J., and S. P. Quigley. 1971. Problems and Programs in the Education of the Multiple Disabled Deaf Child. Institute for Research on Exceptional Children, Urbana, Ill.

Prehm, H. J. 1974. Mental retardation: Definition, classification and prevalence. In P. D. Browning (ed.), Mental Retardation Rehabilitation and Counseling. Charles C Thomas, Springfield, Ill.

Richardson, W. L., and W. P. Higgins. 1964. A survey of handicapping conditions and handicapped children in Alamance County, North Carolina. Amer. J. Public Health 54:1817–1830.

Rittmanic, P. A. 1959. Hearing rehabilitation for the institutionalized mentally retarded. Amer. J. Ment. Defic. 63:778–783.

Robinson, G. J. 1964. Pediatrics and disorders in communication: I. Hearing loss in infants and young preschool children. Volta Rev. 66:314–318.

Robinson, H. B., and Robinson, N. M. 1965. The Mentally Retarded Child: A Psychological Approach. McGraw-Hill, New York.

Robinson, R. O. 1973. The frequency of other handicaps in children with cerebral palsy. Dev. Med. Child Neurol. 15:305–312.

Ruben, R. J., and D. L. Rozycki. 1971. Clinical aspects of genetic deafness. Ann. Otol. Rhinol. Laryngol. 80:255–263.

Schein, J. D., and M. T. Delk. 1974. The Deaf Population of the United States. National Association of the Deaf, Silver Spring, Md.

Schlanger, B. B., and R. H. Gottsleben. 1956. Testing the hearing of the mentally retarded. J. Speech Hear. Disord. 21:487–492.

Siegel, M., J. T. Fuerst, and N. S. Peress. 1966. Fetal mortality in maternal rubella: Results of a prospective study from 1957–64. Amer. J. Obstet. Gynecol. 96:247–253.

Sigenthaler, B. M., and D. F. Krzywicki. 1959. Incidence and patterns of hearing loss among adult retarded population. Amer. J. Ment. Defic. 64:444–459.

Spradlin, J. E. 1963. Language and communication of mental defectives. In N. R. Ellis (ed.), Handbook of Mental Deficiency. McGraw-Hill, New York.

Spriesterbach, D. C., D. R. Dickerson, F. C. Fraser, S. L. Horowitz, B. J. Williams, J. L. Paradise, and P. Randal. 1973. Clinical research in cleft lip and cleft palate: The state of the art. Cleft Palate J. 10:113–165.

Surjan, J., J. Dvald, and L. Palvavi. 1973. Epidemiology of hearing loss. Audiology 12:396–410.

Task Force on the Mentally Retarded and the Deaf. 1973. (November). Report. Office of the Assistant Secretary for Human Development, Office of Mental Retardation, Washington, D.C.

Taylor, E. M. 1961. Psychological Appraisal of Children with Cerebral Defects. Harvard University Press, Cambridge, Mass.

Vernon, M. 1967a. Characteristics associated with post-rubella deaf children: Psychological, educational, physical. Volta Rev. 69(3): 176–185.

Vernon, M. 1967b. Meningitis and deafness: The problem, its physical, audiological, psychological and educational manifestations in deaf children. Laryngoscope 77:1856–1874.

Vernon, M. 1967c. Rh factor and deafness: The problem, its psychological, physical and educational manifestations. Except. Child. 34: 5–12.

Vernon, M. 1967d. Prematurity and deafness: The magnitude and nature of the problem among deaf children. Except. Child. 33:289–298.

Vernon, M. 1969. Sociological and psychological factors associated with hearing loss. J. Speech Hear. Res. 12:541–563.

Webb, C. K., B. Weber, and R. Biddle. 1964. Procedures for Evaluating the Hearing of the Mentally Retarded. United States Office of Education, Cooperative Research Project no. 1731, Washington, D.C.

Weber, H. J., F. J. McGovern, and D. Zink. 1967. An evaluation of 1000 children with hearing loss. J. Speech Hear. Disord. 32:343–354.

Wishik S. M. 1956. Handicapped children in Georgia: A study of prevalence, disability, needs, and resources. Amer. J. Public Health 46:195–203.

Wolf, J. M., and R. M. Anderson. 1969. The multiple handicapped child: An overview. In J. M. Wolf and R. M. Anderson (eds.), The Multiple Handicapped Child. Charles C Thomas, Springfield, Ill.

Wolf, M. M., T. Risley, and H. L. Mees. 1964. Application of operant conditioning procedures to the behavior problems of an autistic child. Behav. Res. Ther. 1:305–312.

3

LANGUAGE ASSESSMENT

Gerald M. Siegel and
Patricia A. Broen

CONTENTS

Dimensions of Language Assessment _____ 76
    Comprehension and expression/77
    Grammar/78
    Concepts and vocabulary/80
    Interpersonal dimensions/81

Use of Language Tests _____ 82
    Test as sample/83
    Objectivity and standardization/84
    Test norms/85
    Reliability/86
    Validity/87
    Test scores/89
    Application to nonstandardized procedures/90

Identification and Screening _____ 92

Specific Assessment Methods _____ 95
    Syntax/95
    Assessment of syntax/99
    In-depth assessment of syntax/103
    Words and concepts/104
    Assessment of vocabulary skills/109
    Interpersonal communication/113

Summary _____ 117

Acknowledgments _____ 118

References _____ 118

Everybody knows what language is—everybody, that is, except for the psychologists, philosophers, linguists, and clinicians who must deal with it in formal and technical ways. For the ordinary person, language is what comes out of the mouth and works its way into the brain, via the ears. Language is disordered when some part of the system is not working; the message is not getting out of the speaker in the proper form or it is not getting through to the listener. These characterizations lack the elegance of formal theory, but it is against such intuitive notions that complex theories and models of language are ultimately measured. The curious paradox in the study of language, and perhaps in all of behavioral science, is that the profoundest mysteries are ensnared in the things best known. Those engaged in the study of normal and deviant language know all that is necessary to be fully competent in the use of the English language. Yet, as Chomsky (1972, p. 26) has ventured, "Only the most preliminary and tentative hypotheses can be offered concerning the nature of language, its use, and its acquisition."

This chapter deals with issues and approaches to language assessment with full awareness that concepts of the nature of language are likely to change profoundly in the next few years. Certainly change and reformulation have been the story of the last two decades. As conceptual systems change, so too will approach to assessment and remediation. Tests that are currently in vogue will seem hopelessly out of touch with new formulations. Basic definitions of what characterizes a "language disorder" will be altered. At one time "language" conjured up visions of vocabulary size, length of response, type-token ratios, parts of speech. More recently, syntax has dominated psycholinguistics and, accordingly, language assessment. Now there are the beginnings of a more semantically oriented linguistics, and this is already evident in certain language assessment approaches (MacDonald and Nickols, 1974).

This chapter reflects a bias about language testing that should be acknowledged at the outset: The most useful and dependable "language assessment device" is an informed clinician who feels compelled to keep up with developments in psycholinguistics, speech pathology, and related fields, and who is not slavishly attached to a particular model of language or of assessment. In the long run, the attributes

Preparation of this chapter was supported by grants to the University of Minnesota Center for Research in Human Learning.

that will serve the clinician best are a willingness to explore new developments, to be experimental in approaching children, and a persevering curiosity about the nature of language that is not too readily sated by some prepackaged procedure.

DIMENSIONS OF LANGUAGE ASSESSMENT

Under the attentive care of linguists, psychologists, and philosophers, *language* has grown so large and amorphous as to resist definition. Still, an intelligent language assessment program must originate with a general concept of language and communication. How else can one decide which aspects deserve attention and which should be ignored? Since there is surely no universally accepted definition of normal and disordered language, each clinician must grapple with the many-headed monster and arrive at a personally satisfying definition. The present authors have found four dimensions of the communication process that are often implicated among children diagnosed as having severe speech or language problems: 1) *articulation* and mastery of the *phonologic* system; discussion of this dimension is omitted in this chapter because it is treated elsewhere by McLean (this volume); 2) understanding and use of *grammatical* structures; 3) understanding and use of certain *vocabulary and concepts;* and 4) the functional or *interpersonal* uses of language. These last three dimensions form the basis for considerations in language assessment. They are not intended to be a theory of language or communication, but such theories as are available tend to be rather narrow, and typically make little provision for disordered language. Linguistic theory ignores the social and interpersonal uses of language. Learning theories ignore the important structural aspects of language, and so on. Even when a test is based upon a specific theoretical model, the practical requirements of test building and administration soon overwhelm any allegiance to the theory. The Illinois Test for Psycholinguistic Abilities (ITPA), for example, was originally (Kirk and McCarthy, 1961) presented as an outgrowth of Osgood's (1957) theory of language, but the most recent version of the test (Kirk, McCarthy, and Kirk, 1968) hardly bears a family resemblance to the original theory. As a matter of fact, the test is now treated as a model of language in its own right.

A number of general treatments of language assessment are available (Johnson, Darley, and Spriestersbach, 1952; Spradlin, 1967; Berry, 1969; Carrow, 1972; Irwin, Moore, and Rampp, 1972; Muma,

1973; Emrick and Hatten, 1974). Carrow (1972) and Irwin, Moore, and Rampp (1972) organized their discussion of assessment procedures in terms of a "taxonomy" of language that is quite similar to the ITPA model. It is more useful to begin with a consideration of the child and the dimensions of his performance that lead to the impression that he is a deviant language user. The various formal models never seem quite adequate to deal with the range of children seen in the clinic, and too much energy is spent trying to fit the child to the model. One works more confidently and with less constraint when dealing with language descriptively within the dimensions of grammar, concepts, and interpersonal use. This chapter first briefly defines these dimensions, along with a discussion of competence and performance, and then discusses them in greater detail.

Comprehension and Expression

Virtually all language assessment procedures distinguish between comprehension and production. Some tests, such as Carrow's (1973) Test for Auditory Comprehension of Language, or the Peabody Picture Vocabulary Test (Dunn, 1965), focus solely on comprehension. Others sample expression and comprehension (the ITPA, for example). The Northwestern Syntax Screening Test (Lee, 1971) evaluates the very same items in both comprehension and production.

The Carrow Elicited Language Inventory procedures (Carrow, 1974) require only that the child imitate sentences and is, therefore, primarily a test of expression. Imitation tests of this sort, however, involve a complex set of assumptions concerning the relationship between imitation, comprehension, and production. Imitation is assumed to involve rote memory for relatively short stimuli. For longer sentences, the child is presumably forced to call on his basic linguistic knowledge to repeat the item. That is, the item is linguistically processed before it is uttered. Thus, imitation of long sentences presumably reflects underlying linguistic skills, and not merely production.

The extent to which imitation necessarily involves linguistic processing is still being argued and investigated (e.g., Fraser, Bellugi, and Brown, 1963; Slobin and Welsh, 1973; Kuczaj and Maratsos, 1975). It is undoubtedly true that imitation does reflect linguistic knowledge in some instances, but certainly not always, and not in any simple way. Imitation is one of those methods that comes out of the research literature and is a useful adjunct to the clinician's skills, but should not be used exclusively or uncritically. One immediate problem with imitation as an assessment technique is that it is impossible to interpret items that are imitated correctly because these may reflect either syntactic knowledge or rote memory. Even though the entire sentence may be too long for the child to memorize, the child may chunk it in various ways and treat the chunks as rote items. Thus, it is not appropriate to assume that a correct imitative response means that the child has mastered the forms that are included in the stimulus item.

Grammar

Speakers of English can call on three basic devices to modulate the meaning of sentences: the selection of particular "bound morphemes" to indicate tense, possessives, number, etc.; the order in which the words of the sentence are arranged; and the choice of particular vocabulary items: "free morphemes." For purposes of discussion, it is convenient to divide grammar into morphology and syntax,[1] and to treat vocabulary as a separate topic.

Morphology   At a surface level, it is possible and often useful to talk about the child's use of bound morphemes. These structures primarily mark tense, number, and possession in English. Many of the "ungrammatical" sentences produced by young children reflect incomplete mastery of these forms. For example, the sentences, *I want two toy, More milks,* and *Yesterday I goed to the park,* reflect three different kinds of errors: omission of the plural morpheme, use of the count noun plural morpheme with a mass noun, and the use of a regular past tense morpheme with an irregular verb. Differences in the use of bound morphemes contribute in part to the special character of black English: *I have live here, This is John mother.* (Dale, 1972).

Mastery of the morpheme system does not come all at once, and failure to understand or use a particular feature does not necessarily mean the child has disordered language. In this, as in all aspects of language acquisition, there is individual variation, although Brown (1973) has found considerable uniformity in the developmental sequence of certain of the morphemes. Failure to produce a proper morphologic form, such as the plural, may signify several things. The child may not understand the concept of more-than-one (numerosity);

---

[1]This division is a simplification that is not entirely consistent with current linguistic usage (Bach, 1974), in which "grammar" subsumes several levels of phonologic, syntactic, and semantic rules.

he may understand the concept, but not know how to use the morpheme system to indicate numerosity; he may know all of the above, but not be able to articulate the necessary sound. In assessing morphology, it is important to determine which of these possibilities is responsible for particular morphologic errors. Following the pioneering work of Berko (1958), who studied morphologic development of normal children, numerous "tests" of morphology are now available. For the most part, these tests are very similar to the procedures Berko devised for her research.

Syntax   Syntax refers to the way in which the words of a language are arranged to create sentences. The problem of linguistic theory is sometimes put in terms of a mythical automaton: Suppose there were a talking robot that could be programmed to produce all of the indefinite number of possible sentences that *could* be uttered in the language. Furthermore, the robot could be spared from human fallibilities and never utter a nongrammatical sentence. What sort of program would be needed to accomplish this feat? First, one would feed in all of the words in the language including information about their phonologic form, their meaning, their grammatical function, and any restrictions on their occurrence. This would be tedious, but not impossible. Then, a more formidable task is faced, in that it is impossible to provide the robot with the entire list of sentences of English. The list would go on forever. Instead, the machine must be provided with a set of rules that "tell" it how words and morphemes may and may not be assembled in English. At present, automata can engage in all kinds of exotic activities, but they cannot carry out the syntactic task just described. The fault lies not with the robot. The problem is that there is not yet sufficient knowledge of the rules of a language to insert that piece of intelligence into the automaton's brain.

Children also must acquire the rule system as well as the lexicon of English. But the child does not wait for someone to insert the program for sentence construction into his nervous system. Somehow the child manages to extract and internalize these rules from the speech he hears around him. It is an awesome accomplishment that places the child well beyond the reach of even the most intelligent computer.

Children do not acquire the rule system as a unitary flash of insight. Linguistic competence develops with time, imperfectly at first, but with increasing scope and precision. Procedures such as Lee's (1974) Developmental Sentence Scoring (DSS) assume that language emerges with a great deal of consistency for all children. In the

DDS procedure, weighted scores are assigned to various morphologic or syntactic features. Irregular past tense verb forms (*ate, saw*) are scored higher than the copula *is:* The modals *can, will, may* are scored higher still. The implication in such a scoring system is that children are all very much alike in developmental pattern. Otherwise, the weighting system would have to be revised for every child. Muma (1973) questioned this implication and pointed out that, even when the sequence of acquisition is comparable across children, rate of development is likely to be extremely variable.

Some grammatical errors occur more frequently than others in the performance of language-disordered children, and Leonard (1972) has suggested that the pattern of errors may help resolve questions of delay versus deviancy in language disorder. The data concerning these patterns are currently very meager, however. Another important question, for which there are virtually no data, concerns which grammatical errors are most likely to catch the attention of listeners. Leonard found that verb and noun phrase omissions were correlated with judgments of deviancy, but the results are quite preliminary and have not been pursued across children of different ages.

Concepts and Vocabulary

Grammar is not the sole determiner of meaning in a sentence. Politicians, humorists, and chapter writers are capable of producing any number of sentences in which the syntax is in order, but the words themselves are largely meaningless.

In order to produce and understand sentences, the child must learn a basic vocabulary. One way to characterize this knowledge is in terms of the number of words the child understands and uses. A more subtle aspect of vocabulary mastery concerns the depth or thoroughness of the child's knowledge. A given word is likely to have several meanings. *He is decent* might mean either that he is fully clothed, or that he is likable and trustworthy. The more meanings and nuances the child can pull from a vocabulary item, the richer his command of the language. Vocabulary assessment requires more than a tally of the number of words the child "knows." It is important to test the depth of the child's knowledge and to describe the particular concepts that are improperly used and understood. One young client had great difficulty understanding prepositions. She would confuse instructions to place an object behind or beside the cup. Her errors were not random, however. She seemed to have a category, "prepositions of place," as distinct from other prepositions. Within that category, however, the items were in virtually free variation. She knew the syntactic but not all of the semantic restrictions on prepositions.

Interpersonal Dimensions

The child also learns to exploit the enormous potential that language offers in human affairs. The infant's earliest vocalizations serve an important communication function. Until he can reach, grasp, and locomote, the child has little direct control over his surroundings. By loud and energetic use of his vocal apparatus, however, he can summon adults from nowhere, cause fallen toys to be replaced, diapers to be changed, and dinner served. Skinner (1957, p. 2) defined verbal behavior as "behavior reinforced through the mediation of other persons." Verbal behavior does not affect the environment directly. Rather, it induces others to make the changes for us. According to Skinner's definition, even cries of pleasure and discomfort from the crib already contain the essentials of verbal behavior. They cause significant personages in the child's environment to operate on the world for him.

Cries and babbling suffice as communicative devices for only a brief period. When words and sentences enter the repertoire, the child becomes ready to undertake the social uses of language. According to Piaget (1926), up until 7 or 8 years, the child's speech is *egocentric* —failing to take into account the attributes and situation of the listener. Regardless of the specific age at which these communication skills emerge, there is little doubt that children get better as they grow, and that certain populations—autistic and severely emotionally disturbed children—are severely handicapped in their communicative use of language. Retarded children also have difficulty with interpersonal communication (Longhurst, 1972), and children from lower-income families are often ineffective in using adults to clarify ambiguities and as sources of information (Cooper, 1972).

These interpersonal abilities are not "language" skills as such, but they are clearly related to communication. Despite their importance, they are rarely included in formal language tests. In order to find methods for tapping these abilities, the clinician must turn to the literature to discover what techniques have been used in studies of children's communication.

In summary, there are three dimensions that are significant for adequate language and communication. The first involves *syntactic structure.* The second is knowledge of the *vocabulary* of one's language and the multiple meanings and nuances that words may have. Finally, there is the matter of *language in use;* language is a powerful social tool for acquiring information and for getting work done. These three dimensions, along with articulation (see McLean, this volume), form the basis for language assessment. Standard tests are used when available, but almost invariably the clinician must collect spontaneous protocols and devise supplemental tests. It is the combination of these approaches and dimensions that defines a thoroughgoing assessment procedure.

USE OF LANGUAGE TESTS

It is hard to imagine a well equipped clinic whose shelves are not filled with a proliferation of articulation and language tests and kits. Often, after the first enthusiastic applications, the tests are allowed to languish and collect dust. There are many reasons for the demise of a particular test. Not all tests are created equal with respect to the care and precision that is lavished on them. No test is likely to cover all of the aspects that a particular clinician has found to be important in therapy. Often there is no logical progression from the test to the therapy room. The test provides a score that tells what was already known—the child is deficient in language—but little beyond that.

Recently, a number of assessment procedures have appeared that do more than yield a language score. They attempt to provide a profile of specific abilities in a way that can lead to therapy programming. The nature of formal assessment devices and the kind of information the clinician must have in order to evaluate and select among various tests are considered in this section. Information about a large number of specific tests and measurement approaches, some published and some in the experimental stages, is included in Appendix A.

Important attributes of tests are discussed here briefly; fuller presentations appear in standard psychometric texts (such as Anastasi, 1968). An important source of information about specific tests can be found in the Mental Measurement Yearbooks edited by Burros (1972). These are published periodically and cover virtually all commercial psychologic, educational, and vocational tests produced in English. The most current yearbook was published in 1972.

Anastasi (1968, p. 21) defined a psychologic test as "an objective and standardized measure of a sample of behavior." The key words in the definition are *sample, objective,* and *standard.*

Tests as Sample

Before a description of a child's language can be offered, there must be some behavior to analyze. The behavior may consist of definitions of a small set of words, or it may involve extensive transcripts of spontaneous speech collected over months and even years, as was done by Brown (1973). In either case, the behavior that is analyzed is really only a sample of the child's total responses. If meaningful interpretations are to be made, the sample must be representative of the child's performance. The approach to data collection used by Brown is impractical for the clinician because it takes an extraordinary amount of time to collect and process the transcripts of speech. In addition, there is no guarantee that all the behaviors of interest will appear, even in extended protocols. Language tests have the advantage of determining in advance the dimensions of performance that will be sampled, even if in a limited way.

Sampling of behavior involves essentially the same considerations that go into sampling of subjects. For example, in a study of stutterers' responses to a therapy method, it is not possible to include all of the stutterers in the universe. Instead, a small sample of stutterers will receive the treatment. In order to generalize the results beyond the particular sample, the stutterers must be similar to clients who are likely to appear for therapy at other times and in other clinics. If the subjects are all college students, there may be reservations about generalizing to noncollege clients, just as methods developed for young adults may not be appropriate for preschool children. Researchers usually describe their sampling methods with care so that it is possible to determine how far the results can be generalized.

In measuring behavior, it is also impossible to include the "universe of relevant behaviors," and so sampling must be used. Ideally, the items included in a language test will be a representative sample, based on a well reasoned definition of language. Since "language" means different things to different people, this poses some difficulties. Sometimes, as in the case of the ITPA or Spradlin's (1963) Parsons Language Sample (PLS), the definition of language is related to a general theory of behavior. In other instances, as with the Houston Test of Language Development (Crabtree, 1963), there is no overarching theory, and so the items themselves must be studied to determine what they represent. The names of tests are often not very helpful. Neither the Parsons *Language* Sample nor the Illinois Test of

Psycholinguistic Abilities includes many items that, by contemporary definition, would be classed as "linguistic."

Given that a test is a sample, it is appropriate to ask, A sample of what? What model of language does the author have? What dimensions are included? Does it have a good range of difficulty? Is the author even aware that the instrument basically provides a sample? In carefully prepared tests, these questions are answered in the accompanying manual. In other cases the user must determine what the test covers. Even in a well designed test, it will be necessary to decode the author's terminology. An item like, *Soup is hot; ice cream is* _____, would be called "intraverbal" on the PLS, and "auditory association" on the ITPA.

No test can sample all aspects of language and communication, and those dimensions that are included will not be tested in depth. This means that the clinician cannot rely entirely on a test or a battery of tests for a comprehensive assessment. To do such a job, the language clinician first must decide what constitutes adequate language. Based on some working definition, the clinician will have to perform reconstructive surgery, creating a coherent and comprehensive approach to assessment by lifting a subtest from one instrument, grafting it to a subtest from a second test, and inventing still other items that appear in no available instrument.[2] Not all children will be tested in the same way. The selection of appropriate devices will depend on the referring complaint and the hints that are generated by general observation and initial assessment.

Objectivity and Standardization

According to Weiner and Hoock (1973, p. 616):

> The use of standardized tests in clinical examinations or in research has a number of advantages over that of more impressionistic methods. Perhaps the value of such tests can best be summarized by the term *objective*. The carefully explicit directions allow for replication of the examination with the same or different individuals. Unwanted and uncontrolled variation can be largely eliminated. Informal measures, usually constructed by the individual examiner, may have the advantage of flexibility. All too often, however, this advantage is outweighed by the subjectivity involved in variable methods of presentation of tasks.

---

[2]When the clinician uses subtests or selected test items in other than standardized test procedure, the norms may no longer be valid.

Weiner and Hoock may have an excessive distrust of the "demon subjectivity" in behavioral assessment. Nevertheless, if a test is presented as a standardized instrument, questions concerning objectivity and standardization are entirely in order. One basis for evaluating such a test is in terms of how well the author succeeds in describing the administration and scoring. If the instructions are vague or incomplete, the scores are likely to be unreliable. The instructions provide a framework of rules for administering and scoring the test items. Among other things, this framework sets the conditions under which the child's performance may be compared to the test norms. If the instructions call for strict timing requirements, the norms are appropriate only when these are adhered to, even though at times it may be impossible to insist on these time requirements—as when testing a physically handicapped child. In this case, the clinician has the option simply of not using the test or of interpreting the results without reference to the original norms.

Test Norms

Test scores are not inherently meaningful. They acquire interpretive value when compared with appropriate norms. Anastasi (1968, p. 24) is rather direct to this point: ". . . without norms, test scores cannot be interpreted," and, "An individual's score can only be evaluated by comparing it with the scores obtained by others." For Weiner and Hoock (1973), norms provide another safeguard against subjectivity.

When norms are used, there are certain precautions that must be kept in mind. In most language tests, the norms are obtained from subjects in a limited geographic area, often from a small community despite the fact that the test is likely to be used mostly in large urban areas. Frequently, minority groups are excluded from the sample, as are children with known deviations or handicaps. All of these factors limit the appropriateness of any set of norms for a given child (Carrow, 1972).

Test norms are generally reported as an average score plus some index of variability, such as the standard deviation. Both the mean and the standard deviation must be considered when norms are used. If there is a great deal of variability (a large standard deviation) in the normative sample, then the fact that a given child deviates substantially from the average may not be terribly noteworthy. For example, the 3-year-old children tested by Templin (1957) obtained a mean articulation score of 93 correct out of 176 items. Should we be alarmed about a 3-year-old who scored only 75? Not when we know that the standard deviation for 3-year-olds was 34 items! Clinicians often accept two standard deviations below the mean as the cutting score for possible clinical attention. In the above example, the child would have to obtain a score of 25 before he was suspected of having a clinical problem. In addition, a test score is not always the best indicator of the presence of a problem. Even a few very distorted sounds may constitute a severe articulation problem, although the speaker might fall well within his age norms for total score on an articulation test.

Finally, the question clinicians most often have to face is not whether the child has a problem, but rather what the nature of the problem is (Leonard, 1972). Norms are not especially useful when the content of performance needs to be described (Muma, 1973), and it is the content that should serve as the basis for developing a therapy program.

Reliability

A minimal requirement for any test is that it be reliable. It must yield scores that are stable, trustworthy indices of performance. Several forms of reliability are usually reported. *Temporal reliability* refers to the stability of performance over some critical period. If the test is readministered after a brief interval, the score on the second administration should approxmiate the first score. Over longer intervals, or after intervention, the correlations may be much lower. In *split-half reliability* two portions of a test are correlated. Because both portions are presumably tapping the same ability, the correlation should be high. Some tests provide *alternate forms,* and these too should correlate highly. *Examiner reliability* involves a comparison between test administrators. This is particularly important when scoring or administration is complex. McCarthy and Kirk (1963) found that an inexperienced tester required more training to prepare him to administer the ITPA than did examiners with psychometric training. This raises questions about the appropriateness of using untrained personnel to administer the test. Spradlin, on the other hand, standardized the PLS with inexperienced testers and obtained very comparable results across examiners.

Experience is not the only relevant dimension. Siegel (1962) compared the articulation scores that were obtained when two advanced speech pathology students tested the same retarded children.

Although the correlations were high, one examiner consistently obtained lower scores than the other. Had these two examiners been used to evaluate a therapy program, the outcome would look variously bleak or encouraging, depending on who administered the pre- and who the posttests.

Test construction is sufficiently advanced that most well standardized tests readily meet reliability requirements and include these data with the test. When reliability data are incomplete, scores must be interpreted with caution. In any case, the decision as to whether a child requires therapy always should be based on more than a tally of the number of errors the child makes.

Validity

A test is valid to the extent that it measures what it purports to measure—that is, that it "does the job." Validity is generally more elusive than reliability. This is particulary true with regard to language, where widely accepted difinitions of what is being tested are lacking. It is relatively straightforward to determine the validity of a test of mechanical aptitude. The subjects would be given the test and then asked to solve some real problems involving machines. In language, however, the validating criteria are as numerous and ambiguous as the definitions.

Technically, validity is usually determined by correlating scores on a particular test with some external criterion, such as another test or performance measure, or a teacher's or clinician's ratings. There are several forms of validity that are discussed in standard psychometric texts. A technical discussion of validity is beyond the scope of this chapter, however. For the purposes of this chapter, it is more important to have an intuitive understanding.

It is often the case that tests present strong evidence concerning reliability and weak evidence for validity. One common method for establishing the validity of a language test is to correlate the scores with age. Because linguistic skills generally improve with age, the correlation should be high. This is a weak measure of validity, however, since so many traits and abilities show a similar course with age, including memory, attention span, ability to follow test instructions, and general intellectual ability. Presumably, a language test is more than, or at least different from any of these, but a high correlation does not establish whether the test is truly measuring language rather than general intellectual or some other skill. Clinician ratings are another frequently used but weak validating criterion. Although a language test should agree with the clinician's ratings of verbal competence, the ratings are generally too diffuse to indicate which aspects of the child's abilities are affecting the judgments. The clinician may be responding to only a tiny segment of the performance tapped by the test.

For the clinician, the most useful assessment procedures are those that lead directly to remedial procedures. Here validity is crucial. If the clinician devises a therapy program based on the strengths and weaknesses revealed by the test, then the components of the test must be valid representations of the child's actual performance skills. The ITPA is often used as a model for therapy, and Bush and Giles (1969) have published a set of exercises based on the components of the ITPA. In this case, the clinician is being invited to take the test model quite seriously as a basic representation of the child's psycholinguistic profile.

Because they are so difficult to obtain, validity data are rarely presented in any detail for most language tests. Indeed, the search for validity often does not even begin until the test has been standardized and published. Of all the current language tests, the ITPA probably has the most complete validity data, but even these are relatively incomplete and not entirely supportive of the test model. Validity studies for the revised edition of the ITPA are not yet available. In summarizing findings for the experimental version, McCarthy and Kirk (1963, p. 40) acknowledged, "It is clear that most validity demonstrations for the ITPA remain to be done." The need is even more pressing for most of the other language instruments.

For the most part, the clinician will have to deal with the question of validity in a subjective way. The tests have to be examined in detail, and the items have to be noted. The clinician ultimately must decide whether the test deals with components of language that are important and whether the items seem to be reasonably related to the abilities presumably being tested. As the clinician surveys a test, a number of useful questions should be kept in mind:

1.   What does the test purport to measure? What is the underlying definition of language?
2.   Do the names of the subtests and the items they subsume go together in a rational and logical way?
3.   Can you understand the definition and selection of items well

enough so that you could generate additional items and exercises that fit the test model?

4. Has the test author addressed the problem of validity at all? In what ways?

5. Is validity considered only in terms of the total test score, or in terms of the components or subtests that comprise the testing instrument?

Test Scores

Percentages One of the simplest forms in which to report test scores is in terms of the percentage of items that are passed. Unfortunately, this is not a very revealing index because it takes no account of the relative difficulty of the items: a score of 50% on test A may indicate better achievement than a score of 70% on test B. When norms are available, relative performance can be stated in relation to them. For example, 50% on test A may be above the mean, while 70% on test B is below the mean. In this example, a higher score does not mean better performance. It is much more convenient to have a system in which higher scores signify better achievement. This is accomplished in many tests by means of *derived* or *transformed* scores.

Age Score The age score is a derived score with some intuitive appeal. A determination is made of the number of items successfully passed at each age level in the normative sample, and that number is then assigned as the typical score for that age. For example, the average mean length of response for 5-year-olds in Templin's data (1957) is 5.7; for 6-year-olds, it is 6.6. A child who scores a mean length of response of 6.0 is performing at a level close to Templin's 5-year-old sample. It is convenient to be able to place the child's accomplishment on such a scale, but it is not easy to decide what constitutes adequate versus problematic performance. For example, what if a mean length of response of 6.0 were obtained from an 8-year-old? To evaluate this score, information is needed concerning the variability of scores in the normative sample. In Templin's data, the mean and standard deviations for 8-year-olds were 7.6 and 1.6, respectively. Thus, our 8-year-old is only one standard deviation below the mean for his peers, and we might regard any score above 4.4 (two standard deviations below the mean) as essentially normal. It sounds rather ominous to say that an 8-year-old is performing like a 5-year-old, until the variability in the original sample is also reported.

Percentiles   Another and somewhat comparable form of recording scores is in terms of percentiles. The 50th percentile corresponds to the median in the normative sample and is the score that separates the distribution into equal halves. A child who obtains a score that falls at the 10th percentile performed poorer than 90% of the normative sample. Percentile ranks are inconvenient because the distance between points on the scale is not constant. On the Northwestern Syntax Screening Test (Lee, 1971), a difference of only four items separates the 10th from the 90th percentile for the 7-year-old children. When expressed in percentiles, a difference between the uppermost and lowest 10% seems formidable, but is not nearly so awesome when one sees how few errors account for that difference. In interpreting percentile rankings, as with age scores, it is important to look at the total distribution and variation in the scores and not simply at the location of the child's score on the percentile scale.

Standard Score   A more complex and sophisticated form of test score entails some sort of standard score. The mathematics of these scores is somewhat involved. What must be kept in mind is that a standard score takes into account the distribution and variation in the normative sample. This is the most satisfactory form for interpreting a given child's performance. To derive standard scores, the mean and standard deviation for the standardization group are first computed. Then, the score obtained by an other child is converted to a standard score by finding the difference between his score and the mean for the standardization group and then dividing that difference by the standard deviation for the normative group. Often, other adjustments or transformations are then made to put the scores in a more convenient numerical form. For example, the ITPA uses standard scores with a mean of 36 and a standard deviation of six for each of the subtests. Thus, a score of 42 is always one standard deviation above the mean on the ITPA, regardless of the subtest being considered or the age of the child. A similar scale is used in the PLS (Spradlin, 1963) and in the Elicited Language Inventory (Carrow, 1974).

Application to Nonstandardized Procedures

Concepts such as sampling, reliability, validity, and norms are crucial for the evaluation of a standardized test. They also have correlates that are relevant to nonstandard procedures. Any technique for obtaining a language corpus necessarily involves sampling, and the impression gleaned from a single situation may not be representative of behavior in other situations. Labov (1970) has shown that the speech of black children is dramatically affected by the style of the interviewer. When the interviewer reduced his imposing 6-foot-plus height by sitting on the floor, and showed a willingness to use the dialect and topics that were familiar to the children, there was a sudden flowering of verbosity, wit, and creativity on the part of children who had earlier seemed sullen and recalcitrant. Any corpus of speech is a sample. There is no less obligation to keep this in mind when using informal procedures than there is when administering a highly standardized test.

Reliability is also relevant to less formal methods of data gathering. The clinician must be assured that the errors observed in one corpus are representative of those that would appear in subsequent samples. Therapy cannot be properly planned on the basis of untrustworthy samples of performance. Rather than formal devices like test-retest correlations or temporal stability coefficients, the clinician may have to use more subjective indices of stability. The child should be observed repeatedly and in depth in a variety of situations so that the patterns of behavior that are observed can be verified. This should be a continuing process, and hypotheses concerning the child's performance constantly must be checked against the data, whether they come from standardized or informal sources.

Similar extensions can be made to validity. In discussing validity, Muma (1973, p. 336) has written:

> With so many variables influencing verbal behavior, how can one be sure he is truly assessing what he intends to assess? There is no absolute assurance, only relative assurance. When a dimension of grammar varies according to a pattern and the pattern (rule) is predictable and relates to or integrates with other patterns, the assumption is made that the observation is valid.

In summary, this section presents a number of formal attributes that go into the evaluation of a standardized test: in particular, the nature and use of norms, reliability and validity, and issues surrounding the test as a sample of behavior. All of these notions have counterparts that apply and are equally relevant to nonstandardized assessment procedures. Whatever the source of data that the clinician uses in describing a child's problem and planning for therapy, the observations must be reliable, and they must relate to the child's basic skills and difficulties. A distinction can be made between "testing" and "assessment." Testing is a relatively narrow and specific method for generating information about a child. Assessment implies the collection of relevant data from all kinds of sources. Formal tests are used when appropriate, though not always precisely as prescribed in the manual, especially when one is not concerned about the test norms. Formal tests may reveal behavioral patterns that deserve fuller exploration. When this is the case, clinicians should not hesitate to devise their own methods and to check their impressions against spontaneous or less formally derived samples. The information obtained from all of these sources constitutes the basis for developing hypotheses about the regularities and patterns in the child's behavior. Subsequent assessment and initial therapy are then based on these hypotheses. Of course, clinicians should be quick to change their suppositions when the child's performance warrants it. Therapy and assessment are continuing, ongoing processes that are closely linked. It is at this level that the clinical and the research dimensions of the field most nearly merge.

IDENTIFICATION AND SCREENING

Clinicians working in school environments are under constant pressure to do more, in less time. In addition to serving school children, clinicians are now assuming responsibility for preschoolers, particularly those with severe language problems. Before therapy can begin, the child with a problem has to be identified, and this in itself is a formidable undertaking. It is not possible to administer extensive tests or to collect large samples of speech from every child. Some form of screening is necessary, but this is more readily stated than accomplished.

The purpose of a screening procedure is to locate children who may have a language difficulty, so that they can be examined more thoroughly at a later time. It seems a modest enough goal. If a test is to be used, it does not much matter what the items are, as long as they successfully identify children. If foot size turned out to be a good predictor of language growth, we would see lines of barefoot children streaming through the speech clinician's office. It would be sufficient unto the task. But, of course, a purely arbitrary measurement of this sort is likely to reveal little about language. What is needed instead is some small set of items that is critically related to language development and can be quickly administered and scored. Unfortunately, no such test exists, and it is questionable whether, in this instance, the old maxim that "necessity is the mother to invention" will be borne out.

Screening seems to work best when some specific sensory or motor system is being investigated. A screening test of vision, for example, is designed to exclude the influence of learning and development, and it does not have to be recalibrated according to the age of the person being examined. In contrast, the definition of "adequate language" changes with the child's age and even with his social circumstance. The criteria for normal vision are unaffected by the passing of years or the hardening of arteries.

Perhaps the greatest difficulty with devising a language screening test lies in the fact that language does not involve a unitary system. There are numerous theoretical approaches and models for language, and they are often quite discrepant. Even within a single model, there are likely to be innumerable components, any one of which could be deviant. Coupled with this is the fact that children do not all develop language at the same rate or even necessarily in the same sequence. The sorts of developmental scales that work in describing specific motor or sensory development are simply not appropriate for language.

Screening for language must take another form. Rather than administer and score innumerable tests, the clinician has to rely on human resources—the parents, physicians, nurses, counselors, social workers, and other teachers who come into frequent contact with the children. A referral system is needed in which the teachers and other professionals form the front line in the initial identification of communication disorder, and the speech and language clinician assumes the responsibility to educate his colleagues about normal and deviant language.

The first step in such a referral system is for the clinician to define *language disorder* in terms that are explicit and can be shared with colleagues. The present authors define language performance in terms of the dimensions presented earlier: grammar, concepts, and interpersonal use. There are no specific scores or exact behaviors that determine deviancy in each of these dimensions, but there are signs and clues to which teachers can be alerted. Some are obvious, and others will come from the clinician's unique experience. It is not necessary that all agree on a particular definition, only that some definition be used.

There are certain children who have so high a probability of language difficulty that they should routinely be referred for language evaluation. In particular, developmentally retarded and hearing-impaired children are "at risk" for language difficulty. In addition, children with behavioral and special learning difficulties should be examined by the speech and hearing specialist. Numerous causes underlie learning problems, including language or hearing deficits. This is not to say that the speech and hearing clinician must be involved in the education of every child in a special school program, but, if nothing else, it should be helpful to the teacher to rule out hearing and language as significant factors for a slow-achieving child.

Language disorders are sometimes quite subtle. For example, a child named Terry was referred to our clinic by an alert teacher who noticed that the child could not carry out simple instructions. When we first listened to Terry she seemed to be a very competent speaker, and we were impressed with her imaginativeness, vocabulary, and apparent control of syntax. It was only when we contrived a series of comprehension tasks for her that we noticed she had marked difficulty understanding directions, especially when these involved subtle differences among prepositions (*Put the doll* near, beside, behind . . . *the table*). Terry is the kind of child who easily might be overlooked or simply written off as not being terribly bright. Her difficulty in understanding certain basic concepts has affected her class performance. Ability to carry out instructions is an important index of language competence and is one of the signs to which teachers should be alerted. Similarly, children who are unusually quiet or withdrawn or who seem confused should be brought to the attention of the clinician.

The clinician serves the role of a specialist who "brings the message" to professional colleagues. There is no prescribed way in which this role is fulfilled. The clinician may want to arrange special in-service sessions in which normal and deviant language development are discussed. Tape recordings, videotapes, or commercial films may be used (see Striefel, Baer, and Douglas, this volume). Some clinicians prepare a pamphlet or brochure for the teachers. All of this should be supplemented by personal contact. Most importantly, when a referral is made, the teacher should be given direct feedback about what was done with the child, what kind of information was obtained, and what impressions were generated. There is probably no better occasion for informing a teacher about the nature of language assessment than when one of his "own" children has been referred. That first referral provides a marvelous opportunity for the clinician to involve the teacher in the speech and language program.

Speech and hearing specialists frequently work in isolation from the mainstream of classroom and other school activities. An adequate referral system requires an additional role, in which the clinician educates the school community about language and solicits help in the important task of identifying children who may require special speech and language services. There are school systems in which all children are routinely given a battery of "language" tests, some of which are of highly questionable reliability and validity. Children who fall below some arbitrary cutoff score on several of the tests are then recalled. This procedure seems like an incredibly inefficient use of the clinician's time. Although the data are lacking, a screening program based upon teacher referrals is likely to be more efficient and accurate, and certainly more satisfying for the clinician.

SPECIFIC ASSESSMENT METHODS

In this section, specific assessment methods are discussed for the three dimensions of language identified earlier.

Syntax

The grammar of a language is the set of rules that describe the relationship between sound and meaning (Chomsky, 1965).[3] The syntax of a language is the subset of rules that specify well formed sentences. These rules are reflected in the surface structure of a sentence by means of: the order in which words occur, the use of bound morphemes, and the use of free morphemes.

In assessing a child's syntactic skill, the clinician is assessing the ability of the child to create grammatical sentences, specifically, the ability to use word order, and bound and free morphemes to express various syntactic rules. To assess syntax appropriately, the clinician needs a model or a characterization of the structure of language that directs attention to the relevant dimensions of language. At this point there is no single model that serves that purpose. There are at least three different models reflected in assessment procedures, and each seems to have its own advantages and disadvantages. Each of these models is considered briefly.

---

[3]Grammar also may be defined more broadly as the set of rules that describe the relationship between meaning and any surface representation, including visual signs, rebus symbols, etc. See the chapters by Woodcock and Clark (this volume) and Wilbur (this volume).

Syntax as Rules   The transformational grammar first proposed by Chomsky (1957, 1965) and later modified by a number of linguists (e.g., Bach, 1974) focuses on syntax as a set of rules. These rules describe the relationship between some deep or underlying representation of a sentence and its surface or spoken form. Transformational grammar is concerned with the rules that create sentences and the rules that relate one sentence to another.

When syntax is considered from this framework, interest centers on certain questions while others are not considered at all. For example, within a transformational model, interrogatives, negatives, and passives are systematically related to declarative sentences. This relationship is illustrated in the following four sentences:

(1) The boy is pulling the wagon. (active-declarative)
(2) Is the boy pulling the wagon? (active-interrogative)
(3) The boy is not pulling the wagon. (active-negative)
(4) The wagon is being pulled by the boy. (passive)

Sometimes children give evidence that they learn these constructions as transformations. For example, children often produce questions with the *sense* of sentence 2 by producing the *form* of sentence 1 with a rising intonation (Klima and Bellugi, 1966). This seems particularly true for certain language-delayed children.

In the case of yes/no questions transformational grammar provides unique insight into the child's problem. Other transformations identified in formal linguistic accounts do not necessarily serve as useful models for language acquisition. A passive sentence such as 4 is, perhaps, a good example here. Most of the current syntax assessment instruments include passive sentences, but there is no evidence that the child learns the passive transformation. In addition, the child who fails to understand or produce passives does not stand out as a language-delayed child. These sentences are included in testing procedures because they are of interest to transformational grammarians, not to speech clinicians.

Transformational grammar has also focused attention on the child's use of other rules and has provided a new and helpful framework in which to consider the child's acquisition of, for example, plurals, verb tense markers, and adjective forms. The questions being asked is, "Does the child have the rule?" (Berko, 1958; Berry, 1966). This is often a useful approach. Sometimes, though, there are grammatical morphemes that cannot be accounted for by the use of rules.

Irregular forms and prepositions do not fit into neat rules. They are also of less interest to the transformational grammarian.

In general, a transformational grammar focuses on the rules of language. It calls the clinician's attention to the regularities that occur and to the child's mastery of those regularities. The child is seen as abstracting the rules of syntax from the speech that he hears.

A transformational grammar is intended as a formal account of the structure of language. It is not intended as a description of language learning or of the processes used by speakers or listeners in actually generating or interpreting speech. The "psychological reality" of transformational accounts of grammar has been questioned for some time (Fodor and Garrett, 1966). It is not surprising that one cannot always map the acquisition pattern or process directly onto a transformational description of language. Nevertheless, where such a formulation does describe the process, transformational descriptions can be useful.

Syntax as Redundancy   In the past, language models were employed that had, as components, input or receptive skills, processing skills, and output or expressive skills (Osgood, 1957; Carrow, 1972). Often, within such a model, syntax was seen as a relatively low level behavior or a set of automatic habits. Viewing syntax in this way calls attention to the redundancy inherent in language. Languages are designed so that the same information is transmitted in more than one way (Shannon and Weaver, 1949). This redundancy has been described rather extensively at the phonologic level; it also occurs at the syntactic level. For example, in the following sentences the form of the missing grammatical morpheme can be predicted from the remainder of the sentence:

(5) The boy run _____.
(6) I would like a cup _____ coffee.
(7) Yesterday I _____ (go) to the store.
(8) I have two flower _____ in my garden.

In sentence 5, boy is singular; therefore, the verb has the singular form *runs*. In 6, the blank can be filled with the preposition *of,* if what is meant is a cup that has coffee in it. In 7, *yesterday* implies past tense, and in 8, *two* modifying the noun indicates that the noun is marked for plural. This redundancy is a part of what makes language so robust in transmission. Adults use this redundancy to fill in portions of speech that have been missed. Children learn to use redundancy in the same way.

Measures of language that focus on redundancy tend to regard syntax in a superficial way. They overlook some of the fundamental rules that must be learned and focus instead on irregular forms, on predicting from syntactic data, and, consequently, on the impression that the speech makes on listeners. Failure to use various irregular forms correctly marks a speaker as different. Most unsophisticated listeners do not distinguish between the child who says *I goed home* because he knows the rule but not the irregular form, and the child who says *I go home* because he knows neither the rule nor the irregular form. Sometimes in working with children it is important to attend to superficial or surface forms.

Syntax as Semantic Relationships   Recently, syntax has been characterized as the expression of a set of semantic relationships (Fillmore, 1968; Chafe, 1970). The primary focus of these models is the meaning or the intent of an utterance. Although these semantic models of syntax are not as well developed as the two previous models, they too have certain advantages.

Brown (1973) and Schlesinger (1971) have found it useful to describe the early productions of children using a semantic based model of syntax. Schlesinger described eight different relationships that can be expressed in early two-word utterances. Here are three typical early sentences (Schlesinger, 1971):

(9) Bambi go. (agent + action)
(10) See sock. (action + direct object)
(11) Sat wall. (X + locative)

Each of these two-word utterances expresses a different syntactic relationship. Both the order of the words and the situational context must be used in interpreting that relationship. Indeed, Bloom (1970) has argued that the structure of children's two- and three-word utterances can be understood only by referring to situational context.

Semantic based models of syntax direct the clinician's attention to the meaning of utterances and provide a rich characterization of the nature of those utterances. At least one assessment procedure and language teaching program uses this kind of model to teach early language skills to retarded children (MacDonald and Blott, 1974; MacDonald and Nickols, 1974).

These models provide the clinician with an interesting characterization of early utterances, but they become less instructive as the child's speech becomes more complex.

Assessment of Syntax

There are several dimensions to the problem of assessing syntactic skills. First, a distinction should be made between an assessment procedure that describes the child's skill relative to other children, and an assessment procedure that describes, in some comprehensive way, the knowledge that an individual has of some aspect of syntax. This section primarily deals with the first dimension of assessment. The comprehensive description of syntax is considered later.

In considering measures of syntax, it is important to inquire into: 1) the model of syntax represented by a test instrument, 2) the nature of its sampling of the domain of syntax, and 3) the relationship of the test items to problems encountered by the population that is of interest. In this section each of these problems is addressed, using as examples the following tests of syntax:

1.   Grammatic Closure subtest of the Illinois Test of Psycholinguistic Abilities (ITPA) (Kirk, McCarthy, and Kirk, 1968)
2.   Developmental Sentence Scoring (DSS) procedure (Lee, 1974)
3.   Test of Auditory Comprehension of Language (TACL) (Carrow, 1973)

Model of Syntax   The model on which an assessment procedure is based can affect both the form and the content of the measure. For example, the ITPA Grammatic Closure subtest concentrates on the redundant aspects of syntactic skills by treating syntax as an automatic overlearned habit. The items in the ITPA provide a framework in which the response is specified both pictorially and by the syntactic form of the question:

> *Here is a dress* (point to a picture of one dress).
> *Here are two* _____ (point to a picture of two dresses).

The form *dresses* is specified by both the picture and the word *two*. Can the child, given these cues, complete the sentence correctly?

The Grammatic Closure subtest of the ITPA is not primarily concerned with the child's ability to use syntactic rules. The test is heavily loaded with irregular forms that could be learned only by rote. Nine of the 33 items in this ITPA subtest are plurals. They are all noun plurals; they all require the plural rather than the singular form; and they all present pictorial and syntactic context that would indicate more than one. Seven of the nine items are irregular plurals.

The TACL contrasts with the ITPA in that it assumes that the child is learning a rule that carries meaning. In this test the child's task is to point to a picture that best represents the examiner's utterance. Redundancy is eliminated by presenting only the syntactic form being tested or a brief and nonredundant phrase containing the form. *Plural* is tested in pronouns, nouns, auxiliary *be,* and main verbs. To determine what is being tested it is necessary to look at the decoy pictures. The item *sleeps* shows one bear sleeping, two bears sleeping, and three bears sleeping. It must be that it is the singular versus plural the form of the verb *sleep* that is being tested rather than *sleep* as a vocabulary item because number is the only error that can be made.

The DSS is an analysis of a sample of spontaneous speech designed by Lee (1974). This analysis provides point values for eight syntactic categories. Some categories correspond to traditional parts of speech (pronouns, main verbs, conjunctions), and some represent sentence types (wh-questions, interrogative reversals, negatives). In each case, Lee has identified a developmental order for the items that occur in the syntactic category.

It is difficult to identify a common theoretical basis for the choice of categories. Within several categories the items selected seem to reflect the development of the auxiliary structure within a standard transformational grammar (Bach, 1974). This seems to be true for the negative and interrogative reversal categories as well as the main verb. The wh-question category probably reflects the semantic development of wh-question words. The secondary verb category probably reflects the development of the use of embedding, although perhaps not in a strict transformational grammar framework. Plurals are never directly assessed in this procedure, but at least two of the categories, pronouns and noun modifiers, consider plural forms to be later appearing and therefore of a higher point value.

Nature of the Sample   Both the ITPA Grammatic Closure subtest and the TACL attempt to sample across syntactic categories and across levels of difficulty so that performance can be placed on a continuum. Consider the three items on the ITPA that test prepositions:

> (12) This cat is under the chair.
> Where is this cat? She is _____. (Item 2)
> (13) There is milk in this glass.
> It is a glass _____. (Item 7)

(14) Here it is night. Here it is morning.
He goes to work first thing in the morning, and he
goes home first thing _____. (Item 9)

These items increase in complexity, or abstraction. Item 2 is logical and simply requires a location preposition. Item 7 is more arbitrary and one of a small set of prepositions is required. Item 9 is idiomatic and only one preposition is acceptable. This range of items probably samples across the range of prepositional usage that occurs in English.

The TACL, on the other hand, tests only locational prepositions. None of the items taps the more idiomatic use of prepositions. The choice of prepositions on the TACL is not broad, but it does reflect the emphasis on the meaning of syntactic forms already observed in this test. The DSS does not include prepositions in its scoring system. Correct use of prepositions would be reflected only in the sentence point that is given for grammatically correct sentences.

Both the ITPA and the TACL attempt to sample across the range of syntactic skills that might be expected of a child. Neither provides a comprehensive description of the child's performance in any one area. These tests allow the child to be placed on some continuum relative to other children.

The DSS allows the child's score to be compared with normative data, and in addition it calls the clinician's attention to certain categories within the sample of spontaneous speech, for example, pronouns or questions. It provides some guidelines as to what might be expected of children at different ages. In this respect it has the potential to sample the child's performance in a more comprehensive way.

The DSS is also subject to all of the difficulties inherent in a sample of spontaneous speech. It may or may not be representative of the child's customary performance. The sample can affect DSS results in another way. Certain categories receive disproportionate weighting. A child who asks a great many questions will obtain a high DSS score. The present authors have data on an 8-year-old mentally retarded child who scored below the 3-year level on the expressive portion of the Northwestern Syntax Screening Test (NSST) (Lee, 1969) and whose sentences were shorter than the average 3-year-old (Templin, 1957). The child scored at the 6-year, 6-month level on the DSS. Half of his sentences were questions and half of the questions were wh-questions. This appeared to be the source of his high DSS score.

Relationship to Disordered Speech   At this point it seems important to raise some questions about all of these measures of syntax, indeed about most of the language tests in general. Do these measures explore the dimensions of syntax with which the clinician is most apt to be concerned? The answer is often no, for a number of reasons. All of these instruments use a developmental scale. They attempt to identify items that are more or less apt to be correct depending on the age of the person being tested. All of the instruments are standardized on a "normal" population. "Normal" is defined as ± 1 SD of the mean on any of a number of measures including IQ, socioeconomic status, and school performance. In using these test instruments with retarded children, or with hearing-impaired, severely language-delayed, or nonnative speakers of English, clinicians are assuming that the developmental progression in normal children defines the difficulty of the syntactic structures for all children, including the various clinical populations. These assumptions may be, and often are, false.

For example, prepositions are treated in various ways in the three measures. The ITPA has a few preposition items that vary in difficulty. The TACL considers only location prepositions, and the DSS does not include prepositions at all. There are two groups of individuals who have a great deal of difficulty with prepositions: nonnative speakers of English and the hearing impaired. These two groups are apt to use the wrong preposition. Consider the following sentences produced by high-school-age deaf students:

(15) I complain of my hip.
(16) My son was disappointed to the outcome of the game.
(17) It was my first time of school.

Prepositions have meaning, but it is often not possible to choose the correct preposition based on rational grounds. Quirk et al. (1972) have developed an elaborate system for explaining prepositional meaning, but to extend such a system to include prepositional use such as *at odds with John, on top of a problem,* or *away on a trip,* is absurd. Many of the uses of prepositions are arbitrary, and the particular preposition is more closely related to the verb or adjective that precedes it than it is to the meaning. All of the sentences above generated by deaf students reflect a choice of the wrong prepositions. There is no logical reason why one could not complain *of* something, but we do not, we complain *about* things. We are *disappointed in, disappointed with,* or *disappointed at* the outcome of a game.

Anyone learning English as a second language must learn which prepositions go with which nouns, verbs, or adjectives. These choices are not only often arbitrary, but they also may be different from the choices made in the speaker's first language. Straightforward translation surely will lead to errors.

In-depth Assessment of Syntax

There is no prepackaged method for describing the syntactic skills and weaknesses of an individual in any kind of detail. The clinician has to devise this kind of assessment. At this point in the assessment process there is no substitute for knowledge of the structures that are of interest. For example, it may appear that a child has difficulty with personal pronouns. Before one can begin to explore this in depth, one must know what the personal pronoun system in English is like. The personal pronoun system in English makes several distinctions that are not generally made with nouns.

Case Distinction   Pronouns make a distinction between the subjective and the objective case:

(18) The *children* gave the book to the *teacher*.
(19) *They* gave the book to *her*.
(20) The *teacher* gave the book to the *children*.
(21) *She* gave the book to *them*.

Note that the form of *teacher* and of *children* does not change from sentence (18) to sentence (20), but the form of the pronouns that take the place of those two words does change. *They* and *she* are in the subjective case while *them* and *her* are in the objective case (see Table 1).

Number Distinction   Most nouns in English are marked to indicate one or more-than-one (boy-boys; man-men). The number distinctions in pronouns indicate both the number and the relationship to the speaker. *I* implies one individual, the speaker. *We* indicates more-than-one, including the speaker. *You* indicates one, or more-than-one, including the hearer but not the speaker. *He, she, it*

Table 1. Personal pronouns

Singular		Plural	
Subjective	Objective	Subjective	Objective
I	me	we	us
you	you	you	you
he, she, it	him, her, it	they	them

indicate one, not including the speaker or the hearer. *They* signals more than one, not including the speaker or the hearer.

Gender Distinction   Most nouns in English do not make a gender distinction, but there is a small set of exceptions that are probably learned as individual vocabulary items (e.g., aunt, uncle; mother, father; actor, actress) or used as indicators of role. The third person singular pronouns *he* and *she* do make a gender distinction (Table 1).

Determiner-Nominal Distinction   There is another distinction that relates to the use of possesive pronouns. Possessive pronouns can function to modify nouns or they can function as independent pronouns, as in "This is *my* book," versus "This book is *mine*." In most cases the nominal form adds -s to the determiner form. The exceptions are *my* and *his* (see Table 2).

It is evident from this analysis that the pronoun system is complex to learn and difficult to teach. It is not uncommon to see children use only one case rather than two. It is less common to see gender errors and even less common to see person errors. The notable exception occurs in children identified an autistic or emotionally disturbed. One characteristic of such children is their use of pronouns, particularly the use of *I* for the hearer, and *you* for the speaker.

This discussion of the pronoun system exemplifies what is meant by a "deep" analysis of a child's syntactic usage and understanding. Similar examples can be developed for other aspects of our language.

Words and Concepts

In recent years the primary focus of language research, testing, and teaching has been on syntax. The introduction of generative grammar presented a new framework for the exploration of children's syntax that both the researcher and the teacher were eager to employ. These same insights have been used to explore the phonologic development of children (Smith, 1973) but not the child's acquisition of words or vocabulary development.

Table 2. Possessive pronouns

Singular		Plural	
Determiner	Nominal	Determiner	Nominal
my	mine	our	ours
your	yours	your	yours
his, her, its	his, hers	their	theirs

If one is interested in the acquisition of language skills in children or, more broadly, in the acquisition of communication skills, the heavy emphasis on syntax is, perhaps, out of focus. The syntax of a language carries a certain amount of meaning, but the bulk of meaning is carried by the words that are assembled and presented within that syntactic framework. The syntactic form NP + V + NP, for example, can represent equally well *Harry loves Sally* and *I hear the air conditioning*. The difference in meaning of these two sentences is carried by the words themselves. The acquisition of words, the assembling of vocabulary, and the concepts that underlie that vocabulary are important aspects of language acquisition.

Generally, it has been assumed that children master the syntactic and the phonologic rules of their language within the first 5 to 8 years of their life. In contrast, humans learn new words throughout their lives. In teaching young children, adults are most aware of teaching the names of objects and actions. It is common to hear adults talk in the following manner to young children: "Doggy. This is a doggy. Can you say 'doggy'? Say 'doggy.' " Although relatively little vocabulary is acquired in this direct, tutorial fashion, a great deal of information regarding syntax and phonology is made available through this kind of patter. Adults seem to talk in this way because they are conscious of the child's need to learn words.

Learning Words: Nature of the Problem   Every language is composed of a lexicon and a set of grammatical rules. Items in the lexicon may be called *formatives* or *morphemes* or *words*. Whatever they are called, these are the units that carry information in speech and that must be learned by the child as he learn his language. These units are called "words" here, even though this is not a wholly adequate term.

When an adult knows a word so that he can use and understand it, he knows a great many things. He knows the phonologic characteristics of that words, how it functions syntactically, a set of semantic markers for the word, and the specific meanings of that word. In addition, most words have more than one meaning. The word *sing* usually requires an animate subject: birds sing, people sing, but rocks and tables do not. But sometimes we talk about singing tea kettles, singing sands, or singing trees, and when a convict *sings,* the song may not be pretty. Adult speakers usually know a variety of meanings and shades of meanings of a word.

In assessing the vocabulary skills of young children one could count the number of different words that the child uses. Jespersen (1922/1964) found that a certain child had three words in his 10th month, 12 words in his 11th month, 106 words in his 15th month, 232 words in his 17th month. By the time the child was 6 years old he was shown to have 2688 words in his expressive vocabulary. The process of documenting those 2688 words was complex and involved enlisting the aid of most of the people in the child's environment, equipping them with pencil and paper, and asking them to record each of the words that the child said. Despite the time and effort put into this documentation, it was probably incomplete. The child probably knew more words than he was given credit for. The occasion to use some words did not occur during the time allotted for recording or in the presence of a recorder. The greatest weakness of this approach, though, is that it fails to capture what the child actually knew when saying those words. It only records instances of the occurrence of various words. It is possible that a child can use a word in a seemingly appropriate manner and still have an incomplete knowledge of it.

In exploring children's mastery of syntax, errors may indicate that a child has indeed mastered a rule and is now applying it broadly. The child who says *goed* or *digged* instead of *went* or *dug* is given credit for mastery of the past tense rule. In a similar way, it is possible to discover what a child does not know about words from the kinds of errors that he makes. A young girl overheard some adults discussing a new channel in a nearby lake. She asked which channel it was, was it four or was it five? She knew the word *channel* only in the context of television. Or, Jespersen (1922/1964) reported a child with a new doll who was asked, "Is that your *son*?" "No," she replied, "that's my *sun*," as she gestured to the window.

Sometimes a child learns a more abstract or a secondary meaning for a word before he learn the primary meaning. This is the case when children agree that *pig* is certainly a good name for that animal . . . Just look at how it lies about in the mud.

An incomplete understanding of the meaning of a word may be the source of cute anecdotes that parents can tell about their children. It also is the source of many comments that are made about the language skills of hearing-impaired and retarded children. For different reasons, children in both of these groups may have a partial understanding of the meaning of words that allows them to use and interpret words, but in a way that is different from that of the adult community. A group of high-school-aged, hearing-impaired students who were preparing for a civics class were asked what was mean by the phrase *to bear arms*. This phrase, in the Bill of Rights, was a part of the day's assignment. Given the context, they were puzzled by the phrase. When one boy smiled and started to roll up his sleeve, everyone laughed. They knew the meaning of those *words,* at least they knew *a* meaning for those words. They also knew that, given the context, their interpretation was incorrect. They did not know the appropriate meaning. The phrase /tu bɛr ɑrmz/[4] is ambiguous. There are as many as 10 different interpretations including the following:

to carry weapons	to uncover weapons	two uncovered weapons
to carry limbs	two animal limbs	two uncovered limbs, etc.

Initially, it was stated that adults were most aware of teaching *words* to young children and that it is probably the case that relatively few words are learned from this sort of tutorial lesson. How, then, are words learned? Children normally learn words by hearing them in context. Initially, that context at least in part, must be situational. The word in some way must be paired with its referent. The very early language learner cannot learn a word in a verbal context. You cannot tell a very young child that, "A dog is a four legged animal with fur that is often kept as a pet." At the time that a child is learning *dog,* he does not understand all of the other words. He does not know *four* or *animal* or *pet.* What usually happens is that the child is given the word in the context of a dog or perhaps a picture of a dog. That provides him with some initial information about the phonetic shape and the syntactic characteristics of the word, as well as its meaning. Adults say, "This is a dog," in the same way that they say, "This is a table" or "This is a cookie." Its use in a sentence helps to describe its syntactic characteristics. It helps group that word with other nouns. One does not say, "This is an *on*" or "This is a *see.*" Nouns are presented in one sort of frame while verbs and verb particles are presented in another.

The Concept of Concept   Underlying almost every word is a concept. This is probably particularly true of the early words that children learn. Words like *in* and *on* and *more* have quite abstract meanings. It is not possible to show a *more* to a child and provide him with

---

[4]For readers unfamiliar with the International Phonetic Association (IPA) Alphabet, a pronunciation key is provided in Appendix B.

the verbal label. But children hear these words in context, and they are among the first words that children use. Words like *chair, dog,* and *car* represent a whole class of objects rather than a single object. Brown (1958) commented that it is just these words that adults choose to teach a young child. They provide the child with the broad term rather than the specific term, with *dog* rather than *Fido,* with *chair* rather than *rocker.* The child, then, must abstract the chairness or the dogness from our examples. He must identify the attributes of a dog that distinguish it from other animals. He makes mistakes. He calls a cow a dog or a male stranger, "Daddy." But he also learns by abstracting relevant information from the physical and the verbal context in which words occur.

The child's task, then, is to abstract relevant information from the speech that he hears and from the physical context in which that speech occurs. He needs to abstract several kinds of information. He needs a phonologic representation of the word so that he can identify and produce it. He needs information about the syntactic characteristics of the word; these are obtained from verbal context. He needs information about the meaning of the word and the semantic restrictions on its use, some of which comes from the situation, some from the verbal context. In a very real sense the first words that children learn are not concrete. They are abstraction. Early words do not stand in a one-to-one relationship with objects (perhaps with the exception of Mamma, Daddy and a few proper names). They are generalizations or concepts. They begin to organize the child's world as his culture organizes the world. For the early language learner, learning about specific words and learning the structure of language occur at the same time. The child learns about the syntactic characteristics of words from their use in sentences. It is through learning the functions of words in language that the child begins to unravel the syntax of his language. Words are specific examples of phonologic rules.

When adults teach words to children, they are generally only aware of teaching the meaning of the words and perhaps their phonologic shape. They are not aware of teaching the syntactic and semantic information that children must have if they are to use the word. Generally this information is not a problem. It is provided and the child learns. It does become a problem when the clinician attempts to assess and to teach language skills to children who have difficulty learning in a normal fashion.

Assessment of Vocabulary Skills

On various occasions the clinician is confronted with the task of assessing the ability of a child to use words, sometimes attempting to identify children who have difficulty in this area, and sometimes describing the relative strengths and weaknesses of a particular child. In either case the clinician is asking, in a broad way, where this child fits, in other words, to compare an individual child to some standard, some yardstick. After completing the measurement, the clinician says, "Yes, this child has adequate skills in this area," or "No, this child does not have adequate word-use skills."

In contrast, sometimes the clinician wishes to obtain a comprehensive indication of the ability of the child to use some specific set of vocabulary items. Does this child understand the words used in first-grade reading materials? Does this child have the vocabulary necessary for daily living within this institution? Does this child know the words that will be used in Driver's Education? Based on this assessment, the clinician teaches the child what he needs to know. This second procedure attempts to identify the particular vocabulary that the child must know to succeed in a particular situation, to assess the child's mastery of those words, and to teach the words that the child does not know.

Standardized Vocabulary Tests   One common way to compare a child to a group of children is through the use of standardized tests. Three common vocabulary tests are presented to illustrate how such tests might be used to assess a child's word-use skills relative to other children of the same age.

The Peabody Picture Vocabulary Test (PPVT) (Dunn, 1965) is probably one of the most widely used tests of receptive vocabulary. The subject is presented with four pictures on a page. The examiner says a word and the subject identifies the picture that represents that word. The words are generally nouns and verbs. They were selected from all of the entries in *Webster's New Collegiate Dictionary (1953)*. From that pool, specific words were chosen because they could be pictured and because there was an age-related increase in the number of subjects who knew the word. To answer an item correctly, a subject must select the referent for a test word from among four pictures. The three decoy pictures vary from dissimilar, at young ages, to thematically similar at older ages.

Compare this to the Auditory Reception subtest of the Illinois Test of Psycholinguistic Abilities (ITPA) (Kirk, McCarthy, and Kirk, 1968). The Auditory Reception subtest was designed to use auditory input and simple verbal output to tap children's vocabulary skills. Word lists from the PPVT and from the Core Vocabulary (Taylor and Frankenpohl, 1960) were used, but the picture pointing task used by the PPVT was rejected because of the visual component. The test uses, instead, a simple sentence frame, *Do Nouns Verb?* (Do dogs fly? Do children climb?).

The results are interesting. Although both tests draw from the same pool of words, the correlation of the PPVT with the ITPA Auditory Reception subtest is low (0.09). Correlations between Auditory Reception and the WISC (Wechsler Intelligence Scale for Children) Similarities test (0.31) and the Paragraph Reading section of the Stanford Achievement Test (0.28) were higher and did reach statistical significance (McCarthy and Olson, 1964). The lack of correlation between Auditory Reception and the PPVT seems to indicate that the subject's task is different. In fact, it is. Instead of matching a word to a pictured referent, the ITPA requires that the subject match one word to another or, perhaps, one set of semantic markers to another. To answer a question like, *Do children climb?*, the listener needs to know that the verb *climb* can take a noun subject like *children*. He needs to know something about *children* and something about *climb* that will let him make the semantic match. Similarly, to answer the question, *Do canines manufacture?*, one needs to know something about *canines* and something about *manufacture* that will allow one to determine if a semantic match is possible.

A third test, the Auditory Association subtest of the ITPA, uses the same word pool and seems to carry this process one step further. In this subtest the child is given a pair of sentences like:

A bee has a hive;
A man has a _____.

The child is asked to complete the second sentence so that the relationship in the second sentence matches the relationship in the first sentence. To answer an item correctly the child must: 1) identify the syntactic and semantic relationship between two words in the first sentence, and 2) find a word that will complete the second sentence so that the same semantic and syntactic relationship exist. In the follow-ign example, taken from this test, two different responses are required to complete the sentence frame *Sugar is* _____.

Grass is green;	Coffee is bitter;
Sugar is _____.	Sugar is _____.
(color)	(taste)

Two different semantic relationships are modeled in the first sentences.

Each of these tests attempts to sample from the whole universe of words that a child might be expected to know. Each assesses a part of the word-use skills of a child. Any one of the tests might be used to place a child relative to other children of the same age, but the placement might differ according to which test is used. A child might be able to identify a referent for a word but not be able to match that word with another semantically. He might be able to make the semantic match but not the referential match.

At this point is seems appropriate to recognize that vocabulary skills are generally seen as a part of general intellectual skills. The PPVT was designed to be a test of verbal intelligence. The ITPA Auditory Association subtest seems to function as an intelligence test (McCarthy and Olson, 1964). This is probably the area of greatest overlap between linguistic and intellectual skill.

Assessing Specific Vocabularies   Often it is more appropriate to ask what a child knows in a given area that it is to ask where he fits with respect to some normative population. The deaf child enrolled in a driver's education class needs to know the words that will be used in the class, in the driving test, and out on the highway. Terms such as *merge left* or *through stop* or *pedestrian* are not necessarily words that he will know. Words like *shoulder* and *yield* have meanings that are specific to driving. In assessing this child's language skills for the purpose of driver's education, one would attempt to identify the words that he will be required to know, assess his knowledge of those words, and teach the words that are unfamiliar to him. The same might be said of an institutional setting, a math class, a civics class, or a cooking class.

There are several common dimensions to these situations. In each case the vocabulary of concern is finite and describable. This contrasts with a test such as the PPVT, which sample from the universe of words that a child might encounter. Many different samples could have been taken. Each would have represented that universe. There is nothing "special" about the words that are found in the PPVT.

Assessing vocabulary for specific needs leads directly to an intervention program. The words that are not known will be needed in a driver's education class or in daily living, or in math. On the other hand, it is not appropriate to teach the words that a child missed on the PPVT or the ITPA subtests.

The Boehm Test of Basic Concepts (Boehm, 1971) is an example of a test that comprehensively explores a specific vocabulary required in a specific situation. It was designed to test a set of terms (concepts, words) that are used in directions given to kindergarten and first-grade children and seldom defined explicitly. These are words that the early school child is assumed to know. The child who does not understand these concepts will have difficulty following directions and will be educationally handicapped. The concepts tested by the Boehm include items such as *below, different, middle, more,* and *last*. The words included in the Boehm are words that the child needs to know to perform well in school. The complete set of words can be assessed in a context that is similar to that in which the child will encounter the word. The test requires that the child respond to sentences such as, "Mark the flower that is in the *middle*." This test has no real norms. It has little application beyond kindergarten and first-grade students, but with these students it is an effective assessment of a part of their vocabulary.

Sometimes students' needs in the area of vocabulary become apparent in a different way. Consider the following sentences, produced by hearing-impaired students in a regular high school:

(22) Will you give me advices?
(23) Are the furnitures small?

In these instances the student fails to recognize that *advice* and *furniture* are mass nouns and must be treated in a manner that is different from count nouns like *books* or *trees*. Mass nouns do not take a plural ending or a plural verb. With that execption, the sentences are well constructed. The students know those words, but incompletely.

Consider the use of the word *differ* in the following set of sentences from the same students:

(24) Is *differ* to live in Crystal or Golden Valley from the City.
(25) We *differed* the money with each other.
(26) We are *differ* from the Europeans.

The verb *differ* is an intransitive verb. In sentences 24 and 26, the students seem to have confused "differ," the verb, with "different," the adjective. In sentence 25, the verb *differ* seems to have been confused with the verb *divide*. However, in sentences 24 and 26 the word *differ* could be used if the sentence were rephrased. One could say:

> (27) Living in Crystal or Golden Valley differs from living in the City.
> (28) We differ from Europeans.

Again, it is possible to analyze the work of students to determine what they need to know to use a word properly. Sentence 25 represents, perhaps, a phonologic confusion. The two words *differ* and *divide* are phonologically similar, and the student may have incomplete phonologic knowledge of the words.

In sentences 24 and 26 the error may be phonologic, since *differ* and *different* are similar phonologically, or the students may have marked *differ* as an adjective rather than as a verb in their lexicon. In any case, it helps to identify the specific errors that the student seems to be making and to address teaching to those errors.

Interpersonal Communication

Only two formal test procedures exist for testing a child's use of language for interpersonal, communicative purposes. The clinician who is interested in these aspects of language also must turn to the research literature for information regarding the kinds of tasks and procedures that have been used. The most rewarding literature deals with the development of role-taking and communication (e.g., Flavell et al., 1968) and of referential skills (Rosenberg, 1972; Glucksberg, Krauss, and Higgins, 1975). It is beyond the scope of this chapter to discuss the substantive areas of role-taking, communication, or referential behavior, but the literature is a source of suggestions for ways to examine children's behavior.

Formal Assessment Methods One of the subtests originally included in the Parsons Language Sample (Spradlin, 1963) was the "mand" subtest. Based on Skinner's (1957) formulation of verbal behavior, the items in this subtest were to examine the extent to which the child would make verbal demands (either vocal or gestural) on his environment in situations that were contrived to create a need or a state of deprivation in the child. Unfortunately, there were problems with the scoring and reliability of this subtest and it was dropped from the test. The mand subtest is unique, however, and deserves further consideration. The five items in the test took the following form:

1.   The examiner holds a wind-up toy in the child's view and lets it run for a few seconds. The child is scored correct if he *requests* the toy, either vocally or by gesture. Reaching for or grabbing the toy is incorrect.

2.   The examiner pounds a peg in a pegboard and then asks the child to do the same, but withholds the mallet. The child has to make a vocal request for the mallet.

3.   A battery-operated car is made to go, and the child is asked to activate it, but the examiner withholds the controls. A correct response is either a vocal or gestural request for the controls.

4.   The examiner secretly puts a number of buttons in his hand and asks the child, "Guess how many buttons I have in my hand." After the child guesses, the examiner puts the buttons away without telling the child whether he was right. A correct response is any vocal or gestural request to know whether the guess was right.

5.   The examiner hands the child a sheet of paper and asks him to write his name, but does not provide a writing implement. A correct response is a vocal or gestural demand for a pencil.

Johnson, Darley, and Spriestersbach (1952) described a procedure for determining the proportion of a child's remarks that may be classed as "egocentric" versus "socialized" speech. The analysis is made from the sample of 50 utterances that serves as the source for determining various measures of verbal output, vocabulary, and language structure. Several sets of norms are included. Johnson, Darley, and Spriestersbach observed that there are very large discrepancies between the norms obtained by later examiners and those proposed originally by Piaget. They attributed the discrepancy to differences in the way samples were obtained in the various studies and suggested that the standard situation for collecting 50 responses is not very revealing because virtually no egocentric utterances are obtained with this procedure. It also should be remembered that Piaget's norms are based on the intensive study of only two children and done almost half a century ago. There is little reason to expect that the specific scores he reported will serve as an exact template for the development of socialized speech.

Neither of these standardized procedures is satisfactory from the point of view of the test requirements discussed earlier. They also tap rather different aspects of language use. In the case of the mand test, the question is whether the child uses language to satisfy his own needs. In the functional analysis, the question is whether the child uses language in a way that satisfies the requirements of his listeners.

Research-Derived Methods   A variety of methods has been devised to study the development of communication skills among children. In many of these, the task is defined as a communication situation involving a speaker and a listener who can hear but not see each other. Both participants have an array of objects, pictures, forms, etc. In the Krauss and Glucksberg (1969) "stack the blocks" game, the listener has a set of four blocks, each of which has an abstract design imprinted on it. The speaker, on the other side of a screen, takes a single block from a dispenser and has to describe it in such a way that his partner can stack the corresponding block on a peg. Communication is measured in terms of how accurately the listener selects the appropriate blocks from the array. In general, the data indicate that the children become more adept on the task with age, and that they are generally better as listeners than as speakers in this communication game (Glucksberg, Krauss, and Higgins, 1975). Longhurst (1972) has used this same procedure to study the communication behaviors of retarded children, and Longhurst and Siegel (1973) created conditions of "communication disorder" with adults by introducing acoustic distortion in the signal presented to listeners and then noting the effect on the speaker's messages. Hanson (1972) used much the same technique with young normal children, except that he substituted familiar objects for the nonsense designs used by Krauss and Glucksberg (1969).

There are a number of variants of this basic procedures, many of which are described in the chapters by Glucksberg, Krauss, and Higgins (1975), Rosenberg and Cohen (1967), and Rosenberg (1972). In all of the variations of the basic procedure, the approach is limited to only one aspect of communicative behavior: the effective transmission of referential information that allows for the identification of a stimulus within some array. Communication in its broadest sense clearly involves more than reference, but this aspect has been studied most extensively.

Flavell et al. (1968) also devised a series of communication tasks to test the development of "role-taking skills" in children. These studies are closely allied to Piaget's concepts of egocentrism and role-taking ability. The tasks are generally very inventive and not nearly as standardized as those used by Rosenberg or Krauss and Glucksberg. The basic strategy is to devise a communication situation in which the listener has some peculiar characteristic that has to be noted by the speaker if adequate communication is to ensue. For example, the listener may be wearing a blindfold, or placed at a peculiar vantage point in the situation, or may be fully familiar versus unfamiliar with the situation, etc.

The procedures in the role-taking and communication studies have almost exclusively focused on the child's sensitivity to his listener's needs. Another important aspect of communication is the child's ability to use language to serve his own needs. This seems to have been studied much less extensively. A doctoral dissertation completed at the University of Minnesota by Cathy Cooper (1972) was designed to teach lower-income children the advantages that result from asking appropriate questions of adults as a means of obtaining information. As part of the program, Cooper devised a number of tasks designed to promote curiosity and questions. She used some simple magician's tricks, in which a kerchief is pulled through a tube and is red at one end of the tube but "magically" becomes blue when pulled through the other end. She did similar things with vials of liquid and colored string. She also constructed a question box in which the child would be asked to place his hand and try to discover what unseen objects were hidden there. These are familiar games for children, but they were used in this instance for a very specific purpose: to measure the child's tendency to use an available adult as a source of information about the various problems and puzzles with which the child was confronted.

Another research approach to interpersonal communication that is relatively unstructured has yielded interesting results in studies involving mothers and their children (e.g., Broen, 1972), and assemblies between pairs of retarded children (Rosenberg, Spradlin, and Mabel, 1961) or of normal adults and retardates of varying verbal abilities (Siegel, 1967). In these assembly studies, the general intent is to determine the extent to which the verbal behavior of each participant is influenced by the behaviors and characteristics of the other participant. This "interpersonal approach" has been summarized in a general way by Siegel (1967, p. 112):

Briefly, this framework suggests that whenever A and B are together in a social situation the behavior of each is at least partially a function of the responses and characteristics of the other. This approach seems especially cogent in the study of communication disorders because speech events are almost always interpersonal, involving both a speaker and a listener. Even if A is a speech clinician and B a child referred to him, not only does the clinician modify the behavior of the child, but the child also exerts some influence over the behavior of the clinician. A child who is very taciturn may evoke different verbal stimulation from the clinician than does a more responsive, talkative child, especially if the clinician is not particularly sensitive to the dynamics of social interactions.

Despite the fact that language and communicative functions are inseparable in the real environment, both formal and informal assessment procedures have generally ignored the child's ability to apply his language skills for interpersonal ends. There are virtually no tests and few experimental methods designed explicitly to inquire into these skills. The methods that have been described here may be useful to the clinician who is interested in the communicative functions of language. To the extent that effective communication is one of the principle goals of therapy, techniques like these may help measure and document the progress of clients who are enrolled in communication therapy.

SUMMARY

This chapter discusses the use of formal tests and of individualized assessment methods in the description of language disorders. Tests are convenient clinical tools. They are especially efficient for generating samples of behavior that then can be compared to some set of norms. But they are necessarily limited. Every test reflects the author's biases about the nature of language, and these biases or underlying concepts are likely to differ from instrument to instrument. Clinicians who use a test as the basis for describing a language disorder are buying more than a kit; they are buying the author's definition of language. In order to interpret the child's performance, each clinician also must be prepared to evaluate the assessment procedures.

No test can solve the complex problems of describing and identifying children with language disorders. Test data provide one source of information about performance, but clinicians must understand the tests that they use well enough so that performance can be probed in greater depth and meaningful therapy procedures can be devised. An assessment procedure may indicate that the child has difficulty with wh-questions. Before using this as the basis for a therapy program, the clinician should explore this much more fully. What kind of errors is the child making? Does he fail to place the wh-word in the correct position at the beginning of the sentence? Does he fail to make the interrogative reversal? Or does he omit the appropriate form of *do* when it is required in the question (e.g., "Where do you want to go?")?

Assessment is a broad concept that includes and goes beyond formal tests. Before an adequate assessment program can be devised, the clinician must have a general notion of what is to be subsumed by language. Language can be thought of in three basic dimensions: grammar, concepts and words, and interpersonal use (see McLean, this volume, for phonology). Formal tests exist that tap the first two dimensions. Tests of interpersonal use are virtually nonexistent. In any case, successful assessment always requires that the clinician go beyond the bounds of specific procedures to the basic language dimensions themselves. As stated at the outset, the most reliable and useful language assessment device is a clinician who has a good grasp of language in its various aspects and a willingness to probe and be inventive in creating new approaches to language assessment.

ACKNOWLEDGMENTS

We are thankful to Judy Bergauer for helping us clarify some of our ideas concerning language screening, and to Shirley Doyle for continually prodding us to think more deeply and creatively about the problems of children with severe language difficulties.

REFERENCES

Anastasi, A. 1968. Psychological Testing. 3rd Ed. Macmillan, New York.

Bach, E. 1974. Syntactic Theory. Holt, Rinehart and Winston, New York.

Berko, J. 1958. The child's learning of English morphology. Word 14:150–177.

Berry, M. F. 1966. Berry-Talbott Language Tests: Comprehension of Grammar. Rockford, Ill.

Berry, M. F. 1969. Language Disorders of Children: The Bases and Diagnoses. Appleton-Century-Crofts, New York.

Bloom, L. 1970. Language Development: Form and Function in Emerging Grammars. MIT Press, Cambridge, Mass.

Boehm, A. E. 1971. Boehm Test of Basic Concepts Manual. The Psychological Corp., New York.

Broen, P. A. 1972. The verbal environment of the language learning child. Asha monogr. 17.

Brown, R. 1958. How shall a thing be called? Psychol. Rev. 65:14–21.

Brown, R. 1973. A First Language: The Early Stages. Harvard University Press, Cambridge, Mass.

Burros, O. K. 1972. The Mental Measurement Yearbook. Vol. 7. Gryphon Press, Highland Park, N.J.

Bush, W. J., and M. T. Giles. 1969. Aids to Psycholinguistic Teaching. Charles E. Merrill, Columbus, Ohio.

Carrow, E. 1972. Assessment of speech and language in children. In J. E. McLean, D. E. Yoder, and R. L. Schiefelbusch (eds.), Language Intervention with the Retarded. University Park Press, Baltimore.

Carrow, E. 1973. Test for Auditory Comprehension of Language. Urban Research Group, Austin, Tex.

Carrow, E. 1974. Carrow Elicited Language Inventory. Learning Concepts, Austin, Tex.

Chafe, W. L. 1970. Meaning and the Structure of Language. University of Chicago Press, Chicago.

Chomsky, N. 1957. Syntactic Structures. Mouton, The Hague.

Chomsky, N. 1965. Aspects of the Theory of Syntax. MIT Press, Cambridge, Mass.

Chomsky, N. 1972. Language and Mind. Revised Ed. Harcourt Brace Jovanovich, New York.

Cooper, C. 1972. Training inquiry behavior in young disadvantaged children. Unpublished doctoral dissertation, University of Minnesota, Minneapolis.

Crabtree, M. 1963. The Houston Test for Language Development. The Houston Test Co., Houston.

Dale, P. S. 1972. Language Development: Structure and Function. Dryden Press, Hindsdale, Ill.

Dunn, L. M. 1965. Expanded Manual for the Peabody Picture Vocabulary Test. American Guidance Service, Circle Pines, Minn.

Emrick, L. L., and J. T. Hatten. 1974. Diagnosis and Evaluation in Speech Pathology. Prentice-Hall, Englewood Cliffs, N.J.

Fillmore, C. J. 1968. The case for case. In E. Bach and R. T. Harms (eds.), Universals in Linguistic Theory. Holt, Rinehart and Winston, New York.

Flavell, J. H., P. T. Botkin, C. L. Fry, J. W. Wright, and P. E. Jarvis. 1968. The Development of Role-Taking and Communication Skills in Children. John Wiley & Sons, New York.

Fodor, J., and M. Garrett. 1966. Some reflections on competence and performance. In J. Lyons and R. J. Wales (eds.), Psycholinguistic Papers. Aldine, Chicago.

Fraser, C., U. Bellugi, and R. Brown. 1963. Control of grammar in imitation, comprehension, and production. J. Verb. Learn. Verb. Behav. 2:121–135.

Glucksberg, S., R. Krauss, and E. T. Higgins. 1975. The development of referential communication skills. In F. D. Horowitz, S. Scarr-Salapatek, and G. M. Siegel (eds.), Review of Child Development Research Vol. 4. University of Chicago Press, Chicago.

Hanson, B. 1972. The effects of communication failure on the subsequent verbal behavior of four-year-old speakers. Unpublished master's thesis. University of Minnesota, Minneapolis.

Irwin, J. V., J. M. Moore, and D. L. Rampp. 1972. Nonmedical diagnosis and evaluation. In J. V. Irwin and M. Marge (eds.), Principles of Childhood Language Disabilities. Appleton-Century-Crofts, New York.

Jespersen, O. 1964. Language: Its Nature, Development and Origin. Norton, New York. (Originally published, 1922.)

Johnson, W., F. L. Darley, and D. C. Spriestersbach. 1952. Diagnostic Methods in Speech Pathology. Harper & Row, New York.

Kirk, S. A., and J. J. McCarthy. 1961. The Illinois Test of Psycholinguistic Abilities—An approach to differential diagnosis. Amer. J. Ment. Defic. 66:399–412.

Kirk, S. A., J. J. McCarthy, and W. D. Kirk. 1968. Examiners manual: Illinois Test of Psycholinguistic Abilities. Revised Ed. University of Illinois Press, Urbana.

Klima, E. S., and U. Bellugi. 1966. Syntactic regularities in the speech of children. In J. Lyons and R. J. Wales (eds.), Psycholinguistic Papers. Aldine, Chicago.

Krauss, R. M., and S. Glucksberg. 1969. The development of communication: Competence as a function of age. Child Devel. 40:255–266.

Kuczaj, S. A., II, and M. D. Maratsos. 1975. What a child can say before he will. Merrill-Palmer Q. 21:89–111.

Labov, W. 1970. The logic of nonstandard English. In F. Williams (ed.), Language and Poverty. Markham, Chicago.

Lee, L. L. 1969. The Northwestern Syntax Screening Test. Northwestern University Press, Evanston, Ill.

Lee, L. L. 1971. A screening test for syntax development. J. Speech Hear. Disord. 36:315–340.

Lee, L. L. 1974. Developmental Sentence Analysis. Northwestern University Press, Evanston, Ill.

Leonard, L. B. 1972. What is deviant language? J. Speech Hear. Disord. 37:427–446.

Longhurst, T. M. 1972. Assessing and increasing descriptive communication skills in retarded children. Ment. Retard. 10:42–45.

Longhurst, T. M., and G. M. Siegel. 1973. Effects of communication failure on speaker and listener behavior. J. Speech Hear. Res. 16:128–140.

MacDonald, J., and J. P. Blott. 1974. Environmental language intervention: A rationale for a diagnostic and training strategy through rules, context, and generalization. J. Speech Hear. Disord. 39:244–256.

MacDonald, J., and M. Nickols. 1974. Environmental Language Inventory (ELI): A Semantic-Based Assessment for Training Early Expressive Language. Ohio State University, Athens.

McCarthy, J. J., and S. A. Kirk. 1963. The Construction and Statistical Characteristics of the Illinois Test of Psycholinguistic Abilities. Photo Press, Madison, Wis.

McCarthy, J. J., and J. L. Olson. 1964. Validity Studies on the Illinois Test of Psycholinguistic Abilities. Photo Press, Madison, Wis.

Muma, J. M. 1973. Language assessment: Some underlying assumptions. Asha 15:331–338.

Osgood, C. E. 1957. Motivational dynamics of language behavior. In M. R. Jones (ed.), Nebraska Symposium on Motivation. University of Nebraska Press, Lincoln.

Piaget, J. 1926. The Language and Thought of the Child. Harcourt Brace Jovanovich, New York.

Quirk, R., S. Greenbaum, G. Leech, and J. Svartvik. 1972. A Grammar of Contemporary English. Seminar Press, New York.

Rosenberg, S. 1972. The development of referential skills in children. In R. L. Schiefelbusch (ed.), Language of the Mentally Retarded. University Park Press, Baltimore.

Rosenberg, S., and B. D. Cohen. 1967. The development of communication skills. In R. L. Schiefelbusch, R. H. Copeland, and J. O. Smith (eds.), Language and Mental Retardation: Empirical and Conceptual Considerations. Holt, Rinehart and Winston, New York.

Rosenberg, S., J. Spradlin, and S. Mabel. 1961. Interaction among retarded children as a function of their relative language skills. J. Abnorm. Soc. Psychol. 63:402–410.

Schlesinger, I. M. 1971. Production of utterances and language acquisition. In D. I. Slobin (ed.), The Ontogenesis of Grammar. Academic Press, New York.

Shannon, C. E., and W. Weaver. 1949. The Mathematical Theory of Communication. University of Illinois Press, Urbana.

Siegel, G. M. 1962. Experienced and inexperienced articulation examiners. J. Speech Hear. Disord. 27:28–35.

Siegel, G. M. 1967. Interpersonal approaches to the study of communication disorders. J. Speech Hear. Disord. 32:112–120.

Skinner, B. F. 1957. Verbal Behavior. Appleton-Century-Crofts, New York.

Slobin, D., and C. Welsh. 1973. Elicited imitation as a research tool in developmental psycholinguistics. In C. Ferguson and D. Slobin (eds.), Studies in Child Language Development. Holt, Rinehart and Winston, New York.

Smith, N. V. 1973. The Acquisition of Phonology: A Case Study. Cambridge University Press, New York.

Spradlin, J. E. 1963. Assessment of speech and language of retarded children: The Parsons Language Sample. In R. L. Schiefelbusch (ed.), Language studies of mentally retarded children. J. Speech Hear. Disord. monogr. suppl. 10.

Spradlin, J. E. 1967. Procedures for evaluating processes associated with receptive and expressive language. In R. L. Schiefelbusch, R. H. Copeland, and J .O. Smith (eds.), Language and Mental Retardation: Empirical and Conceptual Foundations. Holt, Rinehart and Winston, New York.

Taylor, S. E., and H. Frankenpohl. 1960. A Core Vocabulary. EDL research and information bulletin no. 5. Educational Development Laboratories, Inc., Huntington, N.Y.

Templin, M. C. 1957. Certain Language Skills in Children. University of Minnesota Press, Minneapolis.

Webster's New Collegiate Dictionary. 1953. G.&C. Merriam, Springfield, Mass.

Weiner, P. S., and W. C. Hoock. 1973. The standardization of tests. J. Speech Hear. Res. 16:616–626.

4

AUDIOLOGIC CONSIDERATIONS

B. Patrick Cox and
Lyle L. Lloyd

CONTENTS

General Audiologic Programming _____ 125

Identification _____ 128
    Neonates and infants/128
    Children, 18 to 36 months/137
    Preschool and school-age children/140

Audiologic Assessment _____ 141
    Acoustic and other environmental factors/143
    Calibration/143
    Instructions/144
    Response criteria/144
    Response mode/145
    Threshold searching methodology/145
    Stimulus specificity and control/146
    Linguistic variables/146

Basic Battery of Auditory Skills _____ 147
    Pure tone audiometry/148
    Speech audiometry/155

Procedures Used with Children _____ 159
    Usefulness of the procedures/159
    Behavioral procedures/161
    Respondent procedures/166

Aural Habilitation _____ 175
    Speech and language therapy/176
    Hearing and selection and orientation/177
    Auditory training/180
    Training in use of visual cues/181
    Counseling/182

Conclusion _____ 183
References _____ 183

The highly significant relationship between hearing and communication is emphasized by various communication models including the one presented by Sanders (this volume). Indeed, the many processes of audition are vitally linked to the verbal communication system. Myklebust (1960), among others, has stressed the role of hearing in the development of a verbal communication system, pointing out that, ontogenetically, hearing is the primary sensory avenue involved in language acquisition. Among the most important developmental accomplishments of the infant are the acquisition of auditory inner-language and auditory receptive language skills, beginning long before the production of expressive language of any consequence. It follows, then, that any disturbance in the peripheral or central auditory mechanism disrupts to some degree the acquisition and use of normal communication. Hearing impairment occurring in conjunction with other developmental disabilities has an even greater impact. The thesis submitted here is that the effect of the presence of multiple developmental disabilities is not simply additive but results in a complex interaction having extensive effects on the total behavior of the individual. Too often programs designed for hearing-impaired individuals with other developmental disabilities (e.g., mental retardation, cerebral palsy, autism, epilepsy, or severe learning disabilities) focus either on the hearing impairment or on the other disability, as if they were separate entities that may be simply added together.

This chapter discusses various areas of audiologic involvement in the communication assessment and intervention strategies utilized with the developmentally disabled. Initial discussion centers on *general audiologic programming considerations*. After this, the *identification* and *audiologic assessment* aspects of a systematic audiologic program are emphasized. Because several other chapters in this volume are devoted to the *habilitative* aspects, these are considered only briefly. Throughout these sections the role of the audiologist as a member of the interdisciplinary team is emphasized.

GENERAL AUDIOLOGIC PROGRAMMING

Regardless of setting, the comprehensive audiologic program consists of four interrelated but clearly identifiable aspects: 1) identification, including referral systems and screening; 2) audiologic assessment;

3) otolaryngologic consultation; and 4) aural (re)habilitation.[1] In addition, a critical part of such a program is the systematic follow-up necessary to each of these aspects. Figure 1 is a schematic representation of these aspects.

Before discussing the individual aspects of the audiology program, there are administrative factors affecting audiology programs that should be presented briefly. Probably the single most important point about any audiology program is that it conform to appropriate

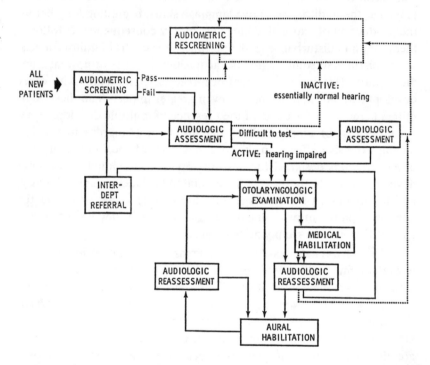

Figure 1. Total audiologic programming. This diagram emphasizes the four major aspects of an audiologic programming: screening and referral, audiologic assessment, otolaryngologic consultation, and aural habilitation. (From Lloyd, L. L. and B. P. Cox, Programming for the audiologic aspects of mental retardation, *Mental Retardation* 10:2, 1972, and reprinted with permission.)

---

[1]The term *(re)habilitation* is hereafter referred to as *habilitation*. Habilitation generally refers to programming, education, or treatment designed to teach a skill to a person who has never had that skill, whereas rehabilitation is the reteaching of a skill. In this chapter habilitation refers to teaching or reteaching activities. Aural habilitation is also referred to as habilitative audiology.

standards in its delivery of services. All such programs should conform as a minimum to the standards and guidelines set forth by the Professional Services Board of the American Board of Examiners in Speech Pathology and Audiology (ABESPA) and by the Accreditation Council for Facilities for the Mentally Retarded (AC/FMR) of the Joint Commission on Accreditation of Hospitals (1971). As described by Lloyd and Cox (1972), although the AC/FMR standards were originally developed for residential programs for the retarded, they are also appropriate to nonresidential programs for persons with developmental disabilities other than retardation. The AC/FMR standards specifically relating to speech pathology and audiology services are provided in Appendix C.

Another consideration concerns the department in which the audiology program is located administratively. Generally the audiology program is within the speech and hearing department. However, it may be located within a medical department (e.g., outpatient clinic, otolaryngology division), an educational department, or in one of the adjunctive therapies devisions depending on administrative prerogative or the facilities themselves. Regardless of the administrative location of the audiology program, the services must be delivered under the supervision of a qualified audiologist. Such an individual must meet the minimal qualifications for an audiologist as described by the American Speech and Hearing Association. These qualifications include as a minimum academic, practicum, and paid professional experience prerequisites in addition to the successful completion of a standardized certification examination.[2]

It also should be noted that an audiology program that delivers quality audiologic services requires specialized equipment. Such equipment is sensitive and forms the basis for audiologic decisions; therefore, it must conform to standards designed for such equipment (ANSI, 1969). This requires periodic calibration checks and maintenance of calibration records. In addition, the program must have available electronic and technical support to perform necessary repairs to diagnostic and treatment equipment and, in some cases, provide hearing aid repair services. Additionally, the audiology program needs testing environments that meet the noise controls specified by

---

[2]The specific requirements for certification as an audiologist can be obtained from the American Speech and Hearing Association, 9030 Old Georgetown Road, Washington, D.C. 20014.

the American National Standards Institute (ANSI, 1969). The program also needs space for habilitative audiology activities.

A final administrative consideration involves the staffing pattern in the audiology program. It is difficult to specify the appropriate number of personnel needed to maintain an adequate program. However, generally the staffing pattern depends on the caseload to be served, logistic and geographic factors, funding, and the use of supportive personnel. At least one audiologist must supervise the audiology program. This individual can make use of supportive personnel to conduct parts of the audiologic screening and assessment procedures under supervision. In addition, supportive personnel can be used in some aspects of treatment activities. Use of supportive personnel facilitates the audiologist's responsibility of providing in-service training of other staff members. In many cases it also provides for carryover from clinical activities to the other aspects of the child's life. The use of supportive personnel is discussed more extensively by Sigelman and Bensberg (this volume).

IDENTIFICATION

The purpose of the identification segment of the audiologic program is to find those individuals who may have a hearing loss. Although identification programs may differ, all have in common the screening of large groups of individuals and the establishment of appropriate referral systems into and out of the program (Darley, 1961). For purposes of discussion, identification audiometry is divided into subsections on neonates and infants, 28- to 36-month-old children, and preschool and school-age children.

Neonates and Infants

It is obvious that one would like to have access to the total population in order to discern those individuals suspected of having a hearing loss. It is unfortunate that presently there is no extensive system for the early detection of developmental disabilities through massive screening programs. One exception to this is the systematic screening that is done in most states for phenylketonuria (PKU), which if untreated causes mental retardation. Even here the screening is for the metabolic disease rather than for the developmental disability. One solution to the problem of not having such a system would be to couple developmental screening, including hearing, with the child's routine well-baby checks and visits for immunizations. (For specific recommendations of how hearing screening might be incorporated in such procedures, see Lloyd, 1976).

With specific regard to hearing, very few communities have active mass screening programs for children below kindergarten age. One exception to this is the group of children covered by federal legislation (Public Law 90-248, Title XIX), which requires hearing screening for those receiving Medicaid services. In addition, very few hospitals have either established registers of infants at risk for hearing impairment, including those whose prenatal or birth histories place them in a suspect category, or have provided for active follow-up of such children.

Besides not having a system that provides the opportunity for mass screening of preschool children, the audiologist is confronted with another dilemma related to the efficacy of mass screening. Mass neonatal hearing screening has been tried (Downs, 1967a) and has been determined to be unsuccessful (Downs and Hemenway, 1969, 1972; Downs, 1970; Goldstein and Tait, 1971). Thus, the audiologist is caught between not having a readily accessible population and the knowledge that, even if it were available, there is currently no truly efficient and reliable mass screening tool to use with the neonatal population.

High Risk Infants In recognition of the absence of a system for mass detection of developmental disabilities and a reliable, efficient hearing screening tool, the American Academy of Ophthalmology and Otolaryngology (AAOO), the American Academy of Pediatrics (AAP), and the American Speech and Hearing Association (ASHA) issued a joint statement recommending the use of a high risk registry rather than only neonatal screening (AAOO, AAP, and ASHA, 1974). Specifically, the joint committee reported (AAOO, AAP, and ASHA, 1974, p. 16):

> . . . since no satisfactory technique is yet established that will permit hearing screening of all newborns, infants AT RISK for hearing impairment should be identified by means of history and physical examination.

Identification by case history of infants at risk involves isolating those aspects of a child's prenatal, birth, and neonatal histories that place the child in a suspect category for hearing impairment. The at-risk categories of the AAOO-AAP-ASHA joint committee include all children who have one or more of the following (AAOO, AAP, and ASHA, 1974, p. 16):

A. History of hereditary childhood hearing impairment.
B. Rubella or other non-bacterial intrauterine fetal infection (e.g., cytomegalovirus infection, herpes infection).
C. Defects of ear, nose or throat. Malformed, low set or absent pinnae; cleft lip or palate (including submucous cleft); any residual abnormality of the otorhinolaryngeal system.
D. Birthweight less than 1500 grams (approximately 3.3 pounds).
E. Bilirubin level greater than 20 mg/100 ml serum.

It has been estimated by one investigator (Downs, 1973) that this categorization puts approximately 7% of the general newborn population at risk. Any neonate who is placed at risk according to these factors should be given a complete audiologic evaluation during his first 2 months of life. In addition, the child should be followed periodically by the audiologist with whom a relationship has been established. These follow-up evaluations can be done as a part of the child's well-baby examination. It is particularly important, because of the possibility of a progressive loss, that the high risk neonate be retested even if the working diagnosis following the initial testing is "normal hearing." Also, false negative errors are more likely than false positive errors because of the relative crudeness of tests for this age group.

In identification activities with the neonate one also can make use of information from parents in addition to the high risk register and audiologic testing. It is advantageous to have parents complete a basic questionnaire regarding the child's auditory behavior and general communication development. Use may be made of a publication from the National Institute of Neurological Disease and Stroke (NINDS, 1969), which poses questions relative to auditory behavior and general communication development and states the average expected behavior for each question. This segment of the publication is reproduced in Table 1. Use of this type of questionnaire, which is easily intelligible for most parents and the various members of the diagnostic and treatment team, enhances the early identification of children with hearing loss. Indeed, in most cases parents are the clinician's greatest source of information relative to a child's development.

Screening Procedures   The audiologic methodologies most frequently used in the actual hearing screening of the neonate are broadly categorized under the heading *behavior observation audiometry*

(BOA). As the name implies, behavior observation audiometry involves presenting the neonate with a sound and observing the response to the stimulus. Although this method is the least reliable and valid of all those used by the audiologist (Goldstein and Tait, 1971; Lloyd, 1975; Lloyd and Cox, 1975; Lloyd and Dahle, 1976), it provides sufficient audiologic information to permit the audiologist to form a tentative hypothesis and to initiate some habilitative procedures.

Screening with the newborn generally involves the presentation of a narrow band signal (i.e., a signal of a specific restricted frequency range) in a sound-treated room at a level that will elicit a response from the average newborn. The response expected of the child is arousal from a light sleep because this has been found to be the most reliable response and infant state (Bench and Boscak, 1970; Northern and Downs, 1973). The level of sound resulting in such arousal depends on the kind of signal used (i.e., noisemakers, speech, narrow band noise). Northern and Downs (1975) have shown that, for this age group, the variability of response ranges from a low of 40 dB hearing level (HL) (ANSI, 1969) for speech stimuli to a high of 78 dB HL (ANSI, 1969) for warbled pure tones. Because of this signal-dependent variability and the variability of individual infants because of developmental differences, the criterion for failure of the neonatal screening is usually established between 70 and 90 dB HL (ANSI, 1969).

Identification procedures with the child of 3 months of age or older become more reliable because the child has a better developed behavior repertoire. One expects the child by this age to begin to localize or seek the source of sound. It is at this age that the child begins to respond less reflexively and more in response to the meaningfulness of sound. Testing hearing by use of sounds that are thought to be meaningful to a child is sometimes called *distraction audiometry*. Ewing and Ewing (1944) were among the first investigators to study the meaningfulness of sounds. They reported that a child of this age is more likely to respond to crinkling paper, a spoon stirred in a cup, and so on, than to less meaningful sounds (e.g., pure tones). In addition, it is noted that the child of this age responds more than the younger child to sounds of less intensity (Ewing and Ewing, 1944; Murphy, 1962; Northern and Downs, 1975). In actual testing, typically the child is placed in a sitting or lying position on the floor or on the parent's lap in a sound-treated area. Various sound toys whose frequency and intensity characteristics are known are presented out of

Table 1. Information for parents concerning the expected auditory and general communication behaviors of children, 3 months to 5 years of age

Average age	Question	Average behavior
3–6 months	What does he do when you talk to him?	He awakens or quiets to the sound of his mother's voice.
	Does he react to your voice even when he cannot see you?	He typically turns his eyes and head in the direction of the source of sound.
7–10 months	When he can't see what is happening, what does he do when he hears familiar footsteps . . . the dog barking . . . the telephone ringing . . . candy paper rattling . . . someone's voice . . . his own name?	He turns his head and shoulders toward familiar sounds, even when he cannot see what is happening. Such sounds do not have to be loud to cause him to respond.
11–15 months	Can he point to or find familiar objects or people, when he is asked to? Example: "Where is Jimmy?" "Find the ball."	He shows his understanding of some words by appropriate behavior; for example, he points to or looks at familiar objects or people, on request.
	Does he respond differently to different sound?	He jabbers in response to a human voice, is apt to cry when there is thunder, or may frown when he is scolded.
	Does he enjoy listening to some sounds and imitating them?	Imitation indicates that he can hear the sounds and match them with his own sound production.

Continued

Table 1—*continued*

Average age	Question	Average behavior
1.5 years	Can he point to parts of his body when you ask him to? Example: "Show me your eyes." "Show me your nose."	Some children begin to identify parts of the body. He should be able to show his nose or eyes.
	How many understandable words does he use—words you are sure *really* mean something?	He should be using a few single words. They are not complete or pronounced perfectly but are clearly meaningful.
2 years	Can he follow simple verbal commands when you are careful not to give him any help, such as looking at the object or pointing in the right direction? Example: "Johnny, get your hat and give it to Daddy." "Debby, bring me your ball."	He should be able to follow a few simple commands without visual clues.
	Does he enjoy being read to? Does he point out pictures of familiar objects in a book when asked to? Example: "Show me the baby." "Where's the rabbit?"	Most 2-year-olds enjoy being "read to" and shown simple pictures in a book or magazine and will point out pictures when you ask them to.
	Does he use the names of familiar people and things such as Mommy, milk, ball, and hat?	He should be using a variety of everyday words heard in his home and neighborhood.

Continued

Table 1—*continued*

Average age	Question	Average behavior
2 years cont.	What does he call himself? Is he beginning to show interest in the sound of radio or TV commercials? Is he putting a few words together to make little "sentences"? Example: "Go bye-bye car." "Milk all gone."	He refers to himself by name. Many 2-year-olds do show such interest, by word or action. These "sentences" are not usually complete or grammatically correct.
2.5 years	Does he know a few rhymes or songs? Does he enjoy hearing them?	Many children can say or sing short rhymes or songs and enjoy listening to records or to mother singing.
	What does he do when the ice cream man's bells rings, out of his sight, or when a car door or house door closes at a time when someone in the family usually comes home?	If a child has good hearing and these are events that bring him pleasure, he usually reacts to the sound by running to look or telling someone what he hears.
3 years	Can he show that he understands the meaning of some words besides the names of things? Example: "Make the car go." "Give me your ball." "Put the block in your pocket." "Find the big doll."	He should be able to understand and use some simple verbs, pronouns, prepositions, and adjectives, such as go, me, in, and big.
	Can he find you when you call him from another room?	He should be able to locate the source of a sound.

Continued

Table 1—*continued*

Average age	Question	Average behavior
3 years cont.	Does he sometimes use complete sentences?	He should be using complete sentences some of the time.
4 years	Can he tell about events that have happened recently?	He should be able to give a connected account of some recent experiences.
	Can he carry out two directions, one after the other? Example: "Bobby, find Susie and tell her dinner's ready."	He should be able to carry out a sequence of two simple directions.
5 years	Do neighbors and others outside the family understand most of what he says?	His speech should be intelligible, although some sounds may still be mispronounced.
	Can he carry on a conversation with other children or familiar grown-ups?	Most children of this age can carry on a conversation if the vocabulary is within their experience.
	Does he begin a sentence with "I" instead of "me," "he" instead of "him"?	He should use some pronouns correctly.
	Is his grammar almost as good as his parents?	Most of the time, it should match the patterns of grammar used by the adults of his family and neighborhood.

From National Institute of Neurological Disease and Stroke (NINDS, 1969).

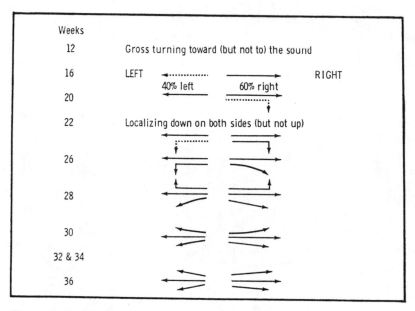

Figure 2. Localization patterns in normal hearing infants and children: responses to a low intensity pure tone delivered through soundfield speakers to the right and left. (Adapted from Murphy, K.P., Development of hearing in babies, *Child and Family* 1:16–17, 1962, and reprinted with permission from Lloyd, L. L. and B. P. Cox, Behavioral audiometry with children, *in* Symposium on Sensorineural Hearing Loss in Children: Early Detection and Intervention, *Otolaryngologic Clinics of North America*, 8:1, 1975.)

the child's field of vision. Observation is made of the behavioral response to the sounds with particular attention being given to the localization responses of the child. Figure 2 shows the expected pattern of localization responses for the various ages as reported by Murphy (1962).

Depending on the setting in which the screening is done, it is possible to enhance the reliability and validity of these procedures by some modifications. Knowledge of the exact intensity at which the child responds is necessary; therefore, the audiologist should present the sound source through a calibrated system.

Because noisemakers and environmental sounds have a wide frequency spectrum, they do not permit screening the child for individual frequencies. Hence it is useful to try using stimuli such as narrow band noise (noise with a restricted frequency spectrum and a known center frequency) or warbled pure tones. Although it is clinically accepted (Ewing and Ewing, 1944; Northern and Downs, 1975) that children in this age range require a higher intensity level before responding to sounds such as these, which may not be meaningful, their use in screening increases the validity of the overall results.

It is expected, then, that a child of 3 to 18 months will orient to sounds in a developmental pattern dependent on the meaningfulness of the sound and the intensity at which it is presented. These relationships are summarized in Table 2. It should be noted that the response levels shown in Table 2 do not represent the actual auditory thresholds of infants. It has been demonstrated through careful application of operant principles that the thresholds of infants as young as 5 months are more sensitive than those shown here (Wilson et al., 1975; Wilson, Moore, and Thompson, in preparation). Is it assumed that the response levels in Table 2 are levels at which infants who have not been trained to listen at threshold respond to the various sounds.

Children, 18 to 36 Months

Audiologic procedures for identification purposes involving children in the age range from 18 to 36 months are somewhat different from those described for the child younger than this. To begin with, children in this age group are more readily available for screening than are infants. With the growth of day care programs and programs such as Head Start, more and more youngsters are accessible for preventive health activities. In addition to being accessible, the normal developing child of this age has a better repertoire of behaviors from which to draw for testing puropses; this makes identification easier.

Like the identification program for younger children, the program for the child of 18 to 36 months old depends on audiometric screening coupled with parent questionnaire and referral by parents and teachers. Pure tone audiometric procedures in this age group usually use some form of play audiometry (e.g., teaching the child to perform a motor act, such as putting a peg in a pegboard, or dropping a block in response to the test sound). For the immature child or one with a developmental disability, the examiner may have to rely on screening techniques involving behavior observation audiometry and/or use of the signals described earlier. Some use has been made of screening tests using speech stimuli such as the VASC (Verbal Auditory Screening for Children) (Zenith Corporation, 1966). This

Table 2. Comparison of two investigations of response pattern and stimulus type of children below 2 years of age

Ewing and Ewing	Age in months	Downs			
Stimulus and response		Noise-makers (dB)	Warbled pure tones (dB)	Speech (dB)	Response
Reflexive responses; more to percussion sounds than voice; some infants began to show more deliberate, learned response	1	40–60	78	60	Eye widening, startle, eye blink
	2				
	3	40–50	70	47	Rudimentary head turn
More responses to voice than percussion sounds; some infants began vocalization response; more attentive to moderately loud voices or sound makers	4				Head turn on lateral plane, "listening attitude"
	5	30–40	51	21	
	6				
Beginning to correctly locate source of sound out of vision	7				
Reflexes found but less easily evoked	8	30–40	45	15	Direct localization of sounds to side or below ear level
	9				
	10				

Continued

Table 2—continued

	Age (mo)				
Turning head and eyes to source of sound most frequent response; highly developed	11	20–30	38	8	As previous and localization indirectly above
Begins to respond appropriately to few simple words and phrases	12				
	13				
	14	20–30	32	5	Direct localization on side, above and below
	15				
	16				
	17				
Simple speech tests suitable; variety of meaningful stimuli needed to meet interests of children in this age group	18	25	25	5	As above
	19				
	20				
	21				
	22	25	26	3	As above
	23				
	24				

Adapted from Ewing and Ewing (1944) and Northern and Downs (1975) and reprinted with permission from Lloyd, L. L. and B. P. Cox, Behavioral audiometry with children, in Symposium on Sensorineural Hearing Loss in Children: Early Detection and Intervention, Otolaryngologic Clinics of North America, 8:1, 1975.

test involves a point-to-the-picture response; pictures are of items with spondaic stress (i.e., two-syllable words with equal stress). Two studies (Griffing, Simonton, and Hedgecock, 1967; Mencher and McCulloch, 1970) have reported problems using this test as a screening tool; the problems were attributable to a high number of false positives and lack of sensitivity to detect losses in the 30- to 40-dB HL (re ANSI, 1969) range. As was pointed out earlier, speech is a broad frequency signal; no matter what words are selected, one runs the risk of failing to identify hearing impairment associated with a sloping audiometric configuration.

In terms of the periodicity of rescreening, the audiologist obviously should see any child who has been identified as having a hearing impairment in earlier screenings. In addition, the audiologist should continue to see children who are at risk (as described earlier) because these children may develop progressive losses. Also, children who have had medical intervention (e.g., tonsillectomy, adenoidectomy, myringotomy) or serious illnesses should be referred for screening and then for an assessment, should this be indicated. Finally, any child who is of concern to his parents, teachers, or other members of the educational or habilitation teams should be referred for screening. This is the age group during which a child's expressive and receptive language should be showing dramatic development. When such development is not evident, the child's hearing should be screened.

Preschool and School-Age Children

A child who reaches this chronologic and developmental age is generally able to respond well to pure tone audiometry. Indeed, hearing screening using pure tone audiometry has been demonstrated to be effective with children as young as 3 years (Belkin et al., 1964). It is the recommendation of the ASHA Committee on Identification Audiometry (ASHA Committee on Audiometric Evaluation, 1975) that all children from nursery school through third grade be given an annual, individually administered, limited-frequency pure tone hearing screening. This recommendation is based on the fact that, if hearing impairment is discovered early, its effects on the development of speech and language and other aspects of development are minimized. Additionally, it is in this age range that progressive hearing impairment may become significant and will be missed if screening is done on a less than annual basis. Finally, children of these ages have frequent significant middle ear pathologies. Screening above grade three is usually done less frequently, but it should meet the demands of the individual system. Children should be referred by teachers, parents, or other individuals who suspect a hearing impairment or in circumstances (e.g., major illness, dramatic behavior change) discussed in the previous section.

In addition to the recommendations regarding the periodicity of testing, the ASHA Committee on Identification Audiometry stipulates that each child should be screened at a 20-dB HL (ANSI, 1969) level at 1000 Hz and 2000 Hz and at a 25-dB HL level at 4000 Hz (ASHA Committee on Audiometric Evaluation, 1975). Any child who fails the screening at these frequencies at the recommended level should be rescreened and, if necessary, scheduled for a complete audiologic assessment.

AUDIOLOGIC ASSESSMENT

The purpose of an audiologic assessment is to describe an individual's auditory abilities and use of these abilities in a way that will facilitate medical and nonmedical habilitation (Lloyd, 1972) As such, the assessment phase is different from the identification phase in that it not only answers the question of whether or not there is a hearing impairment but also specifies the degree and kind of impairment present.

A comprehensive audiologic assessment relies on: 1) case history information; 2) related educational, social, and psychologic information; 3) otologic and general medical findings; 4) audiometric data; and 5) nonaudiometric receptive and expressive communication data (Lloyd, 1972; Lloyd and Cox, 1975). In conducting the comprehensive assessment, the audiologist depends on other members of the interdisciplinary service team to provide input. This is particularly true in terms of the need for information from the otologist, speech pathologist, psychologist, social worker, special educator, and, in the case of the institutionalized person, the caregiver. Of these five kinds of information, the audiologist may rely heavily on information provided by the speech pathologist concerning receptive and expressive communication abilities of the child; the psychologist also may add information in this area. Additionally, the psychologist generally provides information about the child's intellectual functioning and adaptive behavior.[3]

The audiologist depends on the service team physicians, particularly pediatricians, internists, and otologists, to provide information about the child's health history. Of particular note are aspects that affect the child's hearing (i.e., ear infections, congenital malformations, upper respiratory infections). The special educator provides information about the child's academic strengths and weaknesses, including functional language usage and pathways of learning that are more appropriate for the child. The social worker supplies information relative to the child's social history and family. Finally, the caregiver provides information that relates to the child's functional, daily living skills—in essence the aggregate of the child's total adaptive behavior. Further information concerning the role of the various interdisciplinary team members can be found elsewhere (Johnston and Magrab, 1976).

In addition to the information obtained from other specialists, the audiologist must obtain certain case history information that relates particularly to hearing. Most often the information is obtained from the child's parents, his caregiver, or previous records. In addition to the general information obtained, as a minimum the audiologist needs information concerning the presence of speech, language, or hearing problems in family members; the parents' view of whether the child has a hearing impairment, and, it one is suspected, when it was first noticed; child's history of ear infections and how these were treated; child's history of surgery, notably tonsillectomy and adenoidectomy; child's use of amplification; length of use, source of recommendation, and current status; educational placement of child, particularly if there is a known hearing impairment: how the child is progressing academically, method of instruction (e.g., oral, aural-oral, aural or unisensory, manual, or total communication); and the child's auditory behavior at present (Can he localize sound? Does he turn to his name? Can he tell the difference between male and female voices? Does he follow conversation without visual cues?). (For additional information, the reader is referred back to Table 1.) Additional case history information pertinent to the audiologic assessment has appeared elsewhere (Katz, 1972; Northern and Downs, 1975).

---

[3]For more extensive discussion of communication and psychologic assessment, the reader is referred to the chapters by Siegel and Broen (this volume), Vernon (this volume), and McLean (this volume).

With the information obtained from the other service team members and that obtained from the child's parents, the audiologist then turns to the data resulting from the audiometric assessment to complete the audiologic evaluation.

Before presenting the details of an audiometric assessment, it should be pointed out that there are several factors that influence the reliability of the audiometric assessment. As discussed in earlier presentations (Fulton and Lloyd, 1969, 1975; Lloyd and Cox, 1972, 1975), at least eight factors account for reliability of audiometric data: 1) acoustic and other environmental factors, 2) calibration, 3) instruction, 4) response criteria, 5) response mode, 6) threshold searching methodology and criteria, 7) stimulus specificity and control, and 8) in the case of speech audiometry, linguistic variables of the stimulus. A brief discussion of each of these factors with particular reference to the developmentally disabled child follows.

Acoustic and Other Environmental Factors

Audiometric testing as part of an audiologic assessment must be done in a room free of high levels of ambient noise or intermittent noises (e.g., telephone, typewriter). The testing environment must meet standards that specify the ambient noise intensity allowed for particular frequencies (ANSI, 1969). In addition to controlling the acoustic aspects, the test environment also must be free of distracting visual stimulation (Fulton and Lloyd, 1975). Many developmentally disabled children are easily distracted by items such as drawings on the test walls, games stored in the test area, or intricate lighting arrangements.

Calibration

The audiologist must perform periodic calibration checks of all audiometric equipment to be sure that it meets the 1969 ANSI standards. It is advisable to do routine electroacoustic checks of all audiometers at least every 3 months; equipment that is moved from place to place for screening purposes should be checked more frequently. In addition, the clinician should make routine biologic checks of audiometric equipment at least once a day. The clinician can accomplish this by listening to the equipment himself or by having normal hearing persons or persons with stable, known hearing impairments listen to the equipment.

Instructions

Before testing the child, the audiologist or the audiologist's assistant should estimate the child's level of language development and have some knowledge of the child's experiences with audiometric tasks. This information allows the examiner to word instructions most effectively and to build upon the child's prior learning experiences. With the developmentally disabled child it is particularly important to point out how he is expected to respond (e.g., drop a block, put a peg in the pegboard, raise his hand) and what he is expected to hear (e.g., a whistle, a tiny sound).

The area of instructions prior to audiometric assessment is one in which the child's teacher and caregiver may participate. The audiologist who plans appropriately can have persons in the child's immediate environment help with conditioning procedures. Specifically, the child can learn to do the task that he will be expected to perform when tested (e.g., dropping a block in response to sound, raising his hand in response to sound) in the classroom as part of activities there. In addition, the teacher or caregiver can provide invaluable insight, based on day-to-day contact with the child, concerning the child's response repertoire and reinforcement history.

Also, when the audiologist is testing young infants, the developmentally disabled, or difficult-to-test youngsters, nonverbal communication is particularly important. Use of pantomime, demonstration, and exaggerated gesture (i.e., "Oh, I heard it" facial expression) enhance teaching the child the desired task. In addition, when use of nonverbal stimulation is coupled with operant techniques, desirable test behavior increases. Indeed, the success of these nonverbal instructions or procedures is directly proportional to the clinician's ability to apply operant principles such as reinforcement and successive approximation (Lloyd, 1966; Lloyd, Spradlin, and Reid, 1968).

Response Criteria

The audiologist must decide what behavior change (i.e., eye blink, localization to sound source, putting a peg in a pegboard, raising a hand) is consistent enough in the child being tested to be considered an appropriate index of hearing. The behavior that is chosen depends on the developmental level, motor skill level, and interests of the child.

For sensitivity measures (i.e., pure tone air and bone conduction thresholds and speech reception thresholds), the audiologist should have a predetermined number of responses that indicate a reliable measure. Traditionally, audiometric threshold is defined as the lowest decibel level at which the person being tested responds appropriately 50% of the time.

Response Mode

As stated above, the audiologist should decide on a method of response that is within the given child's response repertoire. This choice is limited according to the child's overall developmental level, the presence of physical handicaps, the child's interests, and the child's previous experience with audiometric tasks. The skillful clinician makes sure that the response required of the child is one that is easy for him to produce and is rewarding or reinforcing. For example, the block dropping response in play audiometry is quite successful at the 18-month level or above. It should be noted that infants much younger than this have the eye-hand coordination to make this response, but it is a more elaborate response than is necessary for the test, requiring an excessive amount of time to be brought under stimulus control. Therefore, a simpler response such as pushing a large button can be used with infants as young as 7 or 8 months. For younger infants a localization (or even sucking) response may be more appropriate. It must be emphasized once again that the response and the activity associated with it must be rewarding to the child.

Threshold Searching Methodology

In audiometry the audiologist can use an ascending approach (e.g., approaching the child's threshold from below), a descending approach (e.g., going from a level above the child's expected threshold down to his actual threshold), or the ascending-descending (or "bracketing") approach. Research and experience have shown that consistent use of any one of these threshold searching methodologies results in reliable data (Carhart and Jerger, 1959). However, when testing the developmentally disabled or difficult-to-test child the descending method is frequently preferred (Lloyd, 1966; Fulton and Lloyd, 1975). Use of this procedure allows the clinician to apply reinforcement principles more skillfully. Specifically, the use of the descending procedures provides for: "(a) . . . greater consistency between the training and actual threshold testing segments; (b) more opportunity to administer reinforcement for appropriate responses; (c) the responding to lower and lower decibel levels in the method; and (d) a better approximation of errorless learning" (Fulton and Lloyd, 1975, p. 19).

Stimulus Specificity and Control

Reliable audiometric data depends on the degree to which the stimulus being using to test the child's hearing can be specified and controlled. Although a toy bell or Halloween noisemaker may attract the attention of a youngster more than a pure tone (e.g., signal of a known single frequency) will, the pure tone is more easily specified in terms of its frequency and intensity. Noisemakers and other similar objects used to test are broad frequency in nature and have a varying intensity depending on how they are struck. The audiologist then must decide between using sounds that may be inherently meaningful but hard to specify and those of less meaning but easily specified. This relationship is shown in Figure 3. The sounds that have the highest communicative value are the most difficult to specify and control, and, conversely, the sounds that are of the lowest communicative value are easiest to specify and control. Stated in a different manner, signals with highest face validity (such as speech) are the least reliable; signals with lowest face validity (such as pure tone) are the most reliable.

The audiologist most often uses a combination of such signals as a way out of this dilemma. No clinician should base a diagnosis of hearing loss solely on the results of testing with broad frequency sound resources. Although these results may be used for a working hypothesis, conclusive results depend on responses to signals of known frequencies throughout the range of human audibility.

Linguistic Variables

It already has been noted that the audiologist must pay careful attention to the language level of the child in order to give instructions that are readily understood by the child. The audiologist also must be cognizant of the child's language level when giving test involving speech materials (e.g., speech awareness threshold, speech reception threshold, and speech discrimination). This is particularly true with developmentally disabled children, whose experience base may not be the same as other children of the same chronologic age with no developmental disability. In addition, the materials should be as free of cultural bias as possible.

Relatively easy to
specify and control:
"most analytic"

Low human
communicative
value

Pure tones, clicks, narrow band noise
White noise, "sawtooth" noise
Several bands of noise
    (Environmental sounds)
"Isolated" speech sounds
    (Environmental sounds)
Nonsense syllables
    (Environmental sounds)
Monosyllabic words
Disyllabic words
Phrases and word chains
Sentences and longer word chains
Continuous discourse
"Normal conversation"
"Everyday speech"

Relatively difficult to
specify and control:
"least analytic"

High human
communicative
value

Figure 3. Continuum of acoustic stimuli relative to specificity, control, and human communicative value. Various environmental stimuli may fall at a number of points along the continuum and are therefore shown in parentheses at their three simplest levels. Stimuli from noisemakers, toys, musical instruments, and animals have been omitted to simplify the presentation, but they may be considered with environmental sounds. Synthetic speech, also not included, here would rank higher in specificity and control than human speech. (Reprinted from Lloyd, L. L., The audiologic assessment of deaf students, *in* Report of the proceedings of the Convention of American Instructors of the Deaf, pp. 585–594, Arkansas School for the Deaf, Little Rock, Ark. U.S. Government Printing Office, Washington, D.C., 1971.)

BASIC BATTERY OF AUDITORY SKILLS

In an attempt to evaluate the auditory aspects of communication, the audiologist generally should examine as a minimum the following areas: auditory sensitivity across the frequency range for air- and bone-conducted sounds, stability of the auditory sensitivity, dynamic range and tolerance, recruitment (or loudness distortion), habituation and fatigue, basic auditory discrimination, speech discrimination, and interaural differentiation of any of these measurements (Lloyd, 1972). Information in these areas is obtained primarily by pure tone and speech audiometry.

Pure Tone Audiometry

Pure tone audiometry serves as the fundamental tool of the audiologist and is the single most reliable and valid test available to audiologists. Pure tone audiometry involves use of signals of known single frequencies in the important communication range of human audibility (e.g., 250 to 8000 Hz). These signals are delivered by the air conduction route (via earphones or from soundfield speakers) as well as by bone conduction (via a small oscillator generally placed on the child's mastoid bone behind his ear or on his forehead). Pure tone results provide information about the child's threshold sensitivity at each of the frequencies. From this information the audiologist classifies the child's hearing in terms of the various categories depicted in Figure 4.

Types of Hearing Impairment In addition to providing information concerning the child's sensitivity, pure tone responses provide information about the kind of hearing impairment. Comparison

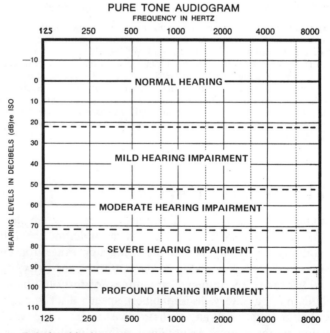

Figure 4. Relationship between pure tone responses and estimated degree of hearing impairment.

of air- and bone-conducted threshold responses signifies whether the loss is conductive, sensorineural, or mixed in nature. *Conductive hearing impairments* are revealed by a separation between the air- and bone-conducted responses, as shown in Figure 5A. This type of impairment is most frequently associated with outer and middle ear problems such as foreign bodies lodged in the external ear canal (including wax and, in the case of youngsters, beans, peas, and assorted objects!), ruptured tympanic membranes, middle ear infections, middle ear deformities (absence of or malformation of ossicles), and poorly functioning Eustachian tubes. The conductive impairment is particularly amenable to medical intervention, or, in cases where such intervention is contraindicated, aural habilitation, including the use of a hearing aid.

It should be noted at this point that another test, referred to as impedance audiometry, provides even more specific information about the nature of the conductive impairment in a given child than does the air conduction–bone conduction relationship. By various tests, which are explained in more detail in the *Procedures* section of this chapter, impedance audiometry assists the audiologist and otologist in pinpointing the specific site of pathology (e.g., tympanic membrane versus ossicles). The use of impedance tests has become such an integral part of testing that many clinics are using it routinely in place of the more traditional bone conduction audiometry. This issue is discussed further in the *Procedures* section.

As Figure 5B shows, the *sensorineural impairment* is characterized by pure tone air- and bone-conducted responses that are superimposed on one another or nearly so. Some of the most common causes of sensorineural hearing impairment in children are summarized in Table 3. This summary is divided into prenatal, perinatal, and postnatal causes of hearing loss. It should be noted that the child with a sensorineural hearing impairment should receive initial and periodic otologic examination to ascertain if there is a conductive pathology superimposed on the basic sensorineural lesion. Unlike what can be done in the case of a conductive loss, it is not possible at this time to remedy or correct the sensorineural impairment medically. However, children with sensorineural impairments respond well to amplification with training, with the possible exception of children with abnormal tolerance problems who may be less successful.

The third kind of hearing impairment, referred to as a *mixed loss,* is depicted in Figure 5C. This impairment is generally char-

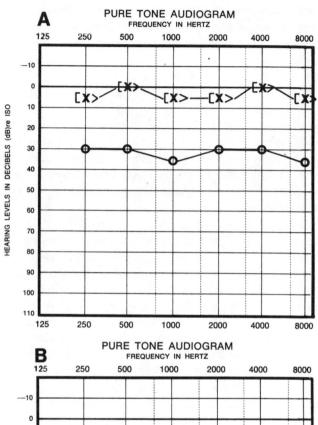

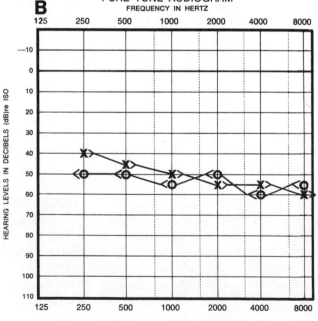

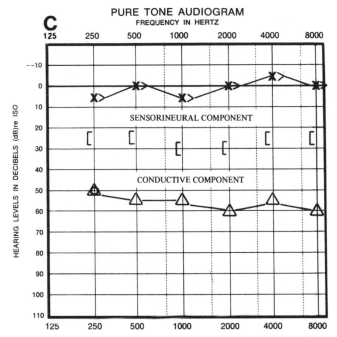

Figure 5. Audiograms showing various types of hearing impairment. The audiograms use the ASHA (1974) *Guidelines for Audiometric Symbols.* Unmarked air conduction results are shown by ○ for the right ear and × for the left ear. Masked air conduction results are shown by △ for the right ear and □ for the left ear. Unmasked bone conduction results are shown by < for the right side and > for the left side placement. Masked bone conduction results are shown by [for the right ear and] for the left ear. *A*: Conductive hearing impairment in the right ear and normal hearing in the left ear. *B*: Moderate, sensorineural hearing impairment. *C*: Unilateral (one ear), mixed hearing impairment in the right ear.

acterized audiometrically by more impairment for air conduction than for bone conduction (sensorineural component), although the bone conduction responses are also depressed; or, it may be characterized by some frequencies with a conductive impairment and some with a sensorineural impairment. This hearing impairment is frequently found in youngsters who have a basic sensorineural impairment with a conductive pathology (e.g., middle ear infection) imposed on this impairment. It is particularly important that a child with a mixed impairment be seen for otologic evaluation so that the conductive pathology can be treated. Resolution of such a problem results in enough change in sensitivity to make a significant difference in the hearing-impaired child's use of his residual hearing.

Table 3. Prenatal, perinatal, neonatal, and early childhood conditions that may lead to sensorineural hearing impairment in children

Prenatal conditions	Perinatal conditions	Neonatal conditions	Early childhood conditions
Family history of deafness	Prolonged labor ($>$ 18 hours, first delivery; $>$ 8 hours, subsequent deliveries)	Birthweight below 1500 g	Infectious diseases (meningitis, encephalitis, measles, mumps, chicken pox)
Maternal rubella or other viruses during pregnancy (including toxoplasmosis and cytomegalic inclusion disease)		Apnea or cyanosis	
	Precipitous delivery	Neonatal infection (meningitis encephalitis)	Ototoxic drugs
Defects involving ear, nose, and/or throat	Maternal hemorrhage, placenta previa	Ototoxic drugs given to neonate	Trauma (skull fracture; other head trauma; prolonged high level noise exposure to excessively loud sound, as in an explosion)
Other non-ear, nose, and throat structural abnormalities	Fetal distress	Bilirubin level, 20 mg/ 100 ml (history of transfusions or phototherapy)	
	Infection in newborn		

Continued

Table 3—*continued*

Prenatal conditions	Perinatal conditions	Neonatal conditions	Early childhood conditions
Ototoxic drugs taken by mother during pregnancy (includes streptomycin, kanamycin, thalidomide)		Evidence of prolonged central nervous system involvement (convulsions, seizures)	Tumors involving auditory pathway
Prematurity			
Syndromes associated with deafness (including achondroplasia, Alport's, Hunter's-Hurler's, Klippel-Feil, long-arm 18 delection, osteogenesis imperfecta, Paget's disease, Treacher Collins, trisomy 13-15, trisomy 18, and Waardenburg's[a]			

[a]The type of hearing impairment associated with each of these syndromes varies; it may be predominantly conductive, predominantly sensorineural, or mixed. In each of these syndromes, sensorineural hearing impairment has been reported.

Finally, it should be noted that a child's hearing impairment may occur at only certain frequencies (e.g., a sloping configuration). Also, the loss may be present in one ear (referred to as a *unilateral impairment*) or in both ears (referred to as a *bilateral impairment*).

In summary, pure tone air and bone conduction audiometry provide a direct index of the degree of hearing impairment at specified test frequencies. In addition, the relationship between air conduction and bone conduction responses is important for determining the site of lesion involved in a given child's hearing impairment.

Information about Communication Skills   Besides these direct sources of information, pure tone audiometry provides inferential data concerning a child's everyday communication abilities. Because it has been shown that a person with normal hearing at the test frequencies of 500, 1000, and 2000 Hz performs fairly well in most communication situations, these frequencies are traditionally called the *speech frequencies*. An arithmetic average of the air conduction responses at these three frequencies is called a *pure tone average* (PTA). This average is generally used to estimate a child's hearing for speech. For example, a PTA of 5 dB HL generally predicts normal hearing for speech whereas a PTA of 55 dB HL predicts a moderate impairment of hearing for speech. Both of these are seen as estimates of the child's overall ability to receive speech for communication. This relationship between air conduction hearing at the pure tone speech frequencies and a child's sensitivity for speech (e.g., speech reception threshold) provides the audiologist a measure of intertest reliability. This relationship between the measures is expected except in the case of a sloping hearing loss. For this configuration, the audiologist expects a good correlation between the average of the two best speech frequencies or, in some precipitously sloping configurations, the single best speech frequency.

In addition to providing information about the child's sensitivity for air- and bone-conducted sounds and the relationship between these measures, pure tone audiometry supplies information about several other basic auditory skills mentioned earlier. The child's dynamic range, the area between the point at which a sound is first heard and where it is uncomfortably loud, is often measured by using pure tones. *Recruitment,* generally defined as the abnormal growth of loudness, is measured by having the child match the loudness of a pure tone in the nonaffected ear to one in the affected ear. This test is referred to as the Alternate Bilateral Loudness Balance Test (ABLB) (Newby,

1964). In this test the child matches two frequencies in the same ear to see if there is loudness distortion for certain frequencies.

Information about a child's dynamic range and the presence of recruitment is particularly important to the audiologist and teacher because these things affect the child's use of amplification. The child who has a dynamic range of 50 dB (e.g., tone detection at 60 dB HL and tolerance level at 110 dB HL) and has no recruitment problems is much more likely to benefit from use of a hearing aid than the child with a 30-dB dynamic range (e.g., tone detection at 60 dB HL and tolerance level at 90 dB HL) and recruitment present. These measures help the audiologist to make appropriate selection and adjustments of the aid.

The audiologist also may make use of other less routinely used procedures involving pure tones in order to assist in differentially diagnosing the site of hearing loss. Specifically, there is a group of procedures used to determine if a loss is cochlear or retrocochlear (i.e., located beyond the cochlea in the auditory nerve or central pathways). These include *Békésy audiometry,* which involves having the child map his threshold for pulsed tones and continuous tones; *tone decay audiometry,* which involves having the child indicate if a continuously on tone, initially presented 5 dB above threshold, is heard for 60 seconds (Rosenberg, 1958) or if an increase in intensity is needed to make the tone continuously audible; and the *Short Increment Sensitivity Index* (SISI) test (Jerger, Shedd, and Harford, 1959), in which the child is presented intensity increments from 1 to 5 dB superimposed on an above-threshold pure tone for some frequency. Detailed explanations of these differential diagnostic procedures and their use with normal and developmentally delayed children may be found elsewhere (Price and Falck, 1963; Fulton, 1967; Fulton and Reid, 1969; Katz, 1972; Fulton and Lloyd, 1975).

Pure tone audiometry also provides information about the child's discrimination of single frequency sounds. The audiologist can determine if the child can tell the difference between a high frequency and low frequency tone. Obviously, such discrimination forms the basis for discrimination of more complicated signals. Finally, pure tone audiometry provides information about any differences in sensitivity between the child's two ears.

Speech Audiometry
Speech audiometry also provides information relating to basic audi-

tory skills. Unlike pure tones, which measure child's skills relative to a single frequency stimulus, speech audiometry relies on a broad frequency signal. Materials were developed for speech audiometry as an outgrowth of work done to test the intelligibility of telephone circuits (Hirsh, 1952). The first researchers to use the speech signal to measure hearing were interested in deriving a quick estimate of the person's speech communication abilities. Consequently, tests have been developed to measure both sensitivity of hearing for speech as well as discrimination of speech at suprathreshold levels. Traditional speech tests include: speech awareness threshold, speech reception threshold, speech discrimination, and dynamic range for speech.

Speech Awareness Threshold   The speech awareness threshold (SAT) or speech detection threshold (SDT) is found by having the child respond in some way (i.e., raising his hand, localizing, dropping a block, etc.) when he barely hears the audiologist call his name, nonsense syllables, or any other speech stimuli. The lowest point, expressed in dB HL, at which the child detects any one of these stimuli 50% of the time is known as the *speech detection* or *speech awareness threshold*. This represents the lowest level speech-auditory task in that the child needs only to detect the signal; no discrimination is involved. It should be noted that, although this measure uses speech, the child may be only responding to it as "sound" and not as "speech."

Speech Reception Threshold   The speech reception threshold (SRT) is that point at which a child can correctly repeat, or identify in some other manner, 50% of a group of test items. Traditionally, the SRT is obtained using two-syllable words that may be pronounced with equal stress on each syllable, referred to as *spondaic words*. These words were first employed because, as a group, they were reported to have fairly equal intelligibility for normal hearing persons (Hirsh, 1952; Hirsh et al., 1952). The initial group of spondaic words was reduced, and there are lists of these words selected for children (Newby, 1964). In addition, for the child who cannot speak, has poor articulation, or is not cooperative, there are pictures of spondaic items (i.e., cowboy, hotdoy, airplane, etc.) (e.g., Lloyd and Melrose, 1966); the child points to the picture named. As an alternative, some audiologists use pictures with nonspondaic names such as the Threshold Identification of Pictures Test (Siegenthaler and Haspiel, 1966). On some occasions the audiologist cannot obtain an SRT by using the full list of spondee words; in such cases, he makes use of a selected list of spondees. In cases where a child cannot respond to even two or three spondees, the audiologist may move to a lower level discrimination task as described by Lloyd (1972). This involves having the child indicate whether two spondees are the same or different. In some cases of children with extremely poor auditory discrimination, the audiologist may even have to use the same-different task with monosyllabic words compared to one-syllable words to see if this discrimination can be made. Obviously, such a discrimination can be made on the basis of the duration difference alone or based on other suprasegmental (nonphonemic) differences.

The SRT, then, provides information about threshold hearing sensitivity for speech. Although the SRT is considered to be a sensitivity measurement, it also may be viewed as a discrimination task at threshold level.

Speech Discrimination   In assessing communicative abilities, even more important than the SRT is the measurement of the child's discrimination of speech at suprathreshold levels. The test words are presented at levels above a person's threshold to answer the question: When speech is made sufficiently loud, how does the child discriminate the finite differences between phonemes such as /f/, /θ/, /s/, /z/, and so on? The level of presentation is a critical factor in such testing. Two levels are particularly useful: 1) average conversational speech level (about 40 dB HL (ANSI, 1969), which may be considered a normative figure); and 2) the individual's optimal listening level. The reader is referred to earlier reports (Hirsh, 1952; Lloyd, 1972) for more extensive information about the effect of presentation level on speech discrimination.

In speech discrimination, a wide range of speech material (e.g., phonemes, syllables, monosyllabic words, connected discourse, synthetic speech) may be used. However, the traditional stimuli are groups of 50 monosyllabic words, initially designed to represent the initial consonant occurrence of English (Hirsh et al., 1952). Lists have been developed for adults as well as for children (Haskins, 1949; Myatt and Landes, 1963). These words were referred to as *phonetically balanced* words. More recent tests have not considered the phonetic balancing to be critical (Giolas, 1975). Typically the child repeats the test word given by the audiologist. For the child who is unwilling or unable to repeat the standard test words, there are several picture tests that are designed to have the child point to one word out of a group of two or more items. The most familiar of these tests are the Discrimination by Identification of Pictures Test (Siegen-

thaler and Haspiel, 1966), the Word Intelligibility by Picture Iden-
tification Test (Ross and Lerman, 1970), the Goldman-Fristoe-
Woodcock Test of Auditory Discrimination (Goldman, Fristoe, and
Woodcock, 1970), and the Goldman-Fristoe-Woodcock Auditory
Skills Battery: Diagnostic Auditory Discrimination Test (Goldman,
Fristoe, and Woodcock, 1974).

Two of these tests have characteristics that make them particularly suitable for assessing the discrimination aspect of communication. The Word Intelligibility by Picture Identification Test is unique
in that it is designed to assess the child's speech discrimination through
the auditory channel, visual channel, and the combined auditory-visual
channel. Information obtained from this test provides the audiologist
and other personnel with an estimate of the relative strengths of the
child's auditory and visual sensory input channels. Knowledge of this
information allows for more appropriate classroom management and
use of amplification. The Goldman-Fristoe-Woodcock tests (1970,
1974) are unique in that they provide for the measurement of the
child's speech discrimination in a competing-noise (including speech)
background. Such measurement provides a more valid estimate of discrimination in an actual communication environment than is obtained
in the quiet, sound-treated room. In addition, the Goldman-Fristoe-
Woodcock tests have a scoring procedure designed to facilitate error
analysis including the distinctive features of voicing, manner of articulation (e.g., stop, continuant) and place of articulation (e.g., bilabial,
velar). This analysis provides more readily usable treatment information about the child's auditory discrimination than does a single score.

Results of any of the speech discrimination tests constitute major
information to the audiologist and teacher. Such information allows
one to plan appropriate educational plans for the child. In addition,
speech discrimination information is vital for establishing an appropriate aural habilitation program.

Dynamic Range   Dynamic range for speech is measured in a
manner similar to that described for pure tones. To obtain the dynamic
range, the audiologist subtracts the child's detection level from the
tolerance level for speech. This usable range of hearing for speech
provides information that aids in determining appropriate amplification.

The foregoing discussion centers on tests designed to provide
information about basic auditory skills that should be measured as a
minimum for each child. These are considered from a pure tone and

speech audiometry standpoint. The following section is concerned with procedures used to measure these skills with children.

PROCEDURES USED WITH CHILDREN

Because any audiometric procedure involves the stimulus-response paradigm, all of those used can be viewed in terms of the response required of the person being tested. Historically, audiometric procedures have used two types of responses: voluntary or operant responses, and reflexive or respondent responses. Audiometric procedures that use operant responses are generally referred to as *behavioral procedures,* while those using reflexive (respondent) responses are frequently referred to as *electrophysiologic procedures.* Table 4 classifies audiometric procedures according to the type of response involved in the procedure.

Usefulness of the Procedures

Before discussing specific behavioral or respondent procedures, it is appropriate to contrast the relative usefulness of each of the two groups. As Lloyd (1976) pointed out, an analysis of audiometric procedures always should include information concerning the reliability, validity, success rate, cost, and subsequent habilitative value of the procedure. It has been generally accepted that respondent procedures are valuable for research purposes (e.g., suprathreshold audi-

Table 4. Audiometric procedures categorized by response

Behavioral (operant voluntary)	Electrophysiologic (respondent, reflexive)
Standard (hand raise, ear choice)	Impedance audiometry
Play	Electrodermal, psychogalvanic skin response (PGSR) audiometry
Visual reinforcement (peep show, conditioned audiovisual reinforcement (CAVR), conditioned orientation response (COR))	Evoked response audiometry Respiration audiometry EKG audiometry
Tangible reinforcement operant conditioned audiometry (TROCA)	Electrocochleography

Behavior observation audiometry (BOA)
uses operants and/or respondents

tory evoked response measurements) and for assessing parts of the total auditory pathway (e.g., impedance audiometry). For clinical utility in assessing the actual threshold of hearing for infants and other difficult-to-test individuals, however, behavioral audiometry seems superior in all of these aspects.

Reliability   In terms of reliability, respondent audiometry is usually considered to be within 10 to 20 dB of the child's actual threshold, whereas operant audiometry has been demonstrated to be reliable within ±5 dB with difficult-to-test children (Nowels, 1971; Yarnall, 1973; Fulton and Lloyd, 1975). The reliability of the operant procedures is attributable to the fact that the child is programmed to respond to a particular stimulus (e.g., pure tones, speech, etc.), resulting in better focus on that one dimension of the incoming sensorium. This may not be the case for many of the respondent procedures, which only attempt to isolate some aspect of audition along the auditory pathway. Because of this factor, electrophysiologic procedures do not identify the child's actual threshold; instead, they provide a suprathreshold response that permits the audiologist to estimate the threshold.

Validity   In terms of validity, whereas respondent procedures measure only the responsivity of a part of the auditory system, operant procedures demonstrate a degree of integration. By definition, operant audiometry goes beyond the reflexive level and provides an index of the functional relationship of an individual to his auditory environment. Thus, operant procedures seem to have greater face validity than respondent procedures.

Success Rate   Success rate is also an important consideration when evaluating various audiometric procedures. Behavioral audiometry has been demonstrated to be highly successful with infants, young children, and difficult-to-test subjects. Studies comparing success of operant and respondent procedures have shown equal or greater success with the operant procedures for a variety of populations (Lloyd, 1970; Fulton and Lloyd, 1975). When this information is coupled with the fact that behavioral procedures generally result in a measurement that is a closer approximation to actual threshold, success rate is further increased. Finally, in clinical application it is generally found that, when a child's hearing cannot be tested successfully with behavioral audiometry, most respondent approaches also fail or give questionable results.

Cost   Cost factors for various audiometric procedures, whether they involve respondent or operant audiometry, include cost of equipment (both initial cost and maintenance), personnel requirements, and the amount of time needed to obtain reliable results. In general, respondent procedures require more elaborate instrumentation, involving higher initial cost and preventive maintenance. Also, many of the respondent procedures require sedation, particularly for infants, young children, and the hyperactive; this involves increased costs for personnel required, for increased time needed, and for the medication.

Subsequent Habilitative Value   The time dimension can be tied to subsequent habilitative value. Although there are occasions with a given child when behavioral procedures may take more than one session, the time spent provides the audiologist with information about the child's learning ability and general adaptive behavior as well as establishing rapport. In addition, such sessions provide the child with an opportunity to learn about the meaningfulness of sound (rudimentary auditory training). This is in contrast to respondent procedures, which often take a longer period of time and do not provide opportunities to observe the ongoing behavior of the child or engage in initial testing or aural habilitation. Indeed, many respondent procedures are aversive enough to the child, so that subsequent interactions with the clinician under these circumstances may be affected negatively.

Behavioral Procedures

Behavior Observation Audiometry   As described in a preceding section, behavior observation audiometry (BOA) involves presenting a sound stimulus and carefully observing any change in behavior. Table 4 shows BOA to be between the strictly operant and respondent procedures. This is because, with the neonate or very young infant, one relies on gross bodily changes that are primarily reflexive, making BOA more like respondent audiometry. However, with individuals above the chronologic or developmental level of 3 to 4 months, the reflexive behavior, such as sound localization, is discriminately reinforced, thereby extending a reflexive behavior through operant conditioning (Spradlin, Karlan, and Wetherby, this volume; Lloyd, 1966, 1976, 1976; Fulton and Lloyd, 1975).

Standard Audiometry   Procedures involving standard audiometry involve teaching the child to raise his hand or push a button in the presence of the test stimulus. Standard audiometry is generally most effective in children at least 2.5 years old. Variations of this approach include having the child raise his hand on the side of the ear in which he hears the test stimulus. This procedure is referred to as the *ear-choice method* (for a description, see Curry and Kurtzrock, 1951; Lloyd, 1966). Additional variations include having the severely orthopedically handicapped individual nod his head when he hears the sounds or say "yes" when sound is heard. Although it involves a different level task, for the child who has the number concept but who cannot raise his hand, one can use a pulsed tone and have him tell how many "beeps" he hears.

Play Audiometry   The audiologist may use a variation of standard audiometry referred to as play audiometry. Generally, play audiometry involves teaching the child to perform a motor task only in the presence of a test stimulus. Play audiometry can be used reliably with children 18 months and older. Frequent tasks include having the child put pegs in a pegboard, clothespins in a milk bottle, blocks in a box, and so on. The basic premise of play audiometry is that it is pleasurable and reinforcing for the child. In addition, play audiometry provides an appropriately structured learning activity for which the child receives reinforcement from the clinician. With this technique one can obtain pure tone thresholds as well as a speech detection threshold. For a further description of the vast number of play audiometry procedures, the reader is referred to detailed presentations reported elsewhere (Utley, 1949; O'Neill, Oyer, and Hillis, 1961; Lloyd, 1966; Fulton and Lloyd, 1975).

Visually Reinforced Procedures   In the event that standard audiometric procedures or play audiometric techniques cannot be employed with a given child, the audiologist may use techniques involving visual reinforcement. Again, these procedures follow the operant procedures described earlier, the reinforcement being something visually pleasant to the child (e.g., a toy or animal plus social reinforcement). Various media have been used as reinforcers, including: pictures (Evans, 1943; Dix and Hallpike, 1947; Kaplan, 1957; Shimizu and Nakamura, 1957; Miller, 1962, 1963; Lloyd, 1965a, b; Weaver, 1965); miniature scenes (Statten and Wishart, 1956); animated toy animals or puppets (Cotton and Hall, 1939; Guilford and Haug, 1952; Waldrop, 1953; Green, 1958; Miller, 1962; Sullivan, Miller, and Polisar, 1962; Moore, Thompson, and Thompson, 1975); toy trains (Ewing, 1930; Keaster, 1951; Ishisawa, 1960; Gaines, 1961); and other mechanical toys (Denmark, 1950; Schwartz, 1952; MacPherson,

1960). Visual reinforcement techniques have been successful with children as young as 5 months (Lloyd and Wilson, 1974; Wilson et al., 1975; Moore, Wilson, and Thompson, in preparation; Wilson, Moore, and Thompson, in preparation) and are particularly useful for a child who is too immature (mentally, socially, and/or physically) for play audiometry, or the child whose neuro-muscular involvement makes a localization response easier than a button-pushing response or any of the responses used in play audiometry.

Suzuki and Ogiba (1960, 1961; Suzuki, Ogiba, and Takei, 1972) noted that one could increase the occurrence of orienting responses by pairing the auditory stimulus with visual reinforcement. These investigators called this procedure the *conditioned orientation reflex* (COR). Many clinicians saw the possibility for use of visual reinforcement and have expanded the orientation reflex to include a variety of localizing response. The power of this approach is that it permits the use of a variety of operant behaviors rather than being limited to respondent (i.e., reflexive) behavior. Therefore, the present authors use COR to mean *conditioned orientation response*. One adaptation described by Redell and Calvert (1967) is called *Conditioned Audiovisual Reinforced Audiometry* (CAVR). More recently, Wilson, Moore, and Thompson (in preparation) have used the term *visual reinforcement audiometry*.

The general clinical procedure for visually reinforced audiometry is to have the child seated in the test environment and engaged in quiet play activities. Signals are then presented through the sound-field at an intensity presumed to be audible to the child. During the auditory signal, the visual reinforcer is presented from the same side of the room, although at a position far enough removed from the child's peripheral field of vision to make it necessary for him to turn his head to see it. After a sufficient number of auditory-visual reinforcement pairings have been presented (i.e., when the child turns fairly rapidly and without prompting by the clinician), the visual reinforcer is presented only after the child responds to the auditory signal. Once the child is under stimulus control, the clinician can find the child's threshold of hearing for tones throughout the frequency range in the soundfield. (Naturally, other stimuli such as narrow bands of noise also can be used in the procedure.) Although this procedure was originally developed to be done in the soundfield, many audiologists have obtained air and bone conduction thresholds for each ear using these procedures. As mentioned earlier, the use of visually reinforced audiometry is generally enhanced by the use of operant procedures. Particular emphasis needs to be given to the use of social reinforcement in concert with the visual reinforcement.

Tangibly Reinforced Audiometry   An additional technique that is useful for both young children and for those with developmental disabilities is *Tangible Reinforcement Operant Conditioning Audiometry* (TROCA) as reported by Lloyd, Spradlin, and Reid (1968) and based on the early work of others using tangible reinforcers (Meyerson and Michael, 1960, 1964; Knox, 1960). Generally speaking, the procedure involves teaching the child to push a button in the presence of an auditory signal. When the child makes an appropriate response, he receives a tangible reward (e.g., an edible reward such as sugar-coated cereal or candy, or a nonedible reward such as a token, trinket, or building block) that is known to have reinforcing value for him.

Equipment used for TROCA includes an audiometer with earphones, soundfield speakers, and a feeder box that has a large button for the child to press. The button has the potential for being lighted with variable intensity.

The TROCA procedure originally described by Lloyd, Spradlin, and Reid (1968) consisted of five steps including: determining a reinforcer, initial training, stimulus generalization, soundfield screening, and bilateral threshold testing. Because these steps continue to serve as the basis for the use of TROCA, their clinical application is discussed next.

Determining a Reinforcer   As with all behavioral audiometry, the audiologist must be certain that the consequence he is using is reinforcing for that particular child. Because a consequence may cease to be reinforcing, the audiologist must be ready to vary consequences within a test session. With some children, the use of edibles may result in rapid satiation. (For a more detailed description of ways to select reinforcers, the reader is referred to Lloyd, Spradlin, and Reid, 1968.)

Initial Training   After the selection of a reinforcer, the audiologist shows the child how to respond. The initial stimulus is a high intensity (i.e., 70 dB HL ANSI) warbled pure tone of 500 Hz delivered through the soundfield speaker and a visual stimulus of the lighted button. Some clinicians have started training with an auditory stimulus only and have found it successful. With the severely hearing impaired, the bone conduction vibrator paired with the lighted response button should be used for initial training. The use of the vibrator at a high intensity and at a low frequency provides a tactile dimension to the signal that facilitates conditioning. One of the major benefits of TROCA is that it can be so easily demonstrated without putting pressure on the child to process verbal directions given by the audiologist. For many young children and for the developmentally disabled, this is particularly useful because their communication ability and motivation for verbal interaction may be limited.

Stimulus Generalization   After the child seems to be under stimulus control for the auditory signal, the 500-Hz tone is reduced in 10-dB steps to approximately 50 dB HL (ANSI, 1969) (or some other suprathreshold level that will maintain stimulus control) for level generalization. Other test frequencies are then presented for frequency generalization.

Soundfield Screening   After the child generalizes the button-pushing behavior to other frequencies, a screening in the soundfield is carried out. Generally, this is done for a wide range of frequencies (e.g., 250 Hz through 8000 Hz) at a level of 20 dB HL (ANSI, 1969).

Bilateral Threshold Testing   After the child's responses to soundfield stimuli are determined, the audiologist tests the child's hearing with earphones for the same range of frequencies. This is generally done using the descending technique. This procedure emphasizes the use of soundfield testing before testing with earphones for two major reasons. First, by getting the child under good stimulus control there are seldom problems when the earphones are introduced. Second, by testing initially in the soundfield the audiologist does not inadvertently attempt to condition the child using an ear that has a severe or profound hearing loss, thus spending more time than is necessary in conditioning the child.

In addition to the foregoing procedure initially described by Lloyd, Spradlin, and Reid (1968), other procedures have been reported (Bricker and Bricker, 1969; Fulton, 1974) that modify the basic procedure, including omitting the use of the lighted button and, or the soundfield screening phase.

As noted for the other behavioral procedures, TROCA is frequently most successful when social reinforcement is paired with tangible reinforcement. Using the TROCA procedure, reliable thresholds can be obtained for any child who is old enough and motorically able to push the button. Children as young as 7 months have been tested successfully with this procedure (Lloyd, Spradlin, and Reid, 1968; Fulton, 1974; Lloyd and Wilson, 1974; Wilson et al., 1975). It is particularly useful for the nonverbal child.

Speech Audiometry   Behavioral techniques are also useful in assessing the child's sensitivity of hearing for speech (e.g., speech awareness, detection, and/or reception thresholds) and speech discrimination. In terms of sensitivity measures, the audiologist uses many of the same techniques discussed in the foregoing sections. Of particular note, the audiologist may obtain the sensitivity threshold using tangible reinforcements (e.g., the TROCA procedure or some variation of it), or visual reinforcement (e.g., conditioned orientation response a visual reforcement audiometry). These approaches are facilitated with social reinforcement from the audiologist as well as the careful use of operant principles for testing (e.g., using an easily heard speech stimulus for initial conditioning so that success is more probable). In addition to the use of the behavioral approach to speech-hearing thresholds or sensitivity measures, there have been reports of the application of operant principles to the assessment of speech discrimination (Berlin and Dill, 1967; Fulton and Lloyd, 1969, 1975; Dahle and Daly, 1972, 1974). A recent development in this area is the use of visual reinforcement of the infant's localization responses made to changes in syllables (Wilson et al., 1975; Eilers, Wilson, and Moore, in preparation).

Respondent Procedures

In addition to the audiometric procedures using operant responses, there are a group of tests involving reflexive, nonvoluntary behaviors. These are referred to as *respondent* or *electrophysiologic procedures*. As shown in Table 4, the respondent procedures include impedance audiometry (the respondent procedure used most routinely), psychogalvanic skin response tests, evoked response audiometry, respiration audiometry, EKG audiometry, and electrocochleography. Although a brief review of each of these is presented, impedance audiometry is discussed at length because of its widespread clinical use.

Impedance Audiometry   The application of acoustic impedance in clinical audiology was first described in 1946 by Metz. However, clinicians concerned with auditory assessment were slow to realize the potential of these measures. Consequently, impedance audiometry was not widely used clinically until the late 1960's or early 1970. Since that time there have been several studies reported that involve the use of impedance tests with children (Robertson, Peterson, and Lamb, 1968; Brooks, 1971; Keith, 1973; S. Jerger et al., 1974). Reports of the use of this procedure with the developmentally disabled have been limited (Lamb and Norris, 1970; Fulton and Lamb, 1972). For an in-depth review of impedance, the reader is referred to other sources (Lilly, 1972; Jerger, 1975; Lamb, 1975).

The basic instrument for impedance audiometry is an electroacoustic impedance meter. It consists of a probe that has three openings: one delivers a probe tone, usually of 220 Hz; a second provides a variable degree of air pressure in the ear canal; and a third is attached to a microphone and picks up the reflected energy from the probe tone. The probe fits snugly in the external ear canal. Also included are meters to monitor air pressure change and compliance change, a tone generator to test the acoustic reflex, and a compliance sensitivity control. Of course, each of the brands of electroacoustic impedance meters has various additional features in addition to these basic necessities.

Impedance audiometry includes three main subtests. These are generally referred to as tympanometry, static compliance, and the acoustic reflex threshold.

Tympanometry   Tympanometry involves placing the probe in the ear to be tested in such a way that a seal is made between the probe and the external ear. A closed space is formed that is bounded on one end by the probe and on the other end by the tympanic membrane. The clinician introduces into this closed space an air pressure that is varied from atmospheric pressure to $+$ 200 mm H_2O and then to -200 mm H_2O pressure. The mobility or *compliance* of the tympanic membrane is measured in terms of the sound reflected back from the eardrum to the probe under these varying pressures. Using this procedure the clinician can detect any abnormality in the movement of the tympanic membrane. In addition, evidence is obtained concerning changes in middle ear pressure, the presence of perforations of the membrane, and the status of ventilation tubes placed in the membrane.

Investigators have identified five basic tympanometric pressure-mobility curves, which are shown in Figure 6 and summarized below:

Type A—found when testing the normal middle ear
Type A_D—associated with large changes in mobility in conjunction
    with small changes in pressure that may be seen when the mid-

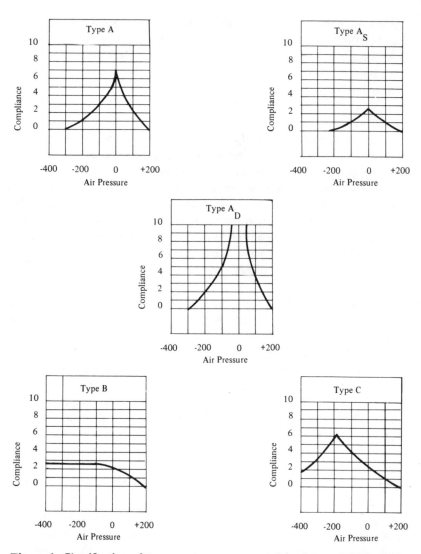

Figure 6. Classification of tympanograms as reported by Jerger (1970). Curve represents the *average* response expected for each type of tympanogram.

dle ear ossicles are disjointed or the eardrum is very thin because of frequent spontaneous ruptures

Type A$_S$—associated with normal middle ear pressure but with relatively small compliance, such as that usually found with cases of otosclerosis (when the smallest ossicle, the stapes, is fixed in the round window leading to the cochlea) or with heavily scarred membranes

Type B—associated with conditions that result in no change in the mobility of the membrane, regardless of pressure changes, such as frequently may be found with serous or suppurative otitis media (middle ear infection), perforations of the tympanic membrane, a cerumen-impacted ear canal, or a ventilating tube that is in place but closed

Type C—associated with normal mobility but obvious negative middle ear pressure, such as that found with serous otitis media and/or poorly functioning Eustachian tubes

Static Compliance   Static compliance involves inspection of the mobility of the middle ear system at rest (Jerger, 1972). Compliance values are based on the fact that the intensity of a sound, or its sound pressure, varies according to the size of the area into which it is introduced, that there is a specific relationship between a tone of a given frequency and intensity, reported in dB SPL (sound pressure level), and cavity volume, reported in cc (cubic centimeters) (Northern and Downs, 1975). Stated in more specific terms, if the area of the space between the impedance bridge probe tip and the tympanic membrane is increased (e.g., because of some change in the middle ear), there is a notable decrease in the pressure of the sound. Conversely, if this same area is decreased, the sound pressure of the probe tone is increased.

The results of this particular subtest of impedance audiometry have shown the greatest clinical variability. Therefore, it has been difficult to develop reliable profiles from group data to be used in interpreting results for an individual. Despite this, it is generally accepted that the middle ear system is abnormally stiffened when the compliance is less than 0.28 cc of equivalent volume and abnormally flaccid if the equivalent volume is greater than 2.5 cc (Northern and Downs, 1975).

Acoustic Reflex Thresholds   The third subtest of impedance audiometry involves measuring the hearing level at which the stapedius muscle contracts. This muscle is one of the two important middle ear muscles. The stapedius muscles in each ear contract in the presence of intense sounds presented to either or both ears, apparently to protect the inner ear(s). Because the stapedius muscle is attached to the stapes (the smallest ossicle located in the oval window leading to the inner ear and attached to the incus), its contraction causes the other ossicles and the tympanic membrane to stiffen. This results in decreased compliance and in attenuation of any intense sound. In normal hearing persons, this contraction occurs somewhere between 70 and 100 dB HL (ANSI, 1969) for pure tone signals. The test is conducted by delivering an intense pure tone signal to one ear and measuring the reflex (present or absent) from the opposite ear as both stapedius muscles contract even when the sound is presented to only one ear if hearing is normal for both ears.

Interpretation of reflex response results is best described in terms of the degree and kind of hearing impairment being studied. In cases where the child has a sensorineural impairment the following may occur: 1) for a unilateral, sensorineural impairment, the reflex is present in both ears; 2) in bilateral, severe to profound impairments —i.e., 80 dB HL (ANSI, 1969)—or greater, the reflex is absent bilaterally; 3) in bilateral, moderate, sensorineural impairments, the reflex will be present in each ear but will be at a reduced sensation level;[4] and, 4) for bilateral, mild, sensorineural impairment, reflexes will be present.

If the child's hearing impairment is conductive, the following responses tend to occur: 1) in the case of a unilateral conductive loss greater than 30 dB HL (ANSI, 1969) with an air conduction–bone conduction difference greater than 10 dB HL, the reflexes are absent bilaterally or, if present, show no decreased sensation level; and 2) for bilateral conductive impairments, the reflexes are absent bilaterally.

Finally, reflex response information contributes to identifying problems involving the auditory neural pathway. If a child has normal hearing for pure tone, speech and tympanometric measures but has bilaterally absent reflexes, there is the possibility of a lesion in the neural pathway.

The use of impedance audiometry, then, plays an important role in the differential diagnosis of hearing impairment in children. The use of tympanometry, static compliance, and acoustic reflex testing make impedance audiometry the most widely used respondent procedure. To summarize the benefits of this procedure, it should be noted that

---

[4]It is this characteristic of response at a lower sensation level, rather than that associated with normal hearing, that suggests cochlear involvement in the child's hearing impairment. This assists the audiologist in determining the presence of abnormal loudness tolerance (recruitment), which may affect the child's use of amplification.

impedance testing takes a relatively short period of test time and is reasonably comfortable for any child. The amount of information provided by the various procedures serves as a valuable adjunct to pure tone audiometry in locating the site of lesion. The procedure is particularly helpful in determining the presence or absence of conductive impairments. Although bone conduction pure tone audiometry provides similar information, the clinician must apply masking (e.g., a narrow band noise delivered to the nontest ear to prevent it from participating in the perception of the test signal delivered to the test ear), which may be distracting or annoying to the child to the point that it makes obtaining reliable behavioral thresholds more difficult. In addition, the use of impedance audiometry is valuable in identifying conductive involvement superimposed on severe to profound sensorineural hearing impairment. In such cases, routine audiograms show no measurable response to bone conduction audiometry because the output limit for this mode is approximately 65 dB HL (ANSI, 1969) in the mid frequencies and approximately 40 dB HL (ANSI, 1969) for the low frequencies. Consequently, a child with an 80-dB HL (ANSI, 1969) loss with no response to bone conduction can have a significant conductive overlay that would be detected by tympanometry but not by bone conduction audiometry.

Finally, impedance audiometry is useful with the very young or difficult-to-test child because it involves no active verbal participation. Assuming that the child will sit relatively quiet for a short period of time and will allow a small probe to be placed in his ear, and that the clinician can achieve an appropriate acoustic seal, impedance audiometry determines the presence or absence of a conductive loss via tympanometry. Acoustic reflex testing, as noted previously, provides information about a possible sensorineural involvement. Finally, the use of a relatively new impedance procedure, the Differential Loudness Summation Test (Jerger et al., 1974), holds promise for providing an estimate of the degree of sensorineural impairment, based on the individual's different acoustic reflex thresholds for broad band noise and pure tone stimuli.

There are several other less frequently used respondent procedures: electrodermal response audiometry, electroencephalographic evoked response audiometry, and electrocochleography.

Electrodermal Response Audiometry   Electrodermal response (EDR) audiometry, also known as psychogalvanic skin response audiometry (PGSR), is based on the principle that one may condition an individual to show changes in skin sweat glands in the presence of an auditory signal. The procedure for accomplishing this involves pairing an auditory signal with a mild electrical shock a sufficient number of times until conditioning occurs. Once the individual is conditioned, he is presented the paired stimuli intermittently to maintain conditioning. In between these presentations, the clinician presents the auditory signal alone, and, because the association has been made, the individual's system responds to the sound and anticipates the shock, causing a detectable change in the sweat glands. The change is detected by electrodes attached to the individual's skin before the testing begins.

This procedure has been used with mentally retarded individuals (Irwin, Hind, and Aronson, 1957; Kodman, Fein, and Mixon,1959; Schlanger, 1961; Fulton, 1962; Webb et al., 1964), but the results of such tests were never better than those obtained with behavioral procedures. In addition, Hogan (1975, p. 279) points out that, "this . . . procedure fails more frequently with difficult-to-test subjects than with normals . . ." probably, in part, because retarded persons tend to "exhibit . . . reduced electrophysiologic responsiveness."

Regardless of the type of developmental disability, electrodermal audiometry is of questionable use with difficult-to-test persons because its success depends on the cooperation of the person during an aversive test session. It is not possible to measure threshold reponses to sound of an individual who is talking, crying, or verbalizing, because the slightest movement causes spurious test results. In addition, this procedure is of questionable value because the noxious nature of the shock oftentimes becomes associated with the clinician. Needless to say, future attempts at testing or habilitation by the clinician or the associated clinical setting may be doomed to failure.

Electroencephalographic Evoked Response Audiometry   Electroencephalographic evoked response audiometry is also known as cortical evoked response audiometry or EEG audiometry. The procedure is based on the observation, first made by Davis (Davis et al., 1939) and supported later by others (Marcus, Gibbs, and Gibbs, 1949; Yamamoto et al., 1953; Giddoll, 1955), that one can measure changes in cortical activity when auditory stimuli are presented. Although this observation was first noted many years ago, the actual procedure was not suited to the measurement of hearing until recently. Because there is so much ongoing activity (sometimes called physiologic noise) in the cortex, early attempts to separate response to sound from ongoing random activity were unsuccessful. With the advent of signal-averaging computers in the early 1960's, however, the instrumentation was available to reliably differentiate response from ongoing activity. Hence, this type of audiometry involves preparing the individual for an EEG, presenting signals of known magnitude and frequency, and interpreting responses via the signal averaging computer. As the names implies, the computer sorts out the responses that are temporally related to the auditory signal and averages these for the signal. Electroencephalographic evoked response audiometry has been demonstrated to produce results within ± 18 dB of voluntary standard audiometry for normal hearing preschool and hearing-impaired children (Derbyshire et al., 1956; Derbyshire and McDermott, 1958) and within ±10 dB for hearing-impaired children (Withrow and Goldstein, 1958). It also has been used with retarded persons (Reneau and Mast, 1968; Nodar and Smith, 1970), brain-damaged individuals (Rapin and Grazini), and deaf infants (Rapin and Grazini, 1967).

Despite the apparent usefulness of this procedure, it has not had widespread clinical use with children and difficult-to-test persons because of the expense of the instrumentation; the time it takes to complete the test (often 3 to 4 hours); the necessity for sedation of many individuals, especially children; the specialized training required to interpret results; and the technical problems, including signal-to-noise ratio, effects of drugs, stimulus dimensions, conditioning procedures, and so on. In the experience of the present authors, evoked response audiometry has been useful with only a small number of children for whom behavioral audiometry provided only gross estimates of hearing sensitivity. In each of these cases evoked response audiometry corroborated the original results. However, it should be noted that the evoked response audiometry findings were never any closer to the child's actual thresholds (obtained later) than were the original behavioral results.

Respiration Audiometry   Respiration audiometry is a respondent procedure that relies on a change in the individual's respiration pattern in response to sound as the basis for hearing assessment. Interest in this procedure as a tool for hearing measurement has grown during the last decade although its clinical use is not widespread. In an initial study of the use of respiration change to measure hearing status, Rosenau (1962) compared the results of children with known normal hearing, children with known mild to severe hearing impairments, and children who were known to be deaf. Results showed that there were changes in respiration near the presumed auditory threshold of the deaf children, but for the two other groups of children, Rousey and Bradford (1971) showed that 85 percent of a group of 498 ears gave threshold agreement within ±15 dB for both behavioral and respiration methodologies.

Although this procedure may be of value in the future, its present clinical usefulness with children, particularly those with developmental disabilities, is questionable. The major disadvantage of respiration audiometry is that it has not been shown to provide actual threshold measures (instead as high as 15 dB above actual threshold) whereas behavioral audiometry does. Furthermore, respiration audiometry depends on changes in the autonomic nervous system. As a result, responses to this procedure do not provide the same functional behavior information that is obtained with behavioral procedures (Hogan, 1975).

Electrocardiograph Audiometry   One of the other physiologic changes that has been studied as a possible aid to differential diagnosis of hearing problems is the change in heart rate that has been observed in response to sound. Such change has been shown in children (Bartoshuk, 1962, 1964; Clifton and Meyers, 1969; Schulman and Wade, 1970; Schulman et al., 1970) and adults (Zeaman and Wegner, 1956). Butterfield (1962) reported that cardiac response audiometry was not successful with a group of mentally retarded individuals. Because of methodologic problems, the role of maturation on the cardiac response, and lack of evidence relative to the use of this procedure with developmentally disabled children, cardiac response audiometry is not a clinically useful procedure at this time (Hogan, 1975).

Electrocochleography   Another technique that may prove useful in determining the degree of hearing loss in a developmentally disabled child is electrocochleography. Presently this procedure is largely used in the experimental study of hearing, although several investigators have reported results with children (Ruben, Lieberman, and Bordley, 1962; Aran and LaBert, 1968; Aran, 1971). It has been used in children as young as 1 month (Aran, 1971).

Electrocochleography attempts to measure the presence of neural activity generated in the auditory system, both within the cochlea in the organ of Corti (referred to as a *cochlear microphonic*) and along the auditory nerve (referred to as an *action potential*). Investigators have measured the neural activity indirectly by placing electrodes on the promontory (a bony structure located between the oval and round windows of the middle ear) via the tympanic membrane (Aran et al., 1969). Other placement locations have included the external ear canal near the tympanic membrane (Solomon and Elberling, 1971; Cullen et al., 1972) and the auricle (Sohmer and Feinmesser, 1967). Electrocochleography, similar to evoked response audiometry, has been made more reliable by the use of the computer averaging response method. In addition, use of computer methodology has made it possible to obtain results at sites more easily reached than the organ of Corti (Northern and Downs, 1975).

Despite the growing experimental evidence, routine clinical use of electrocochleography must await future development. Factors such as the expense of the instrumentation, the question of the most efficient placement of electrodes, the need for sedation of some individuals, the role of the interaction between the cochlear microphonic and the action potential, and the need for appropriately trained personnel to administer and interpret the procedure make the use of electrocochleography of value only as an experimental procedure at the present time. Obviously, there is much potential in the use of this procedure in assisting in the differential diagnosis of sensory, neural, and central auditory disorders.

AURAL HABILITATION

Once the hearing assessment is completed and the audiologist has gathered information about the developmentally disabled child's degree and type of hearing impairment as well as his basic auditory communication abilities, a plan for intervention is formulated. The single most important activity involved in working with the developmentally disabled child who has a hearing impairment is aural habilitation.

Aural habilitation for the hearing-impaired child consists of a wide range of direct care activities based on the child's communication needs. In addition, it includes activities that relate indirectly to the child through the audiologist's participation with other interdisciplinary members of the total habilitation team. Although the aural habilitation program must be tailored to the individual needs of each hearing-impaired, developmentally disabled child, programs usually include: 1) speech and language therapy; 2) hearing aid selection, orientation, and guidance; 3) auditory training; 4) training in the use of visual cues (speechreading, visual speech reception); and 5) counseling regarding the hearing loss. In some cases, aural habilitation also may include the use of manual language and/or manual systems such as those discussed by Wilbur and by Kopchick and Lloyd (this volume). Therefore, in the broadest sense, aural habilitation deals with improving the child's abilities in comprehension and expression. Such programs should meet the minimal criteria previously described in the *Standards for Residential Facilities for Mentally Retarded* of the Accreditation Council for Facilities for the Mentally Retarded, 1971 (also see Appendix C this volume).

Speech and Language Therapy

The speech and language therapy aspects of the intervention plan are discussed in detail by McLean, by Graham, and by Kopchick and Lloyd (this volume) and are not discussed at this point. However, it is important to point out that speech and language therapy is often carried out by someone other than the audiologist (i.e., speech pathologist, psychologist, child development specialist); consequently, the audiologist must carefully relate his findings concerning the child's auditory expressive and receptive abilities to the individual who is delivering the actual therapy. As a minimum, the audiologist should provide the following information about the child: 1) age of onset of hearing loss; 2) the child's major mode of expressive communication (speaking, signing, fingerspelling, and/or cueing); 3) his prior experience with and current status with regard to hearing aids; 4) the child's ability to receive and interpret visual cues; 5) his auditory skills (including auditory sensitivity across the frequency range for air- and bone-conducted sounds, stability of auditory sensitivity, dynamic range and tolerance, recruitment, habituation and fatigue, basic auditory discrimination, speech discrimination, and interaural differences for these measures); 6) the child's abilities to integrate auditory and visual cues simultaneously; and 7) prior educational experiences related to the hearing impairment. In addition to this information, the audiologist should assist the habilitation team in assessing the child's use and understanding of everyday language. Particularly with retarded hearing-impaired youngsters, it is important that all persons on the habilitative team reinforce the use of functional language.

Hearing Aid Selection and Orientation

Once the audiologist has identified a communicatively significant hearing impairment (which is not medically correctable) in the developmentally disabled child, there is a need to see if the use of a hearing aid or aids is appropriate. In cases in which the child already has an aid, it is the audiologist's responsibility to assess the child's current functioning with the aid. This assessment includes one of three recommendations: retaining the present aid with no modifications; making appropriate modifications to the aid, including internal or external adjustments, replacing worn or broken parts (i.e., receivers, cords, batteries, volume control dials); or obtaining a new instrument(s).

Many factors must be considered in the selection of a hearing aid, including: age of the child, degree and type of hearing loss, presence of congenital anomalies that might affect the child's use of an aid (i.e., absence or alteration of the auricle and/or external auditory canal), chronic draining otitis media (which might preclude the use of an earmold), physical disabilities (e.g., cerebral palsy, which might affect the child's ability to manipulate an aid), activity level (which may affect the decision whether to select a body-worn or post-auricular aid), and amount of audiologic information available at the time an aid is selected (in some very young children who are severely developmentally disabled, the audiologist may have to select an aid that offers maximal flexibility so that adjustments can be made as more is learned about the child's loss).

In addition to these factors, the audiologist must be aware of the family's ability to pay for a hearing aid. In the event that the family needs assistance, oftentimes federally or locally supported crippled children's programs can provide funds for prosthetic appliances. In addition, the audiologist (or other members of the habilitation team) frequently can find support from service organizations such as the Lions Club or Rotary Club. This kind of effort frequently leads to a greater appreciation by members of the community of the purposes of the habilitation program. Additional discussion pertaining to the selection of hearing aids is presented in a recent book by Pollack (1975).

Hearing aid orientation refers to direct counseling with the child and parents about the use of hearing aid. It also includes indirect counseling with the other habilitation team members about the child's hearing aid. Hearing aid orientation programs for retarded children have been reported by McCoy and Lloyd (1967) and by Moore, Miltenberger, and Barber (1969).

Although there are individual differences in the orientation programs used with developmentally disabled children, the majority include: description of the child's hearing impairment, supervised use of the hearing aid, care of the hearing aid, and use of the hearing aid in various listening conditions.

Description of the Child's Hearing Impairment to the Child, Parent, and Other Habilitation Team Members   This description includes information on the extent of the loss, the nature of the impairment, and, in cases where the information is available, the cause of the impairment. It should emphasize the effect of the impairment on everyday listening situations. It is critical that the parents and others working with the child understand the effects of a hearing impairment and the advantages and disadvantages of hearing aids in various listening situations. This is best accomplished through demonstrations (e.g., Harford, 1964; Glorig, 1971; Bill Wilkerson Hearing and Speech Center, 1972). Also, the child frequently must be shown the benefits of amplification.

Description, Demonstration, and Supervised Use of the Hearing Aid   This procedure includes identifying the major parts of the hearing aid—*on–off* switch, volume control, microphone, amplifier, receiver, earmold, batteries—and the function of each. Orientation programs must allow time for the child who is mature enough to practice using the various controls and inserting and removing the earmold under supervision.

Care of the Hearing Aid   The child should be instructed in the care of his hearing aid. This can range from instructions on keeping soup or juice out of the microphone for a body-worn aid to keeping the earmold clean. It may include instructions on how often to replace batteries and how to insert and remove them from the aid. A good orientation program also teaches the recognition of symptoms that the aid is not functioning properly. In the case of infants and some of the more severely impaired children, parents or caregivers must take major responsibility to check the aid at least twice a day. Hanners and Sitton (1974) have outlined the major aspects of a daily hearing aid monitoring program. Also, Ross (this volume) provides practical information about hearing aid maintenance.

The child's role involves telling the parent, caregiver, teacher, and/or clinician that something is wrong. In other cases, instruction involves teaching the child how to check the batteries and perform other simple troubleshooting procedures. As with any educational endeavor, involving the child in the responsibility of taking care of his own instrument usually results in greater commitment on the child's part. Behavior modification token systems can be used quite well in such programs.

Use of the Hearing Aid in Various Listening Situations   Before the beginning of the hearing aid orientation session, the audiologist should assess the child's use of amplification for various listening situations and with various stimuli (e.g., nonspeech discrimination such as hearing the difference between a bell and a horn, or between a male and a female speaker; speech discrimination between minimal pairs such as /pæt-pɑt/, tɪn-θɪn/, and /pɪg-pɪt/;[5] open set word discrimination; and phrase discrimination). Each of these types of discrimination can be tested in a quiet and in a noisy environment. In addition, speech-aided discriminations may be checked with and without visual cues using instruments such as the Word Intelligibility Picture Index (Ross and Lerman, 1970) and the Modified Rhyme Test (Pickett et al., 1970). With the developmentally disabled child who has good language development, one can use the Scale for Self-Assessment of Hearing Handicap (High, Fairbanks, and Glorig, 1964).

Based on this information, the audiologist can help the child to use his hearing aid most effectively, both in varying environments and with the myriad of speech and nonspeech stimuli. This portion of the orientation program is essentially tied to the auditory training program described in the next section.

It is important to reinforce again the idea that, although many of the examples given for the four aspects of the orientation program are aimed at direct counseling with the child, there are children whose chronologic age, language level, and general developmental level preclude direct counseling. In these cases, the audiologist works with the parents or other primary caregivers to actualize the orientation program. Additional information concerning hearing aid orientation is available elsewhere (Streng et al., 1958; Downs, 1967b; Davis and Silverman, 1970; Sanders, 1975). The reader is especially referred to the chapter by Ross (this volume) for a better understanding of hearing aids.

---

[5]For readers unfamiliar with the International Phonetic Association (IPA) Alphabet, a pronunciation key is provided in Appendix B.

Auditory Training

Once the child has been fitted with appropriate amplification, the audiologist must design a program that facilitates the child's use of his aided hearing. As was pointed out in the foregoing section, the hearing aid orientation and auditory training sections of the aural habilitation program are oftentimes inseparable, in that both focus on use of hearing. Auditory training, by definition, is designed to help children make maximal use of their residual hearing. Typical activities include having the child identify the sounds made by certain instruments, animals, or environmental sources (e.g., vacuum cleaner, washing machine, doorbell, and so on). The program then progresses to providing the opportunity for the child to learn the differences between phonemes, words, phrases, and sentences. Such programs have been applied to retarded children (Wolfe and MacPherson, 1959; MacPherson, 1960; Schlanger, 1961, 1962; Christensen and Schlanger, 1964; Schlanger and Christensen, 1964).

Although all auditory training is aimed at increasing the child's use of hearing, individual auditory training programs vary in their use of visual cues to enhance the auditory modality. Various methodologies that emphasize the auditory input channel exclusively include the "unisensory method" or the "aural method" (Pollack, 1970; Rupp, 1971). Other methodologies emphasize the importance of auditory input but also make allowances in the total habilitation program for visual and contextual input; these include the traditional "oral-aural method" and the "natural language method" (Groht, 1958). Although some individuals start auditory training with nonspeech stimuli, many teachers and audiologists start with speech stimuli and involve simple sentences and phrases early in the procedures. Many also believe that, regardless of the degree to which the child is allowed to use nonauditory cues in the educational environment, all auditory training activities are directed at heightening the child's use of his hearing as an enhancement to communication. Additionally, programs should utilize every opportunity in the child's daily activities to enhance auditory skills. Auditory training is not an activity that should be relegated to 1 hour per week. While further discussion of this area may be found elsewhere (Streng et al., 1958; O'Neill and Oyer, 1961; Davis and Silverman, 1970; Sanders, 1971; Kretschmer, 1973), one book and one chapter warrant special mention. The Sanders' (1971) book on aural rehabilitation treats auditory training in a practical way within the framework of the communication model presented in the first chapter (Sanders, this volume). Kretschmer's (1973) chapter is an outstanding example of the integration of auditory training into a sound linguistic approach to meet the communication needs of hearing-impaired children. His model for auditory/language training is based upon the following assumptions (pp. 233–234):

> ... (1) the thrust of auditory/language training should be to make the auditory sense as much a part of the language learning process as possible; (2) the linguistic input to the hearing impaired child should be structured so as to approximate the normal language growth pattern found in normally hearing children; (3) work on specific environmental sound recognition will not be emphasized except as such sounds occur as a part of the experiences used to introduce linguistic principles and/or models; (4) linguistic competence and linguistic reception must be the focal point in the language development program and must take precedence over perfection of linguistic performance.

Kretschmer summarizes the critical elements of his approach as (p. 241):

> ... parent participation, aggressive use of amplification, structured linguistic input, emphasis on amalgamation of non-linguistic and cognitive-perceptual experience using direct participation of the child in all learning, and encouragement of the child's attempts at oral language production by rehearsal and expansion of the utterances.

Sanders' approach is based on a broad communication model and Kretschmer's approach is based on a linguistic model (which some may view as narrower than a communication model), but the approaches are compatible because they both: 1) are based on the communication of concepts (semantics) rather than on linguistic structure, and 2) use a multichannel input rather than a strict unisensory or aural-only input. Although they are multichannel, they clearly stress the consistent use of high quality amplification.

Training in Use of Visual Cues

Speechreading, lipreading, visual speech reception, or *visual hearing* are terms often used to describe activities in which the hearing-impaired child watches the face (the lips in particular) and general body language of a speaker in order to facilitate reception of spoken language. In essence, the child must "derive meaning from the partial clues he observes as the articulators pass rapidly from sound to sound, some of which are invisible to him (Streng et al., 1958, p. 166)." This task is not an easy one; it has been shown that only 33% of English speech sounds are readily visible (Hardy, 1970). In addition, it is known that, for hearing-impaired persons, there is a wide range of speechreading abilities. Jeffers (1967) ascribed these differences to three primary factors: 1) perceptual efficiency, the ability to rapidly perceive speech sounds or elements and gain additional information from the cues on the speaker's face; 2) synthetic ability, the ability to identify the essence of words and phrases into a meaningful unit; and 3) flexibility, or the ability to reorder initial perceptions in light of ongoing ones.

Added to all of these factors are the additional variables specific to the speechreading abilities of the developmentally disabled child. It is apparent that a child's speechreading abilities are related to his receptive and expressive language levels. Also, speechreading depends on the child's ability to attend to and derive meaning from very small changes in the speaker's lips. Hence, there are developmental disabilities that affect a child's ability to speechread, including attention span difficulties (hyperactivity); general motor control dysfunctions precluding good focusing posture, such as that seen in cerebral palsy; poor peripheral vision; and/or inadequate visual memory skills.

For a more detailed treatment of speechreading, the reader is referred to books by Berger (1972), Jeffers and Borley (1971), and Sanders (1971).

Counseling

The counseling aspects of aural habilitation include both direct and indirect services for the developmentally disabled child, as was noted in the introductory portion of the aural habilitation section. Discussion up to this point focuses on many of the issues included in direct counseling, particularly the function, care, and use of a hearing aid in various communicative settings. Additional counseling with the child (or his parent or caregiver in the case of the severely disabled, very young child) usually centers on associated issues, including problems with communication in the child's various educational and social situations, specific deficiencies in his school performance, and other areas that the child or his parents may wish to discuss.

Indirect counseling services provided by the audiologist generally include being the advocate of the hearing-impaired developmentally disabled child in the habilitation system. This includes being sure that all professionals and supportive personnel are aware of the child's hearing impairment and its implications. The involvement of parents and the use of supportive personnel described by Baker (this volume) and by Sigelman and Bensburg (this volume) are critical to the successful habilitation of the hearing-impaired child. Therefore, counseling and in-service training activities by the audiologist are imperative for comprehensive communication programming for the child.

CONCLUSION

This chapter presents some of the salient features of the impact of audiology on the developmentally disabled child, particularly those with hearing impairment in addition to other disabilities. With the underlying premise that a child's various developmental disabilities should not be treated as separate entities, aspects of the total audiologic program are presented in the context of the total habilitation program.

Specifically, the chapter considers: screening and identification philosophy and methods, audiologic assessment procedures and their rationale; procedures, both behavioral and electrophysiologic, used with children, with special reference to modifications for developmentally disabled youngsters; and discussion of aural habilitation. Each of these is placed in the context of the role of the audiologist on the interdisciplinary treatment team.

It is the hope of the authors that the reader, regardless of prior formal experience with audiology, will better understand the role of audiology and, as a result, provide better total habilitative care for the developmentally disabled child.

REFERENCES

AAOO, AAP, and ASHA. 1974. Supplementary statement of joint committee on infant hearing screening. Asha 16:160.

Accreditation Council for Facilities for the Mentally Retarded. 1971. Standards for Residential Facilities for the Mentally Retarded. Joint Commission on Accreditation of Hospitals, Chicago. 148 p.

ANSI. 1969. American National Standard Specifications for Audiometers, S3.6-1969. American National Standards Institute, New York.

Aran, J. M. 1971. The electrocochleogram: Recent results in children and in some pathological cases. Arch. Klin. Exp. Ohren. Nasen. Kehlkopfheilkd. 198.

Aran, J. M., and G. LaBert. 1968. Les réponses nerveuses Cochléaires chez l'homme: Image du fonctionnement de l'oreille et nouveau test d'audiometrie objective. Rev. Laryngol. 89:361–378.

Aran, J. M., C. Portmann, J. Delauney, J. Pelerin, and J. Lenoir. 1969. L'électrocochleogramme: Méthodes et premiers resultats chez l'enfant. Rev. Laryngol. 90:615–634.

ASHA Committee on Audiometric Evaluation. 1975. Guidelines for identification audiometry. Asha 17:94–99.

Bartoshuk, A. D. 1962. Human neonatal cardiac acceleration to sound. Habituation and dishabituation. Percept. Motor Skills 15:15–27.

Bartoshuk, A. D. 1964. Human neonatal cardiac responses to sound: A power function. Psychonom. Sci. 1:151–152.

Belkin, M., E. Suchman, M. Bergman, D. Rosenblatt, and H. Jacobziner. 1964. A demonstration program for conducting hearing tests in day care centers. J. Speech Hear. Disord. 29:335–338.

Bench, R. J., and N. Boscak. 1970. Some application of signal detection theory to paedo-audiology. Sound 4:3.

Berger, K. W. 1972. Speechreading Principles and Methods. National Educational Press, Baltimore.

Berlin, C. I., and A. C. Dill. 1967. The effects of feedback and positive reinforcement on the Wepman Auditory Discrimination Test scores of lower-class Negro and white children. J. Speech. Hear. Res. 10:384–389.

Bill Wilkerson Hearing and Speech Center. 1972. A Sound Approach. Bill Wilkerson Hearing and Speech Center, Nashville.

Bradford, L. J. 1975. Respiration audiometry: The indirect assessment of hearing sensitivity. Audiol. Hear. Educ. 1:19–25.

Bricker, W. A., and D. D. Bricker. 1969. Four operant procedures for establishing auditory stimulus control with low-functioning children. Amer. J. Ment. Defic. 73:981–987.

Brooks, D. 1971. Electro-acoustic impedance bridge studies on normal ears of children. J. Speech Hear. Res. 14:247–253.

Butterfield, G. A. 1962. Note on the use of cardiac rate in the audiometric appraisal of retarded children. J. Speech Hear. Disord. 27:378–379.

Carhart, R., and J. F. Jerger. 1959. Preferred method for clinical determination of pure-tone thresholds. J. Speech Hear. Disord. 24:330–345.

Christensen, N. J., and B. B. Schlanger. 1964. Auditory training with the mentally retarded. Ment. Retard. 2:290–293.

Clifton, R. K., and W. J. Meyers. 1969. The heart-rate response of four-month-old infants to auditory stimuli. J. Exp. Child Psychol. 7:122–135.

Cotton, J. C., and J. Hall. 1939. Administration of the 6-A audiometer test to kindergarten and first grade children. Volta Rev. 41:291–292.

Cullen, J. K., M. S. Ellis, C. I. Berlin, and R. J. Lousteau. 1972. Human acoustic nerve action potential recordings from the tympanic membrane without anesthesia. Acta Otolaryngol. 74:15–22.

Curry, E. T., and G. H. Kurtzrock. 1951. A preliminary investigation of the ear-choice technique in threshold audiometry. J. Speech Hear. Disord. 16:340–345.

Dahle, A. J., and D. A. Daly. 1972. Influence of verbal feedback on auditory discrimination test performance of mentally retarded children. Amer. J. Ment. Defic. 76:586–590.

Dahle, A. J., and D. A. Daly. 1974. Tangible rewards in assessing auditory discrimination performance of mentally retarded children. Amer. J. Ment. Defic. 78:625–630.

Darley, F. L. (ed.). 1961. Identification audiometry. J. Speech Hear. Disord. monogr. suppl. 9. 68 p.

Davis, H., P. Davis, A. Loomis, E. Harvey, and G. Hobart. 1939. Electrical reaction of the human brain to auditory stimulation during sleep. J. Neurophysiol. 2:500–514.

Davis, H., and S. R. Silverman. 1970. Hearing and Deafness. Holt, Rinehart and Winston, New York. 522 p.

Denmark, F. G. W. 1950. A development of the peep-show audiometer. J. Laryngol. Otol. 64:357–360.

Derbyshire, A., A. Fraser, M. McDermott, and A. Bridges. 1956. Audiometric measurements by electroencephalography. Electroencephalogr. Clin. Neurophysiol. 8:467–478.

Derbyshire, A., and M. McDermott. 1958. Further contributions to the EEG method of evaluating auditory function. Laryngoscope 68: 558–570.

Dix, M. R., and C. S. Hallpike. 1947. The peep-show: A new technique for pure tone audiometry in young children. Brit. Med. J. 2:719–723.

Downs, M. P. 1967a. Organization and procedures of a newborn infant screening program. Hear. Speech News 35:27–36.

Downs, M. P. 1967b. The establishment of hearing aid use: A program for parents. Maico Audiological Library Series 4. Maico Electronics, Inc., New York.

Downs, M. P. 1970. The identification of congenital deafness. Trans. Amer. Acad. Ophthalmol. Otolaryngol. 74:1208–1214.

Downs, M. P. 1973. Information obtained from seminar on early identification and screening for hearing impairment at the Medical Audiology conference, Vail, Col., March, 1973.

Downs, M. P., and W. G. Hemenway. 1969. Report on the hearing screening of 17,000 neonates. Int. Audiol. 8:72–76.

Downs, M. P., and W. G. Hemenway. 1972. Newborn screening revisited. Hear. Speech News 40:4–5, 26, 28–29.

Eilers, R. E., W. R. Wilson, and J. M. Moore. Developmental changes in infant speech perception. In preparation.

Evans, M. L. 1943. An adaptation of the audiometric technique for use with small children. Unpublished master's thesis. University of Illinois, Urbana.

Ewing, A. W. G. 1930. Aphasia in Children. Oxford Medical Publication, London.

Ewing, I. R., and Ewing, A. W. G. 1944. The ascertainment of deafness in infancy and early childhood. J. Laryngol. Otol. 59:309–338.

Fulton, R. T. 1962. Psychogalvanic skin response and conditioned orientation reflex audiometry with mentally retarded children. Unpublished doctoral dissertation. Purdue University, Lafayette, Ind.

Fulton, R. T. 1967. Standard puretone and Bekesy audiometric measures with the mentally retarded. Amer. J. Ment. Defic. 72:60–73.

Fulton, R. T. (ed.). 1974. Auditory Stimulus-Response Control. University Park Press, Baltimore. 163 p.

Fulton, R. T., and L. E. Lamb. 1972. Acoustic impedance and tympanometry with the retarded: A normative study. Audiology 11:199–208.

Fulton, R. T., and L. L. Lloyd. 1969. Audiometry for the Retarded with Implications for the Difficult-to-Test. Williams & Wilkins, Baltimore. 273 p.

Fulton, R. T., and L. L. Lloyd. 1975. Auditory Assessment of the Difficult-to-Test. Williams & Wilkins, Baltimore. 297 p.

Fulton, R. T., and M. J. Reid. 1969. Bekesy audiometry with the retarded. Amer. J. Ment. Defic. 74:223–230.

Gaines, J. A. 1961. A comparison of two audiometric tests administered to a group of mentally retarded children. Unpublished master's thesis. University of Nebraska, Lincoln.

Giddoll, A. 1952. Quantitative determination for hearing to audiometric frequencies in the electroencephalogram; preliminary report. Arch. Otolaryngol. 55:597–601.

Giolas, T. G. 1975. Speech audiometry. In R. T. Fulton and L. L. Lloyd (eds.), Auditory Assessment of the Difficult-to-Test, pp. 37–70. Williams & Wilkins, Baltimore.

Glorig, A. 1971. Getting Through: A Guide to Better Understanding of the Hard of Hearing. Zenith Radio Corp., Chicago. (33⅓ rpm stereo recording.)

Goldman, R., M. Fristoe, and R. Woodcock. 1970. The Goldman-Fristoe-Woodcock Test of Auditory Discrimination. American Guidance Service, Circle Pines, Minn.

Goldman, R., M. Fristoe, and R. Woodcock. 1974. Goldman-Fristoe-Woodcock Auditory Skills Battery: Diagnostic Auditory Discrimination Test. American Guidance Service, Circle Pines, Minn.

Goldstein, R., and C. Tait. 1971. Critique of neonatal hearing evaluation. J. Speech Hear. Disord. 36:3–18.

Green, D. S. 1958. The pup-show: A simple, inexpensive modification of the peep show. J. Speech Hear. Disord. 23:118–120.

Griffing, T. S., K. M. Simonton, and L. D. Hedgecock. 1967. Verbal auditory screening for pre-school children. Trans. Amer. Acad. Ophthalmol. Otolaryngol. 71:105–111.

Groht, M. A. 1958. Natural Language for Deaf Children. Gallaudet College Press, Washington, D.C.

Guilford, R., and O. Haug. 1952. Diagnosis of deafness in the very young child. Arch. Otolaryngol. 55:101–106.

Hanners, B. A., and A. B. Sitton. 1974. Ears to hear: A daily hearing aid monitor program. Volta Rev. 76:530–536.

Hardy, M. P. 1970. Speechreading. *In* H. Davis and S. R. Silverman (eds.), Hearing and Deafness. Holt, Rinehart and Winston, New York.

Harford, E. R. 1964. How They Hear. Gordon N. Stowe and Associates, Northbrook, Ill. 15 p.

Haskins, H. L. 1949. A phonetically balanced test of speech discrimination for children. Unpublished master's thesis. Northwestern University, Evanston, Ill.

High, W., G. Fairbanks, and A. Glorig. 1964. Scale for self-assessment of hearing handicap. J. Speech Hear. Disord. 29:215–230.

Hirsh, I. J. 1952. The Measurement of Hearing. McGraw-Hill, New York. 364 p.

Hirsh, I. J., H. Davis, S. R. Silverman, E. G. Eldert, and R. W. Benson. 1952. Development of materials for speech audiometry. J. Speech Hear. Disord. 17:321–337.

Hogan, D. D. 1975. Autonomic correlates of audition. *In* R. T. Fulton and L. L. Lloyd (eds.), Auditory Assessment of the Difficult-to-Test, pp. 262–290. Williams & Wilkins, Baltimore.

Irwin, J. V., J. E. Hind, and A. E. Aronson. 1957. Experience with conditioned GSR audiometry in a group of mentally deficient individuals. Train. School Bull. 54:26–31.

Ishisawa, H. 1960. A study on play audiometry. Otol. Fukuoka 6(suppl. 7):397–415.

Jeffers, J. 1967. Process of speechreading viewed with respect to a theoretical construct. *In* Proceedings of International Conference on Oral Education of the Deaf, pp. 1530–1533. Alexander Graham Bell Association for the Deaf, Washington, D.C.

Jeffers, J., and M. Borley. 1971. Speechreading (Lipreading). Charles C Thomas, Springfield, Ill. 392 p.

Jerger, J. 1972. Suggested nomenclature for impedance audiometry. Arch. Otolaryngol. 96:1–3.

Jerger, J. (ed.). 1975. Handbook of Clinical Impedance. American Electronics Corp., Dobbs Ferry, N.Y. 235 p.

Jerger, J., P. Burney, L. Mauldin, and B. Crump. 1974. Predicting hearing loss from the acoustic reflex. J. Speech Hear. Disord. 39:11–22.

Jerger, J., J. L. Shedd, and E. Harford. 1959. On detection of extremely small changes in sound intensity. Arch. Otolaryngol. 69:200–211.

Jerger, S., J. Jerger, L. Mauldin, and P. Segal. 1974. Studies in impedance audiometry. II. Children less than six years old. Arch. Otolaryngol. 99:1–9.

Johnston, R., and P. Magrab (eds.). 1976. Developmental Disorders: Assessment, Treatment, Education. University Park Press, Baltimore. 532 p.

Kaplan, H. F. 1957. A comparison of picture response and hand raising technique for puretone audiometry with young children. Unpublished master's thesis. Pennsylvania State University, University Park.

Katz, J. (ed.). 1972. Handbook of Clinical Audiology. Williams & Wilkins, Baltimore. 842 p.

Keaster, M. J. 1951. A puretone audiometric test for preschool children. Unpublished master's thesis. University of Wisconsin, Madison.

Keith, R. 1973. Impedance audiometry with neonates. Arch. Otolaryngol. 97:465–467.

Knox, E. C. 1960. A method of obtaining puretone audiograms in young children. J. Laryngol. Otol. 74:475–479.

Kodman, F., A. Fein, and A. Mixon. 1959. Psychogalvanic skin response audiometry with severe mentally retarded children. Amer. J. Ment. Defic. 64:131–136.

Kretschmer, R. 1973. Auditory training procedures with hearing-impaired preschool children. In K. Donnelly (ed.), Hearing Aids. Charles C Thomas, Springfield, Ill.

Lamb, L. E. 1975. Acoustic impedance measurement. In R. T. Fulton and L. L. Lloyd (eds.), Auditory Assessment of the Difficult-to-Test, pp. 179–234. Williams & Wilkins, Baltimore.

Lamb, L. E., and T. Norris. 1970. Relative acoustic impedance measurements with mentally retarded children. Amer. J. Ment. Defic. 75:51–56.

Lilly, D. J. 1972. Acoustic impedance at the tympanic membrane. In J. Katz (ed.), Handbook of Clinical Audiology, pp. 434–469. Williams & Wilkins, Baltimore.

Lloyd, L. L. 1965a. A comparison of selected auditory measures on normal hearing mentally retarded children. Unpublished doctoral dissertation. University of Iowa, Iowa City.

Lloyd, L. L. 1956b. The new audiology program at Parsons State Hospital and Training Center. Hear. News 33:5–7, 12.

Lloyd, L. L. 1966. Behavioral audiometry viewed as an operant procedure. J. Speech Hear. Disord. 31:128–136.

Lloyd, L. L. 1970. Audiologic aspects of mental retardation. In N. R. Ellis (ed.), International Review of Research in Mental Retardation. Academic Press, New York. 4:311–374.

Lloyd, L. L. 1972. The audiologic assessment of deaf students. Report of the Proceedings of the 45th Meeting of the Convention of American Instructors of the Deaf, pp. 585–594. U.S. Government Printing Office, Washington, D.C.

Lloyd, L. L. 1975. Behavioral audiometry with children. In D. B. Tower, (ed.), The Nervous System, Vol. 3: Human Communication and Its Disorders, pp. 173–179. Raven Press, New York.

Lloyd, L. L. 1976. Discussion comment: Language and communication aspects. In T. D. Tjossem (ed.), Intervention Strategies for High Risk Infants and Young Children. University Park Press, Baltimore.

Lloyd, L. L., and B. P. Cox. 1972. Programming for the audiologic aspects of mental retardation. Ment. Retard. 10:22–26.

Lloyd, L. L., and B. P. Cox. 1975. Behavioral audiometry with children. In M. J. Glasscock, (ed.), Otolaryngology Clinics of North America: Symposium on Sensorineural Hearing Loss in Children: Early Detection and Intervention, pp. 89–108. Vol. 8(1). W. B. Saunders, Philadelphia.

Lloyd, L.L., and A. Dahle. 1976. Detection and diagnosis of hearing impairment. Volta Rev. Bicentennial monograph (D. R. Frisina, guest editor).

Lloyd, L. L., and J. Melrose. 1966. Inter-method comparisons of selected audiometric measures used with normal hearing mentally retarded children. J. Aud. Res. 6:205–217.

Lloyd, L. L., J. E. Spradlin, and M. J. Reid. 1968. An operant audiometric procedure for difficult-to-test patients. J. Speech Hear. Disord. 33:236–245.

Lloyd, L. L., and W. R. Wilson. 1974. Recent developments in the behavioral assessment of the infant's response to auditory stimulation. Paper presented at the 16th World Congress for Logopedics and Phoniatrics, Interlaken, Switzerland, August 1974.

McCoy, D. F., and L. L. Lloyd. 1967. A hearing aid orientation program for mentally retarded children. Train. School Bull. 64:21–30.

MacPherson, J. R. 1960. The evaluation and development of techniques for testing the acuity of trainable mentally retarded children. Unpublished doctoral dissertation. University of Texas, Austin.

Marcus, R., E. Gibbs, and F. Gibbs. 1949. Electroencephalography in the diagnosis of hearing loss in the very young child. Dis. Nerv. Syst. 10:170–173.

Mencher, G. T., and B. F. McCulloch. 1970. Auditory screening of kindergarten children using the VASC. J. Speech Hear. Disord. 35:241–247.

Metz, O. 1946. The acoustic impedance measured in normal and pathological ears. Acta Otolaryngol. Suppl. 63:1–254.

Meyerson, L., and J. L. Michael. 1960. The measurement of sensory thresholds in exceptional children: An experimental approach to some problems of differential diagnosis and education with special reference to hearing. Cooperative Research Program, Project 418. U.S. Office of Education, Department of Health, Education, and Welfare, University of Houston, Houston.

Meyerson, L., and J. L. Michael. 1964. Assessment of hearing by operant conditioning procedures. Report of the proceedings of the International Congress on Education of the Deaf and of the 41st Meeting of the Convention of American Instructors of the Deaf. U.S. Government Printing Office, Washington, D.C.

Miller, A. L. 1962. The use of reward techniques in testing young children's hearing. Hear. News 30:5–7.

Miller, A. L. 1963. The use of slide projectors in pure tone audiometric testing. J. Speech Hear. Disord. 28:94–96.

Moore, E. J., G. E. Miltenberger, and P. S. Barber. 1969. Hearing aid orientation in a state school for the mentally retarded. J. Speech Hear. Disord. 34:142–145.

Moore, J. M., G. Thompson, and M. Thompson. 1975. Auditory localization of infants as a function of reinforcement conditions. J. Speech Hear. Disord. 40:29–30.

Moore, J. M., W. R. Wilson, and G. Thompson. Visual reinforcement of auditory head-turn responses in infants under 12 months of age. In preparation.

Murphy, K. P. 1962. Development of hearing in babies: A diagnostic system for detecting early signs of deafness in infants. Child and Family 1:16–17.

Myatt, B. D., and B. Landes. 1963. Assessing discrimination loss in children. Arch. Otolaryngol. 77:359–362.

Myklebust, H. R. 1960. The Psychology of Deafness. Grune & Stratton, New York. 393 p.

NINDS. 1969. Learning to talk: Speech, hearing and language problems in preschool children. U.S. Government Printing Office, Washington, D.C. 48 p.

Newby, H. A. 1964. Audiology. Appleton-Century-Crofts, New York. 400 p.

Nodar, R., and J. Smith. 1970. Averaged electroencephalic audiometry applied to medicated mentally retarded adults during sleep. 10:221–225.

Northern, J. L., and M. P. Downs. 1975. Hearing in Children. Williams & Wilkins, Baltimore. 341 p.

Nowels, M. M. 1971. Operant audiometry with two year olds. Unpublished master's thesis. Kansas State University, Manhattan, Kan.

O'Neill, J. J., and H. J. Oyer. 1961. Visual Communication. Prentice-Hall, Englewood Cliffs, N.J. 163 p.

O'Neill, J., H. J. Oyer, and J. W. Hillis. 1961. Audiometric procedures used with children. J. Speech Hear. Disord. 26:61–66.

Pickett, J. L., E. S. Martin, D. J. Johnson, S. B. Smith, Z. Daniel, D. Willis, and W. Otis. 1970. On patterns of speech feature perceptions by deaf listeners. In G. Fant (ed.), Speech Communication Ability and Profound Deafness, pp. 119–133. A. G. Bell Association for the Deaf, Washington, D.C.

Pollack, D. 1970. Educational Audiology for the Limited Hearing Infant. Charles C Thomas, Springfield, Ill. 237 p.

Pollack, M. C. (ed.). 1975. Amplification for the Hearing Impaired. Grune & Stratton, New York. 456 p.

Price, L. L., and V. Falck. 1963. Bekesy audiometry with children. J. Speech Hear. Disord. 6:129–133.

Rapin, I., and L. Grazini. 1967. Auditory evoked responses in normal, brain-damaged, and deaf infants. Neurology 17:881–894.

Redell, R. C., and D. R. Calvert. 1967. Conditioned audio-visual response audiometry. In Proceedings of the International Conference on Oral Education of the Deaf. pp. 502–513. Vol. 1. Alexander Graham Bell Association for the Deaf, Washington, D.C.

Reneau, J., and R. Mast. 1968. Telemetric EEG audiometry instrumentation for use with profoundly retarded. Amer. J. Ment. Defic. 72: 502–511.

Robertson, E. O., J. L. Peterson, and L. E. Lamb. 1968. Relative impedance measurements in young children. Arch. Otolaryngol. 88: 162–168.

Rosenau, H. 1962. Die Schlafbeschallung: Eine Methode der Hörprüfung beim Kleinstkind. Z. Laryngol. Rhinol. Otol. Greüzgebiete 41: 194–208.

Rosenberg, P. E. 1958. Rapid clinical measurement of tone decay. Paper presented at the American Speech and Hearing Association, New York.

Ross, M., and J. Lerman. 1970. A picture identification test for hearing impaired children. J. Speech Hear. Res. 13:44–53.

Rousey, L., and L. J. Bradford. 1971. An indirect hearing sensitivity assessment by respiration in brain-damaged and orthopedically handicapped children as compared to normally appearing children during various states of waking and sleeping. Final Report, Easter Seal Grant N-7010, Menninger Foundation, Topeka, Kan.

Ruben, R. J., A. T. Lieberman, and J. E. Bordley. 1962. Some observations on cochlear potentials and nerve action potentials in children. Laryngoscope 5:545.

Rupp, R. R. 1971. An approach to the communicative needs of the very young hearing impaired child. J. Acad. Rehab. Audiol. 4:11–22.

Sanders, D. A. 1971. Aural Rehabilitation. Prentice-Hall, Englewood Cliffs, N.J. 374 p.

Sanders, D. A. 1975. Hearing aid orientation and counseling. In M. C. Pollack, (ed.), Amplification for the Hearing Impaired, pp. 323–372. Grune & Stratton, New York.

Schlanger, B. B. 1961. The effects of listening training on the auditory thresholds of mentally retarded children. Cooperative Research Program, Project 973 (8936). U.S. Office of Education, Department of Health, Education, and Welfare, University of Houston, Houston.

Schlanger, B. B. 1962. Effects of listening training on auditory thresholds of mentally retarded children. Asha 4:273–275.

Schlanger, B. B., and N. J. Christensen. 1964. Effects of training upon audiometry with the mentally retarded. Amer. J. Ment. Defic. 68: 469–475.

Schulman, C. A., C. R. Smith, M. Weisinger, and T. H. Fay. 1970. The use of heart rate in the audiological evaluation of nonverbal children: I. Evaluation of children at risk for hearing impairment. Neuropediatrics 2:187–196.

Schulman, C. A., and G. Wade. 1970. The use of heart rate in the audiological evaluation of nonverbal children: II. Clinical trials on an infant population. Neuropediatrics 2:197–205.

Schwartz, A. 1952. Supplementary pure tone audiometric screening test for preschool children. Unpublished master's thesis. University of Wisconsin, Madison.

Shimizu, H., and F. Nakamura. 1957. Pure tone audiometry in children with the lantern slide test. Ann. Otol. Rhinol. Laryngol. 66:392–398.

Siegenthaler, B., and G. Haspiel. 1966. Development of two standardized measures of hearing for speech by children. Cooperative Research

Program, Project 2372. U.S. Office of Education, Department of Health, Education, and Welfare, University of Houston, Houston.

Sohmer, H., and M. Feinmesser. 1967. Cochlear action potentials recorded from the external ear in man. Ann. Otolaryngol. 76:427–435.

Solomon, G., and C. Elberling. 1971. Cochlear nerve potentials recorded from the ear canal in men. Acta Otolaryngol. 71:319–325.

Statten, P., and D. E. Wishart. 1956. Pure tone audiometry in young children: Psychogalvanic-skin-resistance and peep-show. Ann. Otol. Rhinol. Laryngol. 65:511–534.

Streng, A., W. J. Fitch, L. D. Hedgecock, J. W. Phillips, and J. A. Carrell. 1958. Hearing Therapy for Children. Grune & Stratton. 354 p.

Sullivan, R., M. H. Miller, and I. A. Polisar. 1962. The portable pup show: A further modification of the pup-show. Arch. Otolaryngol. 76:49–51.

Suzuki, T., and Y. Ogiba. 1960. A technique of pure tone audiometry for children under three years of age: Conditioned orientation reflex (C.O.R.) audiometry. Rev. Laryngol. 1:33–45.

Suzuki, T., and Y. Ogiba. 1961. Conditioned orientation reflex audiometry. Arch. Otolaryngol. 74:192–198.

Suzuki, T., Y. Ogiba, and T. Takei. 1972. Basic properties of conditioned orientation reflex audiometry. Minerva ORL 22(4):181–186.

Utley, J. 1949. Suggestive procedures for determining auditory acuity in very young acoustically handicapped children. Eye Ear Nose Throat Mon. 28:590–595.

Waldrop, W. A. 1953. A puppet show hearing test. Volta Rev. 55: 488–489.

Weaver, R. M. 1965. The use of filmstrip stories in slide show audiometry. In L. L. Lloyd, and D. R. Frisina, (eds.), The Audiologic Assessment of the Mentally Retarded: Proceedings of a National Conference. pp. 71–88. Parsons State Hospital and Training Center, Parsons, Kan.

Webb, C. E., S. W. Kinde, B. A. Weber, and R. K. Beedle. 1964. Procedures for evaluating the hearing of the mentally retarded. Cooperative Research Program, Project 1731. U.S. Office of Education, Department of Health, Education, and Welfare, University of Houston, Houston.

Wilson, W. R., J. M. Moore, T. N. Decker, and L. L. Lloyd. 1975. Behavioral assessment of hearing sensitivity in infants. Scientific exhibit presented at the annual ASHA meeting, November, 1975, Washington, D.C.

Wilson, W. R., J. M. Moore, and G. Thompson. Auditory thresholds of infants utilizing visual reinforcement audiometry (URA). In preparation.

Withrow, F., and R. Goldstein. 1958. Electrophysiologic procedures for determination of threshold in children. Laryngoscope 68:1674–1699.

Wolfe, W. G., and J. R. MacPherson. 1959. The evaluation and development of techniques for testing the auditory acuity of trainable mentally retarded children. Cooperative Research Program, Project 172.

U.S. Office of Education, Department of Health, Education, and Welfare, University of Houston, Houston.

Yamamoto, K., H. Nishikawa, M. Nagata, and S. Itakura. 1953. The objective hearing test in young children and deafness. Nagoya J. Med. Sci. 16:79–84.

Yarnall, G. D. 1973. Comparison of operant and conventional audiometric procedures with deaf-blind, multiply handicapped children. Unpublished doctoral dissertation. George Peabody College, Nashville.

Zeaman, D., and N. Wegner. 1956. Cardiac reflex to tone of threshold intensity. J. Speech Hear. Disord. 21:71–75.

Zenith Corporation. 1966. Verbal Auditory Screening for Children (VASC). Zenith Corp., Chicago.

5

PSYCHOLOGIC EVALUATION OF HEARING-IMPAIRED CHILDREN

McCay Vernon

CONTENTS

Causes of Multiple Handicaps and Mental Retardation in the
Deaf Population ⸻ 197

Nature and Magnitude of Multiple Handicaps and
Mental Retardation ⸻ 199
    Mental retardation/199
    Aphasoid behavior/199
    Emotional disturbance/200
    Visual defects/201
    Others/201

Psychologic Examination ⸻ 202
    General principles/204
    Components/206
    Differential Diagnosis/219

Pragmatics and Psychodiagnostics in Schools ⸻ 220

Summary ⸻ 221

References ⸻ 221

Knowledge about behavioral aspects of deafness and the psychologic evaluation of normally functioning deaf persons is limited. Thus, any discussion of psychodiagnostics with mentally retarded and multiply handicapped hearing-impaired children has about it an inherent and obvious air of presumptiveness. Yet there is great need for such knowledge and for the constructive use of psychologic skills with these children. This chapter presents some basic data on the problem and some suggestions for psychologic evaluation procedures.

The chapter first assesses the scope of the problem by examining some major causes of multiple disabilities in the deaf population. Second, the nature and prevalence of those secondary handicaps are assessed. Third, procedures in evaluation are suggested. Finally, the problem of differential diagnosis and some pragmatic aspects of school psychology are discussed.

CAUSES OF MULTIPLE HANDICAPS AND
MENTAL RETARDATION IN THE DEAF POPULATION

The leading etiologies of deafness frequently leave the child with other disabilities in addition to the hearing impairment. Conditions such as maternal rubella, meningitis, complications of Rh factor, and prematurity, which account for from one-third to one-half of all deafness in school-age children, are also known to be associated with brain damage, learning disabilities, aphasia, mental illness, mental retardation, and other disorders (Bensberg and Sigelman, this volume; Mindel and Vernon, 1971). In the case of the deaf child, the very presence of the hearing impairment is already evidence of major neurologic damage, evidence that increases the probability of other pathologies, especially within the central nervous system.

Genetic factors, which cause from one-fourth to two-thirds of deafness in children, are also associated with other neurologic and physical handicaps (Konigswork, 1971). For example, of the 54 known forms of hereditary transmission of hearing impairment, 30 syndromes are identified, 10 involving vision, hearing, and central nervous system pathology (Danish, Tillson, and Levitan, 1963; Fraser, 1964; Mengel et al., 1967). One of these, Usher's syndrome, which is congenital deafness and progressive blindness, accounts for about 5% of deaf patients in mental hospitals (Vernon, 1969b). Another genetic condition, the Jervell and Lange-Nielson syndrome, involves an inherited heart condition identifiable only by electrocardiographic tests.

It causes death, usually in the early teens—deaths often unexplained because physicians are unaware of the syndrome (Fraser, 1964).

Two important points must be made relative to genetic deafness. First, genetically deaf children are the least likely of all major etiologic groups to be multiply handicapped. In fact, their mean IQ exceeds that of the general population (Brill, 1963). However, there are syndromes in which mental retardation and genetic deafness are components. Second, knowledge about hereditary factors is burgeoning more rapidly than that in any other aspect of deafness. Professionals who work with the deaf are wise to assume responsibility for becoming familiar with this literature.

Of the remaining cases of deafness, unknown factors may account for about 10%. Among these, it could be safely assumed that some are cases of subclinical maternal rubella, recessive hereditary hearing impairment, and certain unidentified diseases originating during the prenatal and neonatal periods (Vernon, 1971).

The balance of childhood deafness, roughly 10%, is attributable to other diseases and conditions, including polio, whooping cough, maternal viral disease, measles, mumps, mastoiditis, scarlet fever, and anoxia. Table 1 reports a current investigation of etiologic factors.

An examination of the etiologic factors in deafness clearly indicates that there is every reason to expect that secondary disabilities will be present among many deaf children. These additional disabilities tend to involve brain damage. Hence, significant numbers of behavioral manifestations, particularly learning disabilities, have to be expected.

Table 1. Leading etiologies of deafness in children

Etiology	Estimated range of prevalence (%)
Heredity	40–60
Rh factor	3– 4
Meningitis	9–10
Rubella[a]	5–85
Prematurity	11–17

Updating of data originally published in Vernon, 1969a. Updating represents a concensus of current literature and available data from the Office of Demographic Studies, Gallaudet College, Washington, D.C.

[a]An epidemic disease. Therefore incidence figures vary greatly from year to year.

NATURE AND MAGNITUDE OF MULTIPLE
HANDICAPS AND MENTAL RETARDATION

In a deaf population, even more than in a hearing population, intellectual, emotional, and learning handicaps are harder to diagnose than are the more gross physical disabilities such as blindness, cerebral palsy, seizures, and orthopedic problems. However, certain types and degrees of multiple handicaps occur more frequently than others among hearing-impaired children.

Mental Retardation

Approximately 50 comparative studies have been made of intelligence of the hearing impaired and that of the general population. The consensus of these findings is that deafness per se does not affect IQ scores on performance-type tests (Mindel and Vernon, 1971). However, among certain etiologic groups where neurologic damage often exists in addition to the hearing impairment, elevated prevalence of mental retardation occurs (Table 2).

Aphasoid Behavior

Aphasia or so-called aphasoid disorders are not always easy to diagnose in any population except when the condition is traumatic in onset and drastic in degree. Among hearing-impaired persons, aphasoid disorders present a crucially important problem because of the already-present language disability resulting from the impaired hearing. Aphasia is also a hundredfold more formidable to diagnose because there is little or no normative information on language

Table 2. Prevalence of mental retardation in five etiologic groups of deaf children

Etiology	No. of cases	Percentage of cases retarded (IQ below 70)[a]
Heredity	62	None
Rh factor	39	5.0
Prematurity	115	16.3
Meningitis	92	14.0
Rubella	98	8.0

Updating of data originally published in Vernon, 1969a.

[a]2.2% of the general population have IQ's below 70.

development and its measurement among hearing-impaired children. Without these data, deviations from the normal become matters of clinical judgment, which is an inadequate measure for such a complex variable. Despite these shortcomings, clinical judgment was the criterion for the data on the prevalence of aphasia reported in Table 3. Classroom teachers and supervising teachers were asked to classify their student as aphasic or aphasoid when the student "presented a marked difficulty with language over and above that expected due to their hearing impairment and IQ." When both raters agreed independently on the diagnosis, the child was categorized as aphasic (Vernon, 1969a).

Based on this acknowledgedly crude diagnostic criterion, it becomes readily apparent that there is a significant amount of language disability present among deaf children that it not simply a consequence of profound hearing loss. It is the result of neurologic lesions associated with the cause of the hearing loss.

Emotional Disturbance

As with aphasia, any statement on the prevalence of emotional disturbance in a deaf population is at best an educated guess because of a similar lack of adequate normative information. Recognizing the problems involved in making such a guess and the tenuous nature of the findings, the author presents some data in Tables 4 and 5. The diagnoses reported were made by psychologists experienced with deaf children and were based on a 1-hour or longer individual diagnostic session and extensive case history data. The criterion for emotional disturbance was that the child have "severe psychological problems which profoundly jeopardized his ability to function adequately in a residential school setting" (Vernon, 1969a).

Table 3. Prevalence of aphasia in five etiologic groups of deaf children

Etiology	No. of cases	Percentage of cases aphasic
Heredity	63	1.6
Rh factor	35	8.0
Prematurity	113	36.3
Meningitis	92	16.3
Rubella	105	21.9

Updating of data originally published in Vernon, 1969a.

Table 4. Prevalence of emotional disturbance in five etiologic groups of deaf children (based on individual psychologic examinations)

Etiology	No. of cases	Percentage diagnosed emotionally disturbed	Percentage diagnosed psychotic
Heredity	63	6.3	2.2
Rh factor	40	12.5	2.5
Prematurity	116	29.3	6.0
Meningitis	91	24.1	3.3
Rubella	103	27.1	7.7

Updating of data originally published in Vernon, 1969a.

Table 5. Prevalence of cerebral palsy in five etiologic groups of deaf children[a]

Etiology	No. of cases	Percentage cerebral palsied
Heredity	79	None
Rh factor	45	51.1
Prematurity	113	17.6
Meningitis	92	9.7
Rubella	104	3.8

Updating of data originally published in Vernon, 1969a.

[a]In the general population there are one to seven cases of cerebral palsy per 100,000 population (Illingsworth, 1958).

Based on this criterion, 34% of deaf children in this sample were judged to have emotional disturbance. Furthermore, 6.3% of them were diagnosed as being psychotic.

Visual Defects

Myklebust (1960) has documented the fact that visual problems are relatively common among deaf children. This is particularly true among those having rubella, prematurity, and complications of Rh factor as etiologies of hearing loss (Vernon, 1969a). Cataracts and ocularmotor problems are especially prominent.

Others

Orthopedic defects and seizures are not uncommon among deaf children (Vernon, 1969a). The former are primarily associated with premature and rubella children unless cerebral palsy is included as an orthopedic problem. Seizures are most frequently found in Rh deaf children or in those who had meningitis. Table 6 summarizes all of the data on prevalence of multiple handicaps among known etiologic groups.

PSYCHOLOGIC EXAMINATION

Certain crucial considerations are fundamental to the psychologic examination of the mentally retarded and multiply handicapped deaf and hearing-impaired child, considerations that are not generally of primary significance with other youngsters. Failure to be aware of these considerations can result in gross psychodiagnostic errors of tragic consequence to the child, the parents, and all involved in the educational or rehabilitative process.

The first of these considerations hinges on the relationship of the child's auditory impairment and other handicaps to his language functioning. In some cases, these hearing-impaired children will appear to the psychologist to be capable of hearing well enough to converse with little difficulty, especially in the relatively quiet one-to-one situation of most clinics or offices. This kind of superficial observation frequently masks the role that the hearing has had in language development of the child. Often, these children are unable to understand well in groups or places where there are background noises, their hearing thresholds may fluctuate, they may have gone through early years (which are crucial for language development) without a hearing aid, or their hearing impairment may have been greater during preschool years. The point in so far as the psychologist is concerned is that even moderate or mild hearing losses often lead to a language deficiency attributable not to a lack of intelligence or some form of personality constriction or withdrawal but simply to a lack of adequate auditory input of language. Hearing-impaired children generally have not had the exposure to language that their peers with normal hearing have. For the deaf child, with or without other handicaps, the language retardation is far more pronounced.

The language problem and its relationship to deaf and hearing-impaired youth is illustrated by the following example. The author was called on to examine a patient at a hospital for the mentally retarded. This youth, who had been in the hospital several years, had received an IQ of 50 on the Stanford Binet, a verbal test, and had been classified mentally retarded. On at least one occasion he also had been di-

Table 6. Prevalence of physical anomalies in five etiologies of deafness

Etiology	Cerebral palsy and/or hemiplegias		Mental retardation (IQ below 70)		Aphasoid disorder		Visual defects		Orthopedic (excluding cerebral palsied)		Seizures	
	No.	%	No.	%	No.	%	No.	%	No.	%	No.	%
Heredity	79	None	62	None	63	1.5	63	20.6	63	1.5	63	None
Meningitis	92	9.7	92	14.1	92	16.3	87	5.7	92	5.4	92	3.2
Prematurity	113	17.6	115	16.5	113	36.2	113	28.3	101	8.9	113	1.7
Rubella	104	3.8	98	8.1	105	21.9	104	29.8	104	4.8	104	None
Rh factor	45	51.1	39	5.1	35	22.8	45	24.4	45	2.2	45	6.6

Updating of data originally published in Vernon, 1969a.

agnosed as sufficiently schizoid and withdrawn to require treatment as mentally ill. When give a nonverbal test, the WISC (Wechsler Intelligence Scale For Children) Performance Scale, the youngster scored above average. Extended interviewing indicated that much of the alleged withdrawal and constriction was actually a failure to understand and a resulting language retardation. Transferred to an educational program for hearing-impaired children, he made rapid academic and social gains. Later he was admitted to college.

Unfortunately, cases of this kind of misdiagnosis are not as unusual as they should be or as one might imagine. The reason underlying the errors is almost inevitably the psychologist's failure to recognize that the language deficiency of the hearing-impaired child is usually unrelated to his intelligence. The deficiency also may give the false impression that a personality pathology is present. For example, flat effect, nonresponsive remarks, and apparent withdrawal may be based on the reality factor of the child not clearly understanding the examiner and/or a history of not being able to grasp speakers' words. The deaf child has often learned to cope by keeping quiet. The hearing-impaired child will either be quiet or try to dominate the conversation in order that he not be forced to try to understand what is unclear to him. Many of these children have learned to handle their hearing loss by becoming masters of the neutral response, smiling, saying yes, and periodically nodding their heads in the affirmative. These techniques are often remarkably effective in unintentionally misleading psychologists and others into thinking there has been understanding and full communication when actually the child has unknowingly used a series of some sort of Rogerian reflective techniques to conceal his inability to understand.

With these introductory concepts as a frame of reference, certain general principles for psychodiagnoses with deaf and hearing-impaired multiply handicapped and mentally retarded children are presented. After this, the eight major components of a full psychologic evaluation are discussed.

General Principles

1. Psychologic tests or interviewing procedures that depend on the use of verbal language to measure intelligence, personality, or aptitude almost inevitably measure the hearing-impaired child's language deficiency caused by his deafness, not his actual mental capacity or psychodynamics. The situation in some cases is analogous to giving

an immigrant whose primary language is German a verbal test battery and interview in English. He could be Einstein, yet test scores probably would indicate retardation and psychopathology. Other handicaps such as aphasia, visual perceptual disorders, and cerebral palsy compound the problems.

Although a few hearing-impaired children function linguistically and in oral communication in essentially the same manner as the normally hearing, in an appreciable number of cases they are psychodiagnostically much more like deaf youngsters. It is, therefore, crucial in a psychologic evaluation that they be given tests appropriate for deaf persons. Tests for persons with normal hearing also can be tried in cases where language development seems normal. Where significant differences appear between the sets of test responses, they often show that the child did better on the nonlanguage measures appropriate for the deaf persons. It is these findings that should be judged valid in such a circumstance.

Whenever possible, instructions and verbal test items should be given to the hearing-impaired child in writing as well as orally. For example, the verbal scales of the Wechsler should be typed on index cards with a separate card for each item. Fingerspelling and sign language should be used in instances where both the hearing-impaired child and the psychologist understand them. These procedures do not in any way eliminate the factor of linguistic skill level, but they do reduce the obstacle that oral communication presents for many hearing-impaired children.

2. Complete and valid psychodiagnostics with deaf and hearing-impaired children, multiply handicapped, and mentally retarded children often require more time than is needed with normal hearing youth (Brenner and Thompson, 1967). Deaf cerebral palsied children are a case in point. Their problems must be accounted for in scheduling and planning. Often several test sessions are required.

3. Test scores on preschool and primary school hearing-impaired children tend to be extremely unreliable. Low scores in particular should be viewed as questionable in the absence of supporting data (Vernon and Brown, 1964; Smith, 1967).

4. Tests given to hearing-impaired children by psychologists not experienced with such youngsters are more often in error than when the service is rendered by one familiar with hearing-impaired children.

5. There are many circumstances that can lead children, especially hearing-impaired multiply handicapped ones, to function below capacity on tests. Thus, there is far more danger that a low IQ is inaccurate than that a high one is invalid.

6. Tests emphasizing timed responses are often not as valid as those that do not. Hearing-impaired youngsters, especially those with other handicaps, frequently want to finish as quickly as possible even if answers are random and therefore meaningless (Hiskey, 1966). In general, their attentive set toward being timed is different.

7. Group testing of hearing-impaired multiply handicapped children is a dubious procedure that at best is useful only as a gross screening device (Lane and Schneider, 1941; Levine, 1960; Myklebust, 1962; Hiskey, 1966).

Components

A complete psychologic evaluation of a deaf or hearing-impaired multiply handicapped or mentally retarded child ideally should include the following information, or at least as much as can be obtained:

1. A measure of intelligence
2. An evaluation of personality structure
3. A test for behavioral symptoms associated with brain damage
4. A measure of educational achievement
5. An appraisal of communication skills
6. Aptitude and interest testing
7. Case history data
8. Report of a physical examination

In many cases all of these data may not be needed or, if needed, can be obtained in part from school records or sources other than the psychologic examination.

Intelligence Testing It is especially important to a deaf or hearing-impaired child that he be given an individual measure of intelligence. Often, his speech and language problems and his inability to understand what is said result in academic retardation and psychosocial problems. These and other handicaps are frequently misconstrued by teachers and other to indicate a lack of intelligence. Hence, a valid measure of the child's intellectual capacity can be of tremendous value.

To obtain an accurate IQ both performance and verbal tests may be administered. However, significant discrepancies between these findings generally involve higher scores on the performance scales. Inevitably, the results on the performance measures are the more valid. The verbal scores often reflect the language handicap resulting from the hearing loss, not from the intelligence level.

Table 7 lists some appropriate performance scales for deaf and hearing-impaired children. Care has been taken to omit tests whose items are nonverbal but require verbal instructions; these are obviously inappropriate. An additional reference of special value is Smith's (1967) discussion of preschool testing with the hearing impaired. Smith has developed an outstanding test that utilizes materials available in most offices and schools. It is based on her years of work as a psychologist at the Tracy Clinic and was standardized on deaf preschool children.

Personality Evaluation   Personality evaluation is inherently a far more difficult task than intelligence testing. With hearing-impaired children, the problem is greatly compounded because almost all psychodiagnostic instruments and interview techniques require verbal and/or oral communication. For a few hearing-impaired children this may present no major obstacle, but for the overwhelming number of the hearing impaired it does. The examiner must be ultrasensitive to this possibility and not misconstrue reactions to communication difficulty as symptoms of psychopathology. For example, the writing of some uneducated deaf youths may reflect confusion and disassociation of marked degree. It may indicate an equally deranged thought process, but it is more likely to be simply a language disability unrelated to mental illness. Misdiagnoses of schizophrenia have been made primarily on the basis of bizarre written communications that actually reflected hearing impairment, not psychosis.

One way to minimize the chance of this kind of error is to administer academic achievement tests. If these tests establish a reading and vocabulary level high enough to permit paper and pencil tests or other verbal measures, then these may be used with some assurance. However, as Rosen (1967) has shown, hearing-impaired youths who have academic achievement scores within the stated reading levels of the personality tests such as the MMPI (Minnesota Multiphasic Personality Inventory) are often not able to understand the test items. This is in part attributable to verbal idiomatic expres-

Table 7. Evaluation of some of the intelligence tests most commonly used with hearing-impaired children with mental retardation or multiple handicaps

Test	Appropriate age range	Evaluation of test
Wechsler Performance Scale for Children (1949)	9–16 years	The Wechsler Performance Scale is presently the best test for deaf children ages 9–16. It yields a relatively valid IQ score and offers opportunities for qualitative interpretation of factors such as brain injury or emotional disturbance (Wechsler, 1955). It has good interest appeal and is relatively easy to administer and reasonable in cost.
Wechsler Performance Scale for Adults (1955)	16–70 years	The rating of the Wechsler Performance Scale for Adults is the same as the rating on the Wechsler Performance Scale for children.
Wechsler Preschool and Primary Scale of Intelligence Performance subtests (Wechsler, 1967)	3 years, 11 months to 6 years, 8 months	This Scale is not as good for use with deaf children as the other Wechsler scales. Picture Completion and Mazes are difficult to explain nonverbally. Other performance subtests are excellent. Standardization seems a little high.
Leiter International Performance Scale (1948 revision)	4–12 years (also suitable for older mentally retarded deaf subjects)	This test has good interest appeal. It can be used to evaluate relatively disturbed deaf children who could not otherwise be tested. This test is expensive and somewhat lacking in validation. In general, however, it is an excellent test for young deaf children. Timing is a minor factor. One disadvantage is in the interpretation of the IQ scores because the mean of the test is 95 and the standard deviation is 20. This means that the absolute normal score on this test is

Continued

Table 7—*continued*

Tests	Appropriate age range	Evaluation of test
		95 instead of 100, as on other intelligence tests. Scores of, for example, 60, therefore do not indicate mental deficiency but correspond more to about a 70 on a test such as the Wechsler or Binet. Great care must be taken in interpreting Leiter IQ scores for these reasons.
Progressive Matrices (Raven, 1948)	9 years to adulthood	Raven's Progressive Matrices are good as a second test to substantiate another more comprehensive intelligence test. The advantage of the Matrices is that they are extremely easy to administer and score, taking relatively little of the examiner's time, and are very inexpensive. They yield invalid test scores of impulsive deaf children, who tend to respond randomly rather than with accuracy and care. For this reason, the examiner should observe the child carefully to assure that the child is really trying.
Ontario School Ability Examination (Amoss, 1949)	4–10 years	This is a reasonably good test for deaf children within these age ranges.
Hiskey-Nebraska Test of Learning Aptitude (Hiskey, 1966)	3–17 years	This is a revision of the earlier (1955) version. Basically it is a sound, useful test, but somewhat weak with children 3 and 4 years old.
Chicago Non-Verbal Examination (Brown et al, 1947)	7–12 years	This test rates fair if given as an individual test, very poor if given as a group test. The scoring is tedious and reliability is rather low.

Continued

Table 7—*continued*

Tests	Appropriate age range	Evaluation of test
Grace Arthur Performance Scale (Arthur, 1947)	4.5–15.5 years	This test is poor to fair because timing is heavily emphasized, norms are not adequate, and directions are somewhat unsatisfactory. The test is especially unsatisfactory for emotionally disturbed children who are also deaf. With this type of subject, this test will sometimes yield a score indicating extreme retardation when the difficulty is actually one of below average intelligence because they often respond randomly instead of rationally.
Merrill-Palmer Scale of Mental Tests (Sutsman, 1931)	2–4 years	The Merrill-Palmer is a fair test for young deaf children, but it must be adapted in order to be used and would require a skilled examiner with a thorough knowledge of deaf children.
Goodenough Draw-A-Man Test (1926)	8.5–11 years	Directions are very difficult to give young children in a standardized manner. Scoring is less objective than would be desired, so that this test is relatively unreliable. It does, however, have some projective value in terms of personality assessment.
Randall's Island Performance Tests (1932)	2–5 years	This is one of the few nonverbal instruments available for measuring preschool children. It consists of a wide range of performance and manipulative tasks which, used by a competent examiner, provide diagnostic and insightful information. This test is relatively expensive, but valuable.

Continued

Table 7—*continued*

Tests	Appropriate age range	Evaluation of test
Dr. Alathena Smith's Test for Preschool Deaf Children	Preschool: 2–4 years	This test is not officially on the market, but the dissertation containing the necessary information can be obtained from Dr. Smith at the Tracy Clinic. The test materials are available in most psychologists' offices, and Dr. Smith gets excellent results with the test. It is the only intelligence test for deaf children in this age range that is well standardized on a large sample.
Vineland Social Maturity Scale	1–25 years[a]	This is a questionable test for deaf children generally, but can be used for very, very difficult-to-test emotionally disturbed youngsters. It is given by asking the parents questions on the development of their child. The norms of this test have to be adapted for the deaf because many of the questions involve items such as onset of speech, length of sentences, vocabulary, etc. This test is inexpensive and can be given to otherwise untestable children.

Updating of a table originally published in Vernon and Brown, 1964.

[a]These age limits are recommended by the author relative to deaf and hearing-impaired youths. The age ranges for hearing children published in the test manuals are wider.

sions used in the MMPI but not usually included in academic achievement tests.

In using personality tests it is advisable with hearing-impaired children to begin with drawing tests such as the Bender Gestalt, House-Tree-Person, or Draw-A-Person and then move into instruments such as the Rotter Completion, Three Dimensional Personality Test, or Make-a-Picture-Story. Clinical observation in play therapy settings is also valuable.

A useful general rule for psychologic evaluation is to start with the least threatening procedures. This means that aspects of the evaluation involving oral communication or verbal functioning should be kept until last. This enables the child to develop a feeling of accomplishment and pleasure in the task, and it gives the psychologist an ideal situation for establishing rapport.

Table 8 provides some specific information on some of the more popular personality tests and their use with the hearing impaired. Brenner and Thompson (1967) offer additional information of value.

Tests for Behavioral Symptoms Associated with Brain Damage
As indicated in a previous section, many of the causes of hearing impairment are also causes of brain damage and resultant learning disabilities. For this reason, a thorough psychologic evaluation of a deaf or hearing-impaired multiply handicapped or mentally retarded child should include psychologic testing for brain damage.

This testing always must be done with full awareness of the severe limitations of psychodiagnostic instruments for detection of brain damage. They are but one of many kinds of data, including neurologic examinations, electroencephalograms, and medical histories, that are usually required to make conclusive findings, except in cases of children where the damage is gross, as in hemiplegias, athetoid cerebral palsies, and advanced chronic brain syndromes. However, neurologic examinations and electroencephalograms are also limited in their diagnostic potentials. Hence, psychologists should use the best instruments available to them, report their findings conservatively, and refer to other disciplines for further clinical investigation when warranted.

The relatively high prevalence of brain damage among deaf and hearing-impaired children is a fact. The development of effective educational and other therapies for these children is contingent on identification and delineation of the problem. Table 9 lists some tests relevant to this purpose.

Educational Achievement Measurement A full psychologic
evaluation of a deaf or hearing-impaired child should include an assessment of educational level. A major reason for this is the prevalence
of academic difficulty in this group, especially in those who are also
mentally retarded. The most appropriate tests for obtaining this information are the Metropolitan or the Stanford achievement tests. Both
have norms for hearing and deaf subjects. They are relatively easy to
administer, but the examiner must make certain that the child understands and successfully completes the sample items for each subtest.
Another critical point in using these or any achievement test is to
choose a battery that is at a level appropriate to the person being tested.

In interpreting results of achievement testing with deaf or hearing-
impaired children, it is important to keep in mind not only the average
achievement levels for the normal hearing but also those for the deaf
and more severely hearing impaired. Only about 5% of graduates from
day and residential schools for the deaf attain a 10th-grade level in
educational achievement, 41% seventh or eighth grade, 27% fifth or
sixth grade, and approximately 30% are fourth grade or below (Vernon, 1971). Most of the last category is termed functionally illiterate
by present governmental standards.

Evaluation of Communication Skills Hearing impairment presents its major handicap in the realm of communication. Thus, an
evaluation should include an assessment of communication skills.

Several dimensions of communication should be appraised in
a hearing-impaired child. First is the ability to read and write because
these determine educational and vocational potential. Achievement
tests provide reading levels. The use of several of the verbal subtests
of the Wechsler yield a reasonably accurate picture of writing skills.
Sentence completion tests can be used also.

Speech and speechreading are other communication skills to
be assessed. These processes have educational and vocational potential to the hearing-impaired child. Psychologists can assess in practical lay terms the intelligibility and pleasantness of the speech. These
should be noted in the psychologic report.

Speechreading skill is a more complex function to measure.
Audiologic skills are needed to do this thoroughly. However,
whether or not the youngster is able to understand most of what is
said in a one-to-one situation is important. It is also helpful if some
note can be made of the extent to which the youngster depends on
visual clues (speechreading) and the degree to which he is able to

Table 8. Personality tests used with hearing-impaired children with mental retardation or multiple handicaps

Tests	Appropriate age range	Evaluation of test
Draw-A-Person (Machover, 1949)	9 years to adulthood	This is a good screening device for detecting very severe emotional problems. It is relatively nonverbal and is probably the most practical projective personality test for deaf children. Its interpretation is very subjective and in the hands of a poor psychologist it can result in rather extreme diagnostic statements about deaf children.
Thematic Apperception Test (TAT) or Children's Apperception Test (CAT) (Stein, 1955)	Can be used with deaf subjects of school age through adulthood who can communicate very well in written language	This ; a test of great potential, if the psychologist giving it and the deaf subject taking it can both communicate with fluency in manual communication. It is of very limited value otherwise, unless the deaf subject has an exceptional command of the English language. This test could be given through an interpreter by an exceptionally perceptive psychologist, although it is more desirable if the psychologist can do his own communicating.
Rorschach Ink Blot Test (Rorschach, 1942)	Can be given to deaf subjects as soon as they are able to communicate fluently manually or if they can communicate with exceptional skill orally	In order for the Rorschach to be used, it is almost absolutely necessary that the psychologist giving it and the deaf subject taking it be fluent in manual communication. Even under these circumstances, it is debatable if it yields much of value unless the subject is of above average intelligence. It would be possible with a very bright deaf subject, who had a remarkable proficiency in English, to give a Rorschach through writing, but this would not be very satisfactory.

Continued

Table 8—*continued*

Test	Appropriate age range	Evaluation of test
H.T.P. Technique (Buck, 1949)	School age through adulthood	This is a procedure similar to the Draw-A-Person test. It requires little verbal communication and affords the competent clinician some valuable insight into basic personality dynamics of the subject.
Rotter Incomplete Sentences Blank (Rotter and Rafferty, 1950)	At least fifth grade reading level	This test is useful with subjects who understand the vocabulary of the test; however, many hard-of-hearing youth do not. Some experienced examiners substitute simple terms for some of the complex ones on the test.
Make-A-Picture-Story Test (MAPS) (Schneidman, 1952)	About same as TAT and CAT above except that it is somewhat less verbal	This test is basically the same as the CAT or TAT except that there are actual figures and a stage that can be moved about and grouped in ways that are indicative of social and personality dynamics.

Updating of a table originally published in Vernon and Brown, 1964.

Table 9. Tests for the indirect measure of brain injury for hearing-impaired children with multiple handicaps

Tests	Evaluation of test
Wechsler Performance Scale	Pattern analysis of these scales is of controversial validity as a diagnostic tool. There is fairly general agreement, however, that in the hands of a capable clinical psychologist a partial qualitative type of diagnosis is possible.
Diamond Drawing from the Stanford-Binet	This test has good validity, is generally available, can be easily administered.
Bender-Gestalt	This test seems to have possibilities, but scoring norms are inadequate and, at present, its interpretation is rather subjective. The Koppitz system is valuable in objectifying scoring.
Goodenough Draw-A-Man Test and Machover Human Figure Drawing Interpretations	Listed together for convenience, these measures, particularly the latter, reveal symptoms such as impulsiveness, rigidity, anxiety, and perceptual difficulties, but here again, scoring for brain injury lacks standardization.
Ellis Test	This test has definite possibilities but lacks validation.
Marble Board	This test is potentially excellent, but very hard to get. Scoring instructions are inadequate.
Hiskey Blocks	These blocks require a great deal of visualization and abstract ability and are of value for this reason.
Rorschach	Its use requires not only competency in the use of the test, but also a fluency in the use of the manual communication used by the deaf. Results reported where these conditions are not met are of highly dubious validity.
Kohs Blocks	These are similar to the block design subtest of the Wechsler but are more extensive. A qualitative diagnosis is possible, but norms are lacking for organic involvement.
Various measures of motor ability and development	Among these would be the railwalking test, tests of laterality, and certain items on the Vineland Social Maturity Scale that pertain to motor development.

Adapted from Vernon and Brown, 1964.

use auditory stimuli; these data give some indication of his ability to communicate in groups. If the psychologist covers his mouth or asks the child to turn his back during conversation, the role of speechreading can be roughly estimated.

The audiologist is usually the primary authority in the area of communication. The psychologist functions only as a lay observer. He must be particularly careful to indicate in his report whether or not his observations were in a relatively quiet one-to-one situation or whether he also assessed communication skills in other settings. The youth's ability to understand speech in a group situation such as a classroom, job, or social setting may be totally different and generally far less effective.

One issue must be made clear in evaluating communication skills. Many extremely intelligent and capable deaf and hearing-impaired youths lack the aptitude and/or ability to speak and speechread fluently. Psychologists must not confuse difficulty in communication with lack of intelligence. Such an error can have drastic consequences. It is also possible that a congenitally deaf or hearing-impaired person may have a very high IQ but a poor vocabulary and inadequate linguistic competence. The psychologist must be keenly aware of these factors in order to be fair and helpful to a deaf or hearing-impaired youngster. A more extensive discussion of the assessment of communication skills is presented by Cox and Lloyd (this volume) and Siegel and Broen (this volume).

Aptitude and Interest Testing   A basic part of a complete psychologic evaluation for older youth is aptitude testing, i.e., finding out the particular abilities that a person may have. As there are hundreds of tests for this on the market, it is not feasible to list or discuss them individually. Levine (1960 and 1971) covered this topic relative to the hearing impaired with excellence and completeness; however, certain information about the following three general areas of aptitude is often of great value because these kinds of aptitudes are directly related to the types of work most deaf and hearing-impaired adults do:

1. Manual dexterity
2. Mechanical aptitudes
3. Spatial relations

In selecting from the many available measures of aptitude it is important to choose some tests that do not primarily depend on language for either their directions or administration.

Interest tests, with one significant exception, are highly verbal. Therefore, they generally cannot be used effectively with hearing-impaired persons. The exception is the Wide Range Interest Opinion Test, which involves choosing interests from among pictures that depict various work- and recreation-related activities.

It would be inappropriate to discuss tests without mention of the General Aptitude Test Battery. As now constructed, this test discriminates against language-impaired persons. With the exception of certain parts, it yields misinformation on the aptitudes of deaf clients because of its verbal makeup.

Case History Data   The past is still the one best predictor of the future. For this reason complete background information on a hearing-impaired child is essential. This is especially important because the child may not be accurately evaluated with regular psychologic procedures. Illustrative of just how essential case history data are, is that the best psychiatric and psychologic evaluations are often based 75% on background information.

Audiologic Reports, Physical Examinations, and Medical History   The findings of the audiologist and the speech pathologist are basic to a comprehensive psychologic evaluation of a hearing-impaired multiply handicapped child. These specialists report in depth on communication, an important part of what is generally integral to the child's problem. As this area is thoroughly covered in other chapters of this volume (Cox and Lloyd; Siegel and Broen), it is not further elaborated here.

It is often extremely beneficial to a psychologist to obtain some data on a hearing-impaired child's physical condition and medical history. Especially useful is information about etiology of hearing impairment. As noted in a previous section, many of the causes of impaired hearing also result in brain damage, learning disability, visual problems, seizures, mental retardation, aphasia, motor deficiency, orthopedic difficulties, cardiac anomalies, and behavior disturbances. These conditions are obviously highly relevant to a child's functioning and to a meaningful psychologic evaluation. Often they are best understood if medical data are available.

All of these eight aspects of psychologic evaluation are not necessary for every hearing-impaired youth, nor is it essential that the psychologist be the one who obtains all of the data that comprise the evaluation. It is important, though, that the psychologist have all of the available data and is able to integrate the diverse information. Every psychologist should have the release and request forms needed to obtain these kinds of information.

By interrelating IQ, educational, and other facts about a hearing-impaired child, it is possible to derive a picture that reveals the role played by the hearing impairment. If the youth's profile is similar to that of his normal hearing peer, his loss and the way it has been coped with is not particularly disabling. By contrast, if the profile is similar to that of a deaf child, then the loss has had major effects on communication, language development, and education. Appropriate planning for the deaf or hearing-impaired child and for the child with normal hearing vary drastically. What would be constructive for one would be devastating for the other. A psychologic evaluation that does not fully address itself to this communication issue has failed to serve one of its major functions. The issue cannot be handled without comprehensive information. Shortcuts will not suffice, and hasty, inadequate evaluations are unethical and wasteful of human resources.

Differential Diagnosis

Differential diagnosis, a popular but somewhat redundant term, is most relevant to the psychologist working with multiply handicapped hearing-impaired children in terms of the problem of distinguishing between deafness, autism, mental retardation, brain damage, and childhood schizophrenia or determining the extent to which aspects of these major pathologies are present. Those with experience in hospitals for the retarded are aware that these facilities often have entire units where there are children with symptoms characterizing one or more of these five considerations yet who cannot be clearly diagnosed. For example, the author once tested the deaf son of a deaf minister who got perfect scores on the WISC Block Designs, who could take apart and reassemble clocks and watches, and who wired his room with all sorts of intricate lighting and switching devices. However, his overall score on a series of six different IQ tests was never over 60, his behavior was bizarre, and he was never accepted for admission to any school. On several occasions he had been in hospitals for the retarded, but his parents always took him out after short stays. He had at various times been diagnosed as retarded, autistic, schizophrenic, brain damaged, and deaf. In any large school for the deaf, at least one extreme case of this type per year is generally seen and a number of similar, but milder cases are evaluated.

The full answer to the problem of differential diagnosis of severely hearing-impaired children lies far beyond the scope of this chapter, and for that matter neither the methods of diagnosis nor the appropriate therapies are completely known. Multidisciplinary technique and full case histories are obviously essential.

PRAGMATICS AND PSYCHODIAGNOSTICS IN SCHOOLS

In addition to the almost overwhelming theoretical problems of psychodiagnostics with multiply handicapped deaf and hearing-impaired children, the school psychologist faces a serious practical dilemma: how to report diagnostic findings in a way that is in both the child's interests and the school's interest, yet that fully conveys the psychologist's knowledge about the child. This very difficult task centers around whether or not to label a person as having a pathology.

Unfortunately, the current stage in understanding human learning and how to teach makes it extremely difficult to cope with deaf children who are aphasic, schizophrenic, autistic, severely brain damaged, etc. Hence, to label youngsters in this way on school reports is unlikely to help them and instead quite often stigmatizes them. Such labels tend to be grasped and clung to by teachers and administrators in order to rationalize failure to provide the best possible academic and vocational opportunity for these "diagnosed children." Rarely are pathologic diagnostic terms used as the basis for constructive therapies or remedial programs because such programs are relatively unknown or are often poorly developed and little understood. Psychologists, though often quick to label children in these ways, too rarely assume responsibility for specifying in operational terms what can be done.

Another example of destructive labeling occurs in the reporting of psychosexual development. Psychologists, especially those who are struggling with their own problems in this area or who are anxious to impress others with their understanding of psychodynamics, often report possible latent homosexuality in a deaf youth or else describe guilt or anxiety over masturbation or fantasy life. Because some of these traits are normal in adolescents, as well as being present in many adults, there is not much constructive value in describing a deaf child to school staffs in these terms. More importantly, when these kinds of descriptions are sent to teachers and administrators, some of whom are repressed inhibited individuals, the child is often perceived of as some sort of depraved sexual monster. As such, the child arouses all sorts of anxieties and resultant hostile rejecting behavior in his teachers.

Ideally, a psychologic report should state in operational terms exactly what kind of treatment and remediation should be instituted. In practice this is rarely possible. However, some specific ways to cope with the problems described in the report should be provided along with referrals to available local services that might be useful in helping the patient. The remaining chapters in this volume focus on intervention strategies rather than labels.

SUMMARY

There is evidence from research, from inductive reasoning, and from the observations of experienced professionals that many hearing-impaired children have disabilities in addition to their hearing impairment. Conditions such as cerebral palsy, aphasia, emotional disturbance, seizures, mental retardation, visual defects, and orthopedic problems are more common among deaf than among the nondeaf. At present, psychodiagnosticians lack the instruments and baseline data to assess adequately most of the behavioral aspects of multiple handicaps, although some tests and a small amount of normative information of value are available.

The importance of extreme care in the use of pathologic labels in describing deaf children in school psychologic reports cannot be overemphasized. Such labels generally have destructive effects and rarely contribute to better care and education.

Although this chapter primarily focuses on the psychologic evaluation of the hearing-impaired child, the major issues of and the approach to the evaluation process can be generalized to most children with communication problems. The most critical of these issues is the effect of language and communication on the psychologic evaluation process and the results obtained.

REFERENCES

Amoss, H. 1949. Ontario School Ability Examination. Ryerson, Toronto.
Arthur, G. 1947. A Point Scale of Performance Tests, Rev. Form II. Psychological Corporation, New York.
Brenner, L. O., and R. E. Thompson. 1967. The use of projective techniques in the personality evaluation of deaf adults. J. Rehab. Deaf 1:17–30.

Brill, R. G. 1963. Deafness and the genetic factor. Amer. Ann. Deaf 108:359–372.

Brown, A., S. Stein, and R. Rohrer. 1947. Chicago Non-Verbal Examination. Psychological Corporation, New York.

Buck, J. 1949. The H.T.P. technique: A qualitative and quantitative scoring manual. J. Clin. Psychol. 4 (1948), 5 (1949).

Danish, J. M., J. K. Tillson, and M. Levitan. 1963. Multiple anomalies in congenitally deaf children. Eugenics Q. 10:12–21.

Doll, E. A. 1947. Vineland Social Maturity Scale: Manual of Directions. Educational Testing Bureau, Minneapolis.

Fraser, G. R. 1964. Profound childhood deafness. J. Med. Genet. 1: 118–151.

Goodenough, F. 1926. Measurement of Intelligence by Drawings. World Book Co., Chicago.

Hiskey, M. S. 1966. Hiskey-Nebraska Test of Learning Aptitude. Union College Press, Lincoln, Neb.

Illingsworth, R. S. 1958. Recent Advances in Cerebral Palsy. Little, Brown, Boston.

Konigswork, B. W. 1971. Hereditary congenital severe deafness syndromes. Ann. Otol. Rhinol. Laryngol. 80:269–289.

Lane, H. S., and J. L. Schneider. 1941. A performance test for school age deaf children. Amer. Ann. Deaf 86:441.

Levine, E. S. 1960. Psychology of deafness. Columbia University Press, New York.

Levine, E. S. 1971. Mental assessment of the deaf child. Volta Rev. 73:80–105.

Leiter, R. L. 1948. The Leiter International Performance Scale. Stoelting, Chicago.

Machover, K. 1949. Personality Projection in the Drawing of the Human Figure. Charles C Thomas, Springfield, Ill.

Mengel, M. C., B. W. Konigsmark, C. I. Berlin, and V. A. McKusick. 1967. Recessive early-onset neural deafness. Acta Otolaryngol. 64: 313–326.

Mindel, E., and M. Vernon. 1971. They grow in silence. National Association of the Deaf, Silver Spring, Md.

Myklebust, H. R. 1960. The psychology of deafness. Grune & Stratton, New York.

Myklebust, H. R., A. Neyhus, and A. Mulholland. 1962. Guidance and counseling for the deaf. Amer. Ann. Deaf 107:383–408.

Randall's Island Performance Series, The. (Manual). 1932. Stoelting, Chicago.

Raven, J. 1948. Progressive Matrices. Psychological Corporation, New York.

Rorschach, H. 1942. Psychodiagnostics. Hans Huber, Berne, Switzerland.

Rosen, A. 1967. Limitations of personality inventories for assessment of deaf children and adults as illustrated by research with the MMPI. J. Rehab. Deaf 1:47–52.

Rotter, J. B., and J. E. Rafferty. 1950. The Rotter Incomplete Sentence Blank. Psychological Corporation, New York.

Schneidman, E. S. 1952. Make a Picture Story (MAPS) Manual. Teachers College (Bur. Publ.), New York.

Smith, A. J. 1967. Psychological testing of the preschool deaf child: A challenge for changing times, pp. 162–181. Proceedings of International Conference on Oral Education of the Deaf. Vol. 1. A. G. Bell Association for the Deaf, Washington, D.C.

Stein, M. I. 1955. The Thematic Apperception Test. 2nd. Ed. Addison-Wesley, Reading, Mass.

Sutsman, R. 1931. Mental Measurement of Preschool Children. World Book Co., Yonkers on Hudson, N.Y.

Vernon, M. 1969a. Multiply handicapped deaf children: Medical, educational, and psychological considerations. Research Monograph, Council for Exceptional Children, Washington, D.C.

Vernon, M. 1969b. Usher's syndrome—deafness and progressive blindness: Clinical cases, prevention, theory, and literature survey. J. Chron. Dis. 133–151.

Vernon, M. 1971. Crises of the deaf. J. Rehab. 37:31–33, 39.

Vernon, M., and D. W. Brown. 1964. A guide to psychological tests and testing procedures in the evaluation of deaf and hard-of-hearing children. J. Speech Hear. Disord. 29:414–423.

Wechsler, D. 1955. Wechsler Intelligence Scale for Children. Psychological Corporation, New York.

Wechsler, D. 1955. Wechsler Adult Intelligence Scale. Psychological Corporation, New York.

Wechsler, D. 1967. Wechsler Preschool and Primary Scale of Intelligence. Psychological Corporation, New York.

6

BEHAVIOR ANALYSIS, BEHAVIOR MODIFICATION, AND DEVELOPMENTAL DISABILITIES

Joseph E. Spradlin,
George R. Karlan, and Bruce Wetherby

CONTENTS

Basic Principles of Measurement and Design _____ 227
    Measurement/228
    Design/229

Basic Principles of Behavior _____ 233
    Types of behavior/233
    Effects of different consequences: reinforcement and punishment/234
    Stimulus control/235
    Contingencies of reinforcement/239

**Behavioral Principles and Analysis of Generalization
and Transfer** _____ 242
    Response classes/243
    Stimulus classes/245
    Functional equivalence in language/250

**Implications for Task Analysis in Development of Complex
Performances** _____ 252
    Selection of useful terminal performances/252
    Organization of materials and procedures to produce terminal
        performances/253

Summary and Conclusions _____ 258

References _____ 259

The term *developmental disabilities* includes a range of disorders resulting from a combination of genetic, prenatal, and postnatal environmental factors. For more information on development disabilities see Bensberg and Sigelman (this volume). The critical features in most developmental disabilities are behavioral. For example, deficiencies of a blind, deaf, congenital aphasic, autistic, or retarded child may be the result of biologic abnormalities, but the problems the child presents are behavioral. Blind children do not respond appropriately to visual stimuli. Thus, special prosthetic training devices and environments must be used to help them develop the behavior necessary to adapt to their social and physical environment. Deaf children do not respond appropriately to auditory stimuli suitable for their hearing peers. If such children are to adapt, they also must be given special training and prosthetic devices. Finally, congenitally aphasic, autistic, and retarded children all show behavioral deficits that set them apart from their peers. These deficits must be remediated if developmentally disabled children are to succeed in the environment of normal children.

Procedures for remediating behavioral deficits or developing compensatory skills almost always involve precise measurement of behavior and teaching or modification of behavior through careful management of the physical and social environment of the child. Therefore, the first section of this chapter covers the basic principles involved in measurement and design. The second section presents the principles of behavior on which effective training programs may be based. The third section extends the basic behavioral principles from the second section to account for the complex organization of human behavior. The final section outlines some of the structural issues involved in behavior measurement, in teaching developmentally disabled children, and in organizing remediation programs for the developmentally disabled.

BASIC PRINCIPLES OF MEASUREMENT AND DESIGN

Measurement provides the means of operationalizing and quantifying behavior so that it becomes possible to measure the effects of a particular modification procedure or technique on behavior. The direc-

This chapter was partially supported by PHS Training Grant HD 00183 and by Grants HD 00870 and HD 02528 from the National Institute of Child Health and Human Development to the Kansas Center for Research in Mental Retardation and Human Development.

tion, magnitude, and stability of change are important in evaluating the significance of treatment effects. The manner in which these three variables are related comprise the issues of measurement. This section describes several methods of measurement, followed by a discussion of research design in behavior analysis.

Measurement

Behavior analysts have, in the past, preferred *rate* measures, which indicate how frequently a person engages in a given behavior in a given situation (Skinner, 1938; Lindsley, 1964). Rate of behavior is determined by observation, permanent records left by behavior, or by mechanical recording.

Discrete behaviors under timed conditions, such as the number of words read aloud correctly in 5 minutes or the number of words written correctly in 5 minutes, are easily recorded. Other behaviors, such as the number of babbling responses made by an infant or a severely retarded child, may be difficult to measure reliably. It may be easier and more reliable to measure the total amount of time the infant or child is engaged in babbling. Moreover, the amount of time the infant babbles may be a much more useful measure. Two children might babble only once during the morning, but one child might babble for 5 seconds while the other might babble for the entire morning. In such a case, *duration,* or the amount of time engaged in babbling, is the most desirable measure.

Another measure may be obtained by breaking a given period of time into intervals and then simply determining whether a given behavior does or does not occur during each interval. This is called *interval recording.* Interval recording is practical for gathering reliable data for behaviors that last for long durations or that occur at such a rapid rate that recording each instance is difficult or impossible. For a more complete discussion of this method, see Hall (1971) and Bijou, Peterson, and Ault (1968).

Rate measures, duration measures, and interval measures are appropriate when the rate at which a behavior occurs depends on the child. However, some behaviors, such as the number of questions a child can answer during a given period, are determined by the teacher or experimenter. In such cases, the *percentage* of questions answered may be a better measure than the number of questions answered. This is especially true if the number of response opportunities varies from day to day. Percentage of correct responses are especially useful in evaluating a child in an educational situation.

Two less frequently used measures are the *force* of a response and the *latency* between the occurrence of a stimulus and the occurrence of a stimulus and the occurrence of the response. Force or intensity is a good measure in a remediation program for a child who speaks at very low voice levels. Latency, like all other measures, has a long history in behavioral experimentation. Changes in latency have been used to evaluate the effects of a behavior modification program for children who show extremely long latencies between the time an instruction is given and the time they comply with it (Fjellstedt and Sulzer-Azarof, 1973). McLean (personal communication, 1969) used latency measurements to evaluate a program for reducing the time it took a young man to reply to questions. Force and latency measures are appropriate measures under certain conditions. Both force and latency can be shaped by applying increasingly stringent contingencies.

Sometimes (in speech) it is useful to measure the variety of words used. A typical measure of variety is the *type-token ratio*. This measure consists of the number of different words used (types) divided by the total number of words used in the sample of words (tokens). This measure is useful in evaluating the effects of procedures that increase or reduce redundancy in speech.

There is no universal formula or rule for selecting a measurement technique. All have a common goal: to define behavior so that it may be reliably and objectively quantified. The technique should be selected to meet the demands of the situation in which measurement will occur and to record accurately the form of the behavior to be measured.

Design

Applied behavior analysis starts with a *baseline observation period*. This baseline observation period is used to evaluate the behaviors in need of treatment. Usually, a subject or group of subjects is observed before introducing a behavioral treatment. Once a specific behavior or set of behaviors has been observed long enough to determine that the behavior under consideration is not changing, a modification procedure is instituted, and the behavior is again observed to determine whether or not it increases or decreases from baseline levels. Such a design is frequently called an *AB design* and is usually not very compelling unless the baseline is extremely stable and the change in behavior immediately follows the introduction of the treatment. Even when the baseline is stable and the change promptly follows the introduction of the treatment, the design does not yield conclusive results because of the possibility of accidental occurrence of confounding variables. Sometimes the treatment can be introduced and withdrawn, as in the introduction and withdrawal of reinforcement of a response. The simple AB design should be extended to an ABAB, or *reversal design,* whenever feasible. Validation then becomes simply a matter of introducing and withdrawing the treatment until the demonstration of control is convincing (Sidman, 1960).

For example, Hall (1970) used a reversal design to demonstrate the effect of contingent reinforcement for appropriate verbalization by a brain-injured child. His results are shown in Figure 1 in which the parts of the ABAB design are labeled ABCD. Hall first took 3 days of baseline measures during which contingent reinforcement was not delivered. The baseline level of behavior was stable and at a low rate. He then introduced his treatment and maintained it for 30 ses-

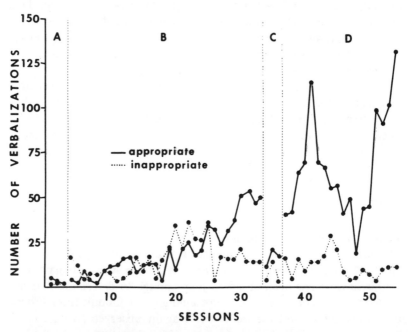

Figure 1. Record of Jackie's appropriate and inappropriate verbalization. A: baseline period before contingent reinforcement; B: reinforcement period, verbalizations reinforced by food, play materials, and the experimenter's attention; C: reversal period, return to baseline conditions of noncontingent reinforcement; D: second reinforcement period, return to procedures of contingent reinforcement. (From Hall, 1970; reprinted by permission.)

sions. The number of appropriate responses per session increased to approximately 50. However, because the rate of increase is very slow, the results in terms of an AB design are far from compelling. However, when the contingency was removed in condition C, the rate of appropriate responses per session quickly returned to a low level. This return to a low rate increases one's confidence that contingent reinforcement is an effective experimental variable. Confidence is increased even more by the increase in rate that occurred when contingent reinforcement was reintroduced in condition D. The application of this design is also discussed by Baker (this volume).

Not all of the effects of experimental treatments are reversible. For example, once a severely retarded child is trained in communication behaviors, these behaviors may (and hopefully do) come under the control of social contingencies in the child's natural environment. This usually prevents a reversal effect from occurring. When behaviors are not reversible or when reversing the treatment has undesirable effects, as it would with most communicative skills, other designs are used. One such design is the *multiple baseline* design (Baer, Wolf, and Risley, 1968). The multiple baseline design involves applying a treatment across conditions that may include changes in settings, behaviors, or subjects. A treatment may be applied to different behaviors of the same subject at different times, or it may be applied to the same behavior of a subject across different settings at different times. A treatment also may be applied to the same behavior of different subjects at different times. A difference in the time of application of a treatment across the conditions is always necessary. This yields the most compelling demonstration of control over behavior by a particular treatment.

A study by Baer, Rowbury, and Baer (1973) included a multiple baseline across different subjects. Initially, a baseline was obtained for percentage of compliance with three subjects, Hannah, Charlotte, and Frankie (see Figure 2). Then, after differing lengths of baseline, a treatment (B), which involved reinforcement of compliance, was introduced. In each case, the percentage of compliance increased when treatment B was introduced. The relative effectiveness of treatment B varied across the three subjects, but the general results suggested that treatment B did increase the desired behavior. As in the case with any baseline study, the results are less convincing when the baseline is unstable and the effects of treatment are not immediate and substantial.

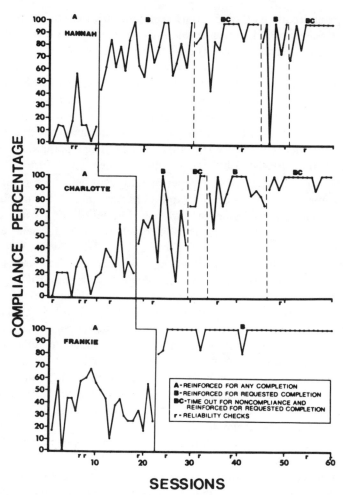

Figure 2. Daily percentage of compliance with invitations received for three children studied, across experimental conditions. A: baseline—subjects received reinforcement for three completions of any task; B: differential reinforcement of compliance—subjects received reinforcement for requested three completions; BC: differential reinforcement of compliance plus time out for noncompliance—a 1-minute time out in a chair for noncompliance added to differential reinforcement of compliance. (From Baer, Rowbury, and Baer, 1973; reprinted by permission.)

In summary, reversal designs and multiple baseline designs are two very useful designs for evaluating behavioral treatment effects with a single subject or small number of subjects (Sidman, 1960;

Risley and Wolf, 1972). Effective treatment evaluation involves: 1) the precise specification and quantification of a specific behavior under study, and 2) the use of a design that allows for comparison of treatment and nontreatment conditions. Only through the consideration of these two issues can the effectiveness of a particular intervention technique or program be evaluated.

BASIC PRINCIPLES OF BEHAVIOR

A powerful technology for changing human behavior currently exists. That technology has been formally designated *applied behavior analysis* (Baer, Wolf, and Risley, 1968). It is based upon well established behavioral principles that have a long history in the field of psychology and that have been explicitly stated by many writers (Skinner, 1938, 1953, 1969; Keller and Schoenfeld, 1950; Lindsley, 1964; Ferster and Perrott, 1967). A central focus for these principles is the notion that the important units of analysis in psychology are behavioral events that can be objectively observed, classified, and measured. These behavioral events are related or controlled by events in the individual's environment. The critical task for experimenters is to determine the functional relations between environmental events and behavior. Hence, experimentation based on these notions is often called the *experimental* or *functional analysis of behavior*.

Types of Behavior

Behavior can be divided into two very broad classes: *respondent behavior* as exemplified in the research of Pavlov (1960), and *operant behavior* as exemplified by the research of Skinner (1938).

Respondent behavior is controlled by an eliciting stimulus that precedes the response. For example, a bite of food in the mouth elicits salivation, or an electric shock elicits changes in skin moisture and resistance. In respondent behavior, an unconditioned "eliciting" stimulus elicits the response. Moreover, an initially neutral stimulus that is repeatedly paired with the unconditioned stimulus soon acquires eliciting properties of its own. For example, a dentist's white coat itself may elicit anxiety or fear responses. Respondent behavior is important because it relates very closely to behavior problems such as phobias. Much of desensitization therapy is based on the extinction and counterconditioning of respondent behavior. A review of this field of therapy and behavior change may be found in Meyer and Chesser (1970).

Although respondent behavior is important in many disabilities involving a strong emotional component, this chapter focuses primarily on operant behavior. Operant behavior is a better analog for the development of skilled behavior, for the remediation of behavioral deficits, and for the assessment and treatment of communication problems. Operant behavior is controlled by its consequences. That is, whether the rate or probability of operant behavior increases or decreases is a function of what stimulus or events occur after the response has occurred. The stimuli or events that follow a behavior may be called the *consequence*.

Effects of Different Consequences: Reinforcement and Punishment

Consequences involve the presentation or removal of stimuli. These stimuli are called *positive reinforcers* and *negative reinforcers*. Positive reinforcers are stimuli that increase the rate or probability of the response on which they are contingent. Negative reinforcers, or *aversive stimuli,* decrease the rate or probability of the response on which they are contingent. The presentation of aversive stimuli contingent on behavior is called *punishment*. Whether a reinforcer is positive or negative depends on its effect on the behavior of the individual. An example of a consequence that is considered a negative reinforcer for behavior but often turns out to be a positive reinforcer is contingent verbal disapproval. Verbal disapproval is a form of social attention, and, for a child who rarely receives encouraging attention at home or school, social disapproval (when contingent on undesirable behavior) may maintain or increase the rate of undesirable behavior. Studies have demonstrated that, when undesirable behaviors no longer result in attention and more desirable forms of behavior result in social attention, the level of undesirable behavior decreases and the level of desirable behavior increases (Zimmerman and Zimmerman, 1962; Harris, Wolf, and Baer, 1967).

What for most children is an aversive event may be for specific children a positive reinforcer, and a customarily positive reinforcer can turn out to be an aversive event for a specific child. For example, swimming is a positive reinforcer for most children, but it is not for one who is afraid of drowning. It is the functional properties of an event that determine whether it is classed as a positive or negative reinforcer, not the preconceived notions of the experimenter, clinician, or teacher.

Just as presentation of a stimulus can increase or decrease the probability or rate of behavior, removing a stimulus can decrease or increase the rate of the behavior on which such removal is contingent. Termination of an ongoing positive reinforcer has been used to eliminate or reduce the probability of a specific undesirable response. Baer (1962) demonstrated that termination of a movie contingent on thumb sucking could be used to reduce the percentage of time that a subject engaged in thumb sucking. Barrett (1962) demonstrated that disruption of music each time a subject exhibited a tic-like response resulted in the reduction of such responses. This procedure of withdrawing a positive reinforcer contingent on behavior is often called punishment.

The termination of aversive stimuli, or negative reinforcers, to increase rates has not been widely used in applied behavior analysis. However, examples of this contingency are readily found in the natural environment. Parents and other caretakers engage in all sorts of behavior to terminate the crying or tantrums of children. Their actions are reinforced by the termination of the child's crying. Children cry or run to their mothers to terminate the threats of the bully or aggressive child. These instances are examples of behaviors that are maintained by the elimination or termination of a negative reinforcer. Unfortunately, in operant terminology, the termination of a negative reinforcer has been labeled "negative reinforcement." The labeling confuses this procedure with punishment. Negative reinforcement is the removal of an aversive event contingent on a response while punishment is the delivery of an aversive event contingent on a response.

A summary of the effects of presenting and withdrawing positive and negative reinforcers contingent on behavior is shown in Table 1.

Stimulus Control

Stimulus control is established by the different reinforcement contingencies occurring under different conditions. Perhaps the simplest example of stimulus control or discrimination is that which occurs when a response is reinforced in the presence of one stimulus and not in the presence of other stimuli. Under such conditions, the response comes to be emitted in the presence of the stimulus under which it is reinforced and not to be emitted in the presence of stimuli that do not result in reinforcement.

Table 1. Effects of various contingencies on rate or probability of behavior

Type of reinforcer	Reinforcer withdrawn	Reinforcer presented
Positive	Decreases rate or probability (punishment)	Increases rate or probability (positive reinforcement)
Negative	Increases probability (negative reinforcement)	Decreases rate or probability (punishment)

No behavior is reinforced in all situations. Behavior that is appropriate in some situations is totally inappropriate in other situations. For example, it might be appropriate for a young deaf child to use manual signs in the presence of adults or older children, but the use of manual signs might not be an appropriate form of communication among normal hearing preschool peers.

A classic example of establishing stimulus control by reinforcing a response in the presence of a stimulus and not reinforcing a response when the stimulus is not present is found in the audiometric testing of difficult-to-test persons (Cox and Lloyd, this volume; Lloyd, 1966; Lloyd, Spradlin, and Reid, 1968; Spradlin et al., 1968; Spradlin, Locke, and Fulton, 1969; Fulton and Spradlin, 1971; Fulton and Spradlin, 1974a, b). Severely retarded individuals in this experiment were required to make a simple button-press response in the presence of a tone. When they made this response the tone terminated, a chime rang, the reinforcement tray lit up, and a bit of food dropped into the reinforcement tray. If they responded when the tone was not present, no observable change in the environment occurred. However, a press of the button when the tone was not there automatically precluded the possibility of the tone occurring for at least 5 seconds. This delay of the onset of the tone obviated the possibility that a response during the absence of the tone would be reinforced by the onset of the tone and subsequent food reinforcement. Operant audiometry made it possible to test the hearing of severely retarded children and other difficult-to-test individuals, like infants as young as 7 months.

Errorless Discrimination Although the above procedure is effective, it does allow the child to make a large number of responses when the tone is not present. For many years extinction of responses to the negative stimulus was considered an essential part of the discrimination learning process. However, Terrace (1963) described a procedure for establishing stimulus control; the procedure has been labeled "errorless discrimination." Terrace conducted the original work with pigeons. However, the procedure is applicable to the type of discrimination used in audiometric testing with difficult-to-test children.

Suppose that a child is brought into a testing situation and a light is presented continuously. When the child presses a button in the presence of the light, reinforcement is delivered as previously described. After the child is consistently pressing the button, the experimenter waits until it seems unlikely that the child will press the button, perhaps when the child is busy retrieving the food. At this point the light is briefly interrupted. The length of time the light is interrupted is gradually increased. However, every effort is made to ensure that the subject does not respond when the light is absent. Using this procedure, it is very likely that discrimination similar to that described above could be established with other responses when the light was not present.

Stimulus Shaping and Stimulus Fading   Errorless discrimination may be used when it is necessary to establish a new discrimination. It is sometimes desirable, however, to refine or extend a discrimination that the child already exhibits. Or perhaps the aim is to establish a new discrimination, using a previously learned discrimination as the basis. Stoddard and Sidman (1967) demonstrated that a complex circle-ellipse discrimination could be established by *stimulus fading* and *stimulus shaping* procedures. They used a match-to-sample apparatus with nine square keys on which forms were projected by a slide projector. Their subjects were severely retarded persons. They initially trained their subjects to press a lighted key located among the eight darkened keys. Next, a circle was presented on the lighted key. They then presented a series of trials in which the unlighted keys were gradually illuminated across trials. The subjects continued to press the key with the circle as the remaining keys were lighted. After all keys were at full illumination, the experimenters begin to "fade in" the ellipses. At first the ellipses were very faint. But across trials the ellipses were gradually increased in darkness until the lines of very flat ellipses were equal in darkness to that of the circle. The stimulus control procedure used was fading, i.e., the light and the ellipses were gradually faded in. The experimenters then began to change the dimensions of the ellipses across trials. As this continued, a more circle-like ellipse was produced. The subject still continued to select the circle during this stimulus shaping procedure. At the end of the training, severely retarded children were making a very fine circle-ellipse discrimination that would be impossible to train using a trial-and-error procedure.

Dixon et al. (1975) taught moderately retarded children to select an object *in front* of an animal from among objects *behind, under,* and *over* using a fading procedure similar to that used by Stoddard and Sidman (1967). They started with only the animal, and the object in the *in front* position, and gradually faded in other objects *under, over,* and *behind.* They were able to teach this concept in two 15- or 20-minute sessions.

Stimulus shaping techniques hold great promise for training. However, they have drawbacks. First, there is no well developed set of principles or procedures for developing effective materials for bringing about discriminations. Second, the development of such programs involves meticulous care and research concerning the effectiveness of each frame of the program.

Time-Delay Perhaps a more practical method for shifting stimulus control from an established stimulus to a new stimulus is the time-delay procedure described by Touchette (1971). This procedure involves first presenting a stimulus that does control a response simultaneously with one that does not control the response. The child is reinforced for making the correct response. On subsequent trials, the new or neutral stimulus is presented first, and then, after a delay that increases on each substantial trial, the old stimulus is presented unless the child has responded to the new stimulus during the delay. This procedure has been used to extend control from a verbal model (as the stimulus for selecting a word) to a picture as the stimulus for selecting a word (Risley and Wolf, 1967) and for shifting control of motor responses from a motor model by a teacher to a verbal instruction from the teacher (Striefel, Bryan, and Aikins, 1974). Unlike the stimulus fading and shaping technique, the delay technique does not require extensive program development and may be used in a wide range of situations by relatively untrained people.

Generalization The discussion of stimulus control thus far is directed toward establishing a discrimination, but stimulus control also involves *generalization.* Even though a response is reinforced in the presence of a specific stimulus while not reinforced in the absence of that stimulus, that stimulus probably will not be the only stimulus that controls the response. For example, the initial discrimination training in audiometric evaluation might be made with a 60-dB, 500-Hz tone. However, subsequent evaluation of tone control might indicate that responding was also controlled by a 40-dB, 2000-Hz tone. Such generalization is of course desirable when giving an audiometric test. However, if a child is trained to label the letter E as [i],[1] but subsequently also labels the letter F as [i] and the number 3 as [i], this generalization would not be desirable, and the trainer would take steps to eliminate it. Development of a finer discrimination could be accomplished by using either a stimulus fading technique or a delay technique such as the one described above.

One point should be made at this time. Just as generalization of behavior is not appropriate in all situations, so a given type of stimulus control is not appropriate in all situations. For example, when Dixon et al. (1975) consistently requested a subject to point to the object in front of the animal, a given type of visual stimulus control was appropriate. However, when the subject was later requested to point to the object under the animal, it was not appropriate for the subject to point to the object in front of the animal. In other words, the aspect of the stimulus that controlled the response was conditional on another stimulus, namely, the spoken command. This type of higher order discrimination is sometimes spoken of as *conditional discrimination* and is, of course, critical to the development of complex behavior such as language.

Contingencies of Reinforcement

To be effective in changing the rate of behavior, reinforcement or punishment must be delivered immediately after the occurrence of the target response. The delayed presentation or withdrawal of stimuli often results in an increase or decrease of a response not selected as the target behavior. For example, if a reinforcing stimulus is selected for presentation after a correct imitation of a raised hand, and the reinforcer is not delivered immediately, the trainer should not be surprised to see an increase in another response, such as turning the head. If this situation is analyzed closely, however, it becomes apparent that the slow trainer has inappropriately reinforced the child's head turning, which was the child's response to not receiving the reinforcer immediately after raising his hand.

---

[1]For readers unfamiliar with the International Phonetic Association (IPA) Alphabet, a pronunciation key is provided in Appendix B.

Sometimes it appears that reinforcement can be delayed and still establish or maintain behavior. This appearance is an illusion. When the primary reinforcement is delayed, there is probably always some immediate change in the environment which signals that such reinforcement is forthcoming. This environmental change is usually called a *conditioned reinforcer*. For example, in audiometric testing, the food may be delayed 0.5 second before dropping into the food tray; however, the light may occur immediately to tell the child that the food is forthcoming. In some cases, the feedback of the child's own behavior may serve as a conditioned reinforcer, or bridging stimulus, between the response and the ultimate reinforcer. This is most apparent when the child's responses result in a permanent product such as occurs in writing and solving arithmetic problems.

Primary reinforcement is sometimes assumed to occur after each response. In reality, such is seldom the case. Only in establishing behavior is it necessary to deliver reinforcement on a continuous reinforcement schedule (CRF). Reinforcement that does not occur every time a target response is emitted is called *intermittent reinforcement*. Intermittent reinforcement, in contrast to CRF, is used to maintain an already established level of responding. Continuous reinforcement, or reinforcement after each response, has certain advantages over intermittent reinforcement. First, early in training, continuous reinforcement may be more efficient in establishing behavior because the person is informed immediately after each response whether or not the criterion has been met. Chances for a drift of the response away from the criterion performance is reduced. Second, if the response requires considerable effort, intermittent reinforcement simply may not be sufficient to maintain the response.

Continuous reinforcement has certain disadvantages. First, the amount of reinforcement may lead to satiation. Second, continuously reinforced behavior shows little persistence during times when the reinforcement is not delivered. To maintain behavior in the face of nonreinforcement, the trainer or teacher should gradually introduce an intermittent schedule.

Intermittent schedules are of two basic types, *time-based* (interval) and *number-based* (ratio). Simple time-based schedules reinforce the person for the first response made after some period of time has elapsed. Number-based schedules reinforce the persons after some number of responses have been made. Ratio schedules typically generate high rates of responding.

Intermittent schedules can be used with either free-operant behavior, such as conversational talking, playing, and singing, or with fixed-trial behavior, such as naming pictures, answering questions, or following commands. The choice of interval or ratio schedules primarily depends on the rate that the teacher, clinician, or experimenter wants to obtain. A teacher who wants to maintain a high rate of responding should use a ratio schedule. For example, the teacher might reinforce a child for naming 10 objects correctly by allowing the child to play with a puzzle. Such a procedure might result in high rates of naming objects. Ratio schedules can be overdone. The teacher may be getting good results with a ratio schedule that requires a few responses for each delivery of reinforcement, but when more responses are required for each delivery of reinforcement, the teacher may find that the child stops responding rather abruptly. If this occurs, the ratio is probably too lean. The teacher should return to requiring fewer responses for each reinforcement.

Time-based schedules should be used when the teacher wishes to maintain the responding at a relatively low rate. For example, the classroom teacher may want a child to talk in class discussion. However, the teacher probably would want talking to occur at low or moderate rates. Thus, a time-based or interval schedule is preferrable to a ratio or number schedule.

Behavior can be maintained by intermittent reinforcement when there is no necessary or planned contingency. Suppose a child consistently exhibits some behavior. Now suppose that reinforcements occur aperiodically whether or not the child is engaged in the behavior. Reinforcements sometimes occur when the behavior is ongoing. The co-occurrence of reinforcement with the behavior strengthens the ongoing behavior because the laws of reinforcement work whether or not the contingency is planned. Hollis (1973) has demonstrated that accidental reinforcement plays a role in the maintenance of stereotyped behavior among retarded children.

In summary, applied behavioral analysis is based on several principles:

1.   The important units of analysis are behavioral events that can be objectively observed and recorded
2.   Behavior is a function of environmental events
3.   A large class of behavior is established and maintained by its immediate consequence

4.   If different consequences follow behavior under different situations, the behavior will have different rates under those different situations

5.   Reinforcement should be delivered on a continuous schedule when behavior is first being established

6.   Behavior need not be reinforced on every occasion to be maintained

7.   Behavior will be more persistent in the face of nonreinforcement if it follows intermittent reinforcement than if it follows continuous reinforcement

BEHAVIORAL PRINCIPLES AND
ANALYSIS OF GENERALIZATION AND TRANSFER

The preceding section analyzes behavior according to stimulus, response, contingency, and consequence. Principles based on these concepts are adequate for developing a technology that: 1) increases and decreases the rate of a response already being emitted, 2) brings an existing response under stimulus control, and 3) develops complex chains of responses. The principles stated in the earlier part of this chapter must be extended if they are to account for the level of organization and integration in complex human behavior.

Researchers who have extended the principles of behavior analysis to complex behavior often use two terms: *stimulus class* and *response class*. These two terms have a long history in the functional analysis of behavior. In 1935, Skinner discussed stimulus and response classes. In that discussion, response classes seem to be based on either topographical similarity or on equivalence in producing an effect on the environment. Stimulus classes were stimuli that were physically similar or stimuli that controlled the same response(s).

Goldiamond (1966) proposed an entirely functional definition of stimulus and response classes. If a set of stimuli control the same response or responses, they were members of the same stimulus class whether or not they had similar physical properties. Goldiamond (1966) gave an example of a stop sign, the spoken word *stop,* a whistle, and a policeman's outstretched arm with the hand extended with the palm away from the body as members of the same stimulus class insofar as each controlled a stopping response. Similarly, such divergent responses, as saying "Could I have another piece of cake," or "That cake is really good," or looking longingly at the remaining cake, may be functionally equivalent in spurring an adult to provide a second piece of cake for a child.

Response Classes

Baer and Guess (1973) defined a response class as a set of responses organized so that an operation that changes the rate of occurrence on some members of the class also changes the rate of occurrence of the remaining members of the class. Nearly all of the experiments in which Baer and his colleagues have introduced this concept of response class have had a common characteristic. The experimenter selects a set of behaviors that is viewed as a class. Then the experimenter begins training specific examples of the class and continues to train these examples until the subject begins to respond appropriately to new examples before direct training is given on those examples. This approach develops a variety of behaviors including imitation, productive and receptive use of morphologic forms in language, expanded sentences, and creative behavior. This research is presented briefly below.

Generalization Imitation   In the late 1950's Bandura and colleagues demonstrated that young children imitated the behavior of a model even though that behavior was not trained or reinforced in the experimental situation (Bandura and Walters, 1963). These demonstration led behaviorists (e.g., Metz, 1965; Lovaas et al., 1966; Baer, Peterson, and Sherman, 1967) to examine whether imitative behavior could be trained in severely retarded and autistic children who did not exhibit the behavior. Baer, Peterson, and Sherman started by teaching a child to imitate responses made by a model. That is, the trainer would say, "Do this," then hit the table with a closed fist. After hitting the table, the trainer would take the child's hand, close it into a fist, and put the child's hand through the hitting motion. Then the child would be reinforced with food. The trainer would continue this procedure, gradually reducing the help until the child was making the response without help whenever the trainer modeled the behavior. At this point, the trainer introduced a new response using the same training procedure. After the subject was correctly responding to the second modeled behavior, the experimenter would start intermixing the two behaviors until the child was correctly responding to each model. Then the trainer would proceed to introduce new behaviors until the child began to imitate new behaviors without direct training.

The number of behaviors that had to be trained before the first generalized imitative response varied across subjects. Baer, Peterson, and Sherman (1967) reported that one of their subjects demonstrated generalized imitation after only eight trained responses, while another subject had to be trained in over 100 different behaviors before exhibiting generalized imitation. Generalized imitation can be trained, and once it occurs, if some imitative responses are reinforced, other nonreinforced imitative responses will be maintained.

Teaching Language Response Classes   The term *response class* also has been used in discussions of studies developed to train children to use specific morphologic forms appropriately. These studies also follow the principle of teaching sufficient examples of the experimenter's class of behaviors to train the subject to respond appropriately to new examples without direct training.

Guess et al. (1968) taught a retarded child who initially did not use the plural morpheme to use that morpheme when two objects were presented. Their procedures followed the same teach-by-example logic used in the imitation experiments. They first presented the child with a single object and made sure that the child labeled the object correctly. Then they introduced a pair of objects. They trained the child to label the pair with the correct name for the plural morpheme. This training was done by presenting the child with the pair of objects. If the child failed to use the plural correctly, they had the child imitate the plural name, and the child was reinforced. Then the experimenter presented the objects again. When the child was consistently labeling the pair of objects with the plural morpheme, presentations of singular and multiple objects were mixed. This procedure was maintained until the child consistently gave the singular label for the single object and the plural label when two objects were presented.

Training was then initiated with another type of object. Once again the single object was presented until the child could give the singular label consistently. Then the pair of objects was presented. If the child did not give the plural label for the pair, training was initiated and continued until the child reached criterion for correctly labeling the single object with the single label and the pair of objects with the plural label. New objects continued to be presented and trained until new pairs of objects were labeled with the plural label before initiating plural training on the new set.

In addition to the Guess et al. (1968) study, this basic line of response class research has been extended to training past tenses, suffixes, and plural allomorphs (Schumaker and Sherman, 1970; Sailor, 1971; Baer and Guess, 1973).

Stimulus Classes

A second term that is often introduced by behavior analysts who study complex behavior is the term *stimulus class*. Although the term frequently has been used to refer to a set of stimuli that control the same or similar response(s) (Osgood, 1953; Goldiamond, 1966; Kendler, 1972; Spradlin, Cotter, and Baxley, 1973), this use is probably too restrictive. More recent uses of *stimulus class* have moved toward a definition in terms of *substitutability* or *equivalence* (Dixon, 1975; Sidman, 1975; Dixon and Spradlin, in press). Dixon and Spradlin (in press) suggested that initially unrelated stimuli can be established as a stimulus class if they are made *functionally equivalent* with regard to reinforcement contingencies. In another article, Dixon (1975) reported that, if a complete set of previously unrelated stimuli is given equivalent functions in some task(s) through direct training, and then a subset of these stimuli is given a new function by direct training in another task, the remaining untrained members of that set will also have that function.

Generalized Match-to-Sample   Generalized match-to-sample is an interesting performance of humans and of great apes. The task involves presenting a specific stimulus to a subject and then having the subject select one like it from an array including one or more non-matching stimuli and one matching stimulus. Several investigators have demonstrated generalized match-to-sample behavior among young, normal children and retarded adolescents (Scott, 1964; Sherman, Saunders, and Brigham, 1970; Saunders, 1973). Match-to-sample can be considered a study of stimulus classes insofar as: 1) the choice stimulus and the sample stimulus are identical, and 2) any pair of identical stimuli can be substituted for any other pair and the matching behavior is still maintained.

These studies have demonstrated that whether children match or mismatch on a particular occasion is a function of the reinforcement contingencies. If a sample stimulus is introduced that has never before been presented to the child, the child very likely will select the stimulus that matches it rather than some other stimulus. Moreover, if that sample stimulus and its choice are presented in the context of other items in which the subjects are being reinforced for matching, the item involving novel stimuli will result in matching responses even though the matching responses to that specific item were never reinforced. In other words, specific matching responses to novel stimuli may emerge without direct training, and they may be maintained even though they are never directly reinforced (Scott, 1964; Sherman, Saunders, and Brigham, 1970; Saunders, 1973).

Further research has demonstrated that such generalized matching is not a result of failure to discriminate nonreinforced from reinforced matching items. However, generalized matching is under the control of higher conditional stimuli. Saunders (1973) reinforced matching under a red light and mismatching under a blue light. He found that his subjects soon came to match when the red light was on and to mismatch when the blue light was on. Moreover, the novel reinforced items were matched or mismatched according to the general contingencies indicated by the red or blue light.

Although match-to-sample behavior has been studied in laboratory settings, it is certainly not restricted to the laboratory. It is very likely that, in the studies described above, the children had learned matching behavior long before they entered the laboratory setting. Young children are frequently shown an object and requested by their parents to find one like it in the home. Whenever children sort objects, they are, in a sense, making a series of match-to-sample responses.

Match-to-sample has many characteristics in common with imitation. In imitation, the correspondence is between the behavior modeled by the experimenter and the behavior emitted by the subject. In match-to-sample, the correspondence is between the sample and the correct choice. In both tasks, certain appropriate responses to novel situations occur and are maintained without direct reinforcements, provided that they are introduced in a series of similar tasks that are reinforced. Moreover, both imitation and match-to-sample behaviors are established by training-by-example.

Stimulus Classes without Common Physical Properties   Stimulus classes consisting of stimuli that have no common physical properties have been established during the last 5 years (Sidman, 1971; Sidman and Cresson, 1973; Sidman, Cresson, and Willson-Morris, 1974; Dixon, 1975). These researchers have demonstrated that, if initially unrelated stimuli are given common controlling properties in one task through training and reinforcement, these common controlling properties are then generalized into new tasks. This principle holds across a variety of common functions. Sidman (1971) conducted a study with a severely retarded microcephalic adolescent. This subject could select pictures of common objects in response to their spoken names. Moreover, he could name the objects. However, he could not select the printed words in the response to their spoken names, nor match the pictures when given printed words as stimuli. After being trained to match the printed word to a spoken word, the subject was able to match the printed names with pictures and to read the printed words, even though he had received no direct training on these two tasks. Sidman's original finding since has been replicated by Sidman and Cresson (1973) and Friedman (1974).

Spradlin, Cotter, and Baxley (1973) demonstrated in a non-identity, match-to-sample task that, if a subject was first trained to select a single choice stimulus in response to two initially unrelated standard stimuli, and then taught to select a second choice stimulus in response to one of the sample stimuli, the subject selected that same choice stimulus whenever the untrained second sample stimulus was presented.

Dixon and Spradlin (in press) demonstrated that, if four initially unrelated visual stimuli were established as a stimulus class within a nonidentity match-to-sample task, and then one or two of them was given a specific name through training, that name was then applied to all remaining stimuli.

It had been long known that, if two initially unrelated stimuli were given the same name and then one of them was used in a discrimination task as the positive or negative stimulus, that other stimulus with the same name would tend to have the same function (Miller and Dollard, 1941; Bialer, 1961; Kendler, 1972; Reese, 1972). Dixon (1975) extended this procedure by conditioning subjects to select four different visual stimuli in response to the same auditory name. When this was done, subjects usually matched these initially unrelated stimuli in a match-to-sample procedure.

Those studies demonstrated that, if initially unrelated stimuli are given equivalent functions in some tasks through training, they also will exhibit similar functions in untrained tasks. Nevertheless, some qualifications are necessary in these extensions of stimulus functions. The organization of stimulus members into stimulus classes is determined by higher order stimuli. For example, in a task requiring that all letters be put together, A,b,c,D,e, and F are equivalent. However, if the instructions specify capital letters, then only A, D, and F are equivalent. Higher level language and academic tasks involve not only functional equivalence but also higher order stimulus classifications that place limitations on that functional equivalence. This conditional equivalence of stimuli is found in language as well as in other educational tasks. The ease with which physically dissimilar stimuli are established as equivalent (under certain conditions), and the ease with which the limitations of stimulus equivalence are placed by higher order stimulus conditions, may be closely related to what is called "intelligent" behavior.

There are several implications of the stimulus class principle to understanding the learning process and to developing teaching programs. The first is that, in any learning task, a great deal more is being learned than is being directly taught. Second, learning develops in a network fashion so that not every person needs to be directly taught the same content to acquire the same repertoire. For example, Sidman (1971), Sidman and Cresson (1973), and Sidman, Cresson, and Willson-Morris (1974) demonstrated in reading tasks that a total repertoire of six reading performances could be developed by training either of two sets of three performances. As shown in Figure 3, the Sidman and the Sidman and Cresson studies were able to establish, without direct training: 1) selecting the printed word as a choice in response to the picture as a sample stimulus, 2) selecting the picture in response to the printed word as a sample stimulus, and 3) naming the printed word by ensuring, through pretesting or training, that their retarded subjects could, a) select a picture in response to a spoken name, b) name the picture, and c) select the printed word in response to the spoken name.

On the other hand, Sidman, Cresson, and Willson-Morris made sure the children were able to: 1) select the picture in response to a spoken word, 2) select the printed word in response to a picture, and 3) name the picture. They then found that the remaining behaviors emerged without direct training.

The stimulus class hypothesis also suggests that not every learner needs to learn the same performances. But it suggests too that certain elements must be taught. For example, in the Sidman studies, at least one equivalence must be trained for each of the three types of stimuli (pictures, spoken words, and printed words). Once these equivalences are taught, by teaching a new function to any one of the three types of stimuli, that new function may be established for the remaining two types of stimuli.

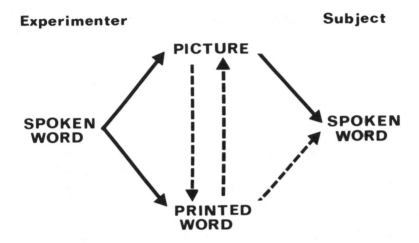

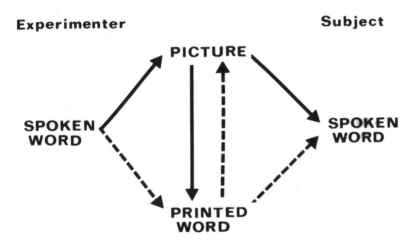

Figure 3. Two separate sequences of trained and generalized reading performances. The solid arrows indicate trained relationships. The dashed arrows indicate relationships that emerged without direct training. *Top:* adapted from Sidman, 1971; *bottom:* adapted from Sidman, Cresson, and Willson-Morris, 1974.

Functional Equivalence in Language

Functional equivalences may be of many types. One type of functional equivalence in language occurs in parts of speech. Parts of speech comprise a class of stimuli that can be combined with other parts of speech (classes) in specific ways. Any element that is a member of one class can be combined in specific ways with any member of another class.

Striefel, Wetherby, and Karlan (in press) established two classes, verbs and nouns, in a receptive language-training task with severely retarded children. They taught the child to respond appropriately to any of 12 verbs combined with any of 12 nouns. They initially taught the child to respond with a specific motor action to each named object when a verb-noun command was given. Once the child responded to each of 12 named objects, a new verb (new action) was introduced and trained in the same manner. Once the child could emit this new behavior with the named object, a mixed sequence was presented in which trials involving the first verb (combined with objects) and the new verb (combined with objects) were mixed. These sequences continued until the child could correctly display the action designated by the verb with the object named by the noun. Training continued across the remaining nouns. A third verb was then introduced and training was given. Once again, after the verb had been trained and combined with one noun, it was presented with a sequence involving the two previously learned verbs combined with the 12 nouns. This training continued with probes conducted before training was begun on a new verb-noun combination. If a generalization criterion was met, the combination was considered learned. As shown in Table 2, after a few verbs had been trained across a series of objects, a new verb was introduced with only one noun to be correctly used with all other nouns. In other words, the child learned that a new verb was a member of a class of words designating actions, and that the designated actions could be combined with any object specified by the noun. The subject had thus learned two stimulus classes, verbs and nouns.

Simple stimulus class and response class extensions presented in this section do not currently constitute a theory to account for all the complex appropriate behaviors found in human activities. However, these simple extensions do suggest that appropriate responses to novel

Table 2. Verb-noun combinations either trained (T) or generalized (G) for subject 1

Verbs	Nouns											
	N1	N2	N3	N4	N5	N6	N7	N8	N9	N10	N11	N12
1. Push	T	T	T	T	T	G	G	G	G	G	G	G
2. Blow on	T	T	T	T	T	T	T	T	T	T	G	G
3. Hold out	T	T	T	G	G	G	G	G	G	G	G	G
4. Drop	T	T	T	G	G	G	G	G	G	G	G	G
5. Point to	T	T	G	G	G	G	G	G	G	G	G	G
6. Wave	T	G	G	G	G	G	G	G	G	G	G	G
7. Tap	T	T	G	G	G	G	G	G	G	G	G	G
8. Pound with	T	G	G	G	G	G	G	G	G	G	G	G
9. Smell	T	G	G	G	G	G	G	G	G	G	G	G
10. Elevate	T	G	G	G	G	G	G	G	G	G	G	G
11. Turn	T	G	G	G	G	G	G	G	G	G	G	G
12. Encircle	T	G	G	G	G	G	G	G	G	G	G	G

Based on Striefel, Wetherby, and Karlan, in press.

situations can be expected, provided that rational and systematic training is given.

In summary, the notions of stimulus and response class are central to the development of generalization and transfer. The integration of these concepts for the remediation of developmental disabilities should result in more learned behavior than is directly trained. Consequently, the development of functional equivalences through the training of stimulus and response classes is a basic step in developing complex human behavior.

IMPLICATIONS FOR TASK ANALYSIS IN DEVELOPMENT OF COMPLEX PERFORMANCES

Knowing the principles of behavior very well does not alone ensure the development of an effective teaching or training program. Developing an effective teaching program requires careful selection of useful terminal performances and organization of materials and procedures to produce such performances.

Selection of Useful Terminal Performances

Much has been written about the selection of educational objectives, behavioral targets, and terminal performances (Gagné, 1970; Brown and York, 1974; Horner, 1975). Most writers agree that the behavioral objectives must involve some specific performance that can be observed and counted or otherwise measured.

The present authors agree that the targets of training must involve specific behaviors. However, with the possible exception of some mundane but socially necessary targets, like toilet training and self-feeding, the specific behaviors themselves are not the aim of training. The aim of training is to prepare a student to perform any one of a class of behaviors. The specific behaviors are simply a sample from that class.

For example, in teaching a child to imitate, the trainer should not stop until the child imitates new responses before direct training is given on those responses. The specific responses selected for demonstrating generalized imitation are not important. What is important is that they are representative members of a class of behavior that the child is capable of performing. In the study by Striefel, Wetherby, and Karlan (in press), what is important is not that the child learned to perform correctly on 20 to 40 trained verb-noun instructional combinations, but that he could respond appropriately to any verb-noun combination for which he knew the meaning of the individual components. The test of effective training is whether the child responds to an untrained sample from a behavioral class.

Organization of Materials and
Procedures to Produce Terminal Performances

The first phase in organizing materials and procedures to produce terminal performances is the determination of the child's current behavioral repertoire in relation to those terminal performances. At first glance, it might seem that, having selected the terminal performance, training would be merely a matter of directly teaching and reinforcing examples of those performances. However, many performances involve such a large number of components that no learning occurs when the whole performance is presented at once (Horner, 1975). In order to develop an adequate training program for the terminal performances, it is necessary to break the total performances into components, and the subsequent ordering of those components is called *task analysis* (Gagné, 1970). Before proceeding to the specifics of task analysis, it might be helpful to make some general observations about the ordering of behaviors derived from the analysis. The result will be a set of component behaviors having an ordered relationship to each other. The ordered relationship derives from the fact that certain behaviors are subordinate to other behaviors and that these in turn are subordinate to others. Subordinate behaviors are prerequisite to behaviors at a higher level. This has been termed a *learning hierarchy* (Gagné, 1970).

Some performances are prerequisites to higher order performances and must be taught in a particular sequence. However, other performances may be parallel and independent but still prerequisite to higher order performances. Still other performances are independent, and when certain parallel performances are taught, even without ordering constraints, another parallel or even higher order performance will emerge without further direct training (Sidman and Cresson, 1973; Friedman, 1974; Sidman, Cresson, and Willson-Morris, 1974). There are some points in which a fixed sequence of training is a necessity. Others may be taught in a sequence that is a matter of choice by the programmer.

Task analysis may be conducted on any task ranging from teaching retarded persons how to feed themselves to teaching astronauts how to handle a trip to the moon. The procedure used in analyzing the task and organizing a training sequence varies with the task. Horner (1975) has developed guidelines for conducting a task analysis for motor behaviors of severely retarded children. He suggested two ways of beginning to analyze a task: 1) proceed through the behavior yourself and attempt to analyze the behavior into components and then determine the sequence in which the components are performed, and 2) observe a number of individuals and attempt to break the total performance into components to determine the sequence in which the components are performed by the individual. The choice of method for analyzing is not critical because this first approximation should be subjected to revision once the training program is tested with a child. If development of one component does not lead to the development of the next component, the trainer knows that a prerequisite behavior has been omitted or that the component complex has not been broken into small enough units.

Regardless of the specific breakdown of behavior or sequence selected, Horner (1975) has suggested that the definition of each behavior should be written in the form of a directly observable action, an object of action, and a performance criterion. Examples of such definitions relevant to chapters in this volume are shown in Table 3.

Once the definition for each behavior has been determined, the behavior (action, object, criterion) is placed in a more extended instructional objective that includes condition, behavior, and overall criterion as shown in Table 4.

Some task analyses in other areas are not so simple. For example, suppose the task is not to teach a simple motor skill but to train a complex skill such as addition. An investigator who gives mature children addition problems, and then simply observes their

Table 3. Examples of behavior definitions used in this volume

Action verb	Object	Criterion	Chapter
Depress	Response button	When tone is on	Cox and Lloyd
Shape	Hand	Into manual sign	Wilbur; Kopchick and Lloyd
Place	Plastic symbol	On stand	Carrier
Place	Bliss symbol	On communicator board or Auto-Com	Vanderheiden and Harris-Vanderheiden

Table 4. Samples of behavior definitions extended to instructional objectives

| Conditions | Behavior | | | | General criterion |
	Action	Object	Criterion	
Given: A presentation of a ball, the child will:	form	the hand	into a manual sign for ball	on at least 90% of all opportunities to do so
Given: A demonstration of "lift block," the child will:	lift	the block	above the head	on 100% of all opportunities to do so
Given: A picture of a boy throwing a ball, the child will:	say	"boy throwing ball"	discernible to a second listener	on at least 85% of all opportunities to do so
Given: A picture of a girl chasing a boy, the child will:	place	the symbols girl, chase and boy	on the response board in the correct order	on at least 90% of all opportunities to do so

terminal performances, certainly would be misled because many of the prerequisites of functional addition are in no way obvious. Fortunately, in the case of addition, one does not have to depend solely on observation of the terminal performances. Empirical studies have been conducted which demonstrate that, if children are able to perform some pre-arithmetic tasks (C, D, and E), they are nearly always able to perform other tasks (A and B); but, children who perform tasks A and B do not always perform tasks C, D, and E. These results provide a rather clear indication that A and B are prerequisite for C, D, and E (Wang, Resnick, and Boozer, 1970; Spradin et al., 1974). These studies, utilizing Lingoes' Multiple Scalogram, involve a survey of a relatively wide range of children at different skill levels (Lingoes, 1963). They provide a basis for a task analysis of pre-arithmetic skills and the development of a curriculum for teaching these skills (Resnick, Wang, and Kaplan, 1973). Their task analysis is rather specific in suggesting which performances are prerequisite to others and which performances may be taught in any of several orders.

.   This discussion of task analysis makes a point of suggesting that, for many performances, programming requires no specific order of arrangement because the component performances are independent or parallel. Moreover, in line with the discussion of generalization, it is suggested that, in some cases, performances emerge without direct training. Viewing Sidman's research in terms of a task analysis, he and his colleagues have done most, if not all, of the task analyses necessary for understanding and producing the six terminal performances, explained below.

In Figure 4, the three lower boxes illustrate three prerequisite behaviors, picture discrimination, printed word discrimination, and spoken word discrimination. Spoken word discrimination is a prerequisite to spoken word production, which in turn is a prerequisite to printed word naming and picture naming. Spoken word discrimination is also a prerequisite to selecting the picture to match a spoken word and selecting a printed word to match a spoken word. It is not a prerequisite to matching a picture to a printed word. Picture discrimination is a prerequisite to four performances: selecting a picture to match a spoken word, selecting a picture to match a printed word, selecting a printed word to match a picture, and picture naming. It is not a prerequisite to selecting a printed word to match a spoken word or printed word naming.

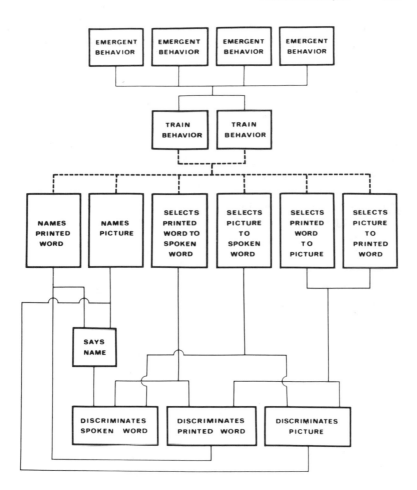

Figure 4. Task analysis of six reading performances. Horizontal relationships indicate that a particular order of training is a noncritical feature. Vertical relationships indicate a critical sequence for training in the order depicted. The four lowest behaviors are prerequisites to the six target behaviors. In addition, if any two of the target behaviors involving all three stimulus classes (spoken word, printed word, and picture) are trained, the remaining four behaviors should emerge without direct training.

A similar analysis can be made for the performances for which printed word discrimination is a prerequisite. In Figure 4, the set of three lower prerequisite behaviors taken together represent the prerequisites to the four, right-most target behaviors. The ability to state the name must be included (as shown in the relationship pictured) as requisite to the two left-most target behaviors. Combinations of the various prerequisite skills then result in six terminal performances.

However, after the prerequisite skills, not all of the six performances must be directly taught. If any two of these target performances involving all three stimulus classes (e.g., picture, printed word, name) are taught, the remaining four will emerge with little or no direct training (Sidman, 1971; Sidman and Cresson, 1973; Friedman, 1974; Sidman, Cresson and Willson-Morris, 1974). In order for training on any two performances involving three stimuli to result in the emergence of the four remaining performances, it must be assumed that there is a reception-to-production transfer. If this is not true, then three performances must be trained. Figure 4 shows (in the upper portion) where training two independent target behaviors (under the stated restrictions) yields the four remaining behaviors. The selection of which two tasks are taught may be solely a matter of preference by the programmer.

In summary, the successful application of behavioral principles to develop complex, meaningful behavior requires a selection or description of the classes of terminal performances to be taught and an analysis of the prerequisite behaviors and components of these performances in order to determine a training sequence in which the various prerequisites and components are to be taught.

SUMMARY AND CONCLUSIONS

This chapter concerns measurement, basic behavioral principles, the extension of behavioral principles to the analyses of complex behavior, and the use of task analysis procedures to plan training programs for developmentally disabled children. The order in which the various topics are introduced is intentional. The authors believe that measurement and design are critical issues—perhaps the most critical issues—in the development of remedial programs for the handicapped. Without careful measurement and designs to evaluate the effects of intervention procedures, workers in the field will not be able to determine whether these procedures improve a child's behavior. Furthermore, they will be unable to improve procedures or to determine which procedure is the most effective. Measurement is the cornerstone of program improvement.

The second area of discussion is directed toward presenting some basic principles of behavior modification. The fundamental principles of behavior are the consequence principles. In short, behaviors that increase in rate are those followed by presentation of a positive reinforcer or the termination of a negative reinforcer. Behaviors that decrease in rate are those followed by no change in the environment, an aversive event, or the termination of a positive reinforcer. Knowledge of these principles, combined with knowledge of measurement, provides the teacher with a sound grasp of the subject matter and the tools for developing effective teaching programs.

However, mere understanding of the principles of reinforcement may not be sufficient. These principles focus very strongly on the reinforcement of specific responses and the training of specific behaviors. Such a focus is often useful because it allows the teacher or clinician to engage in training that is likely to result in change. However, one should not overlook the fact that humans are often asked to exhibit appropriate behavior in situations in which they have had no direct training. Indeed, such generalization is the aim of most training. For this reason, the discussion of generalization and complex behavior is included.

Finally, while the direct application of contingencies on a terminal behavior is often successful, some behaviors are so complex that they must be broken into components and taught in an orderly and sequential manner. Conducting a task analysis is very useful to a teacher or clinician faced with teaching such complex skills.

In conclusion, the teacher or clinician should measure to detect changes in behavior, systematically use consequences to increase appropriate behavior and decrease inappropriate behavior, teach for generalization, and organize teaching into a systematic plan that includes procedures for evaluating the performance of children and the effectiveness of the program.

REFERENCES

Baer, D. M. 1962. Laboratory control of thumbsucking by withdrawal and representation of reinforcement. J. Exp. Anal. Behav. 5:525–528.

Baer, D. M., and D. Guess. 1973. Teaching productive noun suffixes to severely retarded children. Amer. J. Ment. Defic. 77:498–505.

Baer, D. M., R. F. Peterson, and J. A. Sherman. 1967. The development of imitation by reinforcing behavioral similarity to a model. J. Exp. Anal. Behav. 10:405–416.

Baer, A. M., T. Rowbury, and D. M. Baer. 1973. The development of instructional control over classroom activities of deviant preschool children. J. Appl. Behav. Anal. 6:289–298.

Baer, D. M., M. M. Wolf, and T. F. Risley. 1968. Some current dimensions of applied behavior analysis. J. Appl. Behav. Anal. 1:91–97.

Bandura, A., and R. H. Walters. 1963. Social Learning and Personality Development. Holt, Rinehart and Winston, New York.

Barrett, B. B. 1962. Reduction in rate of multiple tics by free operant conditioning methods. J. Nerv. Ment. Dis. 135:187–195.

Bialer, I. 1961. Primary and secondary stimulus generalization as related to intelligence level. J. Exp. Child Psychol. 62:395–402.

Bijou, S. W., R. F. Peterson, and M. A. Ault. 1968. A method to integrate descriptive and experimental field studies at the level of data and empirical concepts. J. Appl. Behav. Anal. 1:175–191.

Brown, L., and R. York. 1974. Developing programs for severely handicapped students: Teacher training and classroom instruction. Focus Except. Child. 6(2), 11 p.

Dixon, M. 1975. Establishing stimulus equivalence by giving stimuli a common receptive label. Unpublished doctoral dissertation. University of Kansas, Lawrence, Kan.

Dixon, M., and J. E. Spradlin. Establishing stimulus equivalence among retarded adolescents. J. Exp. Child Psychol. In press.

Dixon, L. S., J. E. Spradlin, F. L. Girardeau, and B. C. Etzel. 1975. Facilitating the acquisition of an *in front* spatial discrimination. Working paper 317, Parsons Research Center, Parsons, Kan.

Ferster, C. B., and M. C. Perrott. 1967. Behavior Principles. New Century, Meredith, New York.

Fjellstedt, N., and B. Sulzer-Azaroff. 1973. Reducing latency of a child's responding to instruction by means of a token system. J. Appl. Behav. Anal. 6:125–130.

Friedman, M. 1974. Transfer in training preacademic reading and arithmetic skills in preschool children. Unpublished masters thesis. University of Kansas, Lawrence, Kan.

Fulton, R. T., and J. E. Spradlin. 1971. Operant audiometry with severely retarded children. Audiology 10:203–211.

Fulton, R. T., and J. E. Spradlin. 1974a. Puretone threshold measurement. *In* R. T. Fulton (ed.), Auditory Stimulus-Response Control. University Park Press, Baltimore.

Fulton, R. T., and J. E. Spradlin. 1974b. The short-increment sensitivity index. *In* R. T. Fulton (ed.), Auditory Stimulus-Response Control. University Park Press, Baltimore.

Gagné, R. M. 1970. The Conditions of Learning. Holt, Rinehart and Winston, New York.

Goldiamond, I. 1966. Perception, language, and conceptualization rules. *In* B. Kleinmutz (ed.), Carnegie Institute of Technology Annual Symposium on Cognition. John Wiley & Sons, New York.

Guess, D., W. Sailor, G. Rutherford, and D. M. Baer. 1968. An experimental analysis of linguistic development: The productive use of the plural morpheme. J. Appl. Behav. Anal. 1:297–306.

Hall, R. V. 1970. Reinforcement procedures and the increase of functional speech by a brain-injured child. *In* F. L. Girardeau and J. E. Spradlin (eds.), A Functional Analysis Approach to Speech and Language. Asha monogr. 14.

Hall, R. V. 1971. Managing Behavior Part I: The Measurement of Behavior. H & H Enterprises, Lawrence, Kan.

Harris, F. R., M. M. Wolf, and D. M. Baer. 1967. Effects of adult social reinforcement on child behavior. In S. W. Bijou and D. M. Baer (eds.), Child Development: Readings in Experimental Analysis. Appleton-Century-Crofts, New York.

Hollis, J. H. 1973. "Superstition:" The effects of independent and contingent events on free operant responses in retarded children. Amer. J. Ment. Defic. 77:585–596.

Horner, R.D. 1975. Task analysis in instructional programming. Module S of personnel training project, Department of Special Education, University of Kansas, Lawrence, Kan.

Keller, F. S., and W. N. Schoenfeld. 1950. Principles of Psychology. Appleton-Century-Crofts, New York.

Kendler, T. S. 1972. The ontogeny of mediational learning. Child Dev. 43:1–17.

Lindsley, O. R. 1964. Direct measurement and prosthesis of retarded behavior. J. Educ. 147:62–81.

Lingoes, J. C. 1963. Multiple scalogram analysis: A set theoretic model for analyzing dichotomous items. Educ. Psychol. Meas. 23:501–523.

Lloyd, L. L. 1966. Behavioral audiometry viewed as an operant procedure. J. Speech Hear. Disord. 31:128–136.

Lloyd, L. L., J. E. Spradlin, and M. J. Reid. 1968. An operant audiometric procedure for difficult-to-test patients. J. Speech Hear. Disord. 33:236–245.

Lovaas, O. I., J. P. Berberich, B. F. Perloff, and B. Schaeffer. 1966. Acquisition of imitative speech by schizophrenic children. Science 151:705–707.

Metz, J. R. 1965. Conditioning generalized imitation in autistic children. J. Exp. Child Psychol. 2:389–399.

Meyer, V., and E. S. Chesser. 1970. Behavior Therapy in Clinical Psychiatry. Oxford University Press, New York.

Miller, N. E., and J. Dollard. 1941. Social Learning and Imitation. Yale University Press, New Haven, Conn.

Osgood, C. E. 1953. Method and Theory in Experimental Psychology. Oxford University Press, New York.

Pavlov, I. P. 1960. Conditional Reflexes. Dover Publications, New York.

Reese, H. W. 1972. Acquired distinctiveness and equivalences of cues in young children. J. Exp. Child Psychol. 13:171–182.

Resnick, L. B., M. C. Wang, and J. Kaplan. 1973. Task analysis in curriculum design: A hierarchically sequenced introductory mathematics curriculum. J. Appl. Behav. Anal. 6:679–709.

Risley, T. R., and M. M. Wolf. 1967. Establishing functional speech in echolalic children. Behav. Res. Ther. 5:73–88.

Risley, T. R., and M. M. Wolf. 1972. Strategies for analyzing behavioral change over time. In J. Nesselroade and H. Reese (eds.), Life-Span

Developmental Psychology: Methodological Issues. Academic Press, New York.

Sailor, W. 1971. Reinforcement and generalization of productive plural allomorphs in two retarded children. J. Appl. Behav. Anal. 4:305–310.

Saunders, R. R. 1973. An assessment of several variables involved in the maintenance of generalized matching behavior. Unpublished doctoral dissertation. University of Kansas, Lawrence, Kan.

Schumaker, J., and J. A. Sherman. 1970. Training generative verb usage by imitation and reinforcement procedures. J. Appl. Behav. Anal. 3:273–287.

Scott, K. G. 1964. A comparison of similarity and oddity. J. Exp. Child Psychol. 1:123–134.

Sherman, J. A., R. R. Saunders, and T. A. Brigham. 1970. Transfer of matching and mismatching behavior in preschool children. J. Exp. Child Psychol. 9:489–498.

Sidman, M. 1960. Tactics of Scientific Research. Basic Books, New York.

Sidman, M. 1971. Reading and auditory-visual equivalences. J. Speech Hear. Res. 14:5–13.

Sidman, M. 1975. Mental retardation: Basic and applied research. Research grant application HD 05124-96 to the Department of Health, Education, and Welfare, Bethesda, Md.

Sidman, M., and O. Cresson, Jr. 1973. Reading and crossmodal transfer of equivalences in severe retardation. Amer. J. Ment. Defic. 73:515–523.

Sidman, M., O. Cresson, Jr., and M. Willson-Morris. 1974. Acquisition of matching-to-sample via mediated transfer. J. Exp. Anal. Behav. 22:261–273.

Skinner, B. F. 1935. The generic nature of the concepts of stimulus and response. J. Gen. Psychol. 12:40–65.

Skinner, B. F. 1938. The behavior of organisms. Appleton-Century-Crofts, New York.

Skinner, B. F. 1953. Science and Human Behavior. The Free Press, New York.

Skinner, B. F. 1969. Contingencies of Reinforcement: A Theoretical Analysis. Appleton-Century-Crofts, New York.

Spradlin, J. E., V. W. Cotter, and N. Baxley. 1973. Establishing a conditional discrimination without direct training: A study of transfer with retarded adolescents. Amer. J. Ment. Defic. 77:556–566.

Spradlin, J. E., V. W. Cotter, C. Stevens, and M. Friedman. 1974. Performance of mentally retarded children on pre-arithmetic tasks. Amer. J. Ment. Defic. 78:397–403.

Spradlin, J. E., L. L. Lloyd, G. L. Hom, and M. J. Reid. 1968. Operant conditioning audiometry with low-level retardates: A preliminary report. In G. A. Jervis (ed.), Expanding Concepts in Mental Retardation. Charles C Thomas, Springfield, Ill.

Spradlin, J. E., B. J. Locke, and R. T. Fulton. 1969. Conditioning and audiological assessment. In R. T. Fulton and L. L. Lloyd (eds.), Audiometry for the Retarded. Williams & Wilkins, Baltimore.

Stoddard, L. T., and M. Sidman. 1967. The effects of errors on children's performance on a circle-ellipse discrimination. J. Exp. Anal. Behav. 10:261–270.

Striefel, S., K. S. Bryan, and D. A. Aikins. 1974. Transfer of stimulus control from motor to verbal stimuli. J. Appl. Behav. 7:123–135.

Striefel, S., B. Wetherby, and G. R. Karlan. Establishing generalized verb-noun instruction-following skills in retarded children. J. Exp. Child. Psychol. In press.

Terrace, H. S. 1963. Discrimination learning with and without "errors." J. Exp. Anal. Behav. 6:1–27.

Touchette, P. 1971. Transfer of stimulus control: Measuring the moment of transfer. J. Exp. Anal. Behav. 5:347–354.

Wang, M. C., L. B. Resnick, and R. Boozer. 1970. The sequence of development of some early mathematics behaviors. Working paper, Learning Research and Development Center, University of Pittsburgh.

Zimmerman, E. H., and J. Zimmerman. 1962. The alteration of behavior in a special classroom situation. J. Exp. Anal. Behav. 5:59–60.

7

AN APPROACH TO REMEDIATION OF COMMUNICATION AND LEARNING DEFICIENCIES

John H. Hollis,
Joseph K. Carrier, Jr., and Joseph E. Spradlin

CONTENTS

Multiply Handicapped _____ 268

Neurologic Myth _____ 269

Functional Analysis of Learning _____ 270
    Behavioral equation/270
    Behavioral equation component building/271
    Modification of functional equation components/272

Theoretical Orientation _____ 273
    Communicative channels/273
    Input: sensory mode (S)/273
    Integrative process (O): conceptual levels/275
    Output: response mode (R)/277
    Osgood's language model/277
    Language assessment/278
    Related language training/279
    Learning and transfer/279

Functional Analysis of Reading _____ 280
    Word reading lattice/281
    Intramodal equivalence/281
    Intermodal equivalence/281
    Research results/283

Discrimination without Direct Training: Concept Formation _____ 284

Language Learning: Nonspeech Response Mode _____ 285

Dual Structure of Communication Model _____ 285

Response Mode Transfer: Reading and Writing _____ 286

Integrative Processes _____ 288
    Construction (O_3)/288
    Transformation (O_4)/289

Memory Modification _____ 290
    Training/290
    Preliminary research/290

Summary _____ 291

References _____ 292

Since the 1960's, there has been an ever-increasing use of the term *learning deficiencies*. The term is sometimes used to refer to the problems of children who perform within normal limits on intelligence tests but who do not learn academic performances such as reading and arithmetic. However, it is also used to refer to the problems of virtually any child who has problems in learning. There has been a serious attempt to separate learning deficiencies from mental retardation; however, when the term is used in its generic sense there can be little doubt that learning deficiencies are very common among retarded children. Indeed, it seems that the term evolved from the field of mental retardation. A review of the work done by researchers in the area of mental retardation during the 1930's provides a background for the evolution of learning deficiencies (Hallahan and Cruickshank, 1973). The trend of focusing on learning deficiencies continued because, from an educational standpoint, the major problems of all areas of exceptionality involve learning deficiencies. Because learning deficiencies are common to nearly all categories of exceptionality, including mental retardation, it is likely that the close association among them will continue to be maintained. In the final analysis, the same learning theories and principles are applicable to all categories of exceptionality.

Factors such as nutrition and cultural deprivation have been implicated as causative agents in both retardation and learning deficiencies. However, it should be recognized that the teacher or clinician has little or no control over these causative agents. Therefore, from a practical standpoint, both retardation and learning deficiences must be approached from the point of view of environmental programming or teaching.

Historically, learning deficiencies have been subsumed under the rubric of sensory education, and early work was pioneered by such notables as Itard, Seguin, Montessori, and Kephart (Ball, 1971). Thus, it is no surprise that academic programs for learning-deficient children have been orientated toward problems such as perceptual-motor development, attention and motor control, perceptual disorders, and hyperactivity. A gross analysis of these problems suggest that the theorist, researcher, and teacher have focused on three

Preparation of this manuscript has been supported by Grant NICHHD 00870, Bureau of Child Research, University of Kansas, and by Grant B.E.H. OEG-0-74-2766, Kansas Neurological Institute, Topeka, Kansas.

specific factors: sensory input, associative or cognitive processes, and motor output.

Irrespective of a child's handicap or placement within a diagnostic category, deficiencies in communication are a salient characteristic. In order for language intervention specialists or teachers to be effective, they must be able to locate or develop at least one functional communication channel: that is, functional reception (sensory input) and expression (motor output). It is clear that clinicians and teachers have realized the existence of this problem for some time. This, perhaps, is the reason that so many who are concerned with learning deficiencies have elected to use the Illinois Test of Psycholinguistic Abilities (ITPA) as an assessment instrument.

It is not too presumptuous to assume that what clinicians and teachers want is simply that children listen, read, write, and talk. If the child does not have these abilities, then they want an assessment device, in order to pinpoint the specific deficiency, and then a remediation program to eliminate the deficiency.

MULTIPLY HANDICAPPED

Learning deficiencies have no categorical boundaries. They encompass the broad spectrum of children labeled "exceptional" (the gifted excepted). Thus, it is not surprising to discover that many of these children are multiply handicapped. For example, in addition to mental retardation, cerebral palsy, and emotional disturbance, these children also may have visual, auditory, or other impairments. These handicapping conditions serve only to compound the teacher's complex problem of establishing a functional learning environment for the child. It is axiomatic that, as the severity and number of handicapping conditions increases, the more difficult it is to establish functional communication channels and learning situations. Therefore, an attempt is made in this chapter to present ideas, concepts, and research that will be useful to clinicians and teachers and be applicable across the wide spectrum of children with learning deficiencies. The availability of multiple communication channels and prosthetic learning strategies provides many avenues for the elimination of learning deficiencies.

NEUROLOGIC MYTH

Diagnosticians frequently give a child a battery of tests, make electrical recordings from his head (electroencephalograms), poke at him, and then label him "brain damaged," or more recently "minimally brain damaged" (Wender, 1971). This label may result in the child being placed in an institution or a class for exceptional children. This in itself would not necessarily be bad if there were reliable and valid tests for differential diagnosis of brain damage and reliable and valid (effective) differential remediation methods. A case in point is the Strauss-type child who frequently has been diagnosed as brain damaged. Dunn (1965, p. 69) has succinctly stated, "The Strauss-type child is recognized by his *behavior* pattern of hyperactivity, uninhibited actions, perseveration, and perceptual disorders, not by his brain injury." One of the real dangers in labeling a child "brain damaged," for example, is that the labeling may result in a reflexive prediction. He is "brain damaged," therefore he cannot learn X, Y, and Z, and an educational program will be devised that will guarantee that he will not learn X, Y, and Z.

It is almost ludicrous to talk about tests of brain impairment when few of the 50 states have facilities for reliably and validly testing exceptional children for functional visual and auditory impairments (see Bensberg and Sigelman, this volume).

Furthermore, a comprehensive review of primate (monkey) ablation studies (experimental destruction of specific brain areas) by Chow (1967) suggests that, more frequently than not, the learning deficits resulting from brain damage are reversible. That is, with subsequent training the animal's performance level approaches the predamage level or that new tasks are learned as readily as by nondamaged controls. The lesson to be learned is that even if there should be *true* brain damage, behavioral techniques and skills probably exist to reduce the learning deficiency (see Lindsley, 1964; Hollis, 1967). With respect to mental retardation and learning, Estes (1970, p. 69) stated, "It does seem clear that none of the learning or retention processes that have been analyzed in normal human learners in the laboratory differ qualitatively in the mental defective, except perhaps at the most profoundly retarded level (below IQ of 30)."

FUNCTIONAL ANALYSIS OF LEARNING

Even a cursory overview of some recent texts on learning deficiencies suggests that something is missing. Paradoxically, there are few, if any, pages devoted to learning, its theory, methodology, or techniques. This is a sad state of affairs when the name of the game is *learning!* Although the problem cannot be rectified in a single chapter, this chapter presents an outline for a functional analysis of learning. It is anticipated that this analysis will provide the basic tools necessary for assessment and prosthesis of learning deficiencies.

In his discussion of the prosthesis of retarded behavior, Lindsley (1964) presented an operant behavioral equation that translates contemporary learning theory into a functional tool for the clinician or teacher. Estes (1970, p. 62) has succinctly summed up the transition from learning theory to functional techniques as follows: "Operant conditioning techniques are directly translatable into methods for the training of simple habits; thus, in this area there is no sharp line between theoretically oriented research and the development of practical training methods." As a case in point, Lindsley's (1964) behavioral equation provides a method for systematically separating all learning situations into four distinct and modifiable components. Its utility resides in the fact that the behavioral equation is functional for the solution of learning problems across all categories of special education. The behavioral equation components are specified as follows:

$$\text{\textit{Behavioral equation components}}$$
$$S \longrightarrow R \longrightarrow K \longrightarrow C$$
$$\text{Stimulus} \qquad \text{Response} \qquad \text{Contingency} \qquad \text{Consequence}$$

Behavioral Equation

If used, the four-component behavioral equation ($S \rightarrow R \rightarrow K \rightarrow C$) can provide clinicians and teachers with a powerful tool for the establishment of a functional learning situation. If a child is not acquiring new behavior or fails to maintain performance on previously acquired (learned) behavior, the teacher has four specific places to look: 1) the stimulus presentation mode, 2) the child's response mode, 3) the contingency, schedule of reinforcement, or 4) the consequence or reinforcer. The equation ($S \rightarrow R \rightarrow K \rightarrow C$) can be solved for only one unknown at a time; therefore, it is necessary to make sure that all of the components except the one being tested are functional. The process of developing a functional component may be called *component building*.

Behavioral Equation Component Building

The component building strategy has been discussed in detail by Lindsley (1964) and Hollis (1967) and provides the basis for treating crippling learning deficiencies. However, an attempt is made here to present a brief description of component building.

Stimulus Building (S)   Stimulus building gives to nonfunctional environmental events the ability to evoke responses. At the most severe levels of developmental deficiency, this can be accomplished by placing a piece of preferred food in front of the child, an act that normally will elicit reaching, grasping, and flexion movements, and finally, the child consuming the food. After the child has mastered this task, then the food can be paired with a nonfunctional stimulus. For example, a token or symbol can be added (see Premack, 1970). Now the child must respond to the paired food and stimulus object. As training progresses, the food is no longer paired with the stimulus object; i.e., by successive approximations the child is taught to exchange the stimulus object for the food. This technique has considerable generality because it provides a method for establishing stimulus function for otherwise nonfunctional environmental events (Lindsley, 1964).

Response Building (R)   The development of functional limb movements in a child with a deficient operant response is called *response building* (Lindsley, 1964). An example of response building is the external manipulation of limbs by a physical therapist until the child can move the limbs alone. In the case of a child that was unable to extend her left arm but able to flex her forearm, the teacher extended the child's arm away from her body and placed the hand palm down on a piece of food. The teacher then assisted the child in moving her fingers around the object and moving her hand to her mouth. Although this method is similar to that used by physical therapists (which provides proprioceptive stimulation), it differs in that there is an immediate consequence (e.g., food/reinforcer). In this situation, as the child gradually increased her ability to extend her arm and grasp, the teacher gradually faded out physical assistance (see Hollis, 1967).

Contingency Building (K)   Contingency building is concerned with the number of responses per reinforcer, i.e., the schedule of reinforcement. Thus, the schedule of reinforcement might be gradually shifted from continuous reinforcement (one-to-one ratio) to a schedule with a high degree of intermittency (Ferster and Skinner, 1957). In the case of severely handicapped children, it may be necessary to build a reinforcement history, i.e., to provide the child with experience on a variety of contingencies and extinction procedures (Hollis, 1973). Appropriate responding under programmed contingencies and consequences cannot be taken for granted!

Consequence Building (C)   In recent years educators and psychologists have directed considerable attention toward the isolation of reinforcing events or consequences (Ferster and DeMeyer, 1961). For example, nonfunctional events (e.g., verbal statements by teacher) can be established as reinforcing consequences by pairing them with highly reinforcing consequences, such as food. In addition, it is possible to make nonfunctional events into reinforcing consequences by withholding them from the child for varying periods of time (Homme et al., 1963; Baer, Wolf, and Harris, 1964).

Modification of Functional Equation Components

Once a functional operant has been established, the clinician or teacher may wish to change qualitatively or quantitatively the characteristics of an equation component. In order to determine objectively the effect of a change on a child's performance, only one component can be changed at a time (see Lindsley, 1964; Hollis, 1967). At this point, two brief examples are presented, one for a qualitative change in the consequence component and another for a quantitative change in the stimulus component.

Example 1 (Consequence Change)   A functional operant $(S \rightarrow R \rightarrow K \rightarrow C)$ is established in which a child is trained to press a button (R) when the 1000-Hz tone (S) occurs, and this response is reinforced on a one-to-one basis (K) with M & M candy (C). The child develops a steady high rate of responding under this condition. We wish to determine if the child's high level of performance will be maintained on social reinforcement (verbal statement by the clinician). Solving for one unknown, we would substitute social reinforcement for M & M candy and observe to determine if the performance level changed significantly. If it did not, we can then effectively use social reinforcement.

Example 2 (Visual Impairment)   A visually impaired child is trained (i.e., a functional operant equation is established) to read 48-point printed type (one-half inch high), and the teacher desires to establish reading with 24-point type because there are many printed books available in this size type. In this case, the teacher can substitute in the stimulus component (S) 24-point type for 48-point type and determine if the change has a significant effect on the child's reading rate. The teacher might find a lower reading rate acceptable if the child's reading is functional with the smaller print.

THEORETICAL ORIENTATION

Communicative Channels

"I can't get through to this child," is an almost too familiar statement made by clinicians, teachers, and parents at one time or another. What they are really saying is that, "I don't have a communication channel that works or I don't know how to find one." No matter what the handicapping condition(s) may be, the clinician or teacher necessarily must locate or establish a functional communication channel before the acquisition of new or modification of existing behavior can take place. At its most fundamental level, this communication channel consists of *sensory-input* and *response-output*. Thus, in order to teach an exceptional child, a *functional channel* must be found, irrespective of any neurologizing about the "blackbox" or brain (see Sanders, this volume).

Figure 1 presents a schema for the development of several different communication channels; the schema is compatible with the behavioral equation $(S{\to}R{\to}K{\to}C)$. Diagrammatically, it outlines the relationships between recepted sensory information (S), organic process—cognition/association and mediation levels (O), and the expressed response (R).

Input: Sensory Mode (S)

Modern workers tend to forget the work of the pioneers in exceptionality, such as Itard (1801; reprint, 1962) and Seguin (1866; reprint 1971); however, it should be noted that these pioneers were keenly interested in the functional assessment of the senses (Ball, 1971). Today, in the assessment and programming of children,

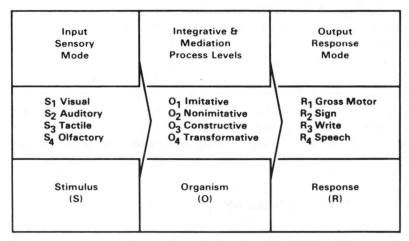

Figure 1. Communication channels. Relationships between recepted sensory information (S), psycholinguistic processes (O), and expressed response (R).

clinicians frequently overlook all the senses except vision and hearing (Montessori programs excepted) and often fail in obtaining a functional assessment for the severely handicapped. Sophisticated methods for audiometric assessment have been developed (Cox and Lloyd, this volume; Fulton and Lloyd, 1975), and initial research has begun in the assessment of vision (see Macht, 1971). Other senses such as tactile (haptic), olfactory, kinesthetic, pain, and so on, are rarely tested, and, when they are, they are not tested objectively. Clinicians or teachers working with severely and/or multiply handicapped children would be well advised to consider, for example, the use of tactile or other sensory input modes.

For instance, a salient factor in the initial selection of a sensory input mode is its degree of stimulus permanency. In other words, how much and what does the child have to remember about the stimulus? Figure 1 lists four common sensory input modes (S): visual, auditory, tactile, and olfactory.

Visual (S_1) Mode   Vision is an important sensory input mode—we live in a visual world. Prosthetic devices and techniques have been developed (Lindsley, 1964). For example, eyeglasses, increased size of pictures or print, and increased levels of illumination all aid the child with a visual handicap. One advantage of working with visual stimuli is their relative degree of permanency. In the case of matching visual stimuli (e.g., pictures or printed words), permanency is not a problem because the stimuli are always present in front of the child (see Clark and Woodcock, this volume).

Auditory (S₂) Mode When one is learning to speak, the auditory input mode is important. Deficiencies in hearing can be overcome by the use of hearing aids (see Cox and Lloyd, this volume; Ross, this volume), by increasing the sound intensity, or by the teacher talking loud enough to exceed the child's auditory threshold. For children with specific types of learning deficiencies, the auditory input mode may present a significant problem. For instance, auditory stimuli are fleeting; i.e., once a word is dictated by the teacher, it is gone. Thus, the child may not remember what the stimulus was and may be unable to make the appropriate response. Clinicians should be aware that deaf children do not learn language and speech without special training.

Tactile (S₃) Mode Tactile stimuli (e.g., braille) are used to teach blind children; however, tactile stimuli are infrequently considered as an input mode for the nonvisually impaired. For multiply handicapped or learning-deficient children, the tactile input mode may prove to be a significant factor in the establishment of a functional communication channel and subsequent cross-modal transfer.

Olfactory (S₄) Mode No matter what the handicapping condition (with the exception of anosmic children), the olfactory sense is the least likely to be nonfunctional. Although Montessori (1965, 1967) incorporated into her programs olfactory discrimination problems, few contemporary educators include this in their programs. Olfactory stimuli present problems in standardization and presentation, and are fleeting in nature. However, in spite of these problems and the problem of memory, when other sensory inputs fail, clinicians might do well with some children by using this sensory mode to attempt to establish a functional channel.

Integrative Processes (O): Conceptual Levels

The center panel of Figure 1 provides a hierarchal list of some integrative and mediation process levels. These are cognitive functions that are traditionally attributed to the "black-box" or brain. Although these process levels currently can be objectively defined and programmed, in the past they have been inferred with respect to sensory input and response output. As pointed out further on in this chapter, they also form a hierarchy with respect to assumed memory requirements. The process levels for the organism (O) are defined as imitative, nonimitative, constructive, and transformative.

Imitative (O₁)   The imitative level refers to imitative or identity matching (matching to sample). In this situation, the sample (input) stimulus and the selected response (output) stimulus are the same, e.g., picture matched to picture, printed word matched to printed word, or dictated word matched by spoken word.

Nonimitative (O₂)   The nonimitative level deals with a non-imitative match, i.e., a symbolic response. Thus, solution of the matching problem requires the selection of a response stimulus that differs from the sample stimulus. For example, matching a printed word to a picture, selecting a printed word that matches a dictated word, or vocalizing the word(s) when presented a picture.

Constructive (O₃)   The constructive level of integration deals with the ability to arrange elements (e.g., objects, pictures, words) in a representational form, in a sequence or specific configuration. For example, given the outline of a face and its elements (eyes, nose, and mouth), a child can place them in their respective positions. In essence, in order to perform at this cognitive level, the child must have developed the concept of face or ability to remember specific environmental events.

Transformative (O₄)   The transformative level is the highest level of integration to be discussed. In transformation, changes occur either in ordered sequences of elements, or in replacement, addition, or subtraction of elements, or both (Warren, 1968): for example, the change of words and/or order in a sentence, or a change in the spatial arrangements of elements (a generative function). In a recent study (Premack, 1975), a young child was provided with pictures of two arms, two legs, a head, and a body. He was asked to construct a male figure. He used the elements as follows: 1) head on body, 2) one leg across chest for arms, 3) the two arms as legs, and 4) the second leg as a genital organ. It should be noted that transformation does not refer simply to an inadequate or different response. It refers to the response of a child who clearly is capable of making a conventional constructive or generative response but then goes beyond this conventional response to transform the output into a creative or original product.

Output: Response Mode (R)

The third segment of Figure 1 concerns the child's response mode. The first three common response modes, gross motor, sign, and write, require an increasing refinement of hand movements and finger dexterity. The last response mode listed is that of speech, and it requires fine motor movements involving quite different anatomical components, e.g., vocal cords, tongue, lips, and so on.

Gross motor (R_1) The first level (R_1) represents gross motor behavior such as grasping, pushing a button, and the like. This level also could include simple sequences such as reach-grasp-pull-drop. Even the most severely handicapped child can learn such simple motor responses (Hollis, 1967) although some children require prosthetic devices (see Vanderheiden and Harris-Vanderheiden, this volume).

Sign (R_2) At the sign level, the complexity of the motor response to that of relatively fine finger movements is increased—for example, in the production of the hand and finger movements required to produce the signs of the American Sign Language, Signed English, or other signed systems (see Kopchick and Lloyd, this volume; Wilbur, this volume; Gardner and Gardner, 1969).

Write (R_3) The third level involves the printing of letters of the alphabet and/or words. Script writing and drawing are also included (see Neisworth and Smith, 1973). It should be noted that normal adults frequently resort to the prosthetic writing device known as the typewriter because their hand movements produce illegible words (see Clark and Woodcock, this volume).

Speech (R_4) Speech, a unique human response mode, is for many retarded children extremely difficult to learn. The speech or the phonologic response mode requires the most complex motor behavior in order to produce the required phonemes (Travis, 1957; also see McLean, this volume). It should be noted that, because a child does not talk or read aloud, it cannot be inferred that he has not developed language or does not have the ability to develop it (Carrier, this volume, 1974; Hollis and Carrier, 1975).

Osgood's Language Model

Language always has been a challenge to the behavior theorist and educator because of its complex organization. Over two decades have passed since Osgood attempted a behavioristic analysis of language (Osgood, 1957), which forms the common thread that emerges in current thinking and approaches to language research. In his original model, Osgood conceptualized language ability in three dimensions:

Channels of communication:
1. Auditory-vocal (Figure 1, S_2-R_4)
2. Visual-motor (Figure 1, S_1-R_1)

Psycholinguistic processes:
1. Decoding or receptive (Figure 1, O; also see Sidman, Cresson, and Willson-Morris, 1974)
2. Associative or organizing (Figure 1, O_1-O_4; also see Premack, 1975)

Levels of organization:
1. Representational, utilization of symbols (Figure 1, O_2; also see Carrier, this volume, 1974; Clark, this volume; Vanderheiden and Harris-Vanderheiden, this volume)
2. Automatic-sequential, reflexive associations (Figure 1, O_3; also see Spradlin, 1973; Sidman, Cresson, and Willson-Morris, 1974)

Language Assessment

Kirk encouraged Osgood to refine his model so that it could be developed into a tool for the assessment of the language behavior of handicapped children. Subsequently, the refined model was used to generate a battery of language tests. This test battery is now known as the Illinois Test of Psycholinguistic Abilities (ITPA— Kirk, McCarthy, and Kirk (1961); revision, 1968). There are probably several reasons why the ITPA has become one of the most commonly used assessment devices in the area of learning deficiencies. Subjectively, some of these are: 1) communication/language is a central problem in learning deficiencies; 2) the test attempts to reduce linguistic behavior into functional parts; 3) it approaches language as if it were just another learned behavior; and 4) by incorporating the concept of input-output channels, it has had a significant appeal to those working with sensory and motor impaired children. The ITPA as a language assessment device presents some problems; for example, some of the subtests seem to be unrelated to language, and some aspects of language such as comprehension and syntactic construction are not directly assessed (Siegel and Broen, this volume; Dale, 1972). Although in the past there has been little experimental evidence to support Osgood's model, there seems to be some recent research that lends support to the model. This research is presented and discussed in the following sections of this chapter.

Related Language Training

The University of Illinois Press (Urbana, Illinois, 61801) has published a number of books by Kirk and his co-workers on the ITPA and related training programs. For example, see *Psycholinguistic Learning Disabilities: Diagnosis and Remediation* (Kirk and Kirk, 1971).

Learning and Transfer

Underlying many educational programs and curricula is the assumption that certain concepts or principles generalize or transfer to new tasks or situations. This phenomenon has been accepted by teachers of normal and handicapped children for a long time. That is, clinicians or teachers do not have to teach everything in order for the child to develop functional language or reading. Traditionally, this ability to generalize to new tasks has been subsumed under the rubric of cognitive processes or integration and mediation process levels (Figure 1). Peters (1935) proposed that ideas A and B could become associated indirectly through a third idea, C. That is, one does not have to teach directly the association between ideas A and B. This concept seems to be an integral part of Osgood's language model at the integration level, and Sidman's (Sidman and Cresson, 1973) reading paradigm at the cross-modal transfer level.

Those who work with learning deficiencies, especially with multiply handicapped children, encounter various types of sensorimotor deficits. Thus, a consideration of processes of cross-modal transfer and sensory equivalence is of utmost importance in the development of educational programs for these children. For example, in the course of development a child normally learns auditory comprehension of words before visual comprehension or reading (Sidman and Cresson, 1973). This in essence is a problem of sensory equivalence or cross-modal transfer (Wright, 1970).

The graphic illustration of communication channels (Figure 1) is intended to provide the reader with a map for delineating various types of intra- and intersensory interactions. Wright (1970) has systematically reviewed studies concerned with cross-modal interactions. These studies generally have been concerned with the question of how sensory information from different modalities (e.g., tactile and visual, or auditory and visual) combine to determine the response output (e.g., gross motor or speech). From a practical educational point of view, it is unlikely that a child would be able to match shape cross-modally (nonimitative match) before he can match shape within both the modalities involved (imitative match). For example, it would be unlikely that a child could match the tactile sensation of a shape to its visual representation before he had learned to match a tactile shape to its identical sample or the visual representation to its identical sample. In like manner, it is unlikely that a child could match his spoken word to a printed word (oral reading) before he was able to match his speech to a dictated word or match a printed word to an identical printed word. As indicated in subsequent sections of this chapter, Sidman's reading program incorporates this basic concept.

FUNCTIONAL ANALYSIS OF READING

Successful reading performance in part requires that a child learn equivalences between auditory and visual stimuli (auditory comprehension). This ability in the normal course of development generally precedes the understanding of written or printed words (reading comprehension). Although during the past decade there has been considerable controversy over how to teach reading, e.g., phonetic versus whole word approaches, in general, these methods have focused on the receptive or expressive aspects of reading. Thus, they have avoided the requirement of undertaking a functional analysis of reading. In recent years there has been a proliferation of labels such as dyslexia for reading problems (Lerner, 1971). These labels have tended to obscure rather than clarify problems encountered in the teaching of reading. In spite of all the interest and controversy surrounding reading, few researchers have attempted a functional analysis of reading. An exception to this point of view is the work of Sidman and Cresson (1973) and Sidman, Cresson, and Willson-Morris (1974), who have attempted a functional analysis of reading and have subsequently conducted research on reading and transfer.

Word Reading Lattice

Figure 2 presents a schema for the functional analysis of reading. The *input* is shown along the abscissa at the bottom of the figure (*stimulus components*). The subject's *output* (*response level*) appears along the ordinate on the lefthand side of the figure. The reading *subobjectives* appear along the ridgeline, starting at the lower left corner (*imitative match*) and moving to the upper right corner (*oral reading*) of the figure. This schema provides an objective method for the assessment of word reading deficiencies and/or the teaching of reading. It should be noted that this is *not* a developmental system; therefore entry and exit can be made at any one of several points. That is, the learning-deficient child may demonstrate deficiencies on one or more of the subobjectives. Using this method of analysis, word reading is reducible to two types of intramodal (within sensory modality) equivalences and four types of intermodal (between sensory modality) equivalences (see Spradlin, Karlan, and Wetherby, this volume, Figure 3).

Intramodal Equivalence

In the analysis of reading, intramodal equivalence refers to stimulus equivalence *within* a specific sensory modality, e.g., visual or auditory. This class of equivalence is achieved through learning or transfer at the imitative and nonimitative process levels (Figures 1 and 2).

Imitative Level (O_1) There are three types of imitative matches in reading (Figure 2). The imitative matches are specified as follows: 1) picture to picture, 2) printed word to printed word, and 3) word dictated by teacher matched by word spoken by child.

Nonimitative Level (O_2) Simple reading comprehension involves learning to make nonimitative matches (Figure 1). These matches take the form of matching a printed word to a picture, or vice versa (Figure 2).

Intermodal Equivalence

The development of stimulus equivalence *across* sensory modalities (e.g., visual/auditory or auditory/visual) may be viewed as intermodal equivalence or cross-modal transfer. Specifically, reading involves four types of intermodal equivalences: 1) auditory comprehension, 2) auditory receptive reading, 3) picture naming, and 4)

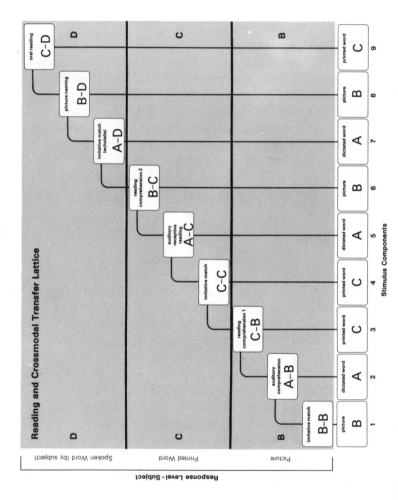

Figure 2. Reading and cross-modal transfer lattice. The lattice presents a schema for the functional analysis of reading. It outlines the interrelationships between classes of input stimuli and the subject's response mode in the development of various specific skills involved in reading. (After Sidman and Cresson, 1973).

oral reading. Proficiency on any one of these equivalences can be achieved by direct training or cross-modal transfer (see Sidman and Cresson, 1973; Sidman, Cresson, and Willson-Morris, 1974).

Auditory Comprehension (A-B)   The auditory comprehension reading skill involves learning equivalences between auditory (input) stimuli and visual (response-output) stimuli. Basically, the task requires that the subject learn to match pictures to words dictated by the teacher or clinician (Figure 2).

Auditory Receptive Reading (A-C)   A second type of equivalence in the nonimitation match between auditory and visual stimuli involves receptive reading. At this level the task requires that the subject learn to match printed words to words dictated by the teacher or clinician (Figure 2).

Picture Naming (B-D)   The picture naming level of equivalence involves the use of the speech mode to respond to picture stimuli (Figure 2). For example, the child produces the appropriate verbal label for the picture stimulus.

Oral Reading (C-D)   The oral reading level of equivalence involves the use of the speech mode to respond to printed word stimuli (Figure 2). For example, the child produces the appropriate verbal label for the printed word stimulus.

Research Results

Sidman and Cresson (1973) undertook a program to teach simple reading skills to two students so developmentally deficient that no IQ could be calculated because they scored below the Binet test's minimum. Before initiation of the reading program they were incapable of matching printed words to their pictures (Figure 2, reading comprehension), or of reading printed words (Figure 2, oral reading). The subjects were trained to match pictures to pictures and words to words (Figure 2, imitative match) and dictated words to pictures and printed words (Figure 2, auditory comprehension and auditory receptive reading). After training, they were able to perform, without specific training, the following: 1) match picture to word (Figure 2, reading comprehension), 2) vocally name the pictures (Figure 2, picture naming), and 3) orally read words (Figure 2, oral reading).

In a second study using similar subjects, Sidman, Cresson, and Willson-Morris (1974) demonstrated that initial training on a different set of subobjectives (Figure 2) would result in the acquisition of the remaining subobjectives without direct training. In another demonstration, the subject was taught to: 1) match upper-case letters to dictated (auditory) letter name, 2) match lower-case letters to upper-case letters, and 3) match upper-case letters to lower-case letters. After this initial training, the subject was able to perform the following: 1) match lower-case letters to the dictated (auditory) letter name, 2) orally name upper-case letters; and 3) orally name lower-case letters.

DISCRIMINATION WITHOUT DIRECT TRAINING: CONCEPT FORMATION

The work of Sidman and his co-workers demonstrated that responding appropriately to new situations may result from what has been learned in prior situations. That is, conditioning two conditional stimuli to control the same response to a third sample stimulus will establish them as a stimulus class or concept. The establishment of stimulus classes in the learning-deficient child has been investigated by Spradlin, Cotter, and Baxley (1973). Using a paradigm similar to that of Peters (1935), they demonstrated, using abstract figures (symbols), that if the subject learned to make a common response (R_1) to different symbols (A and B), and a second response (R_2) is conditioned to one of the symbols (A), the remaining symbol (B) will also control the second response (R_2). They noted that such behavior is especially characteristic of complex academic skills such as language, reading, and reasoning. The implications of their research with learning deficient children were summarized as follows (Spradlin, Cotter, and Baxley, p. 564):

> Usually when persons talk of the importance of concepts, they imply relationships among concepts. It is at this point that the current study has its greatest relevance. The research clearly indicates that if new responses are conditioned to some members of a stimulus class or concept, they will be transferred to other members of the class. For example, if a child is taught to label bananas, apples, and peaches as "fruit," and then taught to say apples and peaches grow on trees, he may, without further training, correctly say that bananas also grow on trees. He may also conclude that since apples and peaches have seeds, bananas do also.

For additional discussion of this area of research, see the chapter by Spradlin, Karlan, and Wetherby (this volume).

LANGUAGE LEARNING: NONSPEECH RESPONSE MODE

Some children during the normal course of development do not acquire speech and language. These children may be deaf, retarded, or have learning deficiencies of unknown origin. This problem suggests that one should look for alternative communication channels (see Figure 1, S-R). Can a channel be found that will circumvent, for example, the auditory input mode (S_2), the speech output mode (R_4), and at the same time require only simple integrative and process levels (O)? Premack (1970), in researching procedures for teaching language functions to chimpanzees, developed a system utilizing visual input (S_1) and gross motor output (R_1). This system, based on *word* units, avoided the problem of speech altogether (Hollis and Carrier, 1975). Carrier (this volume, 1974) modified Premack's procedures in order to make them directly applicable to learning-deficient children and the English language. The prerequisites for entry into Carrier's language program are as follows: 1) ability to use visual input mode, 2) ability to use gross motor output mode, 3) ability to learn imitative matching, and 4) ability to learn nonimitative matching (also see Carrier, this volume).

Dual Structure of Communication Model

Premack's research has demonstrated that communication can be separated into two distinct parameters. The first parameter is delineated by the rules for developing symbols (e.g., speech, writing, or signs) or, in other words, the response mode. Language makes up the second parameter of communication. It in turn consists of two sets of rules and principles.

Semantics   One set of rules consists of those used for establishing symbols to represent different meanings. Thus, a specific symbol may be used to represent *boy* (nonimitative match), a young male human, and another symbol might be used to represent the "action" of running.

Syntax   The other set of rules or principles determines the sequential arrangement of symbols (construction) in a standard grammatical response. For example, in an active declarative sentence, the subject noun precedes the verb.

Program   Procedures for teaching communication behavior to learning-deficient children in the *nonspeech response mode* include a series of programs, each designed to teach some specific parameter of the model, and each carefully integrated into the total goals of the training. (These programs are presented in detail by Carrier, 1974.) The programs in this series all have certain features in common (Hollis and Carrier, 1975):

1.   They are all written in step-by-step sequences
2.   Rather than spoken words, the symbols for various morphemes to be taught are manipulable *geometric* forms of different shapes
3.   Appropriate responses are indicated by placing the geometric forms (words) on a simple tray
4.   Then, to indicate learning of *semantic* or *syntactic* rules, the subject need only to make a gross motor movement

Preliminary Research   Carrier (this volume, 1974) trained 50 severely developmentally deficient children using the Non-Speech Language Initiation Program. Many of the subjects in this initial study had mild sensory and/or motor involvement, but all were able to make gross motor movements. In addition, none of the subjects initially used speech for communication. The results are briefly summarized as follows:

1.   The mean training time for subject noun selection was approximately 1.25 hours
2.   The mean training time for verb selection was approximately 6 hours
3.   The "learning-to-learn" phenomenon was apparent because the time required to learn various constituents became shorter and shorter as subjects progressed through the programs
4.   Analysis of the data suggests that semantic features of the symbols became cues for syntactic sequences
5.   Errors in advanced stages of the program resembled those in the grammar of speaking children

RESPONSE MODE TRANSFER: READING AND WRITING

If a child is taught language using a visual-nonvocal language model such as Carrier's, will his language training transfer to reading printed words or the traditional response modes of speech and writing (Figure 1)? Following up the work of Carrier (1974), Kuntz (1974) attempted to answer this question. The Kuntz study was designed to investigate transfer from the nonvocal communication system of Carrier to traditional reading modes. Fourteen severely developmentally deficient children who had unsuccessfully spent several years in special education classes were used as subjects.

Using abstract symbols, the children were taught left-to-right sequencing (construction), and matching symbols to stimulus pictures (nonimitative matching). In short, using abstract symbols (word units), the children learned communication skills, both semantic and syntactic. That is, they learned to sequence an article, subject noun, auxiliary verb, and verb, and developed a functional semantic comprehension of five nouns and five verbs. All this was accomplished with a mean of approximately 8 hours of training. For example, at the completion of training, the child might be presented with a picture of a boy sitting and an array of meaningful abstract symbols. The child then was able to select and sequence the symbols to write the sentence, *The boy is sitting.* Learning to write (using abstract symbols—Carrier, 1974) took an average of 7 hours, 55 minutes. Most importantly, all children transferred readily from the abstract forms to writing and reading with printed words (also see Sidman and Cresson, 1973). Thus, after the children learned basic semantic and syntactic rules, it was a relatively easy task to establish the normal printed word as an equivalent stimulus. All this suggests that, in developing writing and reading, it is the nature of the program that is crucial, not the configuration of the stimulus element— abstract geometric figure or printed word.

For those children who could print isolated letters and vocalize (produce spoken words in isolation), this program provided them with the ability to transfer learned skills to the speech and writing (printing words) response modes (also see Glass, Gazzaniga, and Premack, 1973). In summarizing her work, Kuntz (1974, p. 119) stated:

> The success achieved through this communication program indicates that a reevaluation of certain teaching procedures may be necessary. The severely mentally retarded children used in this study had been in special education classes from one to nine years. Most had no reading or writing ability at the beginning of this program. Some of the children could recognize their first name and a few common nouns. This is hardly a profitable return for a median of 4 years and 7 months of education. Several of the older subjects had been dismissed from attending special education classes because of not benefiting from the teaching procedures that were employed in the special classrooms.

INTEGRATIVE PROCESSES

Chimpanzees and many children labeled as developmentally deficient do not draw or assemble pieces of existing material to reproduce meaningful events in the natural world.

This chapter points out that even severely handicapped children are able to function at imitative and nonimitative process levels. This conclusion is supported by the research of Sidman and Cresson (1973), Spradlin, Cotter, and Baxley (1973), and Carrier (1974). However, little has been said yet about construction (with the exception of sequencing) and transformational processes. The work of Carrier (1974) and Kuntz (1974) should leave little doubt about the ability of severely developmentally deficient children being able to function as the constructive level (sequence words), when they are programmed adequately. It is logical to ask, as has Premack: Is the lack of visual production attributable to deficiencies in motor, cognitive, or motivational ability, or to some combination of the three (Premack, 1975)?

Construction (O_3)

Premack (1975) addressed the problem of visual production in chimpanzees and children by initially reducing the motor demands to a minimum. That is, the chimp or child was not required to draw (fine motor movements—R_3) but only needed to arrange physical elements (gross motor movements—R_1). His materials consisted of a photograph of a face with the main features blanked out; the photograph was mounted on stiff material. Two eyes, a nose, and a mouth were cut from another photograph and mounted in the same manner (a photograph of the child could be used). Children (ages 2.4 to 10 years) were presented with the blank face and the four pieces scattered randomly and were asked to complete the facial figure, using each of the four pieces at least once. The general results of this study show that the younger children were unable to construct a face, but the older children constructed it without difficulty. Children of intermediate age, in some cases, either constructed or transformed the face. It should be apparent that the task requires an acquisition of the concept of *face,* i.e., memory. In some cases the children, after assembling the face in an appropriate manner, on subsequent trials engaged in simple transformations. For example, they assembled it upsidedown or in some form that resembled modern art.

Transformation (O₄)

Premack hypothesized that the free transforming spirit of the child may be quashed by restrictive socialization. However, he was interested in determining whether children could be induced to be active transformers. It is apparent that normal perception provides only veridical models—intact faces, bodies, animals, trees, and the like. He suggested that transformations must be taught explicitly. He found that the most effective device for increasing the amount of transformation in known transformers was a *self-puzzle,* that is, a mounted photograph of the child cut into pieces. As noted previously, some of the transformations took the form of sexual improvisions. One way to increase the probability of producing a transformation was to repeatedly present the children with the faced puzzle. In his work with chimps, Premack observed Sarah making a facial transformation after playing with a hat and viewing herself wearing it. In one instance she used the mouth piece of the puzzle as a hat, and in another case she used a banana peel as a hat.

Premack's work has important implications for special educators and clinicians because it suggests possible methods for the practical training of learning-deficient children at the integrative and mediation process levels of construction (O₃) and transformation (O₄). His conclusions fit well with the Osgood model and with Sidman's and Spradlin's transfer studies. Premack (1975, p. 235) summarized his research as follows:

> In learning to move the plastic pieces into veridical positions, Sarah acquired visual-motor coordinations analogous in kind to the auditory-motor coordinations of speech. The infant can see the lips of a speaker but not the disposition of the internal speech apparatus, yet learns to produce motor configurations resulting in sounds matching those heard. In both cases the model given the subject supplies only one side of the sensory-motor correlation: the child hears speech sounds and the chimp sees faces. But the child is not shown the motor configurations that produce the sounds nor is the chimp shown the movements that bring the facial pieces into veridical configurations. Although orders of magnitude apart in complexity, these sensory-motor coordinations are analogous in being learned entirely without guidance and indeed without even a complete model.

It should be noted that, in the case of the exceptional child, a functional communicative channel (Figure 1) must be established in order to study construction and transformation. If these processes are found lacking, then it would be appropriate to select one or more of the prosthetic techniques suggested in this volume in order to eliminate the problem.

MEMORY MODIFICATION

Although "memory" is most often viewed as a covert function and most often dealt with indirectly (see Tredgold and Tredgold, 1952; Baumeister, 1963; Vergason, 1964), it is possible to define it operationally and to deal with it in a direct fashion. If a child is taught at one time to make a specific response to a specific stimulus and then at some subsequent time the child makes that same response to the stimulus, memory has occurred. Thus, memory can be objectively measured to the extent that the time interval between the original training and subsequent performance can be objectively measured.

Training

In the same sense that the time interval between successive performances ("memory") can be measured, it can be systematically increased by reinforcing correct responses following gradually increasing time intervals. Thus, if a student learns to emit a response correctly in a situation where intervals between presentation of the stimuli average 2 seconds, but he does not emit the same response to the same stimulus after a 60-minute interval, it is possible to gradually lengthen intervals between trials until he is "remembering" for the full 60 minutes. This might be done by separating trials first by a 2-second interval, then by a 4-second interval, then one with 8 seconds, then 16 seconds, 30 seconds, 60 seconds, 2 minutes, 4 minutes, etc., until the 60-minute interval is established.

Preliminary Research

These procedures have been piloted on children being run on the Non-Speech Language Initiation Program (Non-SLIP). The program is designed to require 24-hour memory, but in many cases it did not originally provide for memory beyond the 24-hour period. It was discovered that behaviors learned at the 24-hour interval and then not reviewed for 3 or more days were retained with only 50 to 60% accuracy. As a result, long weekends, child illness, home visits, etc., nearly always required retraining on previously learned skills. Some children with high illness rates were unable to progress past the first few training steps because of the need to recycle training continually. However, when an interval shaping procedure (1 day, 2 days, 3 days, 5 days, 7 days) was established, children were able to retain learned behavior at accuracy levels ranging from 95 to 100% for periods ranging up to 30 days.

The precise dynamics of the interval shaping are not clearly understood at this time. The concept does seem to have considerable potential and is one that probably deserves careful research into its dynamics and into its application to a variety of problems where memory is important.

SUMMARY

This chapter attempts to synthesize some contemporary ideas relevant to the remediation of learning and language deficiencies. It emphasizes the functional analysis of learning and communication.

The approach has been noncategorical because the authors believe that all children, whether handicapped or nonhandicapped, are subject to the same learning principles. Although the authors are quite aware that many handicapped children have neurologic deficiencies, the approach is environmental because environmental factors can be controlled and modified by the clinician or teacher to produce more adequate performance among handicapped children. The clinician has little control over the neurologic status of the child.

The functional analysis of behavior involves four basic components: stimulus, response, contingency, and consequence. Each of these components can be the subject of manipulation in treatment. The stimulus, contingency, and consequence may be independently manipulated directly. The response is manipulated by the action of these other three variables.

These four components of an operant equation are related to Osgood's input-integration and output model. This model proposes two input modes: visual and auditory, which are well used in training programs. Two other modes (tactile and olfactory) have been used less frequently in training. The chapter suggests that every available mode be investigated in the attempt to establish a functional input channel for handicapped children.

The chapter also notes that in communication there are four common output modes: gross motor acts, signing, writing, and speaking.

Frequently, handicapped children are severely limited in the complex acts of speaking and signing. Deficiencies in these modes should never result in the communication isolation of handicapped children if gross motor modes are made available.

Although currently the conception of the integrative processes such as imitation, nonimitative matching, construction, and transformation is less well understood than the input and output modes, recent experimental work has begun to clarify issues related to integrative processes. Researchers have begun to conduct research that will lead to clear-cut predictions concerning when transfer will and will not occur. Sidman's (1971) research is perhaps the clearest example of such research.

Research by Carrier suggests that even elusive "mental processes" such as memory may be trained.

The studies on integrative processes indicate that the theory of training must be more complex than many once thought, but it also suggests that far less needs to be taught than was once thought. In other words, by teaching some skills, other skills that were never trained may emerge. This fact should be encouraging to those engaged in remediating behavioral deficiencies among handicapped children.

REFERENCES

Baer, D. M., M. M. Wolf, and R. R. Harris. 1964. Effects of adult social reinforcement on child behavior. Young Child. 20:8–17.

Ball, T. S. 1971. Itard, Seguin and Kephart: Sensory Education—A Learning Interpretation. Charles E. Merrill, Columbus, Ohio.

Baumeister, A. A. 1963. Investigations of memory deficits in retardates. Progress Report, MH 07445-01. National Institute of Mental Health, Washington, D.C.

Carrier, J. K., Jr. 1974. Application of functional analysis and a nonspeech response mode to teaching language. Amer. Speech Hear. Assoc. Monogr. 18.

Chow, K. L. 1967. Effects of ablation. In G. C. Quarton, T. Melnechuk, and F. O. Schmitt (eds.), The Neurosciences. Rockefeller University Press, New York.

Dale, P. S. 1972. Language Development: Structure and Function. Dryden Press, Hinsdale, Ill.

Dunn, L. M. (ed.) 1965. Exceptional Children in the Schools. Holt, Rinehart and Winston, New York.

Estes, W. K. 1970. Learning Theory and Mental Development. Academic Press, New York.

Ferster, C., and M. DeMeyer. 1961. The development of performance in autistic children in an automatically controlled environment. J. Chronic Disord. 13:312–345.

Ferster, C. B., and B. F. Skinner. 1957. Schedules of Reinforcement. Appleton-Century-Crofts, New York.

Fulton, R. T., and L. L. Lloyd. (eds.) 1975. Auditory Assessment of the Difficult-to-Test. Williams & Wilkins, Baltimore.

Gardner, R. A., and B. T. Gardner. 1969. Teaching sign language to a chimpanzee. Science 165:664–672.

Glass, A., M. Gazzaniga, and D. Premack. 1973. Artificial language training in global aphasics. Neuropsychologica 12:95–103.

Hallahan, D. P., and W. M. Cruickshank. 1973. Psycho-Educational Foundations of Learning Disabilities. Prentice-Hall, Englewood Cliffs, N.J.

Hollis, J. H. 1967. Development of perceptual motor skills in a profoundly retarded child: Part I—Prosthesis. Amer. J. Ment. Defic. 71:941–952.

Hollis, J. H. 1973. "Superstition": The effects of independent and contingent events on free operant responses in retarded children. Amer. J. Ment. Defic. 77:585–596.

Hollis, J. H., and J. K. Carrier, Jr. 1975. Research implications for communication deficiencies. Except. Child. 41:405–412.

Homme, L. E., P. D. deBaca, J. V. Devine, R. Steinhorst, and E. J. Rickert. 1963. Use of the Premack Principle in controlling the behavior of nursery school children. J. Exp. Anal. Behav. 6:544.

Itard, J. M. G. 1962. The Wild Boy of Aveyron. Appleton-Century-Crofts, New York.

Kirk, S. A., and W. D. Kirk. 1971. Psycholinguistic Learning Disabilities: Diagnosis and Remediation. University of Illinois Press, Urbana.

Kirk, S. A., J. J. McCarthy, and W. D. Kirk. 1968. Illinois Test of Psycholinguistic Abilities. University of Illinois Press, Urbana.

Kuntz, J. B. 1974. A nonvocal communication development program for severely retarded children. Unpublished doctoral dissertation, Kansas State University, Manhattan, Kan.

Lerner, J. W. 1971. Children with Learning Disabilities: Theories, Diagnosis, and Teaching Strategies. Houghton Mifflin, Boston.

Lindsley, O. R. 1964. Direct measurement and prosthesis of retarded behavior. J. Educ. 147:62–81.

Macht, J. 1971. Operant measurement of subjective visual acuity in nonverbal children. J. Appl. Behav. Anal. 4:23–36.

Montessori, M. 1965. Dr. Montessori's Own Handbook. Schocken Books, New York.

Montessori, M. 1967. The Discovery of the Child. Ballantine Books, New York.

Neisworth, J. T., and R. M. Smith. 1973. Modifying Retarded Behavior. Houghton Mifflin, Boston.

Osgood, C. E. 1957. A behavioristic analysis of perception and language as cognitive phenomena. *In* J. S. Bruner et al. (eds.), Contemporary Approaches to Cognition. Harvard University Press, Cambridge, Mass.

Peters, H. N. 1935. Mediate association. J. Exp. Psychol. 18:20–48.

Premack, D. 1970. A functional analysis of language. J. Exp. Anal. Behav. 14:107–125.

Premack, D. 1975. Putting a face together. Science 188:228–236.

Seguin, E. 1971. Idiocy and Its Treatment by the Physiological Method. Augustus M. Kelley, New York.

Sidman, M. 1971. Reading and auditory-visual equivalence. J. Speech Hear. Res. 14:5–13.

Sidman, M., and O. Cresson. 1973. Reading and crossmodal transfer of stimulus equivalences in severe retardation. Amer. J. Ment. Defic. 77:515–523.

Sidman, M., O. Cresson, and M. Willson-Morris. 1974. Acquisition of matching to sample via mediated transfer. J. Exp. Anal. Behav. 2: 261–273.

Spradlin, J. E. 1973. Psycholinguistic training of retarded children. *In* R. M. Allen and A. D. Cortazzo (eds.), Psycholinguistic Development in Children: Implications for Children with Developmental Disabilities. University of Miami Press, Coral Gables, Fla.

Spradlin, J. E., V. W. Cotter, and N. Baxley. 1973. Establishing a conditional discrimination without direct training: A study of transfer with retarded adolescents. Amer. J. Ment. Defic. 77:556–566.

Travis, L. E. 1957. Handbook of Speech Pathology. Appleton-Century-Crofts, New York.

Tredgold, A. F., and R. F. Tredgold. 1952. A Textbook of Mental Deficiency (Amentia). 8th Ed. Williams & Wilkins, Baltimore.

Vergason, G. A. 1964. Retention in retarded and normal subjects as a function of amount of original training. Amer. J. Ment. Defic. 68: 623–629.

Warren, R. M. 1968. Verbal transformation effect and auditory perceptual mechanisms. Psychol. Bull. 70:261–270.

Wender, P. H. 1971. Minimal Brain Dysfunction in Children. Wiley-Interscience, New York.

von Wright, J. M. 1970. Cross-modal transfer and sensory equivalence— A review. Scand. J. Psychol. 2:21–30.

8

AMPLIFICATION SYSTEMS

Mark Ross

CONTENTS

Hearing Aid/Auditory Trainer Components _____ 298

Electroacoustic Dimensions _____ 298
    Gain/299
    Output/300
    Frequency response/301
    Frequency range/302

Types of Hearing Aids _____ 305
    Body-worn aids/305
    Bone conduction aids/307
    Ear-level aids/308
    CROS variations/308
    Binaural aids/309

Auditory Trainers _____ 311
    Hard-wire systems/311
    Radio frequency systems/312

Environmental Considerations _____ 313
    Noise and reverberation/313
    Distance effects/314
    Sound treatment effect/314
    Visual/auditory reception/316

Troubleshooting and Maintenance _____ 317
    Frequency of malfunctions/317
    Visual and auditory inspections/318

Summary and Conclusions _____ 320

References _____ 320

One cannot simply add the disability components in a multiply handicapped person and arrive at a sum total disability. The behavioral configuration seems to be qualitatively and quantitatively different than a simple addition of disabilities would indicate. For the multiply handicapped child with a hearing impairment as one of the component problems, the contribution of the hearing loss to the total behavioral package is difficult, if not impossible, to isolate. Yet, as Kleffner (1973) has pointed out, it makes little sense thereby to ignore the hearing loss as a secondary or trivial matter. Whatever other problems a child manifests, if a significant hearing impairment is evident, it is bound to exert a deleterious influence upon the child's developmental adjustment. Even a partial hearing loss, by itself, without any other compounding problems, can have awesomely severe consequences on the speech, language, educational, and psychosocial status of a hearing-impaired person (Myklebust, 1964; Babbidge, 1965; Quigley and Thomure, 1968; Hine, 1970; Goetzinger, 1972). When other factors enter into the behavioral equation, the resulting problems manifest uniquely new dimensions of severity.

There is also some evidence that the delayed or mismanaged hearing condition may produce secondary emotional and/or language problems, the results of which are a functionally multiply handicapping condition (Merklein and Briskey, 1962; Rosenberg, 1966; Elliot and Armbruster, 1967; Ross and Matkin, 1968). It is necessary, therefore, to take the proper aural rehabilitative measures just as soon as the existence of a hearing loss becomes apparent, both to preclude the emergence and severity of secondary problems and to minimize the impact of the hearing condition on the total behavioral picture.

This chapter is devoted to just one aural rehabilitative measure: the provision of amplified sound. The intelligent use of amplified sound requires some familiarity with the basic electroacoustic dimensions of auditory amplification, their impact upon the reception of speech, the various kinds of amplification systems used in different settings, and the consequences of environmental conditions upon speech perception. It should be noted, however, that the most effective use of amplification requires that this measure be incorporated in a total aural rehabilitative program (Sanders, 1971; Ross, 1972a). Many of the components of such a program are covered elsewhere in this volume (e.g., Cox and Lloyd; Graham; Kopchick and Lloyd).

HEARING AID/AUDITORY TRAINER COMPONENTS

Hearing aids and auditory trainers are essentially public address systems, and no matter how small the hearing aid or how large the auditory trainer, each possesses the same general components and serves the same general function as public address systems. The function of each of these devices is to amplify sound. Each of them includes a microphone, which converts an acoustic signal into an alternating electrical current; an amplifier, which increases the voltage of the electrical current; and a speaker, which converts the increased voltage back to an acoustic signal.

The microphones of wearable hearing aids are usually mounted within the body of the hearing aid, with an aperture to permit the sound to impinge upon the microphone face. The speaker (called the "receiver" in hearing aid terminology) also can be mounted within the hearing aid chassis, in the case of hearing aids worn at ear level, or it can be separated from the chassis and connected to the receiver by a wire, in the case of body-worn hearing aids. The advantages and disadvantages of each of these hearing aid styles are discussed in a later section. Finally, each hearing aid must include an earmold, which couples (connects) the receiver to the person's ear canal. The acoustics of earmolds has received a great deal of attention lately because the total amplification pattern of the hearing aid has been found to be greatly modified, deliberately or inadvertently, by physical modifications of the coupler system (e.g., Lybarger, 1972; Berger, 1974; Langford, 1975).

Auditory trainers are, in effect, large hearing aids for classroom or group instruction. The microphones and the receiver (or earphones) are usually physically separated from the amplifier and connected to it by wires or via radio frequency transmission (Ross, 1969, 1973). An overview of classroom auditory training systems is presented below.

ELECTROACOUSTIC DIMENSIONS

In this section, the basic electroacoustic dimension of auditory amplification devices (hearing aids and auditory trainers) is discussed in as clinical and nontechnical manner as possible. The implications of various modifications on the reception and development of speech and language are stressed. The interested reader is referred to the following references for a detailed, technical coverage of the elec-troacoustics and behavioral aspects of amplification measurements and usage (Katz, 1972; Berger, 1974; Donnelly, 1974; Pollack, 1975; Northern and Downs, 1974).

Gain

The gain of an auditory amplification device (hearing aid and/or auditory trainer) is the difference between the sound pressure level (SPL) of the input and the SPL of the output. The conditions under which the measurements are made must be specified, as well as the frequencies and intensities of the inputs, the characteristics of the room or chamber in which the measurements are made, and the amount of rotation of the gain/volume control. The instrumentation used to measure gain is commercially available and can be found in many speech and hearing centers (Lybarger, 1974). In essence, the gain represents how much the amplification device increases the sound intensity under the particular gain/volume setting specified. Thus, a hearing aid with a gain setting of 50 dB increases a 70-dB SPL speech input signal to 120 dB SPL, while a gain of 40 dB SPL increases the same input to only 110 dB SPL.

It is tempting to relate the gain of a hearing aid to the degree of hearing loss a person manifests. Thus, if someone has a 60-dB hear-ing loss, it seems logical to provide him with a gain of 60 dB, and thereby fully compensate for the hearing loss. Unfortunately, this is not, however, how the ear works. With a gain of 60 dB, an SPL input of 70 dB (or about slightly above average intensity of speech measured 3 feet from a talker) resuults in an output of 130 dB. This figure is just about at the human tolerance limit for intense sounds (Morgan, Wilson, and Dirks, 1974) and, in the example given, is probably about 30 dB greater than someone with this degree of hear-ing loss would find comfortable. A rule of thumb in estimating re-quired gain for a hearing-impaired person is to measure: 1) the SPL at which sound is comfortable; then 2) estimate the most frequent SPL input to which the person will be exposed; and finally 3) sub-tract the estimated input from the SPL at which speech is comfortably loud.

For example, if the comfortable level is 100 dB and the average speech signal is considered to be 60 dB, then a gain of only 40 dB (100 dB — 60 dB) would be required. It is important to remember *what* is being amplified, i.e., the speech signal, and the goal should be to provide sufficient gain to make *this* signal comfortably loud. People tend to understand speech better with a comfortably loud speech signal, and this has to be the primary concern, rather than focusing on the minimal SPL to which a person can respond. When the actual "use" gain of hearing-impaired people has been measured, it has been found to be approximately one-half of their hearing loss. Thus, someone with a 80-dB loss tends to set his gain at 40 dB, while someone with a 60-dB loss sets his gain at 30 dB (Martin, 1973; Byrne and Fifield, 1974).

Output

The electroacoustic dimension of output is often confused with gain. The output refers to the SPL of the amplified signal emitted by the hearing aid. With an input of 70 dB SPL and a gain of 50 dB, the output would be 120 dB. This 120-dB SPL output is delivered to the ear of the hearing-impaired person via earphones or a hearing aid earmold.

The maximum power output (MPO) is the SPL at which no further increase in output is possible, regardless of input or gain. The MPO reflects an engineering decision and is determined by the limitations of the instrument's component parts. If the MPO of a hearing aid is 130 dB, and the gain is set at 60 dB, then an input of 70 dB results in an output of 130 dB (or right at the MPO). Keeping the gain at 60 dB, and increasing the input to 80 dB, does *not* increase the output to 140 dB. The hearing aid cannot exceed its own limitations. The output remains at 130 dB. What occurs for some types of hearing aids is an increase in distortion; i.e., the fidelity of the amplified signal is diminished. A reduction of the actual gain is a by-product of this type of "overloading." In other types of hearing aids, those using an automatic volume control principle, the gain is automatically decreased or increased as the input is intensified or diminished, and thus distortion products are minimized. The point is, however, that no matter what method is used to limit the hearing aid's output, the MPO cannot be exceeded.

An excessively high MPO is a very common reason for unsatisfactory usage of amplification. The SPL that produces a painful sensation in the ear, for both normal and hearing-impaired listeners, is usually about 140 dB (Davis and Silverman, 1970). Discomfort thresholds average about 120 dB. However, there are many individual variations in ability to tolerate intense sounds, and the pain and discomfort thresholds of many hearing-impaired people are frequently much less than these figures. *Satisfactory hearing aid usage cannot be accomplished if the MPO exceeds a person's ability to tolerate loud sounds.*

For example, if someone's tolerance threshold is 120 dB, a not uncommon level, and the gain of the hearing aid is set at 50 dB, then SPL inputs of 70 dB or less would be tolerated, but any input greater than 70 dB would produce an unpleasant auditory stimulus. Sounds of doors slamming, excessively loud speech, playground activities, cafeteria babble, dishes clashing, heavy traffic, and so on, all would probably produce sound inputs greater than 70 dB. The individual's reaction is to reduce the gain of the hearing aid to ensure that these inputs do not cause an uncomfortable or painful auditory stimulus. If the gain is reduced to 30 or 40 dB, then it is quite possible that the person will be unable to efficiently understand speech delivered at an average intensity level. Therefore, the person turns the volume control up, is exposed to loud sounds, and turns the control down. And so on. Under these circumstances, it is unlikely that a successful adjustment to amplification will result. The situation becomes even worse, in the event that the MPO exceeds the tolerance level, for multiply handicapped people who are unable to manipulate or understand the function of the gain control.

For a number of years, much concern has been expressed regarding the effect of high levels of amplified sound on the residual hearing capacity. The question is often asked, if the MPO of a hearing aid is set too high, can this sound produce further decrement in hearing acuity caused by noise trauma? The MPO of hearing aids/auditory trainers far exceeds the maximal sound level that is known to produce, or further exacerbate, hearing losses. Insofar as hearing-impaired individuals are concerned, there is some cause for concern, but not alarm. Research has shown (see Ross and Lerman, 1967, and Markides, 1971, for reviews of the literature) that, although many people may experience temporary threshold shifts, few exhibit permanent losses resulting from hearing aid sound trauma. An active audiology program can detect these instances and take steps to alleviate the problem.

Frequency Response

The frequency response of an acoustic device is an expression of its relative gain across frequency. A range of frequencies of precisely the same intensity is delivered to the microphone, and because few if any hearing aid/auditory trainers can increase the sound precisely to the same proportion at every frequency, the output curve demonstrates different degrees of gain at the different frequencies amplified by the device. A so-called "flat" response is one in which all frequencies present in the output display precisely the same gain relative to the input. A typical hearing aid frequency response curve is shown in Figure 1. Note the unevenness of the curve and the fact that it encompasses a relatively narrow band of frequencies.

Most hearing aids/auditory trainers include adjustments to vary the frequency response curve to a considerable or great extent. One can, for example, emphasize the low frequencies relative to the high frequencies, or the high frequencies relative to the lows. Various degrees of "selective amplification" are possible. This dimension seems to bear an inverse relationship with the pattern of loss demonstrated by the audiogram (which graphically portrays hearing loss as a function of frequency). As with the gain, there is a temptation to compensate for the hearing loss by matching the frequency response to the hearing loss configuration.

There are both problems and merit to this approach. Even if it were possible to engineer a wearable instrument that could match the threshold configuration inversely, it is not the threshold that one is mainly concerned about, but the suprathreshold levels at which the hearing-impaired person actually listens to sound. The listening experiences at these levels cannot be easily predicted by the threshold responses. A certain degree of "selective" amplification does, however, seem to have merit (Ross, 1972b), particularly when it can be accomplished through deliberate manipulation of the earmold acoustics. Thus, a certain degree of low frequency suppression is helpful for individuals with high frequency losses. Currently, though, there is no precise formula for matching a person's hearing loss to the pattern of amplification delivered to his ear (see Ross, 1975, for a discussion of electroacoustic hearing aid selection). Nevertheless, certain modifications are potentially advantageous, and it is not advisable simply to supply every child in a class with a standard frequency response pattern, as frequently occurs when auditory training units are used.

Frequency Range

Hearing aids and auditory trainers do not usually amplify extremely low and high frequencies. The frequency range refers to that band of

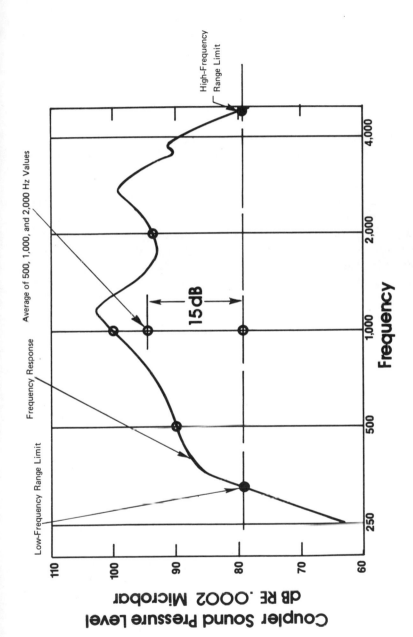

Figure 1. Frequency response curve of a typical hearing aid, including computation procedure for estimating frequency range.

frequencies that *is* effectively amplified by an instrument. The method most often used to assess the frequency range is given in Figure 1. Using a basic frequency response curve, the one that gives 40-dB gain at 1000 Hz to a 60-dB SPL input, the average outputs at 500, 1000, and 2000 Hz are added, averaged, and noted on the 1000-Hz axis. A horizontal line is drawn from a point 15 dB below this average. The lower and upper frequency range limits occur at the points where this horizontal line intersects the frequency response curve.

The electroacoustic dimension of frequency range can be best understood by relating it to the acoustics of speech signals, which is after all what one is most interested in amplifying. Generally speaking, the vowels have lower frequency and stronger intensity than the voiced consonants, with the voiceless consonants showing the highest frequencies and weakest intensities of any speech sounds. The phoneme /s/[1] is the consonant with the highest frequency components, beginning about 4000 Hz and spreading upward to about 7000 or 8000 Hz. The weakest consonant, which also contains most of its energy in the higher frequencies, is the voiceless /θ/. This consonant is 30 dB weaker than the the strongest vowel, /ɔ/ (Whetnall and Fry, 1964; Fletcher, 1970). The intensity of all the other phonemes in the English language thus falls in the intensity range bordered by the voiceless /θ/ on the low end and /ɔ/ on the high end. The implication of this fact is that when amplification delivers a broad spectrum 30-dB sensation level signal, the hearing-impaired listener is provided with the *potential* of perceiving all of the sound elements in our language. For an excellent overview of the relationship between speech acoustics and speech perception, see Ling (1975).

Although the vowels are easiest to hear because of their relatively low frequency and high intensity, they do not contribute as much to the intelligibility of a speech signal as do the consonants, which are usually more difficult to perceive. Perception of consonants is complicated by the fact that, in the vast majority of sensorineural hearing losses, it is the higher frequencies that display the greatest degree of hearing loss. In considering the frequency range of auditory amplifying devices, an attempt must be made to ensure that the device can amplify and present to the hearing-impaired person as many of the higher frequencies as is possible for the person to receive. This is

---

[1]For readers unfamiliar with the International Phonetic Association (IPA) Alphabet, a pronunciation key is provided in Appendix B.

particularly important with children who are attempting to learn or refine their speech and language patterns via amplified sound. Adults with a relatively normal history of speech and language development can predict easily the occurrence of many sounds and words even though they do not actually hear them. This is done repeatedly on the telephone, where the upper frequency range is approximately 3000 Hz, and thus high frequency sounds such as /s/, /θ/, and /f/ are difficult to distinguish auditorially, or in a telegram where many words are deliberately omitted without the primary message being affected. Children with a hearing loss must first develop language competency before being able to make these predictions, but they cannot optimally develop this language competency if too many of the acoustic cues to speech perception are filtered from the amplified speech signal.

In the last few years, a number of wearable hearing aids have been made with very broad frequency ranges, from approximately 100 Hz to 5000 or 6000 Hz. For the individual whose residual hearing range encompasses both the low and high frequencies, it is important to suppress the low frequencies relative to the highs. This is because, at intense sound pressure levels, the amplified low frequencies actually can interfere with the perception of the higher frequencies and thus impede maximal speech intelligibility (Danaher, Osberger, and Pickett, 1973). This is just one example of what should or should not be done with hearing aids and/or auditory trainers. Amplification is not a panacea for any child, but neither is it as ineffective as it sometimes seems to be. With proper concern for the electroacoustic dimensions of hearing aids, much good can be accomplished.

TYPES OF HEARING AIDS

Body-Worn Aids

Until the advent of the transistor circuit, body-worn hearing aids dominated the market. Aids were bulky instruments that required two different types of fairly large batteries to activate the vacuum tube circuitry. The microphone and amplifier of body-worn aids are housed in the same chassis, with wires connecting the amplifier to the receiver (or earphones) at the ear. In the last 20 years, body-worn hearing aids have been drastically modified in terms of circuitry and components, although their ability to serve their basic function (to amplify sound) has not been markedly improved. According to industry sources, body-worn hearing aids comprise only about 10% of the current total hearing aid market. Body-worn aids are useful in four types of cases: the young child, the person with a profound hearing loss, the elderly, and the physically handicapped.

The young child requires an instrument that is sturdy, can deliver high quality sound with a minimum of distortion, permits a prolonged battery life, and incorporates sufficient acoustic flexibility so that modifications can be made as more is learned about the extent and configuration of the hearing loss (Ross, 1975). Although rapid changes are occurring, currently a body-worn aid can best meet these requirements.

The person with a profound loss usually needs a body-worn hearing aid because the instrument can provide more amplification without squeal (acoustic feedback). This factor often limits the effective amplification of a hearing aid. It occurs when amplified sound escaping from the ear is picked up by the microphone, reamplified by the hearing aid, delivered to the ear, and again escapes from the ear, at which time the entire cycle begins again. Acoustic feedback can be reduced by providing an excellently fitting earmold (sometimes, not so easy to accomplish) and by increasing the separation between the hearing aid microphone and the receiver. It is this latter point that gives body-worn hearing aids their major advantage in terms of reducing acoustic feedback, because the microphone is located on the body some distance from the receiver located at the ear.

The need of the elderly and the physically handicapped for a body-worn hearing aid arises from the same factors. It is relatively more difficult with ear-level aids to insert the earmold properly, locate the aid at the ear without crimping the sound tube, manipulate the very small volume control, and change batteries. Getting an ear-level aid properly seated and adjusted can be a frustratingly difficult task for someone whose hand coordination is poor. Sometimes it is simply not possible. When the aid is located on the chest, it is much simpler to insert the earmold/receiver in the ear and to adjust the gain. Battery replacement is also a simple matter with body-worn hearing aids.

One major disadvantage of body-worn hearing aids is the production of "clothing noise," caused by the microphone rubbing against the clothing. This can be quite disturbing and interfere with the understanding of speech. Obviously, "clothing noise" is greater for physically active individuals and is not a major problem for those whose physical mobility is limited. Some body-worn hearing aids produce more clothing noise than others, and obviously the less the better for any hearing-impaired client who requires such a hearing aid.

A Y-cord arrangement is mainly associated with body-worn hearing aids. The output from the amplifier is split in two channels, with one going to an earmold/receiver combination in each ear. This divided output does *not* result in a binaural listening situation. Unless modifications are made in the wire leading to each ear (which is provided for in certain auditory trainers), or if the receivers at the two ears are different, then an identical amplified signal is delivered to each ear. Y-cord arrangements are frequently used with young children when there is insufficient information about the auditory status of the two ears. It is viewed as a temporary expedient until a more permanent recommendation can be made. The splitting of the hearing aid amplifier's output reduces the gain and output by 3 dB or more compared to a single wire arrangement. This can be easily compensated for, because hearing aids should have sufficient amplification reserve to make up for this difference. The understanding of speech with a Y-cord arrangement is about the same that would occur with a monaural arrangement feeding the better ear. An excellent discussion of Y-cord versus monaural and binaural reception is found in a recent book by Northern and Downs (1974). This book is highly recommended as a source for any professional working with hearing-impaired children.

Bone Conduction Aids

The usual route of the amplified sound is through the external auditory meatus (the ear canal), the middle ear, and to the cochlea (where the end organ of the auditory eighth nerve is located). Some medical conditions preclude the insertion of an earmold into the ear canal. Examples of such conditions are atresias of the ear canal, in which there is either no, or just a vestigial opening into the middle ear, or acute otitis media conditions, where effusions from the canal contraindicate the insertion of an earmold. In these instances, the output from the hearing aid amplifier is led to a bone vibrator that is placed behind the ear, at the mastoid process. The vibrations of this device are transmitted directly to the cochlea. The auditory perception that occurs is identical to that perceived through a transmission via the normal ear canal route. It does, however, take somewhat more energy to transmit a sound by bone conduction than by air conduction, and the process is not quite as efficient as that which occurs with the normal method. Some ear-level aids can be adapted to deliver a bone conduction sound, but the usual practice is to utilize a body-worn hearing aid when a bone-conduction aid is necessary.

Ear-Level Aids

Ear-level hearing aids became quite common about 20 years ago, consequent to advances in electronic circuitry miniaturization. With an ear-level hearing aid, the entire electroacoustic package is worn at ear level. Conceptually, ear-level aids that are encased in eyeglass frames or suspended behind the ear are the same and are not further differentiated here.

The major advantage of ear-level hearing aids is that sound is picked up where it should be, at the ear, rather than in a pocket on the chest. The effect of clothing muffling and clothing noise is thus eliminated. Binaural hearing aids (a separate one for each ear) can be worn more advantageously with ear-level aids because the head is now permitted to play its role in the spatial separation of the sound sources. From an electroacoustic standpoint, the current crop of ear-level hearing aids is quite comparable to the larger body-worn hearing aids. As indicated above, however, they tend to be less durable than body-worn aids, they require more frequent battery changes (because the batteries are smaller), and they are somewhat more difficult to seat properly and adjust. Their major disadvantage results from the proximity of the microphone and the receiver, which increases the likelihood of acoustic feedback at lower gain and output levels than would be found with a body-worn hearing aid. Many ear-level hearing aids are now being made with directional microphones, which suppress sounds arriving from the side or the rear relative to frontally arriving signals. This capability can be quite advantageous in noisy locations.

CROS Variations

The acronynm CROS stands for the Contralateral Routing of Offside Signals, and is really more an exploitation of earmold acoustics than it is of hearing aids per se. In its initial use (Harford and Dodds, 1966), the microphone of an ear-level hearing aid was placed next to one ear and the amplified signal was delivered to the other ear. It was meant for individuals with a unilateral hearing loss. The microphone was located next to the nonfunctioning ear, with the amplified signal delivered to the better ear. This enabled the unilaterally hearing-impaired person to improve speech awareness and perception directed to his bad side. It was necessary to modify the standard earmold through which the amplified signal was delivered to the good ear, otherwise it would simply act as an earplug and the good ear would be rendered less effective. In the modification, the earmold served as a frame to anchor the sound tube leading from the hearing aid receiver to the good ear but did not completely occlude the ear canal. Thus, the nonoccluded earmold permitted sound to enter the good ear with no interference from the earmold in that ear.

After some experience with this arrangement, it was found that individuals with a high frequency loss in the better ear could adjust to CROS hearing aids and benefit more easily than the person with a perfectly normal better ear. This was attributed to the acoustic effect of the nonoccluded earmold, which essentially shunted out the amplified low frequencies, so that they were not perceived by the individual, and permitted only the higher frequencies to be perceived. Research with the CROS arrangement has demonstrated that many hearing-impaired individuals can understand speech much better with CROS than they can with traditional earmolds, particularly under noisy conditions (Lybarger, 1972; Ross, 1972b; Langford, 1975). The basic acoustic effect of nonoccluded earmolds has been extensively exploited recently and has proved to be very useful to many hearing-impaired persons who heretofore were not considered hearing aid candidates.

One other common variation of a CROS arrangement should be mentioned, and that is the BICROS variation, the Bilateral Routing Of Signals. The BICROS hearing aid is useful when the poor ear is nonfunctional and when the better ear requires amplification in its own right. Two microphones are used, one placed next to each ear. The signal reaching the microphone by the poorer ear is shunted to the better ear, which also receives an amplified signal from the microphone placed near it. In other words, the better ear receives the signals arriving at both microphones; this permits reception of sounds directed to the poor as well as to the relatively good side. A wire cord, either embedded in the frame of an eyeglass hearing aid, or running under the hairline at the back of the neck in the case of ear-level hearing aids, connects the off-side microphone to the receiver at the better ear.

Binaural Aids

Binaural hearing aids are really two separate instruments, one for each ear. There are two separate microphones, amplifiers, receivers, and earmolds. This should not be confused with the Y-cord arrangements, in which the output from one microphone/amplifier is split and fed to both ears. Many auditory trainers are really Y-cord arrangements; children cover both ears with earphones, but the amplified signal they listen to is that picked up by a single microphone. In a true binaural arrangement, a separate and distinct microphone is electroacoustically connected to each ear.

In binaural hearing, the brain is able to correlate the uniquely patterned signals delivered to each ear and arrive at: 1) a superior ability to localize sound sources in space, 2) threshold and loudness summation (less intensity required in the two ears for comparable unilateral loudness sensations), and 3) enhanced foreground/background differentiation (for extracting the speech signal from a noisy background). In addition, because a microphone is located by each ear, the individual is always favorably situated in regard to detecting speech arriving from various locations (Briskey, 1972). Not every hearing-impaired person is a binaural hearing aid candidate, but for the majority who are, recent research clearly demonstrates the superiority of binaural over monaural amplification, particularly when listening under noisy or reverberant conditions (Dirks and Wilson, 1969; Kuyper and de Boer, 1969; MacKeith and Coles, 1971; Nabelek and Pickett, 1974).

This author and his associates, in their clinical practice, have now begun to recommend binaural hearing aids for all preverbal hearing-impaired children, even when information about the auditory status of the two ears is incomplete. This decision is based on two factors. The first is related to the proved superiority of binaural compared to monaural amplification; it would be better not lose any of the valuable time during the critical early years before proceeding with binaural hearing aids. The second reason is based on an analysis of the hearing losses of the children in our own facility, an analysis that we would expect to be similar in other locations. We have found, after precise auditory measurements were able to be accomplished, that relatively few of the children were not binaural hearing aid candidates. In our estimation, the potential benefits are sufficiently great to warrant risking recommending an occasional superfluous hearing aid (which, in this event, can well serve as an extra, back-up unit). The relatively few experimental studies comparing binaural versus monaural amplification with young children support this practice (Lewis and Green, 1962; Kuyper and de Boer, 1969; Luterman, 1969; Ross et al., 1974; Yonovitz and Campbell, 1974).

AUDITORY TRAINERS

Auditory trainers are hearing aids, rather large ones, to be sure, and quite expensive, but hearing aids, nonetheless. All of them, regardless of the intervening transmission process, present amplified auditory signals to the ears of the hearing-impaired listener. All the electroacoustic dimensions discussed above are also relevant to auditory trainers. Current developments in electronic miniaturization and design are reducing some of the superficial differences between hearing aids and auditory trainers. The major distinction now lies in the classroom and group use of auditory trainers versus the individualized use of hearing aids, although some auditory trainers can encompass both functions (Ross, 1969, 1972a, 1973).

Hard-Wire Systems

The hard-wire auditory training system was the first one developed. Children wear earphones connected to plugs on or by their desks. They hear the teacher, themselves, and each other through one or more microphones. When one microphone is used and is placed close to the teacher, it is possible for the teacher to come through loud and clear. However, with this microphone arrangement the children cannot hear each other or themselves very well. Some hard-wire systems place an open microphone in front of each child, in an attempt to ensure good auditory self-monitoring and child-to-child communication. With this arrangement, however, all the sounds (child or classroom noises) arriving at each microphone are delivered to each child in the room. It takes a very disciplined class to use this type of system effectively.

The restriction of mobility and the necessity for group transmission limits a hard-wire system to relatively stationary and group educational situations. Because of the relatively large size of the system, however, it does have the potential for providing an excellent amplification pattern to the hearing-impaired person. The key to efficient use of a hard-wire system lies in good microphone technique by both the teachers and the children. Briefly, microphone technique refers to the proper positioning of the microphone in front of whomever is speaking. The specific advantages are discussed below. A number of authors have written on the use of hard-wire auditory training systems in some detail (Klijn, 1961; Borrild, 1967; Hirsh, 1968; Damashek and Boothroyd, 1973; Ross, 1973).

Radio Frequency Systems

In the last few years, a large number of developments and changes have occurred in group amplification systems, and a large body of literature has been accumulated (Calvert, 1964; Ling, 1966; Ross, 1969; Matkin and Olsen, 1970a, 1970b, 1973). The latest of these developments, and the one most likely to replace earlier systems, is the radio frequency (RF) auditory training system. The most commonly used RF system operates as a miniature frequency-modulated (FM) radio broadcast station. Teachers wear a microphone/transmitter around their necks. Their speech is broadcast throughout the immediate vicinity via the FM signal. The signal is picked up by what is essentially a radio receiver worn by the child, and which also serves as a monaural or binaural hearing aid.

RF systems are designed to permit a great deal of instructional flexibility. They are completely portable, and no classroom installation of any kind is necessary. The children's and the teacher's mobility is unrestricted because both the microphone/transmitter and receiver/hearing aid are completely self-contained. When engaged in group instruction, the teacher talks in a normal voice, which all the children can receive simultaneously. They can hear each other and themselves directly through the microphones located in the body of the receiver pack they wear. When individual instruction is desired, the teacher's unit is shut off and the teacher communicates directly to each child via these microphones. Research has demonstrated that approximately an average 30% improvement in speech intelligibility can occur when a FM system is used compared to the children wearing only hearing aids under the same conditions of noise and distance (Ross and Giolas, 1971; Ross, Giolas, and Carver, 1973). The major limitation of this system, or any group amplification system, occurs when the instructional setting emphasizes an individual approach for a major part of the day (Ross, 1973). Under this circumstance, when group communication is not desired, the use of binaural, preferably ear-level aids employing directional microphone characteristics, seems to offer the most advantages.

ENVIRONMENTAL CONSIDERATIONS

Noise and Reverberation

The average classroom or institution is a noisy place. The effect that
this noise has on the speech intelligibility of hearing-impaired persons
cannot be easily appreciated by those with normal ears. The effect is
even more marked when such a person is listening to the speech
through a hearing aid. Noise levels that may interfere only slightly
with speech reception of a normal hearing person may completely
obliterate speech comprehension when processed through a hearing
aid and delivered to a hearing-impaired person (Tillman, Carhart,
and Olsen, 1970; Gengel, 1971). Gengel (1971) found that, unless
the speech was at least 10 dB stronger than the noise, the hearing-
impaired person preferred to discard the hearing aid rather than wear
it under the noisy circumstances. Tillman, Carhart, and Olsen's
(1970) findings were even more dramatic. They compared the signal-
to-noise ratio (S/N) levels at which normal hearing and hearing-
impaired subjects could achieve a 40% speech intelligibility score.
Their findings showed a 30-dB difference between the two S/N levels.
They showed that the normal hearing person could achieve this score
when the speech was 12 dB weaker than the noise, but it took a speech
signal of 18 dB stronger than the noise before the hearing-impaired
person could achieve the same score. Unfortunately, the average noise
conditions existing in classrooms result in S/N ratios of +1 to +5
dB on the average (reviewed in Ross, 1972b).

Reverberation, if anything, is even more detrimental to speech
intelligibility than noise, particularly when both co-exist (Nabelek
and Pickett, 1974). Reverberation is defined as the prolongation of
sound after the source has ceased vibrating. The amount of reverberation depends on the type of surfaces in a room. Hard concrete or
wood walls and ceiling reflect most of the sound energy striking them,
while porous surfaces (rugs, drapes, acoustic tiles) absorb much of
the impinging sound energy. Generally, the longer the reflections
continue—in other words, the longer the reverberation time—the
poorer the speech intelligibility score. A good figure to strive for is
an average 0.4-second reverberation time. With durations longer
than this, speech understanding begins to suffer considerably. What
happens is that the strongest elements in the speech signal, usually
the vowels, are prolonged because of the reverberation, and they
overlap in time (and thus mask), the later-arriving weaker, con-

sonantal elements in speech (Nabelek and Pickett, 1974). The actual reverberation time in classrooms has been found to be much longer than this 0.4-second average (Ross, 1972b).

Distance Effects

Possibly the most powerful procedure the teacher/clinician has to assure maximal reception of speech by hearing-impaired children is reduction of the distance between the microphone and the hearing aid or auditory trainer. This apparently simple measure increases the actual S/N ratio at the child's ear and, thus, increases the intelligibility of the speech signal. Every study evaluating this effect has shown an improvement in intelligibility as talker-microphone distance has diminished (reviewed in Ross, 1972b).

The explanation is simple. Assume the ambient noise level in a room to be 60 dB, with the teacher talking in average conversational voice, measured to be approximately 66 dB at a point 3 feet from her. The S/N ratio is thus +6 dB at this 3-foot location. Because the intensity of a sound decreases with increasing distance from the source (at different rates and amounts depending on the dimensions and sound treatment in the room), the S/N ratio becomes poorer as the distance between the speaker and the listener increases. The converse is also true. The intensity of the speaker's voice increases as the distance is diminished. This well documented effect—almost certain to have a positive influence on speech perception—is not really exploited as often as it should be (see Figure 2). Perhaps a concept has to sound complicated before it attains general acceptance and credibility!

Sound Treatment Effect

In many instructional situations, there are many times when it is not possible for a teacher to take advantage of the distance effect at all times during the day. There are many activities when the teacher, the child, or both are moving around during periods of verbal interactions and instructions. Noisy rooms, whether produced by internal activity and sound reflections, or transmitted within the classroom from outside sources, can obliterate effectively any intelligible speech signal. Sound treatment in the classroom can make a substantial difference. This is an obvious point and accords with one's common-sense notions. Unlike many other "common-sense" judgments, this one has been supported by research studies. In the most common paradigm, speech

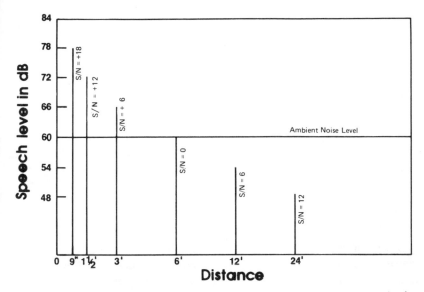

Figure 2. Signal-to-noise ratio relationships in a nonreverberant room having a 60-dB SPL ambient noise level.

intelligibility is measured under exactly the same conditions of speech levels, microphone distance, room dimensions, and subjects, but with sound treatment in one condition and no sound treatment in the other. An invariable finding, hardly surprising, is that speech can be understood more effectively in sound-treated environments (reviewed in Ross, 1972b).

To sound-treat a classroom, the most efficient procedure would be to consult a knowledgable builder who has access to acoustic consultants. Certain measures are obvious, however. Rugs on the floors and acoustic tiles on the walls and ceilings (preferably dropped, low ceilings) make an immediate, discernible difference. The noise sources in the room should be identified, and steps should be taken to reduce or eliminate them (in spite of the occasional temptation, we do not recommend eliminating the primary source of noise in a room—the children). Air conditioners and heating systems are frequent culprits; the noise produced by these devices can be reduced without impairing their operating efficiency. Earphones rather than speakers should be used when an audio medium is employed. The first and most important step to take in reducing noise levels in a room, however, is for the teacher to be sensitized to its detrimental effects.

Visual/Auditory Reception

One of the most consistent findings in speech intelligibility research is the conclusion that hearing-impaired persons can increase their speech perception when they can both hear and see the speaker simultaneously (O'Neil and Oyer, 1961; Dodds and Harford, 1968; Purcell and Costello, 1970; Sanders, 1971; Ross et al., 1972; Erber, 1974).

Each channel provides some unique information that is combined and integrated by the subject. The result is an intelligibility score higher than that obtained when each channel, either visual or auditory, is presented separately. For instance, in one real-life example, the subject obtained a 32% intelligibility score via vision, a 64% score auditorially, and a combined visual/auditory score of 88%.

The reason for this effect becomes clear as one analyzes the phoneme errors made during visual and auditory presentations. In the visual mode, the usual errors are with phonemes having similar places of articulation. Thus, certain groups of consonants, such as /p, b, m/, /t, d, n, l, s/, /f, v/, and /g, k, ŋ/, tend to be confused visually, because of their similar places of articulation, but less so auditorially. In the auditory mode, the hearing-impaired listener is able to distinguish within these place of articulation categories by discriminating between the voice, voiceless, and nasal consonant cognate categories (Erber, 1975). For example, the words /bɛt/, /pɛt/, and /mɛt/ may be confused visually because of the homophonous (look-alike) nature of the initial consonants; however, these three consonants can be distinguished auditorially by most hearing-impaired listeners because of voicing and nasality differences. In this instance, a correct identification can be made when both the auditory and visual information are combined (Hutton, 1969).

Purcell and Costello (1970) pointed out that the addition of another sensory input channel is most necessary when the major input mode can provide only incomplete or distorted information. Thus, when the auditory mode by itself is insufficient, because of noise, a severe hearing loss, or a poorly functioning hearing aid, the additional cues provided by the visual mode are required for efficient communication (Neely, 1956). This effect was illustrated in a study that compared hearing-impaired children's scores on the Boehm Test of Basic Concepts under conditions of hearing aid and RF auditory trainer usage in a classroom. The children performed superiorly with the RF system, as expected. The experimenter made the interesting observation, however, that, when the RF systm was employed, the children concentrated on their paper while listening to the auditory stimulus; when the hearing aids were used, the children carefully observed the examiner, and then made their response. What seemed to be happening was that, with an optimal auditory transmission (these were hard-of-hearing children), the children depended on the auditory event alone for information. When the conditions were less than optimal, as in using a hearing aid 10 or 12 feet from the experimenter in a noisy classroom, they had to use their eyes to supplement the incomplete auditory information arriving via their hearing aids (Kessler, 1974).

What all the above information suggests is that the teacher should *first* optimize the auditory channel, and *then* use vision to supplement the auditory information. This recommendation is most appropriate for hearing-impaired individuals with a significant degree of residual hearing; for the child with very little residual hearing, this author would emphasize a reverse sequence; that is, the optimization of the visual input to be supplemented by whatever auditory information can be made available.

TROUBLESHOOTING AND MAINTENANCE

Frequency of Malfunctions

Regarding hearing aids, one generalization that has withstood the tests of time and experience is that, if anything can go wrong with an aid, it probably will. No area regarding hearing aids and auditory trainers is more frustrating than this. All of the theoretical benefits related to the appropriate use of amplification are minimized or absent when the instruments do not function or when they function improperly. Time and time again one sees children who are either not using hearing aids/auditory trainers, or who are not achieving realistic benefits, because of maintenance problems. Teachers and parents may try to keep the devices working properly, but they frequently give up in disgust. There are perhaps more hearing aids and auditory trainers gathering dust in school storerooms than serving the purpose for which they were designed. Unfortunately, when the potential contribution of amplification is not fully appreciated, then the motivation is lacking to keep on trying to get the amplification devices working properly.

Beginning in 1966, every single study that has evaluated hearing aid performance has found that approximately one-half to two-thirds of aids were either not functioning or functioning improperly (Gaeth and Lounsbury, 1966; Matkin and Olsen, 1970a, 1973; Coleman, 1972; Northern et al., 1972; Zink, 1972; Findlay and Winchester, 1973; Porter, 1973). When one attempts to do the right thing by sending the instruments back for repair, the instruments are returned either unrepaired or with new problems evident (Zink, 1972). *There is simply no chance of maximizing a hearing-impaired child's use of residual hearing under these circumstances.* Some educational programs have instituted a daily check of hearing aid performance to be carried out by parents, teacher, or aides, under the supervision of a trained audiologist. This does not prevent the problems from occurring, but it can minimize the frequency of occurrence (Skalka and Moore, 1973).

Visual and Auditory Inspections

The hearing aid should be examined visually at the inception of each school day. Once the routine is established, such examinations require only a few minutes. Without this precaution, although the hearing aid may be physically present, one can never be sure that it is doing the child any good.

The first step is to look at the case for dents or other disfigurements. Although such occurrences by themselves do not indicate a concomitant electroacoustic problem, physical damage to the hearing aid is frequently associated with a malfunctioning instrument. The battery compartment should be opened and examined for proper battery contact. Occasionally, the battery terminals are warped, corroded, or missing, resulting in an inadequate connection. The cords should be inspected for the residue of chewing, twisting, or other hard knocks. All switches and knobs must be examined to see that: 1) they are present, 2) they are not bent, and 3) they function properly. The cord prongs leading from the hearing aid to the receiver must fit snugly at both ends. For ear-level hearing aids, the tubing must show no cracks or twists. A frequent cause for hearing aid malfunctions is damage to the receiver. The receiver must manifest no cracks, dents, or other sequelae of hard treatment. Finally, the earmold merits an extra-careful inspection. It must be clean and unbroken, with the retaining string at its base able to effect a solid connection to the receiver nub, and it must fit snugly and comfortably in the person's ear.

The auditory inspection can be broken down into two parts. One of the best ways of troubleshooting a hearing aid is simply to listen to it. The experienced listener can detect the presence of a poor amplification pattern and/or changes from previous occasions. If any problems are evident, then an electroacoustic analysis is required. Either a personal earmold or a hearing aid stethoscope (commercially available) is needed to troubleshoot a hearing aid auditorially. One simply listens to the aid as it is worn by the child. One limitation of this procedure is that the normal hearing person cannot easily tolerate the amplified sound at the same level as the hearing-impaired person. It is quite usual for a hearing aid to produce distortion at high sound levels, but not at lower ones. With practice, the normal hearing individual can withstand a surprisingly high degree of amplified sound (but for short periods only!). While listening to the aid, and using one's own voice as input, the teacher should manipulate the external controls and become familiar with their effects upon the amplified sound. (The teacher, however, should always return the adjustments to the ones recommended for the child.) A listening test can detect easily the effects of a weak or dead battery, or other problems that produce an inoperable instrument. The cords leading from the aid to the receiver should be manipulated at the insertion points; any intermittency in the amplified sound indicates a cord problem. Step-by-step procedures for hearing aid troubleshooting are available (McCoy and Lloyd, 1967; Dodds and Harford, 1970; Hanners and Sitton, 1973; Northern and Downs, 1974).

The second part of an auditory inspection is the electroacoustic analysis. This requires specialized equipment and personnel to accomplish (Lybarger, 1974). The analysis should be an integral component of any program that deals with hearing-impaired children. As long as the children use and are expected to benefit from amplification, then the amplification pattern they receive must be the best that present technology can provide. Each time the child is scheduled for a routine audiologic evaluation, an electroacoustic analysis also should be accomplished. Additionally, each time the listening inspection indicates potential or actual problems, of the type that cannot be remedied by a change of batteries, adjustments, tubings, earmold, or cords, then such an analysis is required. This is designed to detect the presence of poor S/N ratios, inadequate gain or output, jagged or inappropriate frequency response curves, and excessive degrees of distortion.

The basic point of visual and auditory inspections is to uncover problems as they occur. An aural rehabilitative program is deficient in a very significant dimension if such inspections do not take place regularly. One eventual goal is to teach the children to assume complete responsibility for the operation of their own hearing aids.

SUMMARY AND CONCLUSIONS

This chapter presents an overview of the electroacoustic dimensions of auditory amplification systems, to describe the types of such devices presently available, to indicate the environmental conditions that limit their most effective utilization, and to relate some of the steps necessary to ensure their proper functioning. It is by no means a complete exposition, and the reader is invited to pursue the topic in more detail by perusing some of the references given at the end of the chapter.

There is no doubt that the auditory channel is the normal route through which speech and language are developed. Other sensory modes are used in a supplementive or substitutive fashion when the auditory avenue is blocked or deficient. Biologically, however, people are programmed to respond to auditory language samples for the optimal development of speech and language. Hearing-impaired children cannot respond maximally to this biologic predisposition unless they are provided with the best possible auditory signal consistent with their hearing loss. Other sensory input then can supply valuable supplemental information, but the basic mode, for most hearing-impaired children, still should be the auditory channel. To accomplish this most effectively, however, requires that teachers, parents, and clinicians be convinced of the potential contribution inherent in the early and effective use of amplification. The technical information contained in this chapter, and in the references that follow, will do little good unless the commitment is present. With such a commitment, and the consequent motivation to pursue the topic, much good can result.

REFERENCES

Babbidge, H. 1965. Education of the deaf. A report to the Secretary of Health, Education, and Welfare by his advisory committee on the education of the deaf. U.S. Department of Health, Education, and Welfare, Washington, D.C.

Berger, K. W. 1974. The Hearing Aid: Its Operation and Development. 3rd Ed. National Hearing Aid Society, Detroit.

Borrild, K. 1967. Electro-acoustic aids applied in the training of deaf and hard of hearing children, pp. 564–576. *In* Proceedings of the 1967 International Congress on Oral Education of the Deaf. Alexander Graham Bell Association for the Deaf, Inc., Washington, D.C.

Briskey, R. J. 1972. Binaural hearing aids and new innovations. *In* J. Katz (ed.), Handbook of Clinical Audiology, pp. 590–601. Williams & Wilkins, Baltimore.

Byrne, D., and D. Fifield. 1974. Evaluation of hearing aid fittings for infants. Brit. J. Audiol. 8:47–54.

Calvert, D. R. 1964. A comparison of auditory amplifiers in the classroom in a school for the deaf. Volta Rev. 66:544–547.

Coleman, R. F. 1972. Stability of children's hearing aids in an acoustic preschool. Final report, Project 522466, Grant No. EG-4-71-0060, U.S. Department of Health, Education, and Welfare, Washington, D.C.

Damashek, M., and A. Boothroyd. 1973. Student to student communication in a group hearing aid. Clarke School for the Deaf, Northampton, Mass.

Danaher, E. M., M. J. Osberger, and J. J. Pickett. 1973. Discrimination of formant frequency transitions in synthetic vowels. J. Speech Hear. Res. 16:439–451.

Davis, H., and S. R. Silverman (eds.). 1970. Hearing and Deafness. 3rd Ed. Holt, Rinehart and Winston, New York.

Dirks, D. D., and R. A. Wilson. 1969. Binaural hearing of speech for aided and unaided conditions. J. Acoust. Soc. Amer. 12:650–664.

Dodds, E., and E. Harford. 1968. Application of a lipreading test in a hearing aid evaluation. J. Speech Hear. Disord. 33:167–173.

Dodds, E., and E. Harford. 1970. Helpful Hearing Aid Hints. Alexander Graham Bell Association for the Deaf, Inc., Washington, D.C.

Donnelly, K. (ed.). 1974. Interpreting Hearing Aid Technology. Charles C Thomas, Springfield, Ill.

Elliott, L. L., and V. B. Armbruster. 1967. Some possible effects of the delay of early treatment of deafness. J. Speech Hear. Res. 10:209–224.

Erber, N. P. 1974. Visual perception of speech by deaf children: Recent developments and continuing needs. J. Speech Hear. Disord. 39:178–185.

Erber, N. P. 1975. Auditory-Visual perception of speech. J. Speech Hear. Disord. 40:481–492.

Findlay, R. D., and R. A. Winchester. 1973. Defects in hearing aids worn by pre-school and school age children. Presented at annual convention of the American Speech and Hearing Association, Detroit.

Fletcher, S. 1970. Acoustics of Speech. *In* F. Berg and S. Fletcher (eds.), The Hard of Hearing Child. Grune & Stratton, New York.

Gaeth, J. H., and A. Lounsbury. 1966. Hearing aids and children in elementary schools. J. Speech Hear. Disord. 31:551–562.

Gengel, R. W. 1971. Acceptable speech-to-noise ratios for aided speech discrimination by the hearing-impaired. J. Aud. Res. 11:219–222.

Goetzinger, C. P. 1972. The psychology of hearing impairment. *In* J. Katz (ed.), Handbook of Clinical Audiology, pp. 666–693. Williams & Wilkins, Baltimore.

Hanners, B. A., and A. B. Sitton. 1974. Ears to hear: A daily hearing aid monitor program. Volta Rev. 76:530–536.

Harford, E., and E. Dodds. 1966. The clinical application of CROS. Arch. Otolaryngol. 83:455–464.

Hine, W. D. 1970. The attainments of children with partial hearing. Teach. Deaf 68:129–135.

Hirsh, I. J. 1968. Use of amplification in educating deaf children. Amer. Ann. Deaf 113:92–100.

Hutton, C. L., Jr. 1969. Aural rehabilitation. *In* J. Griffiths (ed.), Persons with Hearing Loss. Charles C Thomas, Springfield, Ill.

Katz, J. (ed.) 1972. Handbook of Clinical Audiology. Williams & Wilkins, Baltimore.

Kessler, M. E. 1974. Personal communication. University of Connecticut.

Kleffner, F. R. 1973. Hearing losses, hearing aids, and children with language disorders. J. Speech Hear. Disord. 38:232–239.

Klijn, J. A. 1961. The electronic link between teacher and child. *In* H. Huizing (ed.), Proceedings of the 2nd International Course in Paedo-Audiology, pp. 96–102. Groningen University, The Netherlands.

Kuyper, P., and E. de Boer. 1969. Evaluation of stereophonic fitting of hearing aids to hard-of-hearing children. Int. Audiol. 8:524–528.

Langford, G. G. 1975. Coupling methods. *In* M. C. Pollack (ed.), Amplification for the Hearing-Impaired, pp. 81–113. Grune & Stratton, New York.

Lewis, D., and R. Green. 1962. Value of binaural hearing aids for hearing impaired children in elementary schools. Volta Rev. 64:537–542.

Ling, D. 1966. Loop induction for auditory training of deaf children. Maico Audiol. Lib. Ser. 5: report 2.

Ling, D. 1975. Amplification for speech. *In* S. R. Silverman, and D. R. Calvert (eds.), Teaching Speech to the Deaf, pp. 64–88. Alexander Graham Bell Association for the Deaf, Inc., Washington, D.C.

Luterman, D. M. 1969. Binaural hearing aids for pre-school deaf children. Maico Audiol. Lib. Ser. 8: report 3.

Lybarger, S. F. 1972. Ear molds. *In* J. Katz (ed.), Handbook of Clinical Audiology, pp. 602–623. Williams & Wilkins, Baltimore.

Lybarger, S. F. 1974. Electroacoustic measurements. *In* K. Donnelly (ed.), Interpreting Hearing Aid Technology, pp. 40–84. Charles C Thomas, Springfield, Ill.

McCoy, D. F., and L. L. Lloyd. 1967. A hearing aid orientation program for mentally retarded children. Train. School Bull. 64:21–30.

MacKeith, N. W., and R. R. A. Coles. 1971. Binaural advantages in hearing of speech. J. Laryngol. Otol. 85:213–232.

Markides, A. 1971. Do hearing aids damage the user's residual hearing? Sound 5:99–105.

Martin, M. C. 1973. Hearing aid requirements in sensorineural hearing loss. Brit. J. Audiol. 7:21–24.

Matkin, N. D., and W. O. Olsen. 1970a. Induction loop amplification systems: Classroom performance. Asha 12:239–244.

Matkin, N. D., and W. O. Olsen. 1970b. Response of hearing aids with induction loop amplification systems. Amer. Ann. Deaf 115:73–78.

Matkin, N. D., and W. O. Olsen. 1973. An investigation of radio frequency auditory training units. Amer. Ann. Deaf. 118:25–30.

Merklein, R. A., and R. J. Briskey. 1962. Audiometric findings in children referred to a program for language disorders. Volta Rev. 64:294–298.

Morgan, D. E., R. H. Wilson, and D. D. Dirks. 1974. Loudness discomfort level: Selected methods and stimuli. J. Acoust. Soc. Amer. 56:577–581.

Myklebust, H. R. 1964. The Psychology of Deafness. 2nd Ed. Grune & Stratton, New York.

Nabelek, A. K., and J. M. Pickett. 1974. Reception of consonants in a classroom as affected by monaural and binaural listening, noise, reverberation, and hearing aids. J. Acoust. Soc. Amer. 56:628–639.

Neeley, K. K. 1956. Effect of visual factors on the intelligibility of speech. J. Acoust. Soc. Amer. 28:1275–1277.

Northern, J., and M. Downs. 1974. Hearing in Children. Williams & Wilkins, Baltimore.

Northern, J. L., W. McChord, E. Fisher, and P. Evans. 1972. Hearing services in residential schools for the deaf. Maico Audiol. Lib. Ser. 11: report 4.

O'Neill, J. J., and H. J. Oyer. 1961. Visual Communication for the Hard of Hearing. Prentice-Hall, Englewood Cliffs, N.J.

Pollack, M. A. (ed.). 1975. Amplification for the Hearing Impaired. Grune & Stratton, New York.

Porter, T. A. 1973. Hearing aids in a residential school. Amer. Ann. Deaf 118:31–33.

Purcell, G., and M. R. Costello. 1970. Multisensory stimulation and verbal learning. Educ. Hear. Impaired 1:66–68.

Quigley, S., and F. Thomure. 1968. Some effects of hearing impairment upon school performance. Institute of Research on Exceptional Children, University of Illinois, Urbana.

Rosenberg, P. E. 1966. Misdiagnosis of children with auditory problems. J. Speech Hear. Disord. 31:279–283.

Ross, M. 1969. Loop auditory training systems for pre-school hearing-impaired children. Volta Rev. 71:289–295.

Ross, M. 1972a. Principles of Aural Rehabilitation. In H. Halpern (ed.), Monograph Series in Speech Pathology and Audiology. Bobbs-Merrill, New York.

Ross, M. 1972b. Hearing aid evaluation. In J. Katz (ed.), Handbook of Clinical Audiology, pp. 624–655. Williams & Wilkins, Baltimore.

Ross, M. 1973. Consideration underlying the selection and utilization of classroom auditory training systems. J. Acad. Rehab. Audiol. 6:33–42.

Ross, M. 1975. Hearing aid selection for pre-verbal hearing-impaired children. In M. Pollack (ed.), Amplification for the Hearing Impaired, pp. 207–242. Grune & Stratton, New York.

Ross, M., and T. G. Giolas. 1971. Effect of three classroom listening conditions on speech intelligibility. Amer. Ann. Deaf 116:580–584.

Ross, M., T. G. Giolas, and P. W. Carver. 1973. The effect of classroom listening conditions upon speech intelligibility: A replication in part. Lang. Speech Hearing Serv. School 4:72–76.

Ross, M., M. F. Hunt, Jr., M. Kessler, and M. P. Henniges. 1974. The use of a rating scale to compare binaural and monaural amplification with hearing impaired children. Volta Rev. 76:93–99.

Ross, M., M. E. Kessler, M. E. Phillips, and J. W. Lerman. 1972. Visual, auditory, and combined mode presentations of the WIPI test to hearing-impaired children. Volta Rev. 74:90–96.

Ross, M., and J. Lerman. 1967. Hearing aid usage and its effect upon residual hearing. Arch. Otolaryngol. 86:639–644.

Ross, M., and N. D. Matkin. 1968. Rising threshold configuration among children with sensori-neural hearing losses. E.E.N.T. Digest 30:64–66.

Sanders, D. 1971. Aural Rehabilitation. Prentice-Hall, Englewood Cliffs, N.J.

Skalka, E. C., and J. P. Moore. 1973. A program for daily "troubleshooting" of hearing aids in a day school for the deaf. Presented at the annual convention of the American Speech and Hearing Association, Detroit.

Tillman, T. W., R. Carhart, and W. O. Olsen. 1970. Hearing aid efficiency in a competing noise situation. J. Speech Hear. Res. 13:789–811.

Whetnall, E., and D. B. Fry. 1964. The Deaf Child. William Heinemann Medical Books, London.

Yonovitz, A., and I. D. Campbell, Jr. 1974. Speech discrimination in noise: A test of binaural advantage in normal and hearing-impaired children. Presented at the annual convention of the American Speech and Hearing Association, Las Vegas.

Zink, G. D. 1972. Hearing aids children wear: A longitudinal study of performance. Volta Rev. 74:41–51.

9

ARTICULATION

James E. McLean

CONTENTS

**Prerequisite Behaviors Essential to Development of
Sound System** _____ 328
    Sound targets for the severely communicatively delayed/331
    Summary of sound needs for the severely handicapped/338

**Process and Procedures of Articulation Treatment for the
Severely Communicatively Delayed** _____ 341
    Components of articulation learning/344
    Procedures of articulation therapy/347

**Implications for Assessment and Treatment of Articulation
Problems for Severely Communicatively Delayed Children** _____ 360
    Implications for assessment of articulatory behaviors/360
    Implication for treatment of articulatory problems/363

Summary _____ 366

Acknowledgments _____ 366

References _____ 367

It is axiomatic that the human species' most unique behavior is its complex communication system of arbitrary symbols transmitted orally to a listener. This system is basic to the operation of human cultures. People use language to control their world, to get information, to teach their offspring, and to establish and express their deepest attachments to others. Without an oral language, people necessarily lose some part of their membership in society. No matter how well they can function in alternative language modes, people without speech are always functioning in a compensatory fashion. They invariably require extra consideration and accommodation from other members of the culture. Thus, it is easy to understand why it is so compelling to parents and professionals alike to teach speech to their offspring and/or their clinical education clients.

The clinical population that is the subject of this volume includes children for whom an adequate oral mode for language is highly problematic. Whether because of sensory deficits, cognitive deficiencies, or motoric or structural disruptions, these children often require extraordinary attention to the development of the speech sounds by which they will be able to transmit their language.

This chapter discusses sound production and, particularly, the problem found in the speech-sound systems of severely developmentally disabled children, including the sensorially deficient. At first thought it seems a relatively straightforward task. After all, articulation problems have been the most successfully treated aspects of the entire language system. This history of successful treatment is correlated with a history of being the most behaviorally specific of all clinical attempts to modify the language system. In articulation therapy, an overall behavior repertoire has been quantified, the treatment targets specifically prescribed, and treatment success has been routinely accountable by comparison with pretreatment behavioral inventories. Yet, although they are exemplary and effective from a behavioral view, even these relatively successful articulation treatment procedures require continued innovation and refinement if they are to meet the needs of developmentally delayed and multiply handicapped children. It is not so much that current knowledge is inadequate or that treat-

The author's research and development work on articulation programming reported in this chapter was supported by grants to the University of Kansas from the National Institute for Mental Health (NIMH 14877); the National Institute for Child Health and Human Development (NICHHD 05088); and the Office of Education, Bureau for the Handicapped (OEC-0-71-0449 607).

ment methods are ineffective; rather, it is simply that the problems of the severely communicatively delayed require expansion of both the content and the process that characterize current articulation therapy.

PREREQUISITE BEHAVIORS ESSENTIAL
TO DEVELOPMENT OF SOUND SYSTEM

In considering what is needed to attain an oral language system with severely communicatively delayed children, it is necessary first to analyze the characteristics of such a system. For example, it must be realized that oral language is first and foremost a *class* of communication behavior. As such, it has many levels, each of which depends on the other. Sounds alone do not make up an oral language, and a language's meaning units of morphemes and syntactic forms cannot be realized without the phonemes to produce them. The oral language system requires all of these levels of behavior, and each particular language system sets forth definite rules for each level. A language, for example, sets definite constraints on the specific sounds and sound combinations that can be used to create its morphemic components. It requires these sounds to be produced in rapid strings marked by specified suprasegmental patterns in order to create the morphologic and syntactic structures used in human communication. In the sections immediately following, these characteristics of oral language are further examined in terms of their implications for selection of clinical targets and the procedures for attaining these targets.

It is important for professionals in the area of speech and language to renew periodically their awareness of the difference between speech and language. Readers of this volume will know that speech is not necessarily language, and, conversely, that a communicative language system can be attained in modes other than speech. Indeed, this volume contains five chapters concerned with alternative and/or supplemental communication modes (Carrier; Clark and Woodcock; Kopchick and Lloyd; Vanderheiden and Harris-Vanderheiden; Wilbur).

The importance of this awareness lies in its contribution to the identification of behavioral *prerequisites* to an oral language mode. If it is understood that speech sounds are not language, then it also must be understood that teaching speech sounds to children who do not have a basic oral language system is a fruitless endeavor. This is not to say that the development of vocal behavior should be completely ignored before a child has a communicative language system. It does say, however, that the specific phonology of a language should not become a primary focus of intervention until a child has demonstrated some awareness that oral-symbolic behavior can be used to *communicate*. This in turn implies (to paraphrase and expand on a basic construct posited by Miller and Yoder, 1972) that, as a prerequisite to intensive work on a child's phonologic system, the child must have something to say, a reason for saying it, and have indicated a realization that a string of specific speech noises is a *way* of saying it.

The most straightforward interpretation of the perspectives just outlined is one which says that work on the development of a network of specific speech sounds should not begin until a child demonstrates some awareness of speech as a mode of communicative symbolic behavior. This prerequisite demand suggests, then, that *specific* sound development work comes only after a child demonstrates at least some gross oral communication behavior.

In her important investigation of early word learning among children, Nelson (1973) reported that limitations in children's overall phonologic system did not prevent the children from learning words that they wanted to learn. Instead, children make some approximation of a desired word and, apparently, seem uninhibited by any phonemic inaccuracies that occur. It seems clear from Nelson's analyses that children select the early words that they learn for many reasons other than the fact that they can produce the words accurately phonetically. Nelson's work has many important implications for early language programs for developmentally delayed children. Specifically, in terms of sound production, Nelson's observations would obviate the idea that a full repertoire of formal speech sounds is prerequisite to the initial stages of oral language learning among severely handicapped children.

In emphasizing this point, the purpose here is obviously not to suggest that the training of specific speech sounds is never appropriate for developmentally delayed or multiply impaired children. Rather, it is simply to suggest that vocal development work with preverbal communicatively delayed children should not take the form of specific speech sound imitation until a more general vocal repertoire has been established and at least a few components of that repertoire have acquired some consistent meaning or communicative function. By this it is meant that vocal approximations of any topography probably should be the first target with young, communicatively delayed children who have not yet demonstrated any verbal behavior (i.e., symbolic vocalization).

Exactly how to effectively target this early vocalization repertoire is not well defined at this time. Some behaviorists have done specific work relevant to the development of generalized speech imitation with various types of children (Baer and Sherman, 1964; Metz, 1965; Risley and Wolf, 1967; McReynolds, 1970). Others have demonstrated the positive effects of social reinforcement on infant vocalizations (Rheingold, Gerwitz, and Ross, 1959; Weisberg, 1963) and on the overall vocalizations of retarded children (Yoder, 1970). Still other work seeks to quantify the early interactions between mothers and their children, explaining more about the variables that are operational in vocalization development in the normal development context (Wolff, 1969; Beckwith, 1971; Stern, 1974; Strain, 1974).

Effective intervention procedures aimed at the development of the initial vocalization and sound-making repertoires of severely communicatively handicapped children, however, would seem to require an integration of all of these perspectives; but, to this writer's knowledge, this integration has yet to be done on a basis that has provided empirically validated intervention programs. Therefore, at this point, one can only offer the grossest guidelines for a hierarchy of activities directed toward the development of general vocal and sound-making responses among severely handicapped children. Such a hierarchical program consists of at least five general levels of activities:

1.   Reinforcement of all vocalization as a general class of behavior
2.   General refinement of the child's fine motor behavior involving the articulatory mechanism by targeting of chewing, sucking, and swallowing activities
3.   Expansion of the child's vocal repertoire by modeling of simple, but varying, vocal responses of vowel patterns with changes in pitch
4.   Basic imitation of vocal responses, which include consonant-vowel and vowel-consonant-vowel combinations, given with both pitch changes and varying rhythmic patterns
5.   Evocation and development of a repertoire of relatively consistent word approximations

This general vocalization, sound imitation, and word approximation training should provide the prerequisite vocal behaviors that delayed children must have before they are ready for the specific refinements needed for adequate production of all of the standard sounds of their formal language system. After children begin using even relatively gross vocalizations discriminatively to mark some particular events or objects in their environment, it is possible to begin a shift in clinical targets to the more formal aspects of the sound system per se. Because at this point it can be assumed that vocal responses have become, to some degree at least, communicative, one can move into the acquisition of the specific vocal symbolic system of the language being learned. At this point, then, it is possible to move on into a general discussion of the second perspective area in considering true speech-sound development among the targeted population.

Sound Targets for the Severely Communicatively Delayed

The human articulatory system is capable of producing many different sounds; however, each language culture chooses but a few of these sounds to encode meaning among members of that culture. As can be seen from Sander's communication model (this volume), the sound system of a language is traditionally described in terms of the sound families that signal a difference in meaning to a listener. These sound families are called *phonemes,* and they have become the standard unit for analysis and targeting of the sound system within a language. The standard American dialect contains 22 consonant phonemes and 16 vowel and vowel diphthong phonemes. If a standard American dialect is analyzed in terms of actual sounds (phones) produced rather than the sound families used (phonemes), it is found to consist of approximately 44 distinctly different consonant sounds and 18 vowel and vowel combinations (Buchanan, 1963). The difference between the sound families needed and the actual sounds used occurs as a result of the effect that different word environments have on the production of certain individual sounds. For those who desire expansion and/or review of these constructs and the relationship between a language's phones and phonemes, Buchanan (1963) offers a particularly lucid programmed text in this area.

The phone/phoneme comparison is important because the phoneme units have been the restricted, traditional clinical frame of reference in articulation programming. Sound system needs have been analyzed in terms of what phonemes a child can produce compared to what is required by the complete adult language system. This comparison is certainly the ultimate accountability in articulation acquisition; but it leaves the clinician ill prepared to analyze the needs of early emerging language systems and to evaluate fully and choose sound targets for children with severe language delays. Many of the problems in generating appropriate programs for developmentally delayed children result from the singular analysis of a child's sound system in terms of its match with the standard phoneme system of the language. Additional points of view regarding both the assessment and the prescriptions for phonemic development are presented in the following discussion.

Severely communicatively delayed children have extremely limited phonologic systems. That is, such children have sound systems that are far less complex in terms of the phonemes they contain compared to the phonemes required by the total language system. In addition to limitations in their systems, delayed children often demonstrate inappropriate distribution of the phonemes that they do produce. This means that severely communicatively delayed children tested on standard assessment instruments often show patterns of articulation in which consonant phonemes are produced only in certain word positions and are omitted in other positions. Thus, for example, such assessment may show delayed children with patterns of articulation in which consonants are articulated in the word-initial position but are omitted in word-medial and/or word-final positions. The results of these two problems—limited phonologic systems and inadequate distribution of available phonemes—interfere severely with the intelligibility of speech.

It seems, then, that communicative intelligibility is the critical factor in sound system development with this target population. Thus, with obvious delays present in these children and a relatively slow rate of acquisition of new sounds even under ideal clinical conditions, it is necessary to design treatment programs that target intelligibility as a first priority. With problems in comprehension already significant because of delayed morphologic and syntactic structure development, phonologic inaccuracy is even more costly for these children than for those whose other language structures are developing normally. The attainment of a language's *full* phonologic system is a relatively late target in the treatment sequence for severely delayed children. Much of the work discussed in later portions of this chapter is concerned with the final refinement of delayed children's articulation systems. But the major emphasis at this point is on the developmental appropriateness of targeting intelligibility within limited phonologic systems, rather than targeting totally developed phonologic systems among these children, i.e., targeting speech sounds that will contribute the most to improving a child's intelligibility, considering the sounds that already may be present in the child's limited system.

In approaching this need to target better intelligibility of children with severely constrained sound systems, it seems that most traditional perspectives offer little help. The following five factors, for example, are traditionally considered in selecting a sound for remediation:

1.   Developmental order of acquisition of various sounds
2.   Stimulability of various sounds
3.   Contextual value of sounds for child (sound in child's name, pet's name, favorite toy, etc.)
4.   General ease of sounds for teaching (visible focal articulation point, etc.)
5.   Frequency of occurrence of sounds in language

It is difficult to translate the standard developmental order of sound acquisition (Poole, 1934; Templin, 1957) directly into an intelligibility matrix. Because these data represent mean acquisition levels among large populations of children by age, one loses the profiles of individual child's acquisition trends. Thus, although the developmental order reported in the literature does not specifically contradict the distinctive feature development suggested by Jakobson's early work (Jakobson and Halle, 1956), which is discussed further on in this chapter, neither does it specifically target intelligibility.

In a similar vein, the stimulability factor (Milisen, 1954) cannot be considered as a direct factor in intelligibility. The fact that a child can produce a sound in response to an imitative model does not necessarily imply that the sound which is stimulable will improve intelligibility more than some other sound might. And, still further into standard targeting criteria, the contextual values of certain sounds may well improve a child's motivation and a child's more frequent use of a sound in functional communication. Whether a sound targeted on this basis (e.g., sound occurs in child's name) actually contributes to the development of sounds most contributive to intelligibility is a separate question. The relative ease by which sounds might be taught is, similarly, unrelated to whether the sound actually contributes most effectively to early attainment of improved intelligibility.

Of all of the factors usually considered in sound selection, only the relative frequency of occurrence of a sound in a language (Dewey, 1923) would seem to be directly related to a child's intelligibility.

Frequency of occurrence does indicate the relative density of that sound in the language, and, therefore, the implication is there that a highly frequent sound's attainment might improve intelligibility more than another sound might simply because it occurs more often in a child's utterances.

It seems clear, however, that the traditional criteria for sound selection bear, at best, an indirect relationship to the problem of intelligibility. These rather indirect criteria for such an important problem hardly seem satisfactory, however, so that it is beneficial to look for other factors that might be useful in making the clinical decisions in this area. In this regard, it seems that there are four sources of empirical data that may be specifically productive for an analysis of this intelligibility issue: confusion matrices, developmental articulation errors, phoneme contrasts, and phoneme distribution. Each of these sources is identified and discussed in the sections following.

Confusion Matrices for Consonants   In a study of discrimination of English consonants, Miller and Nicely (1955) found that sounds which were similar in voicing and manner of articulation features[1] were the most likely to be confused by adult judges. In a study of kindergarten childrens' ability to imitate English consonants, Bricker (1967) found that children most often confused sounds that had similar manner of articulation features. The confusion matrices generated by both of these studies suggest, then, that the closer two sounds are in voicing and manner features, the higher the probability is that one of them will be heard as the other. Projecting these data to the problem of intelligibility targeting, it seems clear that, if children with severe articulation deficiencies at least substitute sounds of similar manner class for each other, their speech intelligibility may be greater than if they make substitution errors across manner classes.

Developmental Articulation Errors   Although this writer is not familiar with any direct empirical studies to support this assumption, it does seem clear that young children with standard developmental articulation errors of mild to moderate degree do not suffer major intelligibility problems. Adult listeners (and child peers) seem to decode so-called infantile speech rather easily. This type of speech most commonly includes substitutions such as: /f/ for /θ/ and /v/

---

[1]For those not fully conversant with the constructs of manner and place of articulation, recommended is a thorough study of C. A. Buchanan's, *Programmed Introduction to Linguistics: Phonetics and Phonemics* (D. C. Heath, Boston, 1963). Also see S. Singh and K. Singh's *Phonetics: Principles and Practices* (University Park Press, Baltimore, 1976).

for /ð/; /t/ for /k/ and /d/ for /g/; /s/ for /š/ and /z/ for /ž/; /θ-like/ for /s/; and /ð-like/ for /z/[2]. These errors all consist of substitutions *within manner classes.* Even the common /w-like/ for /r/ and /w-like/ for /l/, although not strictly speaking "within-manner" substitutions, show the substitution of a back-glide (which starts from a vowel) for English's two oral resonants, which, in manner of articulation, closely resemble vowels in that they introduce no highly disruptive constrictions in the vocal tract.

Thus, despite the apparent lack of specifically supportive formal research data on this issue, it seems justifiable on the basis of informal empirical observations to at least suggest that the findings of the confusion matrix studies (Miller and Nicely, 1955; Bricker, 1967) do obtain to some extent in real communication events between young children and their peer and adult listeners.

Theoretical Models of Phoneme Contrast Development   In his interpretations of how children acquire a phonologic system, Jakobson (Jakobson and Halle, 1956; Jakobson, 1968) hypothesized a process in which a child develops phonemic "contrasts." In explaining his construct, Jakobson suggested that children first acquire contrasts between vowels and consonants, then between nasal versus oral consonants, and then continue to develop contrasts among sound along a front to back place of articulation continuum (i.e., labials versus dentals; velopalatals versus labials and dentals; palatals versus velars). Among these contrasts between places of articulation, it seems that continuant versus stop contrasts, which first appear in the vowel/consonant contrasts and in nasal/stop contrasts, continue to develop as various manners of articulation are generated at various places of articulation.

Although a full exposition of Jakobson's theories is beyond the scope of this chapter,[3] his construct of the development of phonemic

---

[2]For readers unfamiliar with the International Phonetic Association (IPA) Alphabet, a pronunciation key is provided in Appendix B. However, it should be noted that this chapter deviates from the IPA notation used elsewhere in this book. First, this chapter uses /š/ for /ʃ/, /ž/ for /ʒ/, /ĵ/ for /dʒ/, /č/ for /tʃ/, and /y/ for /j/. Second, the Faircloth (1973) notation of a phoneme plus the word *like* (all within slanted lines) is used to indicate substitutions that are best described by indicating a substitution of one standard English phoneme for another even though the substituted phoneme is not technically correct. Thus, /θ-like/ is used for /s/ even though the substituted sound is not acceptable as a correctly articulated /θ/.

[3]The reader will find a particularly lucid exposition of Jakobson's theories in P. S. Dale's, *Language Development: Structure and Function* (Dryden Press, Hinsdale, Ill., 1972, pp. 175–181).

contrasts across place and manner features seems productive in that it, too, departs from the standard posture of looking at phonologic acquisition on a phoneme-by-phoneme basis. Rather than a phoneme-by-phoneme view, Jakobson's constructs suggest a need to look at development of the manner features of phonemes as they occur at various places of articulation. These ideas, then, lead to perspectives that are very similar to those which the confusion-matrix data suggest and standard developmental misarticulations of normally developing children seem to approximate. That is, all of these perspectives suggest that developing phonologic systems can be analyzed in terms of patterns of phoneme feature development instead of in terms of the more standardly applied normal developmental data (Templin, 1957), which specifies the acquisition sequence of specific, individual phonemes.

The reader will realize, of course, that the contrastive phonemic feature approach being set forth here is a limited representation of the distinctive features approach being widely promulgated in current literature (Menyuk, 1968; McReynolds and Huston, 1971; McReynolds and Engmann, 1975; Singh, 1976). The present writer, at this point, prefers to limit his analysis of distinctive features to voicing, place, and manner rather than move to the fuller system derived from the later work of Jakobson, Fant, and Halle (1963). The three contrastive features being utilized here subsume the richer feature system being applied by others, but, more than that, these three features seem to have immediate reality for specific application in clinical approaches to the emerging phonologic system.

Synthesizing the data and the perspectives suggested by these three sources provides a view of phonologic treatment strategies that differs significantly from that traditionally used in clinical articulation therapy. This modified view focuses on the phoneme features that enable decoding of phonologic information by listeners. These same contrastive features are, naturally, systems that more closely approximate the full system necessary for intelligible expressive language systems.

Phoneme Distribution in Intelligibility At this point, the reader might recall an earlier point about the articulatory behaviors of severely communicatively delayed children showing poor distribution patterns of phonemes that were available in their phonologic system. Faircloth and Faircloth (1970) indicated that syllable integrity in words is a significant factor in their intelligibility. Thus, a speaker whose phoneme distribution patterns allow omissions of consonants in phonemic strings in which they should occur, introduces significant sources of unintelligibility. The Faircloths' findings revealed another point that seems to have major significance. Their research findings indicated that syllable integrity is not necessarily lost by phonemic errors. If, for example, one phoneme is substituted for another in an utterance and yet the basic integrity of the syllable contour is retained, intelligibility may be preserved. In light of the research findings discussed earlier, one must assume that syllable intactness can be best maintained by substitutions that are within manner of articulation classes. These findings by the Faircloths would provide support for and possibly even an explanation of the minimal intelligibility loss that was noted earlier to result from standard developmental misarticulations in which substitutions are largely within the same manner classes.

The general context of the Faircloths' work is also important to consider here. The intelligibility factors that they have been investigating have been generated by their advocacy of a dynamic rather than a static view of articulatory behavior. They have pointed out, for example, that articulation in connected speech is different from that in single-word utterances (Faircloth and Faircloth, 1970, 1971; Faircloth, 1973). This view, then, leads them to question the traditional speech pathologist's construct of initial, medial, and final word positions for phoneme articulation work on isolated words (out of a connected speech context). However, this chapter continues to reflect constructs such as phoneme word position. The reason for this seeming contradiction is a belief that the construct of word position *as applied clinically* is not actually in total opposition to the more technically correct coarticulation perspectives of the Faircloths. It seems that, for one thing, the traditional initial-medial-final position construct simply allows a clinician to generate a number of phonemic environments in which various coarticulation postures are required. Second, considering the effectiveness of articulation therapy over the years, it seems eminently possible that the traditional single-word drill yields some prerequisite responses that are useful to a client in meeting the more dynamic conditions of natural phoneme articulation in connected speech. One must remember, also, that traditional articulation therapy (Milisen, 1954) includes extensive production of a target phoneme in complex configurations of speech-like sentences, extended oral reading, and controlled conversation sessions. Newer, programmed approaches to articulation treatment (Mowrer, Baker, and Schutz, 1970; Irwin and Weston, 1971; Garrett, 1973; McLean, Raymore, and Long, in press) generally ensure dynamic articulation of the target phoneme in complex coarticulation-evoking contexts.

The primary pertinence of the Faircloths' work at this point is not, however, in this issue of relative controversy, but rather in the implications of their findings about syllabic integrity as a basic contributor to intelligibility. These findings about syllables add support to their point that the clinician cannot target just isolated phonemes but must consider their place in strings of phonemes. The fact that traditional procedures do identify the lack of phoneme distribution as a problem does indicate, however, that the artificial analysis of initial, medial, and final word positions for phonemes is sensitive to the same variables that are also revealed in coarticulation contexts. Because the severely communicatively delayed child tends to "omit" word-medial and word-final position consonants, and suffers severe intelligibility loss as a result, the relationship between such omissions and the Faircloths' findings about syllable articulation and intelligibility should be reemphasized.

Whether targeting syllables from phoneme word position perspectives or from more dynamic, coarticulation perspectives, the message for therapy is still clear: *syllable integrity* must be targeted for children with severe articulation disorders. For traditional clinicians, this means that all word positions for phonemes must be sought and the articulation of all words must include at least within-manner-class approximations of all consonants in the word. As words are incorporated into more complex speech configurations such as sentences and connected-speech responses, this distribution of consonants throughout the phoneme strings *must be specifically trained*. If this is done, and if a phoneme repertoire can be developed that represents at least one instance of each manner class, even delayed children with relatively limited systems might approach a reasonable level of intelligibility.

Summary of Sound Needs for the Severely Handicapped

Together, the effect of all of these views has important implications for the task of targeting improved intelligibility for severely communicatively disabled children. By applying the perspectives that emerge from the preceding discussions, one can generate a series of phonemic targets for these children from a much broader base than previously used criteria allowed. The targets generated from this point of view still interact positively with some of the more traditional criteria like stimulability, frequence of occurrence, and ease of teaching. They suggest other criteria as well.

Specifically, these perspectives suggest, first, the following general strategies for targeting phonologic goals for severely communicatively delayed children:

1.   Target the overall development of at least one phoneme in each manner of articulation class
2.   When a phoneme has been developed in a manner class, target another phoneme in that class which has a different place of articulation; in extending place of articulation features, move from the front to the back of the mouth
3.   As phonemes in each class become available, target the voicing versus unvoicing features through cognates of phonemes that have been developed
4.   When one or two phonemes in each manner class are available, including appropriate voicing features, move to more standard phonemic inventories and standard selection criteria

With the general strategies established, attention can be focused on some of the more specific details of the overall process. The translation of the phonemic feature development into a sequence from which to attack actual phone development is suggested by Dale's (1972) excellent synthesis of the work of Jakobson and Ervin-Tripp (1966). This sequence could proceed by targeting:

1.   Contrasts between vowels and consonants; e.g., /a/ versus /p/ or /m/
2.   Contrasts between stops and exemplary continuants (nasals and/or fricatives); e.g., /p/ or /b/ versus nasals like /m/ or fricatives like /f/ or /s/
3.   Contrasts between places of articulation within similar manner classes; e.g., /p/ versus /t/; /t/ versus /k/; /f/ versus /s/; and/or /f/ versus /θ/
4.   Contrasts between voicing and unvoicing in several manner classes; e.g., /p/ versus /b/; /f/ versus /v/; /s/ versus /z/; and/or /t/ versus /d/
5.   Contrasts between other members of the continuant manner classes; e.g., fricatives versus resonants and resonants versus glides; /f/ versus /l/ and /l/ versus /y/

Figure 1 offers a limited representation of three of the constrastive features to be targeted. The manner classes in this figure are limited

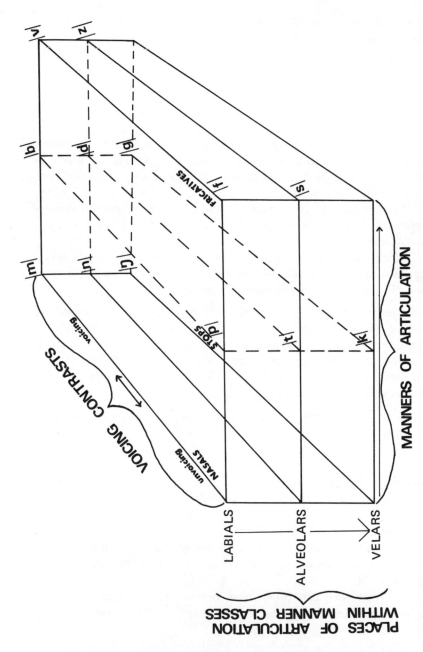

Figure 1. Examples of phonemic contrasts for targeting in early consonant development.

to three (of five), and the voicing feature and the front to back place features are shown in relation to these three manners.

After these contrasts have been established, a return to standard articulation inventories (Templin and Darley, 1960; Goldman and Fristoe, 1969) becomes appropriate. Thus, the later developing phonemes like the affricates (/č/ and /ǰ/), complex fricatives like /š/ and /ž/, and any missing resonants or glides like /r/ and/or /w/ can be targeted.

Figure 2 offers a simple schematic representation of the sequence of targeting and also shows the recycling procedure to new manner features after places within one manner class are attained.

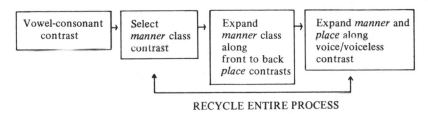

RECYCLE ENTIRE PROCESS

Figure 2. Schematic of sequence of phonemic feature targeting.

Phonemic development should be targeted in the population of severely communicatively delayed children according to the basic feature contrasts needed by children rather than by any other developmental or contextual criteria. Stimulability is still measured (Milisen, 1954) in order to make choices about different sounds that might be suggested by the same feature contrast. Currently, there are no formal empirical data available on the effects of this approach, but this programming, along with a concentration on syllable articulation, seems to have high probability for yielding gains in the early intelligibility improvement of those children who exhibit a limited phonologic repertoire and who indicate that expansion of their repertoires will take an extended period of training.

This area of phoneme need is considered later in the section *Implication for Treatment of Articulatory Problems*. At this point, however, the overall procedures for intervention in the articulation behavior of severely communicatively delayed children are considered.

PROCESS AND PROCEDURES OF
ARTICULATION TREATMENT FOR THE
SEVERELY COMMUNICATIVELY DELAYED

The needs underlying the oral language system have been discussed and an approach to the identification of appropriate sound targets for severely communicatively delayed children has been outlined that should optimize the intelligibility of such children as their phonologic system is systematically expanded. The general principles of the therapy process as they relate to these children are now considered.

Even though it has been pointed out that the severely delayed child requires expansion of the content and the process of articulation therapy when compared to normal developing children, it is important to realize that the needed expansions do not completely alter the basic principles of articulation learning and/or modification. Thus, while it is obvious that seriously developmentally delayed children may not bring the same levels of organismic resources to the articulation learning process that more normally developing children may bring, it is illogical to assume that, at the most basic levels, articulation learning for these children follows a vastly different process than that for normally developing children. McLean (1972) has previously made the point that language and components of the language system make the same demands on delayed children that they make on everyone else. It would seem that the requisite skills and processes, which are essential to any language system as well as to the individual components of such a system, cannot be equivocated to accommodate human deficiencies except in terms of some degrees of loss of relative quality of performance. In a sense, it is this nonaccommodating nature of language that causes the relative quality of it to be such a significant factor in one's judgments regarding the degree to which humans are handicapped and/or delayed. The mentally retarded child who acquires a language system, however, has attained behavior that is basically isomorphic with the behavior acquired by a "normal" child.

Given this awareness that language is language and makes similar demands on whichever human organism seeks to attain it, it must be concluded that the same variables that function for normally developing children in learning language are also critical for delayed children facing the same task. Thus, if severely language-delayed children are to learn the sound system of their language, they must learn the same basic class of behavior learned by their normal peers and they must learn it by processing the same basic input information as their peers. The information that they process may need to be presented in more carefully sequenced ways, made more perceptually salient, and/or presented over more learning trials—but it is still basically the same information, nevertheless. Thus, examining the articulation therapy processes for the delayed and/or multiply impaired child requires looking at those same variables that have been demonstrated as important to articulation learning per se, not just those important to severely communicatively delayed children, including the hearing impaired.

Components of Articulation Learning

It may be concluded that the articulation learning process has two distinct components that direct the design of therapy programs. First, articulation learning requires that the specific individual sounds of the language system be produced within certain acoustic limits. Second, articulation learning requires that a child be able to produce these individual sounds whenever and wherever they are required to produce the desired meaning unit. It seems appropriate to label these components of articulation treatment *response development* and *carryover training*.

The first component, response development, is that portion of the articulation treatment process in which children are exposed to any and all information that help them to make the motor movements of the articulators necessary to produce the desired acoustic product. Because the only means of giving children this information is through their sensory channels, response development procedures naturally call for the presentation of auditory, visual, and tactual stimuli that provide the child with this information as unambiguously and as saliently as possible. Thus, the clinician may produce the sound for the child, demonstrate visually all the place of articulation information that can be made available, and use tactual cues to demonstrate both place and manner of articulation features to the child, e.g., a finger on the alveolar ridge to demonstrate place of articulation and a finger in front of the mouth to demonstrate the aspirated release of the [tʻ]. In the response development component, then, the goal of therapy is for the child to produce the correct acoustic properties of the sound. The information transmitted to the child is that relative to the specific place and manner of articulation characteristics of that sound. The variables that function for carrying that message to the child are auditory, visual, and tactual modeling and cuing stimuli. The criterion behavior target for this component simply seems to be the child's ability to produce this sound in imitation of the clinician's auditory-visual modeling of the sound. When the response is available in simple imitation, the child's production of the acoustic properties of the target sound has been attained. Even though this response still requires an imitative stimulus, it is now in the child's repertoire and is available for the further treatments necessary to get it emitted appropriately in all linguistic and situational contexts. It is now suggested that the movement of a sound response from imitative control to complete linguistic and situational control is all appropriately considered to be carryover training.

This somewhat nonstandard construct of carryover training has been developed in response to a growing awareness that the traditional view of carryover by speech pathologists described a behavioral criterion-referenced assessment of child control of an articulation response more than it described the training process necessary to attain such control. That is, carryover was demonstrated when children produced the target sound in all situations in which they uttered the sound. Thus, carryover actually means that a child has complete control over that sound response and produces it whenever it is appropriate from a linguistic structure point of view. What speech pathologists have done, generally, is to transform criterion for that state of subject control into treatment variables, and, thus, they routinely train a new phoneme response in different *situations*. Although this treatment eventually may produce the desired criterion behavior, it seems obvious that this is not the only way such behavior can be attained. It has been this writer's contention (McLean and Raymore, 1972; Raymore and McLean, 1972; McLean, Raymore, and Long, in press) that subject-control of a response can be attained by systematically extending a phoneme response across a number of evoking stimulus conditions and into a number of increasingly more complex coarticulation contexts, e.g., single words, simple sentences, and complex, sound-loaded sentences. In this approach, the same criterion behavior is sought (production of phoneme in all linguistic contexts and situations), but the treatment variables are within-clinic manipulations of both the evoking stimulus conditions and the linguistic complexity of the response rather than treatment in different situations as is standardly done (Van Riper, 1963; Mowrer, 1971). This modified construct of carryover training, then, is considered to begin as soon as a sound response in imitation is available from a child and is considered to end when a child is producing the sound in complex, spontaneous speech in all situations. Between these two poles, the treatment process systematically works to bring to the child levels of self-control over the phoneme response.

In an initial analysis of this process of targeting child control of the new phoneme response, McLean (1970) developed the construct that the primary behavioral indicator of various levels of child control over the new response was the degree of support that the new response required to be emitted correctly. The support needed for correct articulation was analyzed in terms of the information presented in the stimulus that evoked the sound response. For example, a child who can produce a new phone response only when given an echoic model of the sound to imitate has less self-control over that sound than the child who can produce the sound when presented with only a picture of a word containing that sound. The difference between these two levels of antecedent stimulus support is that the echoic response provides a child with an auditory-visual *model* of that response, and the picture merely sets the occasion for the response to occur without modeling it for the child. Obviously, the less direct modeling information a child needs, the more self-control the child has over that sound.

The contention in this initial work was that the systematic manipulation of the types of antecedent, evoking stimuli in the therapy setting would result in strong subject control over the response. Thus, in the programming that resulted from this hypothesis, a procedure was developed that systematically shifted the response from stimulus conditions that modeled the sound (echoic) to conditions that evoked the sound but did not model it (pictures, graphemes, incomplete sentences that the child completed with the target words containing the target sound). Such programming for new phonemes in the initial position in words was found to be successful with both delayed and nondelayed children (McLean, 1970; Raymore and McLean, 1972).

In probing the results of this type of stimulus shift procedure, however, it was found that children were carrying-over the sounds to untrained contexts only at the specific speech configuration levels in which they were trained, i.e., children trained on single words, with the sound in the word-initial position, produced correct target phonemes only in single words with the phoneme in the word-initial position. They did not generalize the new response into words that contained the sound in the medial or final positions; and, although the newly trained sound did emerge in spontaneous speech, it did so at relatively low levels and in limited word distribution contexts. Thus, even though the validity of the stimulus shift relationship to carryover was established, the data from these children made it clear that subject control established clinically at single-word levels was not enough to attain adequate carryover levels for delayed children. Later research by Garrett (1973) demonstrated basically the same results with a modification of this procedure when it was applied to normal children, and a study by Griffiths and Craighead (1972) also confirmed the limitations of the initial program. The data were clear in their indication that the variable which had not been successfully considered in this early programming was that which concerned the configuration of speech complexity. That is, training in one position within words and training essentially in one-word response levels attained some carryover into spontaneous speech, but it did not attain carryover that was adequate in terms of its appropriate distribution of the phoneme response within connected speech.

As a result of these findings, further development of these training programs extended the attainment of correct articulation of new phonemes in all word positions and, importantly, in complex, sentence-length utterances (McLean and Raymore, 1972; Raymore and McLean, 1972; McLean, Raymore, and Long, in press).

The development of the stimulus shift articulation program has been discussed because the learning data gathered in its development seem to indicate quite clearly the variables that are functional in new articulation learning. In this program, when a target sound was systematically conditioned to "belong" to the child and when the child was required to produce the target sound hundreds of times in phonemic contexts that became gradually more complex from a coarticulation point of view, carryover was attained at extremely high levels with the great majority of both normally developing and developmentally delayed children.

The above discussion outlines a two-component model of articulation therapy. Figure 3 depicts these components of response development and carryover and specifies the general factors involved in the message of therapy, the manipulable variables, and the evaluation criteria for each of these components. The procedures used in these two components of therapy are discussed in the following sections.

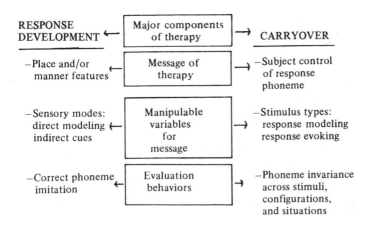

Figure 3. Functional analysis of articulation therapy.

Procedures of Articulation Therapy

If response development and carryover are the basic targets of articulation therapy, and if the message of therapy and manipulable variables are definable, it remains only to analyze the details by which these factors are applied in the therapy process. In analyzing the applications, one necessarily does some hypothesizing about the nature of the basic process of articulation modification as it might be revealed by empirical data obtained on child responses to the various procedures.

Procedures in Response Development   The key to developing effective procedures in response development is, of course, a thorough knowledge of the topography of the sound response being sought. Without this knowledge, the selection of specific variables to be manipulated cannot be adequate. As Figure 3 shows, the message for therapy in the response development component is the specifics of place and manner features for the target sound response. By analyzing these place and manner features, the clinician is able to select the best ways to get this message to the child. It is surprising how little specific information is available about the requirements that different sounds make on clinical procedures. Traditionally, articulation therapy has become strongly biased toward an auditory variable as the primary transmitter of the "message" of threapy. Although the auditory channel is highly appropriate as a transmitter of the model acoustic target of therapy, it seems most apparent that other sensory modes also offer important channels for transmitting certain of these messages. In the consideration of response development programs, both effectiveness and efficiency demand that the procedures stemming from this auditory bias be reassessed and modified by greater exploitation of all other sensory modes.

The first product of reassessment seems to be an awareness that far too little attention has been given to a truly functional analysis of intervention targets and the procedural means to attain those targets. The best example of this lies in the continued commitment to so-called ear training in articulation therapy. Although, of course, a child must have good models of the desired acoustic product, in many response development tasks the acoustic product is the least needy of treatment. For example, a child who is substituting /t/ for /k/ is making a good approximation of the acoustic product being sought. Indeed, /t/ and /k/ both share the same distinctive features in terms of manner of articulation, i.e., unvoiced stops. The message of therapy in developing an appropriate approximation of the /k/ sound is one of placement of the articulators, i.e., movement from an apicoalveolar placement to a dorsovelar contact. If one is objective, one must see that the clinician's production of an acoustic model of the /k/ does very little to tell a child to ". . . move his tongue back and bring the dorsum into contact with the velum." Thus, one sees that attaining this message of therapy requires use of other input. Experienced clinicians know this and provide visual displays of the desired tongue position, provide a motokinesthetic aid (Young and Hawk, 1955) in the form of digital pressure on the fleshy undersides of the mandible to force the tongue dorsum up, and/or directly push the tongue back into a high-back position using a tongue depressor. They also attempt to use visual input by demonstrating the sound with the mouth held open even though they realize that the focal articulation point for the /k/ is still obscured for the child.

In their attempts to attain a good /k/ from a child, clinicians also frequently give verbal cues to the child about tongue position. Likewise, they try to attain appropriate approximations of the desired tongue position by having the child produce sounds, already in the child's repertoire, in which the tongue position is somewhat near the one desired for the /k/, e.g., the vowel /u/, the resonant /r/, and even the high-front vowel /i/; this procedure at least avoids alveolar contact while keeping the tongue high throughout the length of the oral cavity.

These various clinical procedures on the /k/ can be classified according to the sensory mode they use and whether the attempts to give information are *direct* or *indirect* in terms of whether or not they directly model the desired response topography or whether they approach it indirectly. In terms of the examples presented for /k/ the following patterns are evident:

Direct:

1. Auditory modeling
2. Motokinesthetic manipulation
3. Tactual movement of tongue with tongue depressor
4. Visual display of the focal articulation point

Indirect:

1. Verbal descriptions of tongue placement
2. Use of another sound to indirectly attain the place position for /k/

In assessing the relative power of each of these techniques, it should be noted that, taken separately, none of them is particularly powerful in attaining the message of therapy for /k/. Thus, in most cases, clinicians tend to use all of them in combinations and hope that the interactions among all of these inputs allow the child to discover the correct placement and produce the /k/ correctly. Any judgment must hold that the /k/ is a difficult response to develop if it is not immediately stimulable.

Other sounds show highly differential representations of direct and indirect variables that can be used to teach placement. The /l/, for example, is a relatively easy sound to teach because direct visual demonstration of the placement is available and, in combination with the acoustic model, is usually effective in attaining the response. The /s/ is sometimes difficult to attain, particularly if the error is a lateral emission rather than a lingual protrusion. With the focal articulation point obscured by teeth closure, again, direct approaches are inhibited. The finger held in front of the mouth provides a direct demonstration of the central emission of the breath stream and helps a child modify lateral emission. A visual model of the teeth closed often inhibits lingual protrusion. But beyond these, direct models are difficult to attain for /s/ problems.

The point of these examples is simply to demonstrate the variables that must be considered in attempting to attain appropriate response development for required speech sounds. These examples also point out that the traditional auditory bias often masks an awareness of other modes and degrees of direct modeling that can be used to attain new phoneme responses.

Figure 4 graphically represents an overall perspective of the procedures that must be used in the development of new responses. Each feature of the desired sound, i.e., voicing, placement, and manner characteristics, must be assured, and various sensory modes must be utilized to provide both direct models of the placement topography and the acoustic properties of the various target sounds. Thus, in Figure 4 the needed features are specified in the fourth horizontal row; the fact that each feature requires direct and indirect variables directed toward the desired placement, voicing, and/or manner messages is indicated in the third horizontal row; and, then, the sensory modes used to provide the desired therapy information are specified in the bottom two horizontal rows.

The use of this lattice allows an analysis of all of the information necessary for a child to attain a target sound and, by following it in detail, helps in the identification of any and all possible manipulations in the various modes that may be of use in reaching that particular target. Obviously, all modes are not useful for all sound targets.

Two specific examples of sound targets hopefully will help show this process. Response development for the /r/ is discussed first and then a process for /č/ is presented.

Upon examination, the message of the /r/ when it is substituted by a /w-like/ sound in release position is usually described as a "distortion." Even though the /w/ is a glide, it starts from a vowel /u/ and is, as indicated earlier, very similar in manner to the median resonant /r/, which also begins with a relatively unobstructed oral channel created by a high-back tongue position. Thus, the message of therapy is somewhat subtle in that it is a message of tongue placement in which the correct and incorrect tongue positions are not too far apart. The liprounding that accompanies back vowels in English and, thus, accompanies the back glide /w/, actually obscures the real problem in this common and difficult-to-correct substitution.

If, then, the /r/ can be accepted as a placement problem, place features are selected as the primary message of therapy. Although the auditory model is always presented, it usually effects little change in the response. The tongue placement also can be directly modeled for visual instruction, but it very rarely provides change in the sound response of the child. There are few direct tactual manipulations that

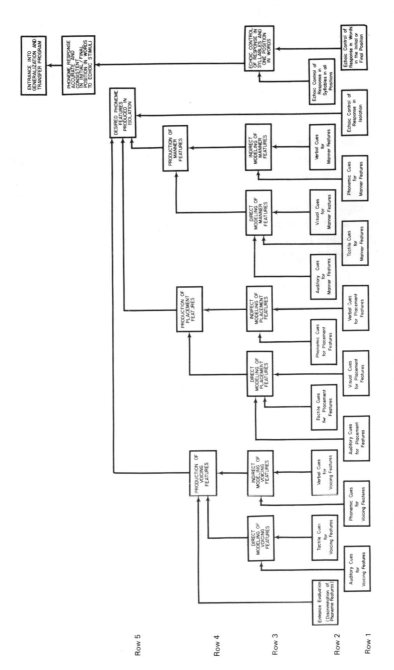

Figure 4. Analysis of variables for phoneme response development.

Row 5

Row 4

Row 3

Row 2

Row 1

can be made and be effective. A tongue depressor can be used to push the tongue back into the mouth, but this generally is not too successful. With direct modeling in the auditory, visual, and tactual modes seemingly ineffective, the next step is to look at indirect ways to give the child placement information.

It has been this writer's experience that verbal instructions about getting the tongue high and back in the mouth to produce /r/ merely seem to move children back to the /u/ position from which they glided into the next vowel and thus produced the /w-like/ rather than extinguishing it as intended. Still, it seemed that indirect use of other phonemic responses would be the most viable method of attaining the tongue position desired for the /r/. Because the aim was for a high-back tongue position from which to attempt the /r/, it was decided to target first one dimension of that placement through another sound and then move to the second aspect of it with still other sounds. The resultant program, then, became:

Initial target: High tongue position that could be well modeled for the child; phonemic approximation of this could be accomplished by evoking the high-front complex syllable /i/ as in *eat* (/it/)

Second target: After attaining a stable imitation of /i/, approximation of the movement of the high tongue position toward the eventually desired back position was begun. To begin this movement back, the /ɪ/ vowel as in the word *it* (/ɪt/) was targeted next. By having a child utter /i/ then /ɪ/, it was possible to visually directly model the high tongue position moving toward the back of the mouth

Third target: In the final procedure, children were asked to utter /i/, move the tongue back one "notch" to /ɪ/, and then move it back one more "notch" and attempt the postvocalic version of the sound /ɚ/

Thus, for /r/, it proved necessary to utilize indirect phonemic approximations to attain correct placements. Other clinicians have observed that they use similar indirect methods by teaching /r/ from /g/ or approach the high-front position with /θ/ and request a quick backward tongue movement from that position. The primary point in this example is that all clinicians use techniques in response development that can be described in rather specific fashion with their process made quite explicit and quantifiable. With developmentally delayed children, clear identification of targets and methods for achieving those targets must be carefully thought through and systematically applied. In this way, new responses can be attained effectively and efficiently.

Without great detail, a similar process can be shown in attacking a nonstimulable /č/ which, also, is often difficult to attain because of its mixing of two manner features (stop plus fricative) and its invisible placement features. With visual, tactual, and auditory direct models relatively inefficient, it was again necessary to move to indirect phonemic approximations. In this case, the program became a coarticulation of two words, *at* (/æt/) and *shoe* (/šu/), in succession. In these cases, the rapid articulation of these words generally produced a good medial /č/, which then could be isolated in both release and arrest syllables and moved into carryover programs.

None of these procedures are novel. McDonald (1964) has emphasized facilitating contexts for some time now, and all clinicians use them to a greater extent than they realize. The primary purpose for this rather labored discussion of these points on analyzing response development programming is simply that few discussions of traditional procedures make them obvious and because most clinicians do not have a full appreciation of their own use of such functional analysis techniques. If successful programs are to be developed for severely delayed children, it is essential that clinicians be more sensitive to the techniques they use and that these techniques be made most specific in clinical approaches to the response development targets for such children.

Such analysis also can increase sensitivity to the factors that must be considered in the treatment of hearing-impaired children. With such children, obviously, nonauditory modes must be exploited to their fullest potential. An analysis directed by the lattice presented in Figure 4 would seem to be productive in this regard. Of even greater potential in response development procedures with hearing-impaired children (and perhaps with severely delayed children as well) is the development and availability of electronic speech aids for such children. Pickett's analysis of these aids (1975) indicates that, of the four primary designs for providing speech aid to hearing-impaired persons, two of these designs transform the speech pattern into sensory stimuli other than acoustic stimuli. One of these two designs transforms the *amplitude-frequency patterns* of sounds into either visual displays or vibrotactile stimuli. The second design, instead of transforming full speech spectrums into other sensory modes, transforms the *articula-*

tory features of a sound into nonacoustic modes. Both of these designs have been applied to produce a number of different devices. To attempt to identify all of them in this chapter would tax both space and competence limitations. Those interested in this important source of technologic aid to the problems of hearing-impaired persons are urged to review the extensive treatment of this area provided in the conference proceedings on this topic edited by Pickett (1968) and other writings by Levitt (1973), Levitt and Nye (1971), Fant (in press), and the aforementioned Pickett (1975) article.

In addition to the nonacoustic stimulus speech aids discussed above, it also seems important to note here the great need to improve the reception of the acoustic stimuli with hearing-impaired clients. While the use of traditional speech amplifying hearing aids may be well known to most readers of this volume, the development of what Pickett (1975) called the auditory recoding design for speech aids to the hearing impaired may not be as familiar. In this design, the frequency characteristics of normal speech are transposed in ways that allow them to be presented in frequency ranges that are more likely to be receivable by hearing-impaired persons, i.e., lower frequencies versus higher frequencies. More information about the application of this design of speech aids can be gotten from the same writings cited above for the other types of speech-aid designs.

In sum, an analysis of response development clinical variables and technologic aids that are available to clinicians will assure the choice of optimal ways to transmit the therapy message to a child. In the case of severely communicatively delayed children, the salience and the power of these treatment techniques are demanded at the highest possible level. These demands are not now well served by the rather vague ideas about what must be done to correct a misarticulated sound. Milisen (1954) stressed a rigorous "integral stimulation" of a sound in his classic work on articulation therapy. It is this author's feeling that only by analyzing the manipulable variables, the sensory modes, and the directness by which information about the target sound can be most specifically delivered to a child, will it be possible to select and apply the most powerful supportive stimulus models for that child's specific articulatory need.

Carryover Treatment Procedures   As indicated earlier, the construct for carryover treatment presented here is not traditional. The data from a program of research in articulation therapy with both delayed and nondelayed children (McLean and Raymore, 1972) and subsequent unpublished data from the field of testing of these programs have demonstrated consistently positive results and, as importantly, have shown surprisingly consistent patterns of variable identification. The analysis of the sum total of all this research and experience with articulation programming has led to the conclusion that the following variables are critical for articulation learning that is adequate for carryover into spontaneous speech:

1.   A systematic procedure in which a child's correct phoneme response is shifted from the support of a direct model of the features of that response to a stimulus that merely evokes the sound but which does not model it, e.g., echoic to picture stimulus

2.   A systematic procedure in which the targeted phoneme is produced by the child in conditions of more and more complex coarticulation interference, e.g., single words, varying word positions for the phoneme within single words, simple sentences containing trained single words that contain the targeted phoneme, and finally, complex sentences in which the target phoneme occurs two or three times in varying word positions

Figure 5 shows the general schematic of the stimulus shift program for the /č/ phoneme. In this graphic presentation, the antecedent stimulus condition changes are indicated, the configuration variables are charted, and the criterion performances on the various steps and conditions are specified.

It has proved interesting that, even with a rigorous attack on this problem in programmatic research and with the modified theoretical base applied to the problem, the therapy programs that finally resulted appear very similar to standard articulation therapy procedures regularly practiced by speech clinicians. The only real difference in the so-called stimulus-shift programs (McLean, Raymore, and Long, in press) is the fact that they are specifically systematic and assure adequate production levels by applying stringent criteria for child performances throughout each step of the program. It is this systematicity that seems particularly required for programming carryover for severely communicatively delayed children. Normally developing children may acquire new learning in the face of unsystematic therapy procedures. There are, of course, limits to even their ability to compensate for inconsistent clinical procedures, and so a systematic ap-

I. INITIAL WORD POSITION

Articulation Context:	Single Word	Simple Sentence (one target word)	Single Word (new)	Complex Sentence (three target words)
Sequence of Stimulus Types	${}_sS^1$ Paired* → ${}_sS^2$ → ${}_sS^2$ Paired → ${}_sS^{3**}$	${}_sS^1$ Paired → ${}_sS^2$	${}_sS^{2*}$	${}_sS^1$ Paired → ${}_sS^2$
Example: Training targets for the phoneme /č/ /***	1. chain 2. cherry 3. cheese 4. chain 5. cherry 6. cheese 7. chain 8. cherry 9. cheese	1. On ice cream, I like a cherry 2. Santa comes down the chimney 3. Mother wrote a check 4–9. (Repeat above sentences two more times)	1. chicken 2. children 3. chin 4. chicken 5. children 6. chin 7. chicken 8. children 9. chin	1. Charles drew a chicken with chalk 2. Chinese children like cheese 3. The chief hurt his chin and cheek 4–9. (Repeat above sentences two more times)

II. FINAL WORD POSITION

Articulation Context:	Single Word	Simple Sentence (one target word)	Single Word (new)	Complex Sentence (three target words)
Sequence of Stimulus Types	${}_sS^1$ Paired* → ${}_sS^2$ → ${}_sS^2$ Paired → ${}_sS^{3**}$	${}_sS^1$ Paired → ${}_sS^2$	${}_sS^{2*}$	${}_sS^1$ Paired → ${}_sS^2$
Example: Training targets for the phoneme /č/ /***	1. branch 2. patch 3. switch 4. branch 5. patch 6. switch 7. branch 8. patch 9. switch	1. On his jeans is a patch 2. Daddy uses a wrench 3. The wind blew away the branch 4–9. (Repeat above sentences two more times)	1. bench 2. sandwich 3. witch 4. bench 5. sandwich 6. witch 7. bench 8. sandwich 9. witch	1. Which coach is on the bench? 2. For lunch, I ate my sandwich at the bench 3. I won't touch the witch too much 4–9. (Repeat above sentences two more times)

Articulation Context:	Single Word			Simple Sentence (one target word) →	Single Word (new) →	Complex Sentence (three target words)
Sequence of Stimulus Types	S^1_2 Paired* → S^2_3 → S^2_3 Paired → S^{3*}			S^1_2 Paired → S^2	S^{2*}	S^1_2 Paired → S^2
Example: Training targets for the phoneme /č/ ***	1. pitcher 2. matches 3. hatchet 4. pitcher 5. matches 6. hatchet 7. pitcher 8. matches 9. hatchet			1. You light fires with matches 2. He cut the tree with a hatchet 3. We buy meat from the butcher 4–9. (Repeat above sentences two more times)	1. handkerchief 2. catcher 3. punchbowl 4. handkerchief 5. catcher 6. punchbowl 7. handkerchief 8. catcher 9. punchbowl	1. Achoo! Achoo! I need a handkerchief 2. The catcher and pitcher are watching the ball 3. The teacher put the punchbowl in the kitchen 4–9. (Repeat above sentences two more times)

IV. MIXED WORD ORDER (OPTIONAL)

Articulation Context:	Simple Sentence (one target word) →	Single Word →	Complex Sentence (three target words)
Sequence of Stimulus Types	S^1_2 Paired → S^2	S^{2*}	S^1_2 Paired → S^2
Example: Training targets for the phoneme /č/ ***	1. On ice cream, I like a cherry 2. Daddy uses a wrench 3. You light fires with matches 4–9. (Repeat above sentences two more times)	1. chicken 2. children 3. chin 4. bench 5. sandwich 6. witch 7. handkerchief 8. catcher 9. punchbowl	1. Charles drew a chicken with chalk 2. Which coach is on the bench? 3. Achoo! Achoo! I need a handkerchief 4–9. (Repeat above sentences two more times)

Key to Stimulus Types

S^1 = Echoic Stimulus
S^2 = Picture Stimulus
S^3 = Intraverbal Stimulus

* Echoic remediation provided if criterion not met with this stimulus.

** S^3 (the Intraverbal stimulus) consists of an incomplete sentence presented by the clinician. The child completes the sentence with the appropriate training word, i.e., "A mouse likes (cheese)."

*** Criterion for all training blocks is 17 correct responses in 18 trials.

Figure 5. Stimulus shift articulation programming. Multiple stimulus control and configuration training for the phoneme /č/.

proach is also productive for normally developing children. Severely delayed children, however, must be given the message of therapy precisely, must be given the most optimal supports for the desired response, and must be given performance opportunities at each level of therapy that are stringent and productive for their integration of the new response into their own internalized control systems.

This quality of systematicity is inherent not only in the stimulus shift program format, but also in most of the recently available programmed approaches to articulation modification. Mowrer's work in articulation programming stresses this feature along with several other features involving the antecedent and consequent events in therapy (Mowrer, 1969a, Mowrer, Baker, and Schutz, 1970; Mowrer, 1973).

Garrett and his associates have developed both an auditory discrimination approach and a production approach to articulation modification that probably represent the ultimate in systematic programming (Garrett and Rigg, 1965; Garrett, 1973).

Weston and Irwin's extensive work developing the paired stimuli technique for articulation modification (Irwin and Weston, 1971; Weston and Irwin, 1971; Irwin and Griffith, 1973) concentrated on developing systematic procedures for attaining both response development and carryover of new phoneme responses. As this program has developed, it too has moved into more consideration of the phonemic environments in which sounds are trained.

Success in applying systematic procedures that program the child to produce a sound in various stimulus conditions and in varying simple-to-complex configurations of phonemic environments (McLean and Raymore, 1972; Raymore and McLean, 1972) speaks convincingly to a perception of articulation as behavior that can be treated at its surface structure level. This, it seems, is not as true of other parts of the language structure, like syntax, for example. In articulation, however, the overall history of success in symptomatologic therapy, and the significantly good results attained in all of the programmed therapy systems attacking the phoneme in coarticulated contexts, clearly seem to indicate that phones and phoneme boundaries are "learned by doing." Thus, by attaining high levels of production in varying levels of environmental complexity, a child can gain the internal control of these responses, enabling the responses to be carried over into any type of utterance. At this time, at least, it does not seem likely that the cognitive understanding of these tasks is adequate to accomplish the end goals. Instead, the spontaneous emission of the correct motor patterns of the desired phone and the coarticulation of these responses in complex phonologic environments are the hard earned products of intensive motor practice in the varying conditions of antecedent stimulus support and configuration complexity discussed here.

All of these empirically suggested perspectives about articulation learning are supportive of the increasing body of empirical data and theory that treats articulation as basically a motor-perceptual behavior dynamically integrated at levels of complexity beyond the single phoneme level. Thus, the motor perception theories of speech and its extensions offered by Liberman, Harris, and Hoffman (1957); the basic realities of both forward and backward coarticulation, indicating that the phone uttered is heavily influenced by other phones in the utterance string (MacNeilage and Sholes, 1964; Kozhevnikov and Christovich, 1966; MacNeilage, 1970); and the perceptual significance of syllables versus single phonemes as reported by the Faircloths (Faircloth and Faircloth, 1970) all contribute to this awareness that articulation is not just a collection of individual phones connected together but are clusters of phones that are integrated at motor levels below the cognitive level. Thus, the empirical data on articulation acquisition that is accomplishd by producing the desired behavior in conditions of increasingly complex coarticulation contexts, as has been done in all articulation programs, seem clearly to vindicate the speech pathologist's attack on this behavior at a surface structure production level. It is certainly not that phonology does not have rules or that children learning language do not learn the rules of the language system. It simply seems to be that, in the case of phonology, the motor production itself contributes heavily to the full learning of the rules of the system.

IMPLICATIONS FOR ASSESSMENT AND TREATMENT OF ARTICULATION PROBLEMS FOR SEVERELY COMMUNICATIVELY DELAYED CHILDREN

The factors inherent in the basic sound system and the acquisition of a functional phonologic system discussed to this point are those which seem to have the most significance for treatment of the severely delayed and/or multiply impaired child. It is hoped that these discussions have indicated, with some intelligibility, the expansion of the content and the process of articulation therapy that seems to be required by severely communicatively disabled children.

The overall implications of the factors discussed herein seem to have important implications for the entire applied area of articulation therapy. In these final pages, the most direct implications of these constructs to applied problems are reviewed.

Implications for Assessment of Articulatory Behaviors

A chapter of this type necessarily precludes an in-depth treatment of all of the topics that are important within the general subject area. Certainly this is the case for assessment in this context. A full discussion of the assessments and evaluations that may be appropriate for severely communicatively delayed children who manifest inadequate speech-sound systems would go far beyond the scope and space resources of this presentation. In discussing assessment in this context, therefore, only factors that are most directly related to the phonologic system per se can be treated. Other important assessment areas related to the evaluation of child-centered problems in the sensory, motor, or higher neurologic domains are not discussed. Thus, the most direct implications of the topics presented in this chapter are related to the quantification of the phonologic system of severely communicatively delayed children and, in turn, to the treatment designs presented herein.

In the face of even limited distinctive feature analysis, new coarticulation perspectives and the requirements of more systematic programming, it is obvious that the current assessment procedures in articulation must be re-reviewed. This review must consider many things, of course, but the most basic assessment issue to be resolved and implemented by new techniques would seem to be that of the nature of the articulation responses from which judgments about the child's phonologic system will be made. In this perspective, rather than get into a negativistic review of current procedures and test contexts, it seems more productive to consider the kinds of data that will provide the information most helpful to therapy design for delayed children. In this regard, previous discussions indicate that, initially, the following factors should be served by phonologic assessment procedures:

1. All of the phonemes that are expressed in a child's speech system should be quantifiable
2. All of the phonemic features of (at least) voicing, manner of articulation, and place of articulation that are available in a child's speech system should be identifiable

3. The status of the available phonemes in syllables both in release and arrest functions should be quantifiable where appropriate

4. The status of phonemes in coarticulation contexts that represent the highest complexity-configuration used by the child in communicative speech should be discernible

5. The child's general representation of the syllabic structure of words uttered in his/her highest utilized complexity-configuration level should be quantifiable

A review of these needs should convince most clinicians that the traditional picture articulation test, which evokes single-word responses in three word positions, does not provide adequately for the information needed. Although the more standard tests do seem to provide information that has high correlation with the factors listed above, they, most often, do not provide direct quantification of them. Faircloth (1973) indicated that, for many reasons in addition to those listed here, the only "test" that adequately assesses phonemic adequacy in all of its appropriate dimensions is a carefully analyzed *spontaneous speech sample*. In her paper, Faircloth cites research by Dickerson (1971) indicating that samples of 60 to 90 word segments in connected, spontaneous speech provide an adequate sample of a child's phonologic system. Obviously, the spontaneous speech sample would yield information pertinent to the five factors listed above.

In addition to the information given by Faircloth (1973) and reported by Dickerson (1971) when considering spontaneous speech samples, the reader might wish to investigate the general procedures of language sampling used in psycholinguistic research. Slobin (1967) has the most complete procedural guide to this type of sampling, but the published works of Bloom (1970), Bowerman (1973), and others contain typescripts of language samples that can be used to guide this procedure. Obviously, the sample size required for in-depth sampling of language structures of syntax is far larger than that needed for articulatory inventories. Thus, one working with language structures as well as articulatory responses obviously may utilize the samples collected for language analysis to serve for articulation analysis too.

Such speech samples provide directly quantifiable data about a child's available phonemic repertoire; these data then can be analyzed from the several points of view that underlie the selection of treatment targets for severely delayed children. The phonemic distinctions being produced can be subjected to feature analysis to show the voicing, manner, and place distinctions already being made by the child.

The child's general performance in regard to the syllabication that appears so important to the child's intelligibility can be readily evaluated. In addition, spontaneous speech samples, by their very existence, indicate that a child is a communicator in the oral mode and, thus, an appropriate candidate for articulation therapy. Beyond this most basic indicator of an orally communicating child are the spontaneous speech data that show the level of complexity-configuration to which new phoneme responses must be trained. As previously mentioned, research findings (McLean and Raymore, 1972) indicate that, for the carryover of new phoneme responses to occur optimally, systematic training on them must occur up through the level of linguistic complexity that the child uses in spontaneous speech (e.g., single words, two- to three-word phrases, five- to six-word sentences, etc.).

In addition to the speech samples and other tests that indicate the general content of a child's available phonologic system, one also must assess the general viability of the child's system for modification and/or expansion. In this context, then, stimulability testing (Milisen, 1954) should be utilized to probe a child's ability to use clinician-presented models to produce modified or totally new phone responses. For severely communicatively handicapped children, however, this type of evaluation should be extended considerably beyond the auditory-visual stimulus model usually applied in this procedure. The effectiveness of as many as possible of the direct and indirect modes for providing information about the desired response change should be evaluated. Naturally, the goal is, as it always has been, to identify the phone responses that have the highest probability for effective modification at that time.

Still another area of assessment pertinent to the general phonologic system of delayed children is that of receptive performance at the phonologic level. Auditory tests with at least rudimentary distinctive feature representations are becoming available to test children's receptive *phonemic* discriminations as opposed to their *sound* discrimination, e.g., Goldman, Fristoe, and Woodcock (1970) as compared to Wepman (1958). Although the relationship of receptive performance and expressive performance at the phonologic level is not totally clear at this point, it does seem intuitively desirable to attempt to teach a phoneme that a child discriminates as a communication receiver in preference to a phoneme that is not receptively communicatively contrastive for the child. This is, of course, when all other targeting factors seem to be equal.

In sum, it seems apparent that assessment of articulation for the severely communicatively delayed child is well served only by careful and detailed analysis of the child's available expressive and receptive phonemic repertoire. For many reasons, both of these performance areas would be most ideally evaluated in spontaneous communication contexts. It is most important that, at least, the expressive system of a child be described from spontaneous speech samples. The child's available phonemic feature system can be quantified and the needed targets of place and manner can be specified. The need for targeting of syllable articulation also can be determined from these data as can the availability of specific phonemic features in both release and arrest functions. In addition to these assessments of the available sound system of a child, extended testing of the child's responses to modeling stimuli in all sensory modes can be undertaken as in traditional stimulability testing procedures.

Implications for Treatment of Articulatory Problems

Speech and the speech sounds are but one mode of transmitting a language system. This mode is the most basic, the most effective, and the most generic to a language's creation—but it is still only one of the modes. Thus, before one thinks of teaching the phonologic system per se, one should ensure that a child has the basic rudiments of a *communication* system. These rudiments are well covered in other parts of this volume (e.g., Graham; Sanders; Siegel and Broen; Wilbur) and include representational and symbolic behavior, interactive relationship with both the world of things and the world of people, cognitive/conceptual development adequate to generate the semantic intent of communicative utterances, and a basic drive to communicate orally with others in one's world. With these underpinnings of language and communicative functioning available, the refinement of a child's sound system becomes meaningful and productive. Simply teaching the imitation of speech sounds does not seem to be productive if the other indicators of communicative behaviors and/or their prerequisites are not present.

Thus, with severely communicatively delayed children, one must ensure that the prerequisites of *communication* and *language* exist before initiating intensive efforts to shape specific phonemic acquisition. When these prerequisites are unavailable, attention to the sound system should be directed toward the general class of vocal noisemaking and oral practice that is generally referred to as babbling and vocal play. The attention to these general oral responses probably should take the form of reciprocal vocal play between an adult and a child with the specific topography of the child's approximations being rather loosely judged and, thus, allowed to develop without stringent attention to the child's attainment of specific speech phonemes.

During this vocal reciprocal play, the adult caregiver or teacher should be working to develop the child's receptive abilities for oral language and to encourage the child's oral approximations of words. As indicated earlier, when a child begins to approximate oral language topographies, work should be directed toward the attainment of specific speech sounds that are not initially available in the child's repertoire.

When a child becomes an oral language user in the expressive mode, intelligibility should guide the development of the child's sound system. In a preceding discussion, it was argued that optimal intelligibility can be attained by targeting phoneme development along phonemic feature lines. The attainment of feature contrasts between vowels and consonants is suggested as a first target; the attainment of the feature representations of sounds within all manner classes as a second goal; and the development of different places of articulation within manner classes as the third consideration.

The specific process of sound system modification with severely communicatively delayed children demands the most rigorous therapy programs that can be devised. The target or message of therapy for each child must be specified in precise behavioral terms. The variables that are most functional and effective in attaining the message(s) must be identified with specificity and behavioral precision. The procedures by which the functional variables are presented to the child must be systematic and perceptually salient for the child's use. This means, again, a rigor and precision applied to the development of such procedures.

The research reviewed herein indicates that articulation change can be effected by attention to the surface structures represented by the phone or phoneme response being targeted. The research indicates, however, that a static view of the sound units is probably not productive. Instead, articulation behavior must be viewed both as dynamic and as controlled at motor integration levels below the cognitive level. This means that the desired responses are most effectively acquired by producing them in contexts and conditions that assure both their appropriate topography and their eventual control by the subject's own internal monitoring and production mechanism. Both of these demands require a perspective of therapy that does not seem to be clearly represented in traditional therapy procedures. The construct of a two-stage therapy process of response development and carryover seems justifiable and productive.

In response development, there is a need for a more functional analysis of the "message" of therapy and the sensory modes and techniques by which information specific to that message is carried to the child. This means a careful analysis of the actual utility of various sensory modes for various therapy messages—something seemingly not adequately represented in the approaches currently available in most training programs. A lattice-directed review of all the direct and indirect manipulations that can be made in all sensory modes in order to carry the needed information to the child is presented in the foregoing discussions to help in the analysis of response development targets and procedures.

In carryover training, the view presented is that the targeting of invariance of phoneme production begins immediately after a sound is available in imitation of an auditory-visual model presented to the child. All therapy procedures after this imitation state seem directed toward attainment of child-control of the sound and, thus, its carryover into spontaneous speech. To accomplish this state of child-control, systematic programming across various levels of antecedent stimulus conditions and careful programming through a steadily more complex configuration of coarticulation contexts, ranging from single words to complex, sound-loaded sentences, is generally necessary and successful.

The early targeting of approximations of the syllable properties of words along with phonemic acquisition is also recommended. Approximations of the syllable properties seem to add significantly to a child's intelligibility, particularly if the syllables contain consonant productions that are at least within the same manner classes of the sounds included in the target word(s).

Continued integration of new research data on coarticulation and distinctive feature analysis undoubtedly will alter some of the targets and procedures outlined in this chapter. The clinician/teacher working with these children, then, must be constantly aware of the research in articulation behavior and incorporate new empirically validated perspectives as rapidly as possible. Even without immediate new data, however, the current knowledge of articulation behavior and articulation acquisition provides significant bases for innovation in traditional therapy procedures—innovations that should allow more effective management of articulation deficiencies among children who a few years ago would have been summarily rejected as valid clinical subjects for such therapy.

SUMMARY

This chapter sets forth some basic perspectives for aiding clinicians in planning programs for enhancing the acquisition of a speech sound system by severely communicatively delayed children. The key points are:

1. A phonemic-feature approach that allows an orderly approach to early phonemic development

2. A dichotomization of articulation therapy that stresses and outlines a systematic, functional analysis approach to:
    a. Development of nonstimulable phone responses
    b. Attainment of carryover of new phonemes

ACKNOWLEDGMENTS

The author wishes to acknowledge the significant contributions that Lee K. Snyder, Research Associate, George Peabody College for Teachers, made to the preparation of this manuscript.

REFERENCES

Baer, D. M., and J. A. Sherman. 1964. Reinforcement control of generalized imitation in young children. J. Exp. Child Psychol. 1:37–49.

Beckwith, L. 1971. Relationships between infant's vocalizations and their mother's behaviors. Merrill-Palmer Q. 17:211–226.

Bloom, L. M. 1970. Language Development: Form and Function of Emerging Grammars. MIT Press, Cambridge, Mass.

Bowerman, M. 1973. Early Syntactic Development: A Cross-linguistic Study with Special Reference to Finnish. Cambridge University Press, Cambridge, England.

Bricker, W. A. 1967. Errors in the echoic behavior of preschool children. J. Speech Hear. Res. 10(1):67–76.

Buchanan, C. D. 1963. A Programmed Introduction to Linguistics: Phonetics and Phonemics. D. C. Heath, Lexington, Mass.

Dale, P. S. 1972. Language Development: Structure and Function. Dryden Press, Hinsdale, Ill.

Dewey, G. 1923. Relative Frequency of English Speech Sounds. Harvard University Press, Cambridge, Mass.

Dickerson, M. V. 1971. An investigation of a method of sampling spontaneous speech for the evaluation of articulatory behavior. Unpublished doctoral dissertation, Florida State University, Tallahassee.

Ervin-Tripp, S. 1966. Language development. In L. W. Hoffman and M. L. Hoffman (eds.), Review of Child Development Research, pp. 55–105. Vol. 2. Russell Sage Foundation.

Faircloth, M. A. 1973. Articulation for communication. Paper presented at the Special Study Institute on: Articulation disorders in School Children Revisited, April-May, San Diego.

Faircloth, M. A., and S. R. Faircloth. 1970. An analysis of the articulatory behavior of a speech-defective child in connected speech and in isolated-word responses. J. Speech Hear. Disord. 35:51–61.

Faircloth, S. R., and M. A. Faircloth. 1971. Delayed language and linguistic variations. In W. C. Grabb, S. Rosenstein, and K. R. Bzoch (eds.), Cleft Lip and Palate. Little, Brown, New York.

Fant, G. Speech and hearing defects and aids. In G. Fant (ed.), Proceedings of the Stockholm Speech Communication Seminar. Vol. 4. Royal Institute of Technology, Stockholm. In press.

Garrett, E. R. 1973. Programmed articulation therapy. In W. D. Wolfe and D. J. Goulding (eds.), Articulation and Learning. Charles C Thomas, Springfield, Ill.

Garrett, E. R., and K. E. Rigg. 1965. Automated self-correction of functional misarticulation in the public schools. Paper read at the American Speech and Hearing Association 1965 National Convention. Abstracted in Asha 7:442.

Goldman, R., and M. Fristoe. 1969. Goldman-Fristoe Test of Articulation. American Guidance Service, Circle Pines, Minn.

Goldman, R., M. Fristoe, and R. Woodcock. 1970. Test of Auditory Discrimination. American Guidance Service, Circle Pines, Minn.

Griffiths, H., and W. E. Craighead. 1972. Generalization in operant speech therapy for misarticulation. J. Speech Hear. Disord. 37:485–494.

Irwin, J. V., and F. A. Griffith. 1973. A theoretical and operational analysis of the paired stimuli technique. In W. D. Wolfe and D. J. Goulding (eds.), Articulation and Learning, pp. 156–194. Charles C Thomas, Springfield, Ill.

Irwin, J. V., and A. J. Weston. 1971. A Manual for the Clinical Utilization of the Paired-Stimuli Technique. National Educator Services, Memphis.

Jakobson, R. 1968. Child Language, Aphasia, and Phonological Universals. Mouton, The Hague. (Translated from the German by A. Keiler).

Jakobson, R., C. G. M. Fant, and M. Halle. 1963. Preliminaries to Speech Analysis: The Distinctive Features and Their Correlates. 2nd Ed. MIT Press, Cambridge, Mass.

Jakobson, R., and M. Halle. 1956. Fundamentals of Language. Mouton, The Hague.

Kozhevnikov, V. A., and L. A. Christovich. 1966. Speech: Articulation and perception. Joint Publications Research Services, Washington, D.C., 30:543. (Translated from the Russian 1965 article).

Levitt, H. 1973. Speech processing aids for the deaf: An overview. IEEE Trans-Audio Electroacoust. Au-21:269–273.

Levitt, H., and P. W. Nye (eds.). 1971. Sensory Training Aids for the Deaf. Proceedings of a Conference, National Academy of Engineering, Washington, D.C.

Liberman, A. M., K. S. Harris, and H. S. Hoffman. 1957. The discrimination of speech sounds within and across phoneme boundaries. J. Exp. Psychol. 54:358–368.

McDonald, E. T. 1964. Articulation Testing and Treatment: A Sensory-Motor Approach. Stanwix House, Pittsburgh.

McLean, J. E. 1970. Extending stimulus control of phoneme articulation by operant techniques. In F. L. Girardeau and J. E. Spradlin (eds.), A Functional Analysis Approach to Speech and Language Behavior, pp. 24–27. Asha Monogr. 14.

McLean, J. E. 1972. Developing clinical strategies for language intervention with mentally retarded children. In J. E. McLean, D. E. Yoder, and R. L. Schiefelbusch (eds.), Language Intervention with the Retarded, pp. 1–14. University Park Press, Baltimore.

McLean, J. E., and S. Raymore. 1972. Programmatic research on a systematic articulation therapy program: Carry-over of phoneme responses to untrained situations for normal-learning public school children. Kansas Center for Research in Mental Retardation and Human Development Report 6, Parsons, Kans.

McLean, J. E., S. Raymore, and L. Long. Stimulus Shift Articulation Program. Edmark Assoc., Belleview, Wash. In press.

MacNeilage, P. F. 1970. Motor control of serial ordering of speech. Psychol. Rev. 77:182–195.

MacNeilage, P. F., and G. N. Sholes. 1964. An electromyographic study of the tongue during vowel production. J. Speech Hear. Res. 7:209–232.

McReynolds, L. V. 1970. Reinforcement procedures for establishing and maintaining echoic speech by a nonverbal child. In F. L. Girardeau and J. E. Spradlin (eds.), A Functional Analysis Approach to Speech and Language Behavior. Asha monogr. 14:60–66.

McReynolds, L. V., and D. L. Engmann. 1975. Distinctive Feature Analysis of Misarticulations. University Park Press, Baltimore.

McReynolds, L. V., and K. Huston. 1971. A distinctive feature analysis of children's misarticulations. J. Speech Hear. Disord. 36:155–166.

Menyuk, P. 1968. The role of distinctive features in children's acquisition of phonology. J. Speech Hear. Res. 11(1):138–146.

Metz, J. R. 1965. Conditioning generalized imitation in autistic children. J. Exp. Child Psychol. 2:389–399.

Milisen, R. 1954. The disorder of articulation: A systematic clinical and experimental approach. J. Speech Hear. Disord. monogr. suppl. 4:1–86.

Miller, G. A., and P. E. Nicely. 1955. An analysis of perceptual confusions among some English consonants. J. Acoust. Soc. Amer. 27(2): 338–352.

Miller, J., and D. Yoder. 1972. A syntax teaching program. In J. E. McLean, D. E. Yoder, and R. L. Schiefelbusch (eds.), Language Intervention with the Retarded, pp. 191–211. University Park Press, Baltimore.

Mowrer, D. E. (ed.). 1969a. Modification of Speech Behavior: Ideas and Strategies for Students. Arizona State University Bookstore, Tempe.

Mowrer, D. E. 1969b. Evaluating speech therapy through precision recording. J. Speech Hear. Disord. 35:239–244.

Mowrer, D. E. 1971. Transfer of training in articulation therapy. J. Speech Hear. Disord. 36(4):427–446.

Mowrer, D. E. 1973. A behavioristic approach to modification of articulation. In W. D. Wolfe and D. J. Goulding (eds.), Articulation and Learning. Charles C. Thomas, Springfield, Ill.

Mowrer, D. E., R. Baker, and R. Schutz. 1970. S-PACK: Modification of the frontal lisp. EPRA, Tempe, Ariz.

Nelson, K. 1973. Structure and Strategy in Learning to Talk. Monographs of the Society for Research in Child Development, Vol. 38. nos. 1 and 2. University of Chicago Press, Chicago.

Pickett, J. M. (ed.). 1968. Proceedings of the conference on speech analyzing aids for the deaf. Amer. Ann. Deaf 113:116–330.

Pickett, J. M. 1975. Speech-processing aids for communication handicaps: Some research problems. In D. B. Tower (ed.), The Nervous System. Vol. 3: Human Communication and Its Disorders, pp. 299–304. Raven Press, New York.

Poole, I. 1934. Genetic development of articulation of consonant sounds in speech. Elem. Eng. Rev. 11:159–161.

Raymore, S., and J. E. McLean. 1972. A clinical program for carry-over of articulation therapy with retarded children. In J. E. McLean, D. E. Yoder, and R. L. Schiefelbusch (eds.), Language Intervention with the Retarded, pp. 236–253. University Park Press, Baltimore.

Rheingold, H. L., J. L. Gerwitz, and H. W. Ross. 1959. Social conditioning of vocalizations in the infant. J. Comp. Physiol. Psychol. 52:68–73.

Risley, T., and M. Wolf. 1967. Establishing functional speech in echolalic children. Behav. Res. Ther. 5:73–88.

Singh, S. 1976. Distinctive Features: Theory and Validation. University Park Press, Baltimore.

Slobin, D. (ed.). 1967. A Field Manual for Cross-Cultural Study of Communicative Competence. University of California Press, Berkeley.

Stern, D. N. 1974. Mother and infant at play: The dyadic interaction involving facial, vocal and gaze behaviors. In M. Lewis and L. A. Rosenblum (eds.), The Effect of the Infant on its Caregiver, pp. 187–213. John Wiley & Sons, New York.

Strain, B. A. 1974. Early dialogues: A naturalistic study of vocal behavior in mothers and three-month-old infants. Unpublished doctoral dissertation, George Peabody College for Teachers, Nashville, Tenn.

Templin, M. 1957. Certain Language Skills in Children. University of Minnesota Press, Minneapolis.

Templin, M., and F. Darley. 1960. The Templin-Darley Tests of Articulation. Bureau of Educational Research and Service, University of Iowa, Iowa City.

Van Riper, C. 1963. Speech Correction: Principles and Methods. 4th Ed. Prentice-Hall, Englewood Cliffs, N. J.

Weisberg, P. 1963. Social and nonsocial conditioning of infant vocalizations. Child Dev. 34:377–388.

Wepman, J. M. 1958. Auditory Discrimination Test: Manual of Directions. Language Research Associates, Chicago.

Weston, A. J., and J. V. Irwin. 1971. Use of paired-stimuli in modification of articulation. Percept. Motor Skills 32:947–957.

Wolff, P. H. 1969. The natural history of crying and other vocalizations in early infancy. In B. M. Foss (ed.), Determinants of Infant Behavior, pp. 81–110. Vol. 4. Methuen, London.

Yoder, D. E. 1970. The reinforcing properties of a television presented listener. In F. L. Girardeau and J. E. Spradlin (eds.), A Functional Analysis Approach to Speech and Language. Asha Monogr. 14:10–19.

Young, E. H., and S. S. Hawk. 1955. Moto-kinesthetic Speech Training. Stanford University Press, Palo Alto.

10

LANGUAGE PROGRAMMING AND INTERVENTION

Louella W. Graham

CONTENTS

Prelinguistic and Extralinguistic Considerations _____ 373
    Prelinguistic behaviors/374
    Extralinguistic behaviors/375

Early Intervention _____ 377

Goals for Programming _____ 380

**Approaches to Language Intervention with the Retarded and
  Other Groups** _____ 382
    Developmental approaches to language intervention/383
    Nondevelopmental approaches/390
    Manual approaches/393
    Use of parents and peers in intervention strategies/395

Programming for the Hearing Impaired _____ 397
    Parent involvement/401
    Early detection and amplification/403
    Integration of the hearing-impaired child/404
    Programs for the multiply handicapped hearing impaired/405

**Communication Systems for the Nonoral Physically
  Handicapped** _____ 410

Conclusion _____ 412

References _____ 413

Although the normal child acquires language relatively rapidly and without any special assistance, many developmentally disabled children acquire only a rudimentary form of language and some, even as adults, are essentially without language. For the mentally retarded group, the degree of mental retardation is usually closely related to the level of language deficiency, and the absence of language or deficiencies in language define retardation to a great extent. Staats (1974) has suggested that the correlation between intelligence and language holds because the two are essentially the same thing.

The ability to communicate with others in one's environment is a critical aspect of human behavior. When this ability does not develop spontaneously, the clinician's task is to intervene. Weiner (in Ruder, 1972) has suggested that one probably will not find a single language disorder within a given developmentally delayed group, but rather a number of different types of language disorders. Consequently, few fully developed programs for language intervention have been designed to establish sequentially a full system of language in the developmentally delayed child. There are, however, several strategies for language intervention that enable the clinician to eliminate or develop various responses within the individual's behavioral repertoire.

Fristoe (1975, 1976) has recently completed a national survey of language intervention programs used with the retarded. She identified 229 programs or systems and cataloged detailed information on 187. Thirty-nine of these are published in kit form; 31 are reported in journals and/or commercially published books; 66 are published privately or as experimental editions; and 51 are in preparation or not currently available. Most of these approaches to language intervention are equally applicable for use with other types of developmental disabilities. Appendix D provides a brief report on this project and summaries of the programs that have been published in kit form.

This chapter is not intended as a "cookbook" for clinicians. Rather, it is intended to familiarize clinicians with various approaches to language intervention and to guide them to sources for more specific programmatic content.

PRELINGUISTIC AND EXTRALINGUISTIC CONSIDERATIONS

There seem to be several forms of behavior that must exist in the child's behavioral repertoire or that must be brought under control before the process of language learning can be fully realized. These forms of behavior can be thought of as those that are prerequisite to the process of language learning (prelinguistic) and those that may compete or interfere with the process of language learning (extralinguistic).

During the prelinguistic period many developmental tasks face the young child. Perhaps the most important of these in terms of later language development is the need for the child to organize his or her environment conceptually. Within the last few years, particularly in the study of normal language acquisition and also to a lesser degree in approaches to language intervention (see Bricker and Bricker, 1973, 1974), the cognitive bases for language have received considerable attention. There is increasing support for the notion that the emergence of language in the child cannot be attributed simply to the presence of certain innate linguistic factors, but that language is the logical outgrowth of the child's development of certain cognitive skills. That is, the process of acquiring language is seen as more than just the acquisition of words and their subsequent use in various combinations. Rather, the child is said to acquire language as a result of various interactions with his or her environment, and these interactions are thought to precede and directly influence the acquisition of language (Cromer, 1974b).

Prelinguistic Behaviors

The cognitive theorist specifically bases his views on those of Piaget concerning the development of the sensorimotor stages of intelligence and the subsequent emergence of language at about the age of 18 months. That language appears at this time and not before is said to result from the necessity for the prior formation of certain cognitive schemas. It is just these schemas that are developed during the sensorimotor period. In Brown's view (1973a, p. 200): ". . . the first sentences express the construction of reality which is the terminal achievement of sensorimotor intelligence."

The sensorimotor period extends from birth to 24 months and is divided into six substages. The first substage begins at birth with the infant being merely a reflexive organism. As infants develop, a number of changes occur in their cognitive behavior until they acquire the symbolic function wherein they possess the ability to represent one thing with another. The symbolic function is considered to be one of the most important prerequisites for the acquisition of language (Cromer, 1974b), and its appearance depends on the child's prior perceptual organization of his environment. Within the context of Piagetian theory (Piaget and Inhelder, 1969; Piaget, 1970), the emergence of language depends on specific underlying cognitive constructs, and the subsequently observed language reflects the child's thought processes as they are facilitated by these structures during different stages of development.

However, as Cromer (1974a) has pointed out, although the development of certain cognitive constructs seems to be necessary for the acquisition of language, there is some evidence that cognitive advances by themselves are not sufficient to explain language acquisition. Thus, there is some question concerning what implications cognitive theory has for training in the case of the language-delayed child. The application of cognitive theory within specific training strategies, such as those described by Bricker and Bricker (1973), should yield some evidence with respect to the importance of training in prelinguistic cognitive skills for the language-delayed child.

Extralinguistic Behaviors

In addition to the view that there may be prelinguistic behaviors or skills that are prerequisite to the emergence of language, there are behaviors that may compete or interfere with the process of language learning. These extralinguistic factors have been described as limiting the language learning ability of the retarded in particular. In a now classic study, Zeaman and House (1963) found that moderately and severely retarded individuals displayed deficits in attention within the context of visual discrimination learning tasks. Specifically, Zeaman and House reported that their retarded subjects were unable to utilize all of the stimulus dimensions available to them, with their attention being limited to one or a few of the stimulus dimensions. The more recent literature has further defined this attentional deficit. Crosby (1972) differentiated the ability to attend to relevant stimuli from the characteristic he referred to as "distractibility"—the inability to inhibit responses to irrelevant stimuli. In general, his findings did not support the view that, as a group, the retarded are more distractible than their normal counterparts. His observations indicated that the degree of distractibility is a highly individualized characteristic rather than a group characteristic.

Several writers have suggested methods of clinical management for the child with attentional deficits. Zeaman and House (1963) recommended the "engineering" of the child's attention by manipulating the training situation so that the relevant dimensions of the stimulus would be most salient to the child. In suggesting methods by which this might be done, they referred to the work of Montessori (1964). The basis of Montessori's program was to focus the child's attention on a specific dimension of the thing to be taught, while reducing the importance of other dimensions. Teaching materials used in a Montessori type of program were specifically designed to accomplish this. Richardson (1967) also has advocated the use of the Montessori approach with retarded children; although, as she points out, use of the Montessori materials without proper training should be avoided.

Strauss and Lehtinen (1947), in their work with brain-injured children, cited hyperactivity as the source of the observed learning difficulties. Consequently, they advocated the elimination of distracting stimuli from the learning environment. On the basis of a review of experimental evidence and his own research, Lucker (1970) concluded that such educational practices cannot be justified. Crosby (1972) also noted that there is no evidence to support the belief that brain-injured individuals, as a group, are more distractible than the non-brain-injured retarded. Furthermore, in differentiating between attending behavior and distractibility, he noted a wide range of individual differences in the degree of distractibility. He suggested that increasing the level of sensory stimulation might increase the performance of individuals with low activity states, while increasing the level of sensory stimulation might further impair the performance of already highly aroused individuals. Crosby also suggested that stimulus modality might affect performance in the retarded and suggested that the clinical management of distractibility needs to be highly individualized. Douglas (1974) also discussed the situation-specific behavior of hyperactive children along with several programmatic approaches. She recommended that the choice of the approach should be based on the individual's behavioral response in the learning situation.

In addition to specific deficiencies in attention, the retarded, as well as other developmentally disabled groups, display other extralinguistic behaviors and inappropriate responses that seem to be incompatible with the language learning process. These are perhaps the most discouraging elements of the child's behavior with which the clinician must deal. Some individuals wander randomly around the therapy room, often engaging in stereotypic and/or self-destructive motor patterns such as repetitive and apparently meaningless hand movements, and head-banging (commonly seen in the older institutionalized retarded). Some exhibit severe withdrawal and failure to relate to other people (characteristic of autistic and autistic-like groups). Jargon (vocalizations that have the inflectional, temporal, and phonemic patterns characteristic of spoken English, but that are unintelligible) and echolalia (a pattern in which the child repeats in an echo-like fashion what was just heard, or develops and inappropriately uses repetitive phrases) occur commonly. To make matters worse, many developmentally disabled individuals display some of these characteristics in combination, presenting a seemingly impossible situation for the clinician.

In fact, however, clinicians have several sources to which they can turn in developing procedures for extinguishing behaviors that are incompatible and in competition with the ones they wish to teach or in controlling and refining specific patterns of behavior. Such procedures typically rely heavily on the principles and techniques of behavior modification and are often included as the earliest components of a total language programming sequence.

Differential reinforcement and shaping procedures have been used very successfully in bringing under control undesired behaviors, such as rocking and other incompatible behaviors as described above, and in establishing appropriate attending behaivors. Hegrenes, Marshall, and Armas (1970), Kent (1972), Marshall and Hegrenes (1970, 1972), and Sulzbacher and Costello (1970), for example, have described techniques for developing appropriate sitting and visual attending behaviors as well as for eliminating a variety of competing motoric patterns. Sulzbacher and Costello (1970), in addition to describing the use of these procedures in the clinical setting, presented detailed procedures by which their subject's program was extended to the home and to the school setting with a high degree of success. Baker (this volume) and Spradlin, Karlan, and Wetherby (this volume) also offer considerable assistance in this area. Sigelman and Bensberg (this volume) consider this area relative to the role of supportive personnel.

EARLY INTERVENTION

The importance of early intervention when sensory deficits are a factor in the developmental disability has been recognized for some time. The presence of impairment in auditory or visual function is often recognized early because of the uneven attainment of developmental milestones by the child. In many cases, identification can be accomplished during the first year of life. Educators of the deaf have stressed the importance of early identification in order to provide amplification and to design environments that facilitate the development of communication skills as early as possible (Sanders, 1971). It has been suggested that early sensory stimulation for children with hearing and visual impairments may result in a reduction of the self-stimulation in which the child engages (Baltzer, 1973). It has become increasingly apparent to educators of the blind and the partially sighted that early acquisition of spatial and relational concepts are crucial to the later acquisition of educational and vocational skills (Lydon and McGraw, 1973).

With other developmentally delayed groups, however, the typical practice has been to wait until there is evidence of a significant delay in the development of communication skills before intervention is attempted. By this time, the language problem is often so complicated by serious emotional overlay or severe behavior problems that delineation of the language deficit within the total behavioral pattern is difficult. There are perhaps several reasons for the delay in intervention with such groups, particularly for the mildly and moderately language delayed. For example, governmental agencies have made few attempts to establish developmental screening programs earlier than just before the point of entry by the child into the formal educational system or to establish criteria for at-risk populations and to provide the necessary programs for early identification within such populations. As Lloyd (1976) has pointed out, some states that require education for handicapped children as young as 3 years, while thinking of themselves as progressive, have still failed to meet the need for early intervention programs that should be applied during infancy.

The recommendation that early intervention programs are a necessity if one expects to attain optimal results is not new (Richardson, 1967). When heeded at all, implementation of this recommendation has taken various forms. Recent discussions of the role of early cognitive development and the relationship between cognition and language development have resulted in the formulation of several early intervention programs designed to provide developmental environments that are structured to maximize the acquisition of specific cognitive behaviors and linguistic structures. For the most part, these programs are administered in at least a quasi-experimental context with application of the program yielding further information concerning what it is that children acquire when they acquire their language system. Such information then leads to refinements in the program based upon more complete data about developmental processes.

Bricker and Bricker (1974) have suggested that an early intervention program actually may serve a preventative function in addition to a corrective function because early stimulation patterns and early sensory and perceptual training may prevent the moderate to severe language delay seen in older developmentally disabled groups. It has been suggested also that early intervention for the mentally retarded may be effective in facilitating the learning of later skills that are important in social and vocational situations (Schiefelbusch, Copeland, and Smith, 1967). A project reported by Heber et al. (1972) has been directed at determining whether an early language intervention program may serve in a preventative capacity for infants at risk. Preliminary results have indicated substantial gains for the experimental group in comparison to the control group in the areas of imitation, comprehension, and production.

Early intervention programs for hearing-impaired children have for several years viewed the parents and the home situation as central mediators of training. Early projects carried out at the John Tracy Clinic in Los Angeles and at the Central Institute for the Deaf in St. Louis, demonstrated the effectiveness of parents as trainers within the everyday living environment. Intensive parent involvement is now seen as central to early programs for the hearing impaired (Lowell, 1965; Simmons, 1967; Northcott, 1971; Horton, 1974; McConnell, 1974).

Typically, one finds in the literature statements to the effect that the language-delayed child, specifically the retarded child, cannot be expected to acquire certain language skills until his mental age corresponds to that of the normal child who is acquiring these skills. This view has been expressed as the maturational concept by Lenneberg (1966), who stated that the child's capacity to acquire language is a result of maturation and that there is no evidence that intensive training procedures can produce various levels of language development before the child is at the appropriate maturational stage.

This concept more recently has been discussed in terms of critical periods for the acquisition of prelinguistic and linguistic skills (see Cromer, 1974a). Nevertheless, the relative success of early stimulation and intervention programs, particularly with the retarded, must be taken to indicate that it is possible, in some sense, to provide what has been called a prosthetic environment (Turton, 1974) and to structure the early experiences of the child at least to facilitate the acquisition of prelinguistic and linguistic skills (Haviland, 1972; Heber et al., 1972; Bricker and Bricker, 1974; Horton, 1974).

At present, there are theories that argue for and against the efficacy of early intervention programs, particularly for the retarded child. No one, however, has argued that such programs will have an adverse effect on the child. The limited data now available suggest that, when programs are appropriately designed, the results will be positive (Bricker and Bricker, 1973).

GOALS FOR PROGRAMMING

Regardless of the form of the language training program, the terminal goal is not necessarily to teach the fully developed adult system of communication to every child. Many factors may restrict the level of language acquisition that the developmentally disabled child can achieve. Although a fully developed adult language system may not be attainable, one goal of any training program should be to provide a system of communication that is both effective and functional for that individual within his own environment (Miller and Yoder, 1974; Shaffer and Goehl, 1974). The result of the training program should be a communication system that is appropriately used and socially useful (Lillywhite and Bradley, 1969). Furthermore, the language system that is selected for the individual should be one that, through use, allows for facilitation of further acquisition. With such a system the child's use in daily activities of those language forms that have been taught in the training sequence will allow him to incorporate additional expressions of these forms into his repertoire. Marshall and Hegrenes (1972) have referred to the motivational effects of language usage as the language-learning child discovers the power of language for manipulating his environment. This realization by the child results in the consequences of language usage becoming reinforcing in themselves. Thus, the overall goal is for the child to use a spontaneous language system that is effective within his environment and that contains more than just those expressions that were specifically programmed during the language-training sequence.

Lloyd and Cox (1972) have noted that individuals vary in their language needs. Vocabulary that is functional for one child may have little or no relevance for another child because the specifics of each child's expressive needs are determined by differences in the kinds of relationships experienced with other people and with objects in the everyday living environment. For example, what the institutionalized retarded child needs to be able to talk about may be limited, or at least very different, in comparison to what the retarded child living at home needs to be able to talk about. With the present emphasis on deinstitutionalization, the institutionalized population of the future probably will tend to be more developmentally limited, in comparison to those who have not been institutionalized, than is the case today. The communication needs of the retarded child in an institutional setting may be limited to getting personal needs fulfilled and to low-level social interactions with peers. Several studies have shown that verbal interaction between adult caregivers and residents within institutions tends to be relatively infrequent (Butterfield, 1967), suggesting that institutionalized retarded children likely experience fewer situations in which they interact linguistically with adults. Retarded children living at home, on the other hand, can be expected to have a much broader range of situational contexts within which they need to be able to communicate. Although the above has been true historically, several writers have provided alternatives that, when fully implemented, can provide the institutionalized individual with a broader and richer communication environment (Kopchick and Lloyd, this volume; Haviland, 1972; Wilson, 1974).

Although the prognosis for attaining more than a rudimentary language system may be poor for many institutionalized children, the language training program for the institutionalized retarded child should not be designed simply to maintain the child in that environment. Recognition of the differences between the communication needs of the institutionalized and the noninstitutionalized child should assist the language trainer in developing appropriate priorities for more relevant, functional communication behavior in these children. As Schiefelbusch, Copeland, and Smith (1967) have noted, the goal for any language training program should be to eliminate, or at least to reduce, the differences between the skills that the child has and the language requirements that are operative within the child's specific environment.

Once the goal of a language training program for a given child is formulated, the design of the program can begin. The program design includes a series of intermediate goals that can be viewed as successive approximations of the desired terminal behavior. The selection and sequencing of these intermediate goals should be based on the designer's belief as to the most efficient way in which the terminal behavior can be acquired. Thus, one's theoretical viewpoint is of major importance in structuring the training program. For example, as Bateman (1974) noted, if one views the nonlanguage or language-delayed child as one who acquires the language system in the same manner as the normal child but at a slower rate, the intermediate goals will be to establish those successive linguistic behaviors evidenced in the normal child as he progresses through the stages of language acquisition. If, however, one views the nonlanguage or language-delayed child as an individual who has failed to acquire the language code in the normal manner and thus must be limited in some sense, the intermediate goals that are established need not correspond to the developmental sequence of language as it is acquired by normal children.

APPROACHES TO LANGUAGE INTERVENTION WITH THE RETARDED AND OTHER GROUPS

The language interventionist may approach language training from several different perspectives. Regardless of the approach used, however, the clinician must answer at least two basic questions before beginning. The clinician must decide both what to teach and how to teach it. Although there is considerable variation in the choice of what to teach and the sequence in which to teach it, there is somewhat less disagreement concerning the choice of the instructional procedure. Most language training programs make use, formally or informally, of the techniques of behavior modification. This is particularly true in programs designed for the older or more severely retarded and the emotionally disturbed individual where the programs heavily rely on the use of imitation and differential reinforcement (Bricker and Bricker, 1970; Hartung, 1970; Sulzbacher and Costello, 1970; Kent, 1972).

The response to the question of what to teach and how to sequence this content seems to depend on several factors. One of these factors, as noted by Bateman (1974) and described earlier, is the way in which the nonlanguage or language-delayed child is viewed by the trainer. Another factor that seems to strongly influence the form of intervention strategies is the extent to which the interventionist has participated in what has been called the rediscovery of Piaget (Morehead and Morehead, 1974) and the extent to which it is felt that descriptions of early cognitive development are adequate or relevant in the design of intervention strategies. Furthermore, although not longitudinally or programmatically derived, there is some evidence to indicate that at least some subgroups of retarded children acquire language in the same manner as normal children, but at a slower rate (Lenneberg, 1967; Lackner, 1968; Graham and Graham, 1971). Such reports have had some influence on specifying the form of language-training programs.

Developmental Approaches to Language Intervention

The particular programs described in this section synthesize psycholinguistic and behavioral models, in which psycholinguistic data are used to determine what will be taught and the principles of behavioral technology determine what instructional procedures will be used to teach the program content. The rationale for this approach has been described by Lynch and Bricker (1972), Miller and Yoder (1972a, b, 1974), and Stremel and Waryas (1974). The use of descriptions of the normal developmental sequence of language acquisition as a basis for language intervention strategies has been suggested frequently (e.g., Lillywhite and Bradley, 1969; Bloom, 1972; MacDonald and Blott, 1974).

In an applied example, W. Bricker (1972) described a training sequence for establishing the production of pivot-open phrases in the speech of retarded children. This program was designed to train those structures described by Braine (1963) in accounts of the young normal child's early utterances. According to Braine, the child's earliest two-word combinations are not random, but conform to simple patterns in which words are selected from generalized grammatical classes and are ordered in specific sequences. Braine termed these early grammatical classes "pivot" and "open," with the pivot class having few members in comparison with the open class. Furthermore, pivot words were said to be used more frequently, with the pivot class acquiring new members more slowly than the open class. Braine's characterization of these early utterances has been questioned with respect to a number of theoretical issues (McNeill, 1966) and, as seen in the recent literature, is no longer considered to be an acceptable construct (Bloom, 1970, 1972; Ruder, 1972; Brown, 1973a). However, the programmatic approach used by Bricker is an example of a syntactic or structural intervention strategy based on one description of what it is the normal child acquires as in learning language and is one possible form of a developmental approach to language intervention.

Since the appearance of Bloom's (1970) description of what is being acquired by the child learning language, the area of normal language acquisition has undergone a change in emphasis from a syntactic explanation to a semantic explanation of early child language. That is, much of the recent literature considers the semantic intent of a child's early utterances in addition to specifying the structural form of these utterances. During the past few years, several researchers have studied normal language acquisition longitudinally (Bloom, 1970; Brown, 1973a). In each case, these researchers have found that purely syntactic or structural explanations fail to account for the knowledge that children demonstrate as they use their language to talk about what is going on around them. These findings have led to an increasing emphasis on semantic explanations of early child language, an approach that is exemplified by the work of Bloom (1970). The children that Bloom studied produced combinations of words that could be described in terms of pivot-open constructions. However, in considering the semantic intent of the utterances, Bloom noted that the same expression could be serving different grammatical functions if meaning were taken into account. In the text of one of the children studied by Bloom, the utterance, *Mommy sock*, occurred twice, but was identifiable as expressing two different relationships. When the child produced *Mommy sock* as the mother was putting the child's sock on her, the utterance was interpreted as expressing a subject-object relationship, but when the child picked up a sock belonging to her mother, the utterance, *Mommy sock,* was interpreted as a possessional expression.

From such data, Bloom concluded that children's earliest utterances code what they know about the world and express relationships between objects and events in their environment. In her description of the development of negation, Bloom provided further evidence for children's use of the same form to express different semantic functions. In the utterances of the children she studied, she found that children first use negation to indicate nonexistence, while later the form is used to express rejection, and then denial. Although not completely parallel, a study by McNeill and McNeill (1968) showed the same general pattern for the emergence of negation in Japanese. Indications of such regularities and similarities across languages are used as further support for the semantic basis of language acquisition.

Several developmentally based language-training strategies have appeared in the last few years. Some are syntactically based, and the intent is to train specific utterances in a certain order under the assumption that these utterances express the syntactic relationships observed by children as they are exposed to the language they are learning. However, the trend has been to design programs that assimilate the more recent developmental information such as that described above. These programs are said to be semantically based (MacDonald and Blott, 1974).

Because these programs are based on the proposition that, through the use of language, the child is expressing certain conceptual notions about objects, events, and relationships within the environment, the cognitive and perceptual development of the child is seen as being of central importance to the overall program. Within the various intervention strategies, however, the degree to which cognitive development is considered to be directly programmable differs.

Working in the context of the Infant, Toddler, and Preschool Research and Intervention Project, the Brickers and their colleagues heavily relied on cognitive theory in specifying the early elements of their training program (Bricker and Bricker, 1973, 1974). The early aspects of the program were based on the assumption that possession of certain cognitive strategies may be necessary prerequisites to the development of language. The project was designed to discover and to demonstrate early instructional techniques that facilitate cognitive development and result in those behaviors thought to be necessary for the acquisition of language and that need to be established before formal language-teaching procedures are implemented.

In line with Piagetian theory, the Brickers and their colleagues have constructed what they call a sensorimotor lattice structure, which specifies a sequence of behaviors including prerequisites for each

(Bricker and Bricker, 1973). A screening instrument is used to locate the child in developmental space, and it provides the basis for a test-teach system. For example, a sequence of behaviors has been tentatively specified with respect to the object permanence concept, extending from the point where a child does not search for an object removed from view to the point where the child indicates wanting an object and actively searches for it even though it is hidden. By systematically varying conditions that fall between these two points and noting the behavior of the child in attempting to locate an object, it is possible to discover strategies that the child uses in acquiring the concept of object permanence and thus to develop teaching procedures to move a child through this sequence.

Through the Toddler Project, the Brickers have acquired preliminary data that indicate that young children classify and conceptually structure their environments in specific ways and that such prelinguistic behaviors are prerequisite to the learning of language. When there is evidence that the children in this project have acquired at least some of these prelinguistic skills, the program moves to specific language-training procedures, such as those described in the Brickers' earlier work (Bricker and Bricker, 1970).

In a series of papers describing a developmentally based language-teaching program, Miller and Yoder (1972a, b; 1974) stressed the importance of the child's nonlinguistic experiences and the cognitive aspects of his development in relation to the learning of the linguistic code. These writers agreed that abilities on the part of the child, such as being able to use one object to represent a second, are essential to the expression of such relationships in the form of verbal language. However, Miller and Yoder argued that whether or not one can discover specific training procedures to enhance the early stages of cognitive development is, at this point, an unanswered question. Rather than developing specifically ordered training strategies such as those in the Brickers' program, Miller and Yoder stressed the importance of pairing the environmental experiences of the child with the appropriate linguistic referents. For example, they reported success in developing the understanding and expression of the concept of recurrence with a severely retarded child by structuring the training activities so that they were highly motivating for the child and by sequencing the training so that the activities were continued only if the child demanded "more" (Miller and Yoder, 1974). Their intervention strategy provided for the manipulation of a child's environment in order to provide him with an array of experiences that enabled him to discover and, ultimately, to talk about relationships within his environment.

Developmental approaches to language intervention are based on the assumption that, because the task is to teach the child an effective language system rather than to eradicate deficiencies in a deviant system, the data available on normal language acquisition should form the bases for the design of a language teaching program. This has been stated in the form of an operating principle for the design of a program (Miller and Yoder, 1972b, p. 9): "The content for language training for retarded children should be taken from the data available on language development in normal children, and this content should be taught in the same sequence that it is acquired by the normal child." This approach is most fully in evidence in the program described by Miller and Yoder that appeared in 1974, and which is an extension and refinement of their earlier writings (Miller and Yoder, 1972a, b; Yoder and Miller, 1972).

On the basis of developmental data as reported by Bloom (1970, 1973), Brown (1970, 1973a, b), and Schlesinger (1971a, b), Miller and Yoder (1974) constructed a sequence of semantic concepts or functions that they considered would provide a relevant basis for a language-teaching program. The content of the program included those functions expressed in the early speech of normal children, such as recurrence and nonexistence, and the later expression of semantic functions, such as agent-action-object sequences, as children progress beyond the single-word utterance stage. The program content is similar to what Brown (1973a) has described as Stage I in the language development of normal children. The content as described was ordered to follow the sequence in which forms expressing various functions appear in normal children's speech. For example, the ordering of "no" to first express the function of nonexistence, then rejection, and still later to express denial, is consistent with the normal developmental sequence described by Bloom (1970). By designing the program in a developmentally sequenced form in which the first utterances of the child express semantic functions, Miller and Yoder pointed out that, although it will be limited, meaningful communication will occur as the child uses his first words in specific contexts and that, even if the retarded child stops learning language at some point, he still will be able to communicate to some extent within his environment.

Stremel and Waryas (1974) have presented a detailed language training program that is similar to the Miller and Yoder approach described above. The Stremel and Waryas program is divided into three major sections: 1) early language training, 2) early-intermediate language training, and 3) late-intermediate language training. Training strategies are sequenced on the basis of data from the acquisition of language in the normal child including the data of Bloom (1970) and Brown (1973a). Training is accomplished through the use of behavior modification techniques. The Stremel and Waryas (1974) paper is recommended to clinicians because it provides a detailed description of program content.

In constructing their Environmental Language Intervention Strategy, MacDonald and his associates also have utilized normal developmental data to specify the form of a language-training program (MacDonald and Blott, 1974; MacDonald et al., 1974). This is one of several programs based on the agent-action-object characterization of children's early multiword utterances (Schlesinger, 1971b). Descriptions of the normal child's early utterances indicate that what children talk about in their early use of language is considerably uniform across languages (Brown, 1973a) and that this is the result of the similarity in the early experiences of all children. The agent-action-object description is an attempt to characterize the semantic intent of children's early utterances in consideration of the environmental context in which the utterances occur. Although some training programs treat the agent-action-object sequence and the subject-verb-object string as equivalent, Stremel (1972) and Bowerman (1973) provide theoretical discussions of the differences between these sequences.

The Environmental Language Intervention Strategy is a program that utilizes the realization rules described by Schlesinger (1971b) in a training sequence to move the child with severe language delay from the one-word utterance stage to the expressive use of multiword utterances. The program directly addresses the problem of generalizing learned structures from the training setting to a more natural setting in that sequences are trained in imitation, conversation, and play. When the child has learned to express the functions in the imitation phase, the conversational and play environments of the child are specifically structured to elicit the trained forms (MacDonald et al., 1974). Positive reinforcement for use of the structures proceeds from verbal praise and token rewards during the imitation stage to the more natural reinforcement provided by the ability to control events in the conversation and play stages. In similar approaches to training the agent-action-object sequence with language-delayed children, Bricker et al. (1973) and Stremel (1972) described an imitation training procedure that subsequently programs for generalization of the learned sequence to new situations by structuring the environment to elicit the learned responses.

At present, there are only a few reports of experimental applications of programs designed to develop the agent-action-object sequence, and these have dealt with small subject populations. However, the available data indicate that children do acquire the structures programmed and further generalize the use of these structures to new situations (Stremel, 1972; MacDonald et al., 1974).

In summary, developmental language teaching programs such as those described base their strategies on the way in which the normal child is thought to acquire language. For the most part, this includes consideration of the level of cognitive development as a prerequisite to the emergence of expressive language. The particular programs described in this section synthesize psycholinguistic and behavioral models, in which psycholinguistic data are used to determine what will be taught and the principles of behavioral technology determine what instructional procedures will be used to teach the program content. Furthermore, these programs are concerned with the generalization of trained structures to new situations as well as with the spontaneous development of new structures not specifically trained.

Several criticisms or questions have been directed toward developmental approaches to language intervention. Some researchers have felt that there are insufficient developmental data on which to base language intervention strategies (Guess, Sailor, and Baer, 1974), while others have expressed the reservation that psycholinguists' descriptions of what the child is acquiring when acquiring language have undergone so many changes over a short period of time, that it is difficult to discover a consistent theoretical base to use in planning intervention strategies (see Bateman, 1974). Furthermore, as Guess, Sailor, and Baer (1974) have noted, simply because descriptions of the normal language acquisition process indicate that children acquire language in a certain way does not necessarily mean that this is the necessary or the most effective means of teaching the system to the language-disordered child. Bloom (1972) also has expressed some reservations about the strict application of data on normal development to intervention programs for children with language disorders.

Nondevelopmental Approaches

In contrast to developmentally based programming approaches, a number of language training strategies have been described by those who view the nonlanguage or language-delayed child as one who, by virtue of not having acquired the language code in the normal manner, should be managed in ways that differ from the normal developmental sequence. As noted by Baer at the Chula Vista Conference (quoted by Bateman, 1974, p. 608): "A deviant population by definition demonstrates the inappropriateness of the developmental sequence for that group." Gray and Ryan (1973) expressed a similar view, and Cromer (1974a) hypothesized that the very fact that language is delayed may indicate that older, subnormal individuals utilize different processes in the acquisition of language than do young normal children.

Generally, nondevelopmental strategies are not based on considerations of prerequisite cognitive skills or any necessity to consider developmental sequence in the ordering of the structures to be trained. Programs in this category do not deal with a hierarchy of language skills, each prerequisite to the following. Therefore, rather than teaching language in the sequence in which the normal language-learning child acquires it, these programs train language forms and skills that are seen as most useful to the child in order for him to control and interact with his environment. Central to these language training strategies is the use of imitation and reinforcement techniques to establish the desired responses on the part of the child. Rather than being used as a means for accomplishing the language teaching program, as tends to be the case in the developmental strategies, such techniques are often viewed as the processes of language learning rather than as instructional procedures, and many reports of success using such strategies are presented simply to demonstrate the power of behavioral technology.

The use of imitation, in particular, has received a great deal of criticism as being a departure from the way in which the normal child acquires language. This criticism has been generated in a long-standing debate between linguists and psycholinguists on the one hand, and behaviorists on the other hand (Jakobovits and Miron, 1967). Behaviorists hold that the acquisition of language can be explained by principles of learning theory (Skinner, 1957), while statements in the psycholinguistic literature hold that processes such as imitation cannot possibly explain the emerging linguistic sophistication evidenced by the child as he becomes a language user (Brown and Bellugi, 1964; Ervin, 1964; Miller, 1967).

More recently, the view has been expressed that, while imitation may not be a necessary element in normal language acquisition, the techniques of imitation and differential reinforcement together can be very successfully applied in establishing some form of verbal behavior in the individual who has not acquired language in the normal manner (W. Bricker, 1972; Bricker and Bricker, 1974; Gray and Ryan, 1973), and that, perhaps the inherent differences between a language acquisition model and a language intervention model should be acknowledged (Risley, Hart, and Doke, 1972; Ruder, 1972; Gray and Ryan, 1973).

Many of the programs considered in this section are directed toward individuals who, in addition to language delay or total absence of language, also present severe and disruptive behavior problems and lack of an attentional component in their behavioral repertoire. Consequently, many of these programs contain an early component designed to establish behavioral control before attempts are made to establish verbal language.

Kent (1972) has described a language program for severely retarded institutionalized individuals. The program contains a preverbal section and a verbal section. The preverbal section of the program contains a phase specifically designed to develop appropriate attending behaviors, and completion of this phase is seen as necessary before beginning other phases of the program. In the preverbal section, through the use of positive reinforcement for appropriate behavior and the use of shaping procedures to elicit desired behaviors, the child is taught to attend to the language trainer, to sit in a chair, to attend to objects presented to him, and to initiate visual contact with the trainer. The attending phase also includes a component designed to eliminate behaviors that are incompatible with the training situation. These behaviors include body rocking, stereotypic movements of the extremities, and a variety of other competing motoric patterns.

Marshall and Hegrenes (1972) referred to children who present the types of behavior patterns listed above, whether considered to be mentally retarded or emotionally disturbed, as "cognitively disorganized," and their therapy model includes what they refer to as "spatial organizers." Spatial organizers are procedures intended to develop an appropriate set of clinical behaviors in the child before specific language training begins. These procedures have been discussed and utilized by others as well (Hartung, 1970; Hegrenes, Marshall, and Armas, 1970; Marshall and Hegrenes, 1970; Sulzbacher and Costello, 1970; Stark et al., 1973).

Once the child is able to sit in a chair and attend to the language trainer, the development of imitation skills is initiated. While some programs begin with vocal or verbal imitation, a number begin with motor imitation. Although it has not been demonstrated that the development of a motor imitative repertoire is a necessary prerequisite for the development of verbal imitation, some researchers have implied that the establishment of motor imitative responses facilitates a later verbal imitative repertoire (Peterson, 1968; Bricker and Bricker, 1970). For the severely retarded or autistic child, beginning with motor imitation seems to be effective because the child can be physically guided through the required imitative movements and reinforced for appropriate responses. Strategies using motor imitation typically begin with gross imitative movements, and these are refined as the program progresses until the child is imitating articulatory movements (Marshall and Hegrenes, 1972). At this point, vocal and verbal imitation are introduced, usually in the form of labeling (Bricker and Bricker, 1970). Other strategies have omitted the motor imitation phase and initiated training in vocal imitation. Risley and Wolf (1967) and Sulzbacher and Costello (1970) have described this procedure as they applied it to autistic children. Some children, of course, are already imitating words or phrases from the speech of others or perhaps from television when the intervention process is initiated. Whether initial motor imitative training is necessary before vocal and verbal imitative training, or whether the former facilitates the latter, still seems largely to be an unanswered question (Garcia and DeHaven, 1974).

The later phases of nondevelopmental language training strategies differ with respect to the content taught, but all of the strategies train specific sequences of verbal output, beginning with single words and then combining words into phrases. Some teach noun-verb sequences followed by longer phrases (Marshall and Hegrenes, 1972). Gray and Ryan (1973) presented a comprehensive language curriculum containing a set of 41 programs beginning with identification of nouns and ending with an articulation program. For each grammatical form to be taught, they developed a separate program of instruction.

Typically, the nondevelopmental strategies discuss the importance of generalization, in which generalization refers to the child's use of the trained skills in situations other than the training setting. Bricker et al. (1973) described an attempt to program generalization. Most of the strategists at least assume that training a set of language skills will result in the spontaneous acquisition of other skills not specifically trained. However, that this acquisition occurs has not been demonstrated to any significant extent. For those who disagree with the behavioral approaches to language intervention, these aspects are those with which they most often take issue. As Bloom (1972) and Miller and Yoder (1974) pointed out, the process of acquiring language involves more than simply learning new words and learning to produce them in various combinations. As Miller and Yoder observed, an operant approach to language training may be more appropriate in some instances than it is in others, but no such program can possibly teach all of the language that a child requires.

Manual Approaches

Rather than attempting to program oral language, some individuals, working with severely retarded groups or with children who present autistic types of behaviors in addition to retardation, have chosen to program some form of manual communication (see Kopchick and Lloyd, this volume; Wilbur, this volume). Shaffer and Goehl (1974) have reported that some nonlanguage children, who seem to have intact sensory systems, may refuse to relate to their environment through the use of oral language. According to these writers, some children may respond to the use of signs when they are apparently unable or unwilling to respond to oral language. Furthermore, Shaffer and Goehl have reported that these children often become more manageable from a behavioral standpoint when an initial system of manual communication is established and that some children eventually acquire oral language. For the nonverbal child, teaching manual signing or some form of gestural system seems to be accomplished more easily than attempting to program oral language because signs and gestures can be shaped through physical manipulation with relative ease in comparison to training the fine movements of the oral structures that are required for speech.

D. Bricker (1972) demonstrated experimentally with low functioning children that the use of imitative-sign training facilitated subjects' word-object association abilities. Other clinicians reported that training in manual or total communication seemed to facilitate the development of oral language in nonverbal children (Creedon, 1974; Shaffer and Goehl, 1974). It also has been reported that the introduction of such a means of communication results in a decrease in behavior problems and an increase in appropriate responses to others in the environment (Shaffer and Goehl, 1974; Wilson, 1974). Recently, Topper (1975) presented a case report of the successful use of a gestural communication system with an older, institutionalized individual functioning in the high-profound to low-severe range of retardation. Rather than teaching the fine motor movements typified by a standard sign language, Topper taught her subject gross motor gestures that imitated the natural action as closely as possible. She recommended the application of such a program for essentially nonverbal, profoundly and severely retarded individuals and suggested that the use of a gestural communication system may at least reduce frustration levels and perhaps may result in increased receptive language levels.

Although it has been demonstrated that, through structured classroom teaching procedures, it is possible to establish some level of manual communication skills in individuals who have failed to acquire verbal language, the use of these skills also must be extended beyond the classroom to the individual's daily living environment if a truly usable communication system is to be a reality for these individuals. Wilson (1974) reported considerable resistance to the use of signing by others in the institution and a generally negative attitude toward signing as a means of communication. Certainly, in programs designed to develop manual or gestural communication systems for normal hearing individuals, this is an obstacle that must be overcome. Kopchick and Lloyd (this volume) present one approach to solving the problem.

The results reported to date of programming manual or gestural systems for low functioning individuals have been encouraging, and the use of such programming seems to be increasing (Fristoe, 1975). It would seem, therefore, that more widespread use of such systems with nonlanguage or language-delayed individuals is warranted. For further discussions of manual and gestural communication systems, as well as other nonspeech systems, the reader is referred to other chapters in this volume (Carrier, Kopchick and Lloyd, Vanderheiden and Harris-Vanderheiden, Wilbur).

Use of Parents and Peers in Intervention Strategies

Although for several years parents have been considered to play an important role in training programs for hearing-impaired and deaf children, a specific role for parents in language training programs for other developmentally disabled groups has been defined more recently. The general supportive role for parents has a long history (Barnard and Powell, 1972). More recently, many programs have begun to utilize parents more specifically as trainers. The primary reasons for this seem to be the amount of time required for most structured language teaching programs and the difficulty in extending trained skills from the clinical setting to the child's everyday living environment. There seems to be a growing feeling that, if parents are not involved in the intervention process, the ways in which they relate to their child outside of the formal teaching situation may not encourage the use of skills that the child is learning and may even negate what the child is being taught. The training given to parents varies in extent and form, but several reports have documented the success of parents as clinicians, not only in the teaching of language and language-related skills (Bricker and Bricker, 1972; Gray and Ryan, 1973; MacDonald et al., 1974), but in teaching motor, self-help, and social skills (Bricker and Bricker, 1973) and in extending the management of behavior problems to the home (Sulzbacher and Costello, 1970; Bricker and Bricker, 1973). Robinson and Filler (1971) have described a "Maternal Teaching Style Assessment Scale," which is designed to assess the extent to which mothers use appropriate techniques in interacting with their children during training sessions. The intent is to develop specific and effective training programs for parents.

One of the most successful programs utilizing parents as teachers has been the Portage Project (Shearer and Shearer, 1972), an early childhood education program that was developed out of the need to serve a number of handicapped children who were distributed across a wide geographic area in rural Wisconsin. Because it was not feasible to transport the children to various central locations for educational programs, the Portage Project was designed so that it could be implemented directly in the home. The Project's home trainers visit families once each week to assess the progress made during the previous week and to teach the parent how to teach skills to be trained during the following week. The program is directed at five areas: cognition, self-help, motor, language, and socialization. Results from the Portage Project have demonstrated that children enrolled in the program have progressed significantly beyond a comparable group enrolled in a classroom program (Shearer and Shearer, 1972, 1976). For further discussion of parental involvement in language intervention, the reader is referred to Baker (this volume).

Some language interventionists also integrated peers into the training setting. Gray and Ryan (1973) suggested that programming children in groups may result in children learning from each other, particularly when they are at different levels in the training sequence. Jeffrey (1972) reported successfully using peers specifically as trainers in a language training program for a retarded child. In order to promote extension of the child's trained language skills from the specific training setting to the classroom, two of the child's retarded peers were taught how to use teaching materials with her and to reinforce her socially for correct responses.

Bricker and Bricker (1971, 1972, 1973, 1974) reported the integration of delayed and nondelayed children in the Infant, Toddler, and Preschool Research and Intervention Project. The nondelayed children received specific developmental training and were reported to demonstrate at least the expected levels of developmental progress. In addition to the training they received, the nondelayed children served several other functions within the project. They provided a developmental model for the delayed children because they were reported to play more appropriately and spontaneously than their delayed counterparts. Furthermore, the nondelayed children provided the teachers with a sort of perspective in relation to their expectancies for the delayed children, and observations of the ways in which the nondelayed children acquire skills serve as a basis for teaching strategies employed with the delayed children. Observations of nondelayed children also provide further developmental data related to the acquisition of cognitive and linguistic skills by the normal child.

The Toddler Project attempted to equalize the numbers of delayed and nondelayed children within the program. However, in summarizing a discussion of the role of normal children in intervention programs, Turton (1974) reported various recommended ratios of nonhandicapped to handicapped children in such projects. From the discussion, Turton concluded that the role of the nonhandicapped child within the intervention program seems to be the most important variable in determining what the ratio should be. According to the discussion, if the nonhandicapped child is considered to be a member of the treatment group, the ratio is not significant. When the role of the nonhandicapped child is seen as a model and a facilitator of acquisition for the handicapped child, however, the ratio between the two becomes important, although the optimal ratio remains undetermined.

PROGRAMMING FOR THE HEARING IMPAIRED

It is virtually impossible to discuss language programming for the hearing impaired without reference to the mode or methods controversy. The oral/manual controversy within the general field of deaf education has been long standing, emotionally charged, divisive, and still remains as one of the central issues in considering educational provisions for the hearing impaired. Few would quarrel with the statement that language is central to the child's intellectual and educational development. Yet, relatively current textbooks can be found that virtually ignore language and focus almost entirely on techniques for speech training (see Connor, 1971).

There are two primary approaches to oral programs. The most common includes training in reception through all possible sensory modalities, referred to as the multisensory approach with auditory and visual channels usually being emphasized. In this approach, the hearing-impaired child is provided with amplification, and the program components include auditory training to develop and teach the child to utilize whatever residual hearing is present. In addition to auditory training, structured training in speechreading is included (Sanders, 1971).

In contrast to the multisensory approach, Pollack (1964, 1967), Niemann (1972), and others have advocated the use of a unisensory approach called acoupedics. This approach specifically avoids training in speechreading and stresses early amplification and the training of the function of hearing. All training given to children is directed at teaching them to interpret the sounds they hear around them. Daily experiential situations are used as training contexts, and the program emphasizes intensive parent involvement. Because of the program's concentration on the auditory modality, this approach is most often referred to as the aural method.

In contrast to such oral or aural approaches, many have concentrated on one of a variety of manual approaches. For an in-depth discussion of manual systems, see Wilbur (this volume).

Several arguments have been used to negate the use of the oral approach on the one hand, and the use of the manual approach on the other hand. Those who support the oral approach argue that any use of a manual system by the child will suppress the development of speech and result in his inescapable placement in the "deaf ghetto" (van Uden, 1970). Others, who support the use of manual systems, argue that to deprive the child of such a system of communication will result in irreversible educational and emotional damage because of his limited communication abilities. Although the oral/manual dispute is by no means resolved, there is some evidence one may use for guidance.

In the early 1950's, educators of the deaf in the Soviet Union concluded that use of the traditional pure oral method had been unsuccessful in providing young deaf children with a functional communication system. Therefore, a number of studies were conducted in order to examine alternate methods for providing a communication system for these children. These experiments, reported by Morkovin (1968) and Quigley (1966), demonstrated that, when oral and written forms of speech were combined with fingerspelling, children acquired a significantly larger vocabulary than when the oral method alone was used. Furthermore, they discovered that use of the new method, called Neo-oralism, facilitated the development of speechreading and oral language because the children were equipped with early language and a vehicle for communication.

Stuckless and Birch (1966) also reported that hearing-impaired children who learned to communicate manually from a very early age demonstrated significant advances in reading, speechreading, and written language in comparison with children who did not begin manual communication early in their lives. More recently, Schlesinger and Meadow (1972) reported that, for very young children who were exposed to signs and fingerspelling in addition to speech, there were concomitant gains in the number of spoken words and speechreading facility as sign language was acquired.

In 1969, Moores and his colleagues at the University of Minnesota began a longitudinal project designed to evaluate the effectiveness of seven preschool programs for hearing-impaired children. Moores, Weiss, and Goodwin (1974) reported the first four years of the project. The seven programs were chosen as being representative of differing educational and communication methodologies, including the oral method, the Rochester method (see Wilbur, this volume), and total communication (see Kopchick and Lloyd, this volume). Results have shown that when children communicated with each other, the most frequently used means of communication was sign language, regardless of the program's espoused communication system. Generally, the use of fingerspelling in addition to signing increased as the children matured. In child-to-teacher communication, the most frequently used method was sign language, while in teacher-to-child communication, oral communication was most frequently used. Programs evaluated as being most effective exposed children to signs very early and used techniques that combined the use of residual hearing, speechreading, and signs (Moores, 1974).

Although reports such as those above generally support the use of some form of manual communication in combination with oral language, several writers have suggested that the choice of mode of communication should be individualized for each child (Lynch and Tobin, 1973; Moores, 1973; Northern and Downs, 1974). As Lynch and Tobin pointed out, the fact that the oral-manual controversy persists provides some support for the suggestion that there is no one best communication mode for all hearing-impaired children. Many would perhaps agree that, for children with minimal hearing impairment, the mode should be oral, while for severely and profoundly hearing-impaired children, language should be taught by a system that includes some form of manual instruction. Even the notably oral Alexander Graham Bell Association for the Deaf in a recent reexamination of its purpose and mission (Flint, 1975), while reaffirming its oral philosophy, allowed that for some individuals an auditory-oral program may not be the most appropriate and that a total communication program including auditory-oral components may be the choice for some hearing-impaired children.

If the choice of mode is, in fact, to be individualized, it is not yet clear just how this is to be done. Northern and Downs (1974) addressed the problem by attempting to develop what they have termed a *deafness management quotient* (DMQ). The DMQ is derived from a 100-point scale based on five factors: 1) amount of residual hearing, 2) degree of central intactness, 3) intellectual factors, 4) degree of family support, and 5) family socioeconomic level. Although the scale, as it presently exists, has not been tested with young deaf children, Northern and Downs presented two retrospective applications of the scale to young deaf adults, and, in their opinion, the scale was effective in telling them what should have been done when these individuals were infants. Although such an approach offers the promise of a useful method of determining educational placement, many would question the factors and the weightings assigned in the present format of the DMQ, and most would be reluctant to apply the scale without more extensive information about its validity.

Several trends in language programs for the hearing impaired have been in evidence in the past few years. The use of total communication as a means for developing language has been more readily applied and more accepted than was previously the case for systems involving some manual component. The general public, through exposure to certain television programs (primarily newscasts and religious programs) where signs and fingerspelling are usually used with speech, has tended to accept this variant of standard communication, and, therefore, parents have not been as reluctant as in the past to place their children in programs where total communication is used. However, in many cases, such programs have not truly employed a total communication approach. As has been noted (Lloyd, 1973, p. 61): ". . . the failure of some so-called total communication approaches has been an overemphasis on the manual with a corresponding de-emphasis of the oral-aural aspects. In some cases, total communication has really been a euphemism for the manual method. Those using the manual method usually say they are using the simultaneous method. Unfortunately, the signs and fingerspelling many times communicate a different message than does the oral presentation, if any spoken words are presented. In other words, simultaneous and total communication are often misnomers."

Moores, Weiss, and Goodwin (1974) noted similar discrepancies between what is claimed and what is done. They noted that, within the seven programs they studied, there were no "pure" programs of any type. In programs committed to a simultaneous or a total approach, teachers often spoke without the use of signs or fingerspelling. On the other hand, in programs committed to a totally oral approach, teachers often used gestures to a great extent in com-bination with speaking. Moores, Weiss, and Goodwin suggested that oral-only programs significantly restrict the amount of communica-tion within the classroom and, at the same time, give rise to inefficient gesture systems.

Another trend in language and educational programs for the young deaf child has been a shift from programming that consists of unstructured and random verbal stimulation, with an emphasis on socialization, to programs that stress cognitive development and the acquisition of preacademic and early academic skills (Horton, 1974). Programs developed for populations other than the hearing impaired, such as those described by Karnes, Hodgins, and Teska (1968) and Spicker (1971), have had considerable impact on the restructuring of early programs for hearing-impaired children. Working in the context of early intervention programs for economically and socially disadvantaged children, Karnes, Hodgins, and Teska and Spicker compared the effectiveness of various types of preschool programs. Each found that, in contrast to the traditional nursery school curric-ulum models, programs involving a high degree of structure with emphasis on the development of cognitive skills and language devel-opment through specific instruction resulted in significantly greater gains in intellectual functioning and in verbal expressive skills.

Several projects are underway at the Research, Development, and Demonstration Center in Education of Handicapped Children at the University of Minnesota that are designed to develop and to test such programs with young hearing-impaired children. In their report of an evaluation of programs, Moores, Weiss, and Goodwin (1974) stated that children in programs that stress articulation skills and social adjustment routinely fall behind children who are in programs emphasizing cognitive and academic skills in conjunction with socialization.

Some trends in language programs for the hearing impaired have been described earlier. Other major trends discussed in the following sections include parent involvement, early detection, and the early and consistent use of amplification.

Parent Involvement

Parents of a young deaf child require a considerable amount of emotional support in the beginning and ongoing guidance as they become active participants in their child's language development program (Northcott, 1971). With the increasing utilization of parents in programs for young hearing-impaired children, the need has been expressed for emphasis on more direct and relevant training for parents, in contrast to traditional classroom demonstrations and lectures (Parsons, 1967; Horton, 1968, 1974). There are many excellent guides available to parents, most of which include information on general child development in addition to specific routines to facilitate language development on the part of the young hearing-impaired child. Most of these publications are orally oriented. They include John Tracy Clinic publications such as the *John Tracy Clinic Correspondence Course for Parents of Little Deaf Children* (John Tracy Clinic, 1961), which is sent to parents in installments, and *Getting Your Baby Ready to Talk* (1968), and other parent-oriented manuals such as those developed by Alpiner and Amon (1972) and Northcott (1972).

An even more specific approach to parent education was initiated by the John Tracy Clinic in Los Angeles in 1965. Since its goal for parent training was to teach the parents what to do in the home to stimulate language development, rather than training the parent in a clinic situation, the John Tracy Clinic established its home teaching facility. This facility was a simulated home with the furnishings, utensils, and facilities normally found in a home. The parents and their child came to the home and were shown how everyday activities and routines within the home atmosphere could be used as vehicles for teaching language and for general child development. Several similar facilities were subsequently established at the Central Institute for the Deaf in St. Louis, at the University of Kansas Medical Center, and at the Bill Wilkerson Hearing and Speech Center in Nashville. As Horton (1968, 1974) reported, such programs have been demonstrated to be effective, and parents respond positively because they play an active role in their child's program. As a part of the model home program of the Bill Wilkerson Hearing and Speech Center (Nashville, Tenn.), a series of *Rules of Talking* have been developed to assist in teaching parents how to talk with their child. These *Rules of Talking* are reprinted in Appendix E to this volume.

All of the programs mentioned above are oral programs. A similar program at the University of Denver, called Project Parent-Child, operates in much the same manner except that it allows parents a choice of the communication system their child will use. Amon (1972) has concluded as a result of her experience in the program that the parents must make the choice of the communication system because the parents' commitment to the system has considerable effect on the success with which they carry out the program. Of course, if the parents choose some form of manual communication for the child, it is imperative that all family members and anyone who has ongoing direct contact with the child be skilled in the use of the system as well. In addition to programs that bring parents and child to a simulated home for instructional purposes, there are several reports of programs in which teachers or clinicians go to the child's home to offer instruction and guidance to parents (McCrosky, 1967; Shearer and Shearer, 1972, 1976; Stack, 1973). This approach is further discussed by Baker (this volume).

Early Detection and Amplification

With recent technologic advances and advances in procedures for testing hearing in infancy, the identification of the hearing-impaired child is possible very early in life. Once the child has been identified as having a significant hearing loss, the provision of amplification becomes the immediate question. Most clinicians, particularly those committed to an aural approach, subscribe to a philosophy of providing amplification as soon as possible after identification of the hearing impairment. Pollack (1967) stressed the importance of fitting a hearing aid no later than the age of 6 months. Such amplification is usually quite powerful. Van den Eeckhaut (1967) summarized two points of view concerning the age at which amplification should be provided. One point of view is that amplification should be provided as early as possible because early amplification is seen as central to the overall development of the hearing-impaired child. The second point of view is that the provision of amplification should begin at about 3 or 4 years of age because the amount of residual hearing and thus the effective level of amplification is difficult to determine before that time. Cox and Lloyd (this volume) and Fulton and Lloyd (1975) clearly demonstrate that the second point of view is no longer a defensible position. As pointed out in a position paper of the American Organization for the Education of the Hearing Impaired (1975), today's technology makes possible the early determination of the amount of residual hearing that a child has, and the subsequent provision of early and consistent amplification will have a profound effect on the extent to which the child will develop auditory-oral communication skills.

An issue that has been argued for a number of years concerns whether or not wearable amplification can result in traumatic hearing loss as a result of overamplification. Northern and Downs (1974) discussed this issue in detail and cited several reports, studies, and opinions to the effect that, in fact, overamplification can result in additional hearing loss. However, because of the extreme importance of the child's early experiences and training and because the child who is left to wait may develop behavioral and emotional problems in addition to the hearing impairment, amplification should be provided as early as possible. As Northern and Downs (1974) pointed out, additional hearing loss resulting from amplification is probably the result of the use of extremely powerful aids; therefore, they recommended the use of aids with a maximum power output of less than 130 dB SPL (sound pressure level). In conjunction with providing wearable amplification, Northern and Downs stressed frequent and periodic hearing reevaluation and hearing aid evaluation to provide for adjustment in type and level of amplification as more information is gained about the child's hearing status. In their program, children who wore hearing aids were reevaluated every 6 months. Ross (this volume) presents a detailed description of the characteristics of wearable amplification.

Along with provision of wearable amplification for the child must go training for the parent in assisting to orient the child to the hearing aid and in maintenance of the aid. Northern and Downs (1974) have described such a program in detail. Excellent booklets also have been provided by Ronnei and Porter (1965) and by Dempsey (undated). Hanners and Sitton (1974) have described an innovative and successful program for ensuring optimal hearing aid function through daily hearing aid checks performed within the child's school program and a training program for parents that teaches them how to monitor hearing aid maintenance within the home. Hearing aid orientation programs are further discussed later in this chapter with specific reference to the multiply handicapped.

Integration of the Hearing-Impaired Child

Integration of the hearing-impaired child with normal hearing children in an educational setting, or "mainstreaming," is one of the most important goals of aural-oral programs for hearing-impaired children. The emphasis on integration gives rise to one of the oralists' major objections to any manual system of communication: a child who does not speak the language of the community cannot be integrated with normal hearing peers.

In 1963, Motto and Wawrzaszek reviewed a number of studies concerning the integration of hearing-impaired children into regular classrooms. One of the primary reasons given for integration has been that, as a result, hearing-impaired children will develop more nearly normal communication abilities as a result of their response to the model presented by normal children. Motto and Wawrzaszek stated that there is a lack of evidence to support or reject this position. An interesting issue is raised by these writers, that of pace of integration. According to them, integration should be accomplished by a gradual and increasing exposure to normal hearing children rather than in an abrupt manner. Motto and Wawrzaszek also noted that there is no substantial evidence to support the argument that, as a result of integration, the hearing-impaired child will make significant gains in educational achievement. Along these lines, Moores, Weiss, and Goodwin (1974) reported the results of one of the preschool programs they studied that included integration of hearing-impaired children with younger normal hearing children, rather than with children of their own age. They suggested that such a practice actually may tend to reverse early progress on the part of the hearing-impaired child.

Traditionally, it has been assumed that integration is probably accomplished more easily with hearing-impaired children who have relatively good hearing and oral language. Recently, however, Rister (1975) has reported that severity of hearing impairment is not the only factor determining the degree of success of the hearing-impaired child in regular educational placement. Both Rister (1975) and the American Organization for the Education of the Hearing Impaired (1975) have argued that early detection, early amplification, and early training will contribute significantly to the successful integration of the hearing-impaired child. Although there can be no doubt that this is true, the total effect of integration on the academic achievement of hearing-impaired children and the full spectrum of prerequisites for their success in the regular classroom have not been completely determined.

Programs for the Multiply Handicapped Hearing Impaired

In addition to the hearing-impaired child who is intellectually and behaviorally normal, an increasing number of individuals present other disabilities in addition to hearing impairment. As Lloyd (1973) has noted with respect to the dual handicaps of hearing impairment and mental retardation, problems seem to increase exponentially as they appear in combination, and there seems to be an interaction between the handicaps. This is undoubtedly true with respect to the combination of other disabilities with hearing impairment. The presence of multiple handicaps presents considerable management problems for those who must develop and implement programs for these individuals. Although the tendency has been to establish one disability as the priority disability from a management standpoint, there is no consistent basis for doing so, neither has it been determined whether this procedure is necessary or productive in an educational sense. The practice probably has been the result of the lack of teacher preparation in the area of the multiply handicapped, so that it has been necessary to label the disabled individual in order to determine in what kind of educational setting to place him.

In reality, the multiply handicapped hearing impaired are found in residential programs for the hearing impaired, residential programs for the mentally retarded, programs for the emotionally disturbed, and a number of other special education programs servicing a wide variety of disabled individauls. Mitra (1970) reported that mental retardation appears in combination with hearing impairment more frequently than any other single handicap, although Jensema and Trybus (1975) reported that the emotionally disturbed hearing impaired constitute a large portion of the multiply handicapped group. Jensema and Trybus attributed the high incidence of emotional disturbance in conjunction with hearing impairment, at least in part, to the high incidence of maternal rubella which, in addition to hearing loss, also can result in brain damage that may later give rise to emotional and behavioral disorders. Mitra (1970) also reported that the majority of the hearing-impaired retarded population is found in state residential facilities for the mentally retarded. Consequently, the teachers of these individuals tend to be trained in the field of retardation and know little, if anything, about communication programming for the hearing impaired.

Anderson and Stevens (1969), reporting the results of a survey of several residential schools for the deaf whose populations included mentally retarded individuals, found that hearing loss is considered to be the most disabling condition from an educational standpoint. Consequently, programming tends to be that typically applied to the intellectually normal hearing-impaired child. Vockell, Vockell, and Mattick (1973) stated that, because hearing impairment can be considered to be the major problem of the hearing-impaired mentally retarded, teaching methods applicable to hearing-impaired children should be the primary procedures used with these children, although they recommended adapting these procedures to meet particular individual needs. In an example, Vockell, Vockell, and Mattick reported the successful use of the Project LIFE program, which was originally developed for the intellectually normal hearing impaired (Wooden and Willard, 1965), with the hearing-impaired mentally retarded. The Project LIFE program emphasized cognitive and perceptual skill development as prerequisite to specific language instruction.

Only recently have there been reports of programs specifically developed for multiply handicapped hearing-impaired children. Naiman, Schein, and Stewart (1973) have described a day program for emotionally disturbed hearing-impaired children, and Lennan (1973) has described a residential program for the emotionally disturbed hearing impaired, some with additional physical disabilities. Both programs, although primarily oriented toward behavioral control, emphasize communication skills within their curriculum. The goal of both programs is placement of these children in regular classes for the hearing impaired, and both programs use modifications of procedures typically used with emotionally disturbed individuals.

Perhaps the most sophisticated of the programs that have been developed for the multiply handicapped is the one developed by Berger (1972a, b) for the hearing impaired mentally retarded within the context of a residential facility for the mentally retarded. The program is structured to establish response development within a sequence of language modes beginning with gross motor responding and proceeding through specific motor responding, signing, fingerspelling, writing, and speaking. Behavioral technology defines the teaching procedures used within the program. Throughout the program sequence, verbalization is used in conjunction with all manual language given to the child, and all manual language given by the child is verbalized by the teacher. Although manual language is not the terminal goal of the program, some individuals do not progress beyond this level, and those who exit the program with a manual system are seen as benefitting from the program in terms of improved social and emotional interaction in conjunction with a system of communication.

In addition to the work of Berger, there have been other reports of the successful use of manual communication systems with the hearing-impaired mentally retarded (Kopchick and Lloyd, this volume; Hall and Talkington, 1970; Hoffmeister and Farmer, 1972). Fristoe (1975) has recently reported on the increased use of manual and gestural systems in programs for all types of retarded persons throughout the United States.

Although it has been demonstrated that the hearing-impaired mentally retarded can acquire a manual communication system and the evidence suggests that they do so more rapidly than they acquire oral language as an initial means of communication, it has been reported that manual communication systems are not widely used with hearing-impaired mentally retarded individuals within state institutions for the mentally retarded (Brannan, Sigelman, and Bensberg, 1975). The difficulty seems to be one of grouping of the residents because the language instruction presented during the relatively small number of hours spent in the clinic or classroom is not reinforced by the use of that language system in the total daily environment where individuals spend the majority of their time (Berger, 1972a; Brannan, Sigelman, and Bensberg, 1975). It is difficult, and probably impossible, to train all personnel in a large institution to use manual communication consistently with these residents, yet this is what is required when the hearing-impaired mentally retarded are dispersed across the facility. Although the *Standards* of the Accreditation Council for Facilities for the Mentally Retarded (1971) discourage grouping clients according to disability, Brannan, Sigelman, and Bensberg (1975) and Kopchick and Lloyd (this volume) recommend grouping some residents for programmatic reasons and establishing a 24-hour program in which there is complete consistency with respect to communication mode. At the present time, this seems to be the only logical approach, and, unless a workable alternative is found, consideration should be given to rewording the *Standards*.

The provision of amplification for the multiply handicapped hearing impaired seems to be as important as with otherwise normal but hearing-impaired individuals, although perhaps it is more difficult, or even impossible in some cases. Rittmanic (1959) reported that, in an institutional setting for the mentally retarded, providing wearable amplification, along with auditory training programs, resulted in a reduction in emotional and behavioral problems for some of the hearing-impaired mentally retarded residents. However, Brannan, Sigelman, and Bensberg (1975) reported that the majority of hearing-impaired mentally retarded individuals within state residential facilities are not provided with hearing aids, apparently because these residents have difficulty in caring for their hearing aids. In one program for the hearing-impaired mentally retarded in a residential setting, such problems were reportedly reduced when a single staff member was designated responsibility for individuals who wore hearing aids. This staff member, the "hearing aid consultant," made daily checks of all hearing aids (Brannan, Sigelman, and Bensberg, 1975).

Another approach to the problem of hearing aid use by the hearing-impaired mentally retarded within an institutional setting is described by McCoy and Lloyd (1967) and Moore, Miltenberger, and Barber (1969). These writers advocated a program of intensive hearing aid orientation. Their respective programs were conducted within residential institutions for the mentally retarded. McCoy and Lloyd (1967) stressed the importance of involving direct-care staff members as well as the training of the residents who are the prospective hearing aid wearers. In the McCoy and Lloyd program, direct-care staff were given specific training with respect to hearing aids, including the reasons for their use, and were involved in the monitoring process as the user gradually became a full-time hearing aid wearer.

In comparison, the program described by Moore, Miltenberger, and Barber (1969) seems to place less emphasis on specific training for direct-care staff, while the prospective hearing aid wearers receive intensive training including prehearing aid orientation followed by specific training in care and use of the aid. Direct-care staff assumed a primary role in advising the audiologic staff with respect to residential living conditions that may or may not be conducive to successful hearing aid use and in monitoring the individual wearer's behavioral progress in the daily living environment as a result of the use of the aid. On the basis of a 2-year evaluation of their program, Moore, Miltenberger, and Barber (1969) reported success with respect to the use of hearing aids, less breakage of aids than was previously the case, and, interestingly, the elevation of hearing aids to the level of a status symbol as other residents asked that they also be given a "radio." For further discussion of amplification systems and hearing aid orientation or guidance considerations, the reader is referred to Ross (this volume) and Cox and Lloyd (this volume).

With respect to the multiply handicapped hearing impaired, there seems to be a long overdue recognition of just the existence of such a population, even if efforts to program these individuals have been sporadic and usually without any apparent a priori rationale. Cooperative, cross-disciplinary efforts are crucial to the development of effective programs. A relatively early, positive step in relation to the hearing-impaired mentally retarded was the creation of the AAMD-CEASD Joint Committee on the Deaf-Retarded, which was established in 1970 and which has facilitated communication among professionals concerned with the mentally retarded and those concerned with the hearing impaired. (AAMD stands for the American Association on Mental Deficiency; CEASD stands for the Conference of Executives of American Schools for the Deaf. For a brief historical sketch on the development of cooperative efforts between educators of the hearing impaired and speech pathologists and audiologists concerned with habilitation of the mentally retarded, see Lloyd, 1972). The need for teacher preparation curricula that cross traditional disciplinary lines is in evidence throughout the recent literature (Lennan, 1973; Ortiz, 1973; Brannan, Sigelman, and Bensberg, 1975).

COMMUNICATION SYSTEMS FOR THE NONORAL PHYSICALLY HANDICAPPED

Approaches to the development of oral language for the severely physically handicapped individual have emphasized a close working relationship between the physical therapist, the occupational therapist, and the speech pathologist (Mysak, 1959; Crickmay, 1970). Such cooperative therapeutic approaches have been successful in establishing intelligible oral communication for many motorically handicapped individuals. However, some physically handicapped individuals with normal hearing and appropriate receptive language ability are unable to develop an oral system of expression even after prolonged therapy. In addition to the respiratory, phonatory, and articulatory dysfunctions that preclude establishing usable speech, these individuals exhibit a general neuromuscular disorder that also precludes the use of signs or fingerspelling as an alternate mode of communication. Although this group is a very special population in which the lack of an expressive language system is primarily the result of physical limitations, it is unnecessary and irresponsible for the clinician to insist on oral language as the immedate goal for a training program and thereby deprive these individuals of other possible means of communication.

Although the development of alternate methods of communication for the physically handicapped has been in process for several years, only recently have clinicians and researchers begun to exchange information and to coordinate their efforts in the development of nonoral communication systems. As in oral language development programs for the physically handicapped, the development of nonoral (nonvocal) communication systems for this population requires a team approach in order to meet physical, emotional, and educational needs. In addition to the traditional team members, the development of nonoral systems requires input from other specialists, such as carpenters and mechanical and electrical engineers, who can assist in the design and construction of the necessary devices through which nonoral communication can be established.

There is often considerable resistance to the use of nonoral communication systems, usually from those who argue that use of a nonoral system suppresses or permanently negates the development of oral language. There are indications that this suppression does not occur, but that, in fact, as the pressure on the individual for oral language is decreased, spontaneous vocalization and verbalization often increase along with the use of the nonoral system (McDonald and Schultz, 1973; Seligman, 1973). It also has been suggested that, as success is realized in nonoral communication, the inherently slow rate of communication with such systems acts as a stimulus for increased efforts toward oral expression (Vicker, 1974b).

Nonoral communication devices range from relatively simple, nonmechanical devices to highly sophisticated electronic devices. Perhaps the most widely used nonoral system is the communication board, with which the individual uses some sort of pointing response to indicate his choice of various characters that are located on the board. The characters may be pictures, words, specialized symbols, or simply letters of the alphabet used to spell out what the individual wishes to communicate. The design and construction of a communication board is usually individualized for each user because the choice of characters, their arrangement on the board, and factors such as positioning of the individual and the board are highly dependent on the individual's intellectual level, educational level, and physical capabilities. Although such systems have been developed predominantly for the intellectually normal, physically handicapped, they have been used with at least some degree of success with mentally retarded, physically handicapped individuals who are non-oral (Hagen, Porter, and Brink, 1973; Vanderheiden et al., 1975). There are several good descriptions of nonmechanical, nonoral communication systems available, including those provided by the Ontario Crippled Children's Centre group (1973) pertaining to the use of the Bliss symbol system, and by McDonald and Schultz (1973) and Vicker (1974a). Kladde (1974), Sayre (1963), and Schurman (1974) present good descriptions of the physical design and construction of communication boards.

In addition to nonmechanical devices such as communication boards, a number of other communication aids have been developed for the nonoral physically handicapped. Since these devices are usually considerably more expensive to design and construct, they are developed so that they are applicable to a relatively larger number of users. For a more complete description of nonoral systems of communication and their use, see Vanderheiden and Harris-Vanderheiden (this volume).

CONCLUSION

It is hoped that, through reading this chapter, clinicians will gain further appreciation for the communication problems of the developmentally disabled and will have at least begun to come to terms with the nature of the task they face, as each clinician must do, when confronted with individuals without language or with language delay. It is hoped also that they will have developed some further insight into the nature and extent of available programs and strategies for the developmentally disabled.

There should be the realization that there is probably no single developmental disability from a communication standpoint, or even any clear-cut combinations of disabilities. Each child, adolescent, and adult must be viewed as an individual who presents problems that are perhaps unique to that individual.

Throughout this chapter the writer has intentionally avoided any pedantic discussion of terms such as *communication, language, speech, hearing impairment, emotional disturbance, developmental disability,* and so forth. It is hoped that, in the absence of any such definitions, clinicians will adopt the view that getting developmentally disabled individuals interacting with their environment ("communication") should be the first objective. A highly organized, standardized, and systematic way of doing so ("language") should be the second objective after the first has been realized. The third and ultimate objective, in cases where intellectual, sensory, and physical capabilities allow, should be the most widely used and most accepted system of communication ("speech"). For some developmentally disabled individuals, attainment of this final objective is truly the "icing on the cake."

REFERENCES

Accreditation Council for Facilities for the Mentally Retarded. 1971. Standards for Residential Facilities for the Mentally Retarded. Joint Commission on Accreditation of Hospitals, Chicago.

Alpiner, J. G., and C. F. Amon. 1972. Talk To Me. A Home Study Program of Language Development for Hearing Impaired Children: Infancy to Preschool. Department of Speech Pathology and Audiology, University of Denver, Denver.

American Organization for the Education of the Hearing Impaired. 1975. A position paper of the American Organization for the Education of the Hearing Impaired, May 1, 1975. Volta Rev. 77:330–334.

Amon, C. 1972. Project Parent-Child: A model for prescriptive intervention. Paper presented at the American Speech and Hearing Association annual convention, San Francisco.

Anderson, R. M., and G. D. Stevens. 1969. Practices and problems in educating deaf retarded children in residential schools. Except. Child. 35:687–694.

Baltzer, S. 1973. Auditory training and early management of the child with auditory and visual impairments. *In* C. A. Tait (ed.), Audiological Considerations with Acoustically and Visually Impaired Children. Institute for the Study of Mental Retardation and Related Disabilities, University of Michigan, Ann Arbor.

Barnard, K. E., and M. L. Powell. 1972. Teaching the Mentally Retarded Child: A Family Care Approach. C. V. Mosby, St. Louis.

Bateman, B. 1974. Discussion summary—Language intervention for the mentally retarded. *In* R. L. Schiefelbusch and L. L. Lloyd (eds.), Language Perspectives—Acquisition, Retardation, and Intervention. University Park Press, Baltimore.

Berger, S. L. 1972a. A clinical program for developing multimodal language responses with atypical deaf children. *In* J. E. McLean, D. E. Yoder, and R. L. Schiefelbusch (eds.), Language Intervention with the Retarded: Developing Strategies. University Park Press, Baltimore.

Berger, S. L. 1972b. Systematic development of communication modes: Establishment of a multiple-response repertoire for non-communicating deaf children. *In* Report of the Proceedings of the 45th Meeting of the Convention of American Instructors of the Deaf. U.S. Government Printing Office, Washington, D.C.

Bloom, L. 1970. Language Development: Form and Function in Emerging Grammars. MIT Press, Cambridge, Mass.

Bloom, L. 1972. Semantic features in language development. *In* R. L. Schiefelbusch (ed.), Language of the Mentally Retarded. University Park Press, Baltimore.

Bloom, L. 1973. One Word at a Time. Mouton, The Hague.

Bowerman, M. 1973. Structural relationships in children's utterances: Syntactic or semantic? *In* T. E. Moore (ed.), Cognitive Development and the Acquisition of Language. Academic Press, New York.

Braine, M. D. S. 1963. The ontogeny of English phrase structure: The first phase. Language 39:1–14.

Brannan, A. C., C. K. Sigelman, and G. J. Bensberg. 1975. The Hearing Impaired/Mentally Retarded: A Survey of State Institutions for the Retarded. Research and Training Center in Mental Retardation, Monograph 4, Texas Tech University, Lubbock.

Bricker, D. D. 1972. Imitative sign training as a facilitator of word object association with low-functioning children. Amer. J. Ment. Defic. 76: 509–516.

Bricker, D., and W. Bricker. 1971. Toddler Research and Intervention Project Report: Year I. IMRID Behavioral Science Monograph 20, Institute on Mental Retardation and Intellectual Development, George Peabody College, Nashville.

Bricker, D., and W. Bricker. 1972. Toddler Research and Intervention Project Report: Year II. IMRID Behavioral Science Monograph 21, Institute on Mental Retardation and Intellectual Development, George Peabody College, Nashville.

Bricker, D., and W. Bricker. 1973. Infant, Toddler, and Preschool Research and Intervention Project Report: Year III. IMRID Behavioral Science Monograph 23, Institute on Mental Retardation and Intellectual Development, George Peabody College, Nashville.

Bricker, D., L. Dennison, L. Watson, and L. Vincent-Smith. 1973. Language Training Program for Young Developmentally Delayed Children. IMRID Behavioral Science Monograph 22, Institute on Mental Retardation and Intellectual Development, George Peabody College, Nashville.

Bricker, W. A. 1972. A systematic approach to language training. *In* R. L. Schiefelbusch (ed.), Language of the Mentally Retarded. University Park Press, Baltimore.

Bricker, W. A., and D. D. Bricker. 1970. A program of language training for the severely language handicapped child. Except. Child. 37: 101–111.

Bricker, W. A., and D. D. Bricker. 1974. An early language training strategy. *In* R. L. Schiefelbusch and L. L. Lloyd (eds.), Language Perspectives—Acquisition, Retardation, and Intervention. University Park Press, Baltimore.

Brown, R. 1970. The first sentences of child and chimpanzee. *In* R. Brown (ed.), Psycholinguistics. The Free Press, New York.

Brown, R. 1973a. A First Language: The Early Stages. Harvard University Press, Cambridge, Mass.

Brown, R. 1973b. Development of the first language in the human species. Amer. Psychol. 28:97–106.

Brown, R., and U. Bellugi. 1964. Three processes in the child's acquisition of syntax. Harvard Educ. Rev. 34:133–151.

Butterfield, E. C. 1967. The role of environmental factors in the treatment of institutionalized mental retardates. *In* A. A. Baumeister (ed.), Mental Retardation: Appraisal, Education and Rehabilitation. Aldine, Chicago.

Connor, L. E. (ed.). 1971. Speech for the Deaf Child: Knowledge and Use. Alexander Graham Bell Association for the Deaf, Washington, D.C.

Creedon, M. P. (ed.). 1974. Appropriate Behavior Through Communication: A New Program in Simultaneous Language for Nonverbal Children. Unpublished manual, Dysfunctioning Child Center, Michael Reese Medical Center, Chicago.

Crickmay, M. C. 1970. Speech Therapy and the Bobath Approach to Cerebral Palsy. Charles C Thomas, Springfield, Ill.

Cromer, R. F. 1974a. Receptive language in the mentally retarded: Processes and diagnostic distinctions. *In* R. L. Schiefelbusch and L. L. Lloyd (eds.), Language Perspectives—Acquisition, Retardation, and Intervention. University Park Press, Baltimore.

Cromer, R. F. 1974b. The development of language and cognition: The cognition hypothesis. *In* B. Foss (ed.), New Perspectives in Child Development. Penguin Books, Harmondsworth, Middlesex.

Crosby, K. 1972. Attention and distractibility in mentally retarded and intellectually average children. Amer. J. Ment. Defic. 77:46–53.

Dempsey, C. (undated). Caring for a Child's Hearing Aid. Zenith Hearing Aid Sales Corp., Chicago.

Douglas, V. I. 1974. Sustained attention and impulse control: Implications for the handicapped child. *In* J. A. Swets and L. L. Elliott (eds.), Psychology and the Handicapped Child. U.S. Department of Health, Education, and Welfare Publication (OE) 73-05000. U.S. Government Printing Office, Washington, D.C.

van den Eeckhaut, J. 1967. Hearing aids in children. Int. Audiol. 6: 293–295.

Ervin, S. M. 1964. Imitation and structural change in children's language. *In* E. H. Lenneberg (ed.), New Directions in the Study of Language. MIT Press, Cambridge, Mass.

Flint, R. W. 1975. A. G. Bell Board re-examines the Association's purpose and mission. Volta Rev. 77:152–154.

Fristoe, M. 1975. Language Intervention Systems for the Retarded: A Catalog of Original Structured Language Programs in Use in the U.S. State of Alabama Department of Education, Montgomery, Ala.

Fristoe, M. 1976. Language intervention systems: Programs published in kit form. J. Child. Commun. Disord. Vol. 1.

Fulton, R. T., and L. L. Lloyd (eds.). 1975. Auditory Assessment of the Difficult-to-Test. Williams & Wilkins, Baltimore.

Garcia, E. E., and E. D. DeHaven. 1974. Use of operant techniques in the establishment and generalization of language: A review and analysis. Amer. J. Ment. Defic. 79:169–178.

Graham, J. T., and L. W. Graham. 1971. Language behavior of the mentally retarded: Syntactic characteristics. Amer. J. Ment. Defic. 75:623–629.

Gray, B., and B. Ryan. 1973. A Language Program for the Nonlanguage Child. Research Press, Champaign, Ill.

Guess, D., W. Sailor, and D. M. Baer. 1974. To teach language to retarded children. In R. L. Schiefelbusch and L. L. Lloyd (eds.), Language Perspectives—Acquisition, Retardation, and Intervention. University Park Press, Baltimore.

Hagen, C., W. Porter, and J. Brink. 1973. Nonverbal communication: An alternate mode of communication for the child with severe cerebral palsy. J. Speech Hear. Disord. 38:448–455.

Hall, S. M., and L. W. Talkington. 1970. Evaluation of a manual approach to programming for deaf retarded. Amer. J. Ment. Defic. 75:378–380.

Hanners, B. A., and A. B. Sitton. 1974. Ears to Hear: A daily hearing aid monitor program. Volta Rev. 76:530–536.

Hartung, J. R. 1970. A review of procedures to increase verbal imitation skills and functional speech in autistic children. J. Speech Hear. Disord. 35:203–217.

Haviland, R. T. 1972. A stimulus to language development: The institutional environment. Ment. Retard. 10:19–21.

Heber, R., H. Garber, S. Harrington, and C. Hoffman. 1972. Rehabilitation of Families at Risk for Mental Retardation: Progress Report. Rehabilitation Research and Training Center in Mental Retardation, University of Wisconsin, Madison.

Hegrenes, J. R., N. R. Marshall, and J. A. Armas. 1970. Treatment as an extension of diagnostic function: A case study. J. Speech Hear. Disord. 35:182–187.

Hoffmeister, R., and A. Farmer. 1972. The development of manual communication in mentally retarded deaf individuals. J. Rehab. Deaf 6:19–26.

Horton, K. B. 1968. Home demonstration teaching for parents of very young deaf children. Volta Rev. 70:97–101, 104.

Horton, K. B. 1974. Infant intervention and language learning. In R. L. Schiefelbusch and L. L. Lloyd (eds.), Language Perspectives—Acquisition, Retardation, and Intervention. University Park Press, Baltimore.

Jakobovits, L. A., and M. S. Miron (eds.). 1967. Readings in the Psychology of Language. Prentice-Hall, Englewood Cliffs, N.J.

Jeffrey, D. B. 1972. Increase and maintenance of verbal behavior of a mentally retarded child. Ment. Retard. 10:35–40.

Jensema, C., and R. J. Trybus. 1975. Reported Emotional/Behavioral Problems Among Hearing Impaired Children in Special Educational Programs: United States, 1972–73. Office of Demographic Studies, Gallaudet College, Washington, D.C.

John Tracy Clinic. 1961. John Tracy Clinic Correspondence Course for Parents of Little Deaf Children. John Tracy Clinic, Los Angeles.

John Tracy Clinic. 1968. Getting Your Baby Ready to Talk. John Tracy Clinic, Los Angeles.

Karnes, M. B., A. Hodgins, and J. A. Teska. 1968. An evaluation of two preschool programs for disadvantaged children: A traditional and a highly structured experimental preschool. Except. Child. 34:667–676.

Kent, L. R. 1972. A language acquisition program for the retarded. In J. E. McLean, D. E. Yoder, and R. L. Schiefelbusch (eds.), Language Intervention with the Retarded: Developing Strategies. University Park Press. Baltimore.

Kladde, A. G. 1974. Nonoral communication techniques: Project summary 1, August, 1967. In B. Vicker (ed.), Nonoral Communication System Project 1964/1973. University of Iowa, Iowa City.

Lackner, J. R. 1968. A developmental study of language behavior in retarded children. Neuropsychologia 6:301–320.

Lennan, R. K. 1973. The Deaf Multi-Handicapped Unit at the California School for the Deaf, Riverside. Amer. Ann. Deaf 118:439–445.

Lenneberg, E. H. 1966. The natural history of language. In F. Smith and G. A. Miller (eds.), The Genesis of Language: A Psycholinguistic Approach. MIT Press, Cambridge, Mass.

Lenneberg, E. H. 1967. Biological Foundations of Language. John Wiley & Sons, New York.

Lillywhite, H. S., and D. P. Bradley. 1969. Communication Problems in Mental Retardation: Diagnosis and Management. Harper & Row, New York.

Lloyd, L. L. 1972. You've come a long way baby, but—. Ment. Retard. 10:2.

Lloyd, L. L. 1973. Mental retardation and hearing impairment. In A. G. Norris (ed.), PRWAD Deafness Annual. Vol. 3. Professional Rehabilitation Workers with the Adult Deaf, Washington, D.C.

Lloyd, L. L. 1976. Discussant's comments: Language and communication aspects. In T. D. Tjossem (ed.), Intervention Strategies for High Risk Infants and Young Children. University Park Press, Baltimore.

Lloyd, L. L., and B. P. Cox. 1972. Programming for the audiologic aspects of mental retardation. Ment. Retard. 10:22–26.

Lowell, E. 1965. Parental skills and attitudes, including home training. The Young Deaf Child: Identification and Management. Acta Otolaryngol. suppl. 206.

Lucker, W. G. 1970. The Effects of Environmental Stimulation on the Perceptual Thresholds of High-Active and Low-Active Mentally Retarded Persons. IMRID Behavioral Science Monograph 15, Institute on Mental Retardation and Intellectual Development, George Peabody College, Nashville.

Lydon, W. T., and M. L. McGraw. 1973. Concept Development for Visually Handicapped Children. American Foundation for the Blind, New York.

Lynch, J., and W. A. Bricker. 1972. Linguistic theory and operant procedures: Toward an integrated approach to language training for the mentally retarded. Ment. Retard. 10:12–17.

Lynch, L., and A. Tobin. 1973. The development of language-training programs for postrubella hearing-impaired children. J. Speech Hear. Disord. 38:15–24.

McConnell, F. 1974. The parent teaching home: An early intervention program for hearing impaired children. Peabody J. Educ. 51:162–170.

McCoy, D., and L. L. Lloyd. 1967. Hearing aid orientation program for mentally retarded children. Train. School Bull. 64:21–30.

McCrosky, R. L. 1967. Progress report on a home training program for deaf infants. Int. Audiol. 6:171–177.

McDonald, E. T., and A. R. Schultz. 1973. Communication boards for cerebral palsied children. J. Speech Hear. Disord. 38:73–88.

MacDonald, J. D., and J. P. Blott. 1974. Environmental language intervention: The rationale for a diagnostic and training strategy through rules, context, and generalization. J. Speech Hear. Disord. 39:244–256.

MacDonald, J. D., J. P. Blott, K. Gordon, B. Spiegel, and M. Hartmann. 1974. An experimental parent-assisted treatment program for preschool language-delayed children. J. Speech Hear. Disord. 39:395–415.

McNeill, D. 1966. Developmental psycholinguistics. *In* F. Smith and G. A. Miller (eds.), The Genesis of Language: A Psycholinguistic Approach. MIT Press, Cambridge, Mass.

McNeill, D., and N. B. McNeill. 1968. What does a child mean when he says "no"? *In* E. M. Zale (ed.), Proceedings of the Conference on Language and Language Behavior. Appleton-Century-Crofts, New York.

Marshall, N. R., and J. R. Hegrenes. 1970. Programmed communication therapy for autistic mentally retarded children. J. Speech Hear. Disord. 35:70–83.

Marshall, N. R., and J. R. Hegrenes. 1972. A communication therapy model for cognitively disorganized children. *In* J. E. McLean, D. E. Yoder, and R. L. Schiefelbusch (eds.), Language Intervention with the Retarded: Developing Strategies. University Park Press, Baltimore.

Miller, G. A. 1967. Some preliminaries to psycholinguistics. *In* L. A. Jakobovits and M. S. Miron (eds.), Readings in the Psychology of Language. Prentice-Hall, Englewood Cliffs, N.J.

Miller, J. F., and D. E. Yoder. 1972a. A syntax teaching program. *In* J. E. McLean, D. E. Yoder, and R. L. Schiefelbusch (eds.), Language Intervention with the Retarded: Developing Strategies. University Park Press, Baltimore.

Miller, J. F., and D. E. Yoder. 1972b. On developing the content for a language teaching program. Ment. Retard. 10:9–11.

Miller, J. F., and D. E. Yoder. 1974. An ontogenetic language teaching strategy for retarded children. In R. L. Schiefelbusch and L. L. Lloyd (eds.), Language Perspectives—Acquisition, Retardation, and Intervention. University Park Press, Baltimore.

Mitra, S. B. 1970. Educational provisions for mentally retarded deaf students in residential institutions for the retarded. Volta Rev. 72: 225–236.

Montessori, M. 1964. The Montessori Method. Schocken Books, New York. (Translated by A. E. George.)

Moore, E. J., G. E. Miltenberger, and P. S. Barber. 1969. Hearing aid orientation in a state school for the mentally retarded. J. Speech Hear. Disord. 34:142–145.

Moores, D. F. 1973. Early Childhood Special Education for the Hearing Handicapped. Research, Development and Demonstration Center in Education of Handicapped Children, Occasional Paper 13, University of Minnesota, Minneapolis.

Moores, D. F. 1974. Nonvocal systems of verbal behavior. In R. L. Schiefelbusch and L. L. Lloyd (eds.), Language Perspectives—Acquisition, Retardation, and Intervention. University Park Press, Baltimore.

Moores, D. F., K. L. Weiss, and M. W. Goodwin. 1974. Evaluation of Programs for Hearing Impaired Children: Report of 1973–74. Research, Development and Demonstration Center in Education of Handicapped Children, Research Report 81, University of Minnesota, Minneapolis.

Morehead, D. M., and A. Morehead. 1974. From signal to sign: A Piagetian view of thought and language during the first two years of life. In R. L. Schiefelbusch and L. L. Lloyd (eds.), Language Perspectives—Acquisition, Retardation, and Intervention. University Park Press, Baltimore.

Morkovin, B. V. 1968. Language in the general development of the preschool deaf child: A review of research in the Soviet Union. Asha 10:195–199.

Motto, J., and F. J. Wawrzaszek. 1963. Integration of the hearing handicapped: Evaluation of the current status. Volta Rev. 65:124–129, 160.

Mysak, E. D. 1959. Significance of neurophysiological orientation to cerebral palsy habilitation. J. Speech Hear. Disord. 24:221–230.

Naiman, D., J. D. Schein, and L. Stewart. 1973. New vistas for emotionally disturbed deaf children. Amer. Ann. Deaf 118:480–487.

Niemann, S. L. 1972. Listen! An acoupedic program. Volta Rev. 74: 85–89.

Northcott, W. H. 1971. Infant education and home training. In L. E. Connor (ed.), Speech for the Deaf Child: Knowledge and Use. Alexander Graham Bell Association for the Deaf, Washington, D.C.

Northcott, W. H. (ed.). 1972. Curriculum Guide: Hearing Impaired Children—Birth to Three Years—and Their Parents. Alexander Graham Bell Association for the Deaf, Washington, D.C.

Northern, J. L., and M. P. Downs. 1974. Hearing in Children. Williams & Wilkins, Baltimore.

Ontario Crippled Children's Centre. 1973. Symbol Communication Research Project, Project Report 1972–73. Ontario Crippled Children's Centre, Toronto.

Ortiz, E. R. 1973. Teacher training program for deaf-blind. In C. A. Tait (ed.), Audiological Considerations with Acoustically and Visually Impaired Children. Institute for the Study of Mental Retardation and Related Disabilities, University of Michigan, Ann Arbor.

Parsons, M. B. 1967. The improvement of techniques in parent guidance for parents of pre-school deaf children. Int. Audiol. 6:151–158.

Peterson, R. F. 1968. Some experiments on the organization of a class of imitative behaviors. J. Appl. Behav. Anal. 1:225–235.

Piaget, J. 1970. Piaget's theory. In P. H. Mussen (ed.), Carmichael's Manual of Child Psychology. Vol. 1. John Wiley & Sons, New York.

Piaget, J., and B. Inhelder. 1969. The Psychology of the Child. Basic Books, New York. (Translated by H. Weaver.)

Pollack, D. 1964. Acoupedics: A uni-sensory approach to auditory training. Volta Rev. 66:400–409.

Pollack, D. 1967. The crucial year: A time to listen. Int. Audiol. 6: 243–247.

Quigley, S. P. 1966. Language research in countries other than the United States. In S. P. Quigley (ed.), Language Acquisition. Alexander Graham Bell Association for the Deaf, Washington, D.C.

Richardson, S. O. 1967. Language training for mentally retarded children. In R. L. Schiefelbusch, R. H. Copeland, and J. O. Smith (eds.), Language and Mental Retardation: Empirical and Conceptual Considerations. Holt, Rinehart and Winston, New York.

Risley, T. R., B. Hart, and L. Doke. 1972. Operant language development: The outline of a therapeutic technology. In R. L. Schiefelbusch (ed.), Language of the Mentally Retarded. University Park Press, Baltimore.

Risley, T. R., and M. M. Wolf. 1967. Establishing functional speech in echolalic children. Behav. Res. Ther. 5:73–88.

Rister, A. 1975. Deaf children in mainstream education. Volta Rev. 77:279–290.

Rittmanic, P. A. 1959. Hearing rehabilitation for the institutionalized mentally retarded. Amer. J. Ment. Defic. 63:778–783.

Robinson, C., and J. Filler. 1971. Maternal Teaching Style Assessment Scale. In D. Bricker and W. Bricker (eds.), Toddler Research and Intervention Project Report: Year I. IMRID Behavioral Science Monograph 20, Institute on Mental Retardation and Intellectual Development, George Peabody College, Nashville.

Ronnei, E. C., and J. Porter. 1965. Tim and His Hearing Aid. Alexander Graham Bell Association for the Deaf, Washington, D.C.

Ruder, K. F. 1972. A psycholinguistic viewpoint of the language acqui-
sition process. *In* R. L. Schiefelbusch (ed.), Language of the Mentally
Retarded. University Park Press, Baltimore.
Sanders, D. A. 1971. Aural Rehabilitation. Prentice-Hall, Englewood
Cliffs, N.J.
Sayre, J. M. 1963. Communication for the non-verbal cerebral palsied.
C. P. Rev. 24:3–8.
Schiefelbusch, R. L., R. H. Copeland, and J. O. Smith. 1967. Introduc-
tion. *In* R. L. Schiefelbusch, R. H. Copeland, and J. O. Smith (eds.),
Language and Mental Retardation: Empirical and Conceptual Con-
siderations. Holt, Rinehart and Winston, New York.
Schlesinger, I. M. 1971a. Learning grammar: From pivot to realization
rules. *In* R. Huxley and E. Ingram (eds.), Language Acquisition:
Models and Methods. Academic Press, New York.
Schlesinger, I. M. 1971b. Production of utterances and language acqui-
sition. *In* D. I. Slobin (ed.), The Ontogenesis of Grammar: A Theoreti-
cal Symposium. Academic Press, New York.
Schlesinger, H. S., and K. P. Meadow. 1972. Sound and Sign: Childhood
Deafness and Mental Health. University of California Press, Berkeley.
Schurman, J. 1974. Custom designing communication board frames:
The role of the occupational therapist. *In* B. Vicker (ed.), Nonoral
Communication System Project 1964/1973. University of Iowa, Iowa
City.
Seligman, J. 1973. Speech pathology progress report. *In* Symbol Com-
munication Research Project, Progress Report 1972–73. Ontario Crip-
pled Children's Centre, Toronto.
Shaffer, T. R., and H. Goehl. 1974. The alinguistic child. Ment. Retard.
12:3–6.
Shearer, D. E., and M. S. Shearer. 1976. The Portage Project: A model for
early childhood education. *In* T. D. Tjossem (ed.), Intervention
Strategies for High Risk Infants and Young Children. University Park
Press, Baltimore.
Shearer, M. S., and D. E. Shearer. 1972. The Portage Project: A model
for early childhood education. Except. Child. 39:210–217.
Simmons, A. A. 1967. Home demonstration teaching for parents and
infants at Central Institute for the Deaf. *In* Proceedings of Interna-
tional Conference on Oral Education of the Deaf. Vol. 2. Alexander
Graham Bell Association for the Deaf, Washington, D.C.
Skinner, B. F. 1957. Verbal Behavior. Appleton-Century-Crofts, New
York.
Spicker, H. H. 1971. Intellectual development through early childhood
education. Except. Child. 37:629–640.
Staats, A. W. 1974. Behaviorism and cognitive theory in the study of
language: A neopsycholinguistics. *In* R. L. Schiefelbusch and L. L.
Lloyd (eds.), Language Perspectives—Acquisition, Retardation, and
Intervention. University Park Press, Baltimore.
Stack, Sister P. M. 1973. In our program—Everyone gets into the act.
Volta Rev. 75:425–430.

Stark, J., R. L. Rosenbaum, D. Schwartz, and A. Wisan. 1973. The non-verbal child: Some clinical guidelines. J. Speech Hear. Disord. 38:59–72.

Strauss, A. A., and L. E. Lehtinen. 1947. Psychopathology and Education of the Brain-Injured Child. Grune & Stratton, New York.

Stremel, K. 1972. Language training: A program for retarded children. Ment. Retard. 10:47–49.

Stremel, K., and C. Waryas. 1974. A behavioral-psycholinguistic approach to language training. In L. V. McReynolds (ed.), Developing Systematic Procedures for Training Children's Language. Asha Monogr. 18. Interstate Press, Danville, Ill.

Stuckless, E. R., and J. W. Birch. 1966. The influence of early manual communication on the linguistic development of deaf children. Amer. Ann. Deaf 111:499–504.

Sulzbacher, S. I., and J. M. Costello. 1970. A behavioral strategy for language training of a child with autistic behaviors. J. Speech Hear. Disord. 35:256–276.

Topper, S. T. 1975. Gesture language for a non-verbal severely retarded male. Ment. Retard. 13:30–31.

Turton, L. J. 1974. Discussion summary—Early language intervention. In R. L. Schiefelbusch and L. L. Lloyd (eds.), Language Perspectives—Acquisition, Retardation, and Intervention. University Park Press, Baltimore.

van Uden, A. 1970. A World of Language for Deaf Children. Part 1: Basic Principles. Rotterdam University Press, Rotterdam, The Netherlands.

Vanderheiden, D. H., W. P. Brown, P. MacKenzie, S. Reinen, and C. Scheibel. 1975. Symbol communication for the mentally handicapped. Ment. Retard. 13:34–37.

Vicker, B. (ed.). 1974a. Nonoral Communication System Project 1964/1973. University of Iowa, Iowa City.

Vicker, B. 1974b. The communication process using a nonoral means. In B. Vicker (ed.), Nonoral Communication System Project 1964/1973. University of Iowa, Iowa City.

Vockell, K., E. L. Vockell, and P. Mattick. 1973. Language for mentally retarded deaf children: Project LIFE. Volta Rev. 75:431–439.

Wilson, P. S. 1974. Sign Language as a Means of Communication for the Mentally Retarded. Paper presented at the Eastern Psychological Association meeting, April, Philadelphia.

Wooden, H. Z., and L. Willard. 1965. Project LIFE: Language improvement to facilitate education of hearing impaired children. Amer. Ann. Deaf 110:541–552.

Yoder, D. E., and J. F. Miller. 1972. What we may know and what we can do: Input toward a system. In J. E. McLean, D. E. Yoder, and R. L. Schiefelbusch (eds.), Language Intervention with the Retarded: Developing Strategies. University Park Press, Baltimore.

Zeaman, D., and B. House. 1963. The role of attention in retardate discrimination learning. In N. R. Ellis (ed.), Handbook of Mental Deficiency. McGraw-Hill, New York.

11

THE LINGUISTICS OF MANUAL LANGUAGE AND MANUAL SYSTEMS

Ronnie Bring Wilbur

CONTENTS

Linguistics of Manual Languages _____ **427**
    Language/427
    American Sign Language as a language/430
    Notational conventions/434
    Research on Sign Language/434

Linguistics of Manual Systems _____ **450**
    History/451
    Relationship between manual systems and English/452
    General comments on the systems/456
    Paget-Gorman Systematic Sign/458
    Signing Exact English/459
    Manual English/462
    Signed English/463
    Fingerspelling and Cued Speech/465

Practical Considerations of Manual Communication _____ **471**
    Acquisition of language/472
    Speech skills/478
    Socialization, achievement, and emotional development/479
    Memory/481
    Use with other populations/486

Summary _____ **490**

Acknowledgments _____ **491**

References _____ **491**

A profound hearing loss disrupts the language acquisition process to such an extent that most deaf people never achieve the level of linguistic competence of a hearing 10-year-old child. Thus, whereas normal hearing children acquire their native language without formal instruction and in a relatively short time span, in the deaf person the acquisition of English language structure and reading is impaired and delayed. For hearing children, most language structures are learned considerably earlier than reading skills, and reading skills are generally acquired within the regular classroom framework. On the other hand, the entire formal educational system for deaf people primarily hinges on the teaching of English, with reading and language structures taught more or less simultaneously. Other impairments that affect the acquisition of language (autism, aphasia, mental retardation, etc.) produce difficulties of a greatly different kind than those found with the deaf, and yet people who work with these different types of disorders are united in a common goal—to enable the person with a language disorder to reach the highest possible degree of fluency in English. People have turned to the use of one form or another of manual communication in the hopes that, where aural/oral language has failed, manual language may succeed.

The disruption of the auditory speech signal by a profound hearing loss can result in a switching of the perceptual, coding, and memory processes from an auditory to a visual modality. Although it might seem that the use of manual language might best fit the compensatory adjustments to the visual mode, and although deaf adults use manual communication among themselves, the use of any kind of sign language *in the classroom* has been the subject of a long and heated controversy. Sign language instruction was used in a school founded by the Abbé Charles Michel de l'Épée in 1775. He took the sign language used by deaf adults, which he believed to be the "true" language of the deaf, and used it with some modification in the classroom. More recently, objections have been raised against the use of manual communication because of the belief that abstract thinking is not possible without speech and that the use of manual communication impairs the development of speech. (For evidence to the contrary, see the discussion below.) Most of the formal education of the deaf in the United States purports to be orally conducted although the trend now is toward increasing use of some form of manual communication.

The term *manual communication* refers to several types of signing. American Sign Language (ASL) or Ameslan (Stokoe, 1960; Fant,

1972a) is, in the United States, the native language of many deaf people who have deaf parents and is the language used by deaf adults among themselves. Nearly 500,000 deaf people and an unknown number of hearing people use ASL, making it the third most widely used non-English language in the United States (Spanish, 4.5 million; Italian, 600,000) (O'Rourke et al., 1975). Schlesinger and Meadow (1972) reported that most of the deaf children whose native language is not ASL acquire some form of signing on entering school, where they come in contact with other children who know it. Performance on the *Test of English as a Foreign Language* indicates that many deaf students learn English more as a second language than as a first (Charrow and Fletcher, 1973). For educational purposes, several systems have been developed that put signs into the framework of English syntactic structure, on the (as yet untested) assumption that signs in English word order would make the transition from ASL to English easier for the student. These systems include: Systematic Sign Language, also known as the Paget-Gorman Sign System (Paget and Gorman, 1968); Signing Exact English (Gustason, Pfetzing, and Zawolkow, 1972); Seeing Essential English (Anthony, 1966, 1971); Linguistics of Visual English (Wampler, 1971, 1972); Signed English (Bornstein, 1973; Bornstein et al., 1973) also called Siglish (Prickett, 1971; Fant, 1972a, b); and Manual English (Stokoe, 1970a, b; Washington State School for the Deaf, 1972). Not included in this group are fingerspelling, which is a manual code for the letters of the alphabet, or Cued Speech, which is a manual code for the pronunciation of the phonemes of English (both discussed separately further in the chapter).

The proliferation of alternate names, e.g., Ameslish (Bragg, 1973), Siglish, etc., implies discrete languages to the uninitiated and is likely to be extremely confusing when attempting to choose a method of manual communication to use in an educational program (Woodward, 1974d). In the deaf community, there seems to be a dialect continuum (Moores, 1972, 1974; Woodward 1973a, b), with dialects of ASL at one end and dialects of Manual English at the other, because of the coexistence of ASL with the majority language, English. Woodward (1973d) has demonstrated that the intermediate dialects bear strong resemblance to pidgin languages on linguistic and sociolinguistic grounds. Pidgin languages are characterized by the fact that they are a partial mixture of two or more languages (in this case, ASL and English) but also contain reduced structures that are not common to any of the languages that they combine. Pidgins are not the native language of any group; their use is restricted to communicative necessities in certain environments (for example, at work) and not for socially integrative or expressive purposes. Pidgins are generally accompanied by negative attitudes toward their use (Woodward, 1974c). Woodward suggested that the naming situation could be simplified by using Sign for the American Sign Language (ASL, Ameslan) end of the continuum, (Manual) English for the other end (the parentheses indicating that the end of the signing continuum is Manual English but the end of the language continuum is English, spoken and written), and that Sign-English can be used for the intermediary forms (Ameslish, Signed English, Siglish). In spite of the variation, there are only two distinct language poles on the continuum—ASL and (a manual representation of) English; everything else partially overlaps, but is describable in terms of current variation theory (Woodward 1973a, b, c, d, 1974 a, b).

The linguistic consideration of American Sign Language (ASL or Ameslan) and several manual systems in this chapter concentrates on: 1) the linguistic structure of ASL and its formal definition as a language, 2) the similarities and differences of the linguistic structures of the several manual systems with respect to each other, to ASL, and to English, and 3) other psycholinguistic, sociolinguistic, and educational considerations that necessarily must enter into any decision to adopt a particular form of manual communication in an educational setting. The discussion relates primarily to the deaf, but many of the issues discussed are generalizable with appropriate modifications to other language disorders.

LINGUISTICS OF MANUAL LANGUAGES

Language

A primary cause of the controversy and the resultant hesitation to use manual communication in the education of the deaf is the confusion of *language* with *speech,* a confusion attributable to the fact that many people have only an obscure notion of what *language* is. Also involved is the failure to distinguish between verbal use of the hands (sign) and nonverbal use (gestures), again stemming from an imprecise understanding of the nature of language. It is necessary to consider why speech and language are not the same and why the title of this chapter distinguishes between manual languages and manual systems. It seems appropriate to start by considering some formal (linguistic) features of *language*.

Most animals have some method for communicating among themselves. Their "discussions" generally are, so far as is known, restricted to the topics of food, mating, emergency survival, and group cohesiveness. They do not discuss the weather, the state of the nation, yesterday's football game, or how to form past-tense verb forms. These may seem like trivial topics, but they reflect a difference in capability between animal and human forms of communication. Although it is, unfortunately, not possible to give a definition of *language* that all linguists would agree on, a number of basic criteria distinguish human language from animal communication. Four of the most important (Hockett, 1958) are creativity, language use, displacement, and language learning.

Creativity   Creativity refers to the fact that languages are not limited in either the number of possible sentences or the length of any sentence. New sentences may be produced by different combinations of lexical items and syntactic structures. Any sentence can be lengthened by combining it with another sentence using *and* or *but* (or others) or by adding modifiers to the noun or verb. Computer languages, talking parrots, bee dances, flag or smoke signals do not have creativity because they are limited to a small set of syntactic structures or lexical items. A parrot may learn a large number of sentences, with a variety of syntactic structures and different words, but it can only repeat the sentences that it has actually heard; it cannot take apart the sentences that it "knows" and make new ones that it has not heard and has never said before.

Language Use   Although many cultures and religions do not believe this, the relationship between a word and its meaning is essentially arbitrary. Language may be used independently of the objects it refers to. There is nothing about the word *white* that binds it to any physical object which is white, and no required relationship between the notion "white" and the way the word *white* is put together. In fact, this is the reason why the color "white" may be referred to by different names in different languages. There are usually a small number of words in a language that are not completely arbitrary with respect to their meaning. For example, *chug-chug* is a word that "sounds like" what it means. These words are called *onomatopoetic,* and their relationship to their meaning is more iconic than usual. Because words are generally arbitrary in meaning, new words can be made up (new inventions do not come prenamed, names are created for them), and the meanings of words are subject to changes. Consider how quickly words can become specialized in meaning, how quickly they become taboo or slang, how dialects differ, or how a particular word is used (*bucket/pail, soda/pop, bag/sack,* and so on).

Displacement   Because the meaning of words is essentially arbitrary, words can refer to objects and events that are not immediately present or do not even exist (e.g., *unicorns*). In this way, languages can be used to refer to things and events that are remote in time or space, so that with language people can: 1) report on the past and future, 2) communicate about communication, and 3) form hypotheses and lie (displacement). Bees cannot lie, parrots cannot decide whether a sentence they have just learned is ungrammatical or not, and questions like, "What shall we do tomorrow?," are outside the domain of known animal communication systems.

Language Learning   Another feature of language is the fact that the structures of language and the physiology of man are sufficiently universal that a speaker of one language can learn any other. People are capable of learning several languages, and young children learn language very easily and in a relatively short amount of time. Furthermore, a particular individual can be both sender and receiver of language.

Components   On a formal linguistic basis, languages are composed of several subcomponents. There must be a *syntactic* component that includes the rules for putting together new sentences. (Only certain combinations of words are grammatical in a particular language, so that each language has different sentence formation rules.) The syntactic component is in large part responsible for the infinite number of sentences required to meet the criterion of creativity. There also must be a *semantic* component, which includes words and their meanings and the special restrictions on their use. There is a *morphologic* component, which includes the rules for creating new words (derivational morphology) and for making tenses and plurals and marking other parts of speech (inflectional morphology). There is a *phonologic* component, which specifies the actual representation of words and word parts; e.g., the plural of nouns is [s] for words that end in voiceless stops, [z] for words that end in voiced stops, [əz] for words that end in fricatives.

With this very brief introduction to what is formally meant by *language,* it is now possible to look at ASL, the different manual systems that have been created for classroom use, and other forms of communication, such as fingerspelling and Cued Speech, and to compare them in terms of linguistic components.

American Sign Language as a Language

American Sign Language is the language used among deaf adults in the United States. It is not related to the sign language used by the American Indians (Kroeber, 1958) but is descended from Old French Sign. The French Abbé de l'Épée took the signs used by the deaf and expanded them, changed the syntax to parallel French, and used the signs in his school. Thomas Gallaudet studied at the school and, together with Laurent Clerc, brought signs to the United States. In 1817, they founded the American Asylum for the Education and Instruction of the Deaf and Dumb, now the American School for the Deaf in Hartford, Connecticut. The French signs combined with signs that were already in use by deaf adults in the United States, and American Sign Language has been on its own since, changing as do all natural languages (see further discussion below).

Sign language is occasionally mistaken as universal and, therefore, somehow tied to a basic set of human communicative gestures. This is not in fact the case. Different sign languages have different signs, different sign formation rules, and different sentence formation rules. There is no reason to expect that a user of American Sign Language will be any better at communicating with a user of Israeli Sign Language than a speaker of French with a speaker of Russian.

Syntatic Structures   The syntax of ASL contains a set of rules from which an infinite number of different sentences can be created. This means that it is not possible to memorize all the sentences of ASL or to learn all of the sentence "patterns." This is also true of other languages. Because ASL is descended from Old French Sign, its syntactic rules are quite different from English rules. A number of English constructions do not occur in ASL, thus leading people to conclude erroneously that ASL is not a language. Difficulties in representing signs by the use of English words have led people to believe that ASL is telegraphic, or simplified, or restricted. Again, it should be pointed out that these conclusions are drawn by people who are using English as their frame of reference, because it is their native language, and who are 1) erroneously equating *English* with *language,* and 2) translating what little they know of ASL into English.

As indicated, *language* can be defined formally, and English is only one example of it. Many languages do not pattern at all like English, and it is only when ASL is compared to languages of the world, rather than just English, that its status can be determined. Furthermore, it should be remembered that the problem of translating from one language to another has plagued linguists, interpreters, and book translaters for many years. It is a simple fact that certain words in one language do not have exact translations in another, and that when certain expressions are translated word for word into another language, the idiomatic meaning is completely lost. Because the syntax of ASL is different in many respects from English, it is unfortunate that traditional descriptions of it have to rely so heavily on comparisons to English (Fant 1972a).

For example, Fant (1972a) lists among the features of ASL syntax that it has no passive voice, no sign for the verb *to be,* and no determiners. This gives the impression that ASL is incomplete. A brief survey of the syntactic structures that are "missing" from ASL and that are also "missing" from other languages should illustrate the point. ASL does not have a passive: neither do Kwa (African) languages, Melanesian, Tzeltal, nor Thai. ASL has no special marking of gender on nouns: neither do Malagasy and Maori, to name just two. ASL marks the tense not on the verb, like English, nor necessarily on the sentence, like Walbiri and Luiseño, but on the conversation, so that tense is marked once and does not have to be marked again (although it *may* be) until the time reference is changed, as for example in Malay. ASL does not have articles to mark the definiteness or indefiniteness (*the* and *a/an*) of nouns: neither do Russian, Czech, Yoruba, Japanese, nor Hindi. But one is not tempted to suggest that the millions of people who speak Russian, Hindi, or any of the others are speaking a "less complete" language. Furthermore, the fact that a particular syntactic structure is missing from a language does not mean that the language does not have some other syntactic structure for conveying the meaning. One of the functions of the passive voice, for example, is to place emphasis on the object of the action by moving it to the front of the sentence. ASL has several mechanisms for indicating emphasis, including facial expression, repeating (reduplicating) the sign, and moving the hands more deliberately. These are discussed in greater detail below. The point is that, what needs to be indicated sequentially in auditory languages, by using markers and word order, often can be indicated simultaneously in ASL. This should be no more surprising than that some auditory languages use word order to indicate a particular meaning, others use markers, and still others use nothing. ASL then, has a syntax of its own, different from English, but not unlike other languages of the world. With these syntactic rules, and with the rules to create new signs to be discussed below, ASL has the capability of creating an infinite number of sentences, just like other languages.

Linguistic Rules   As indicated, one of the main features of *language* is that the relationship between the word and its referent is essentially arbitrary. One of the frequent criticisms of ASL is that it is "situation-bound," an inference that is drawn from the fact that a number of the more common signs look suspiciously similar to the objects or events that they are supposed to represent. Some signs do in fact look too iconic for comfort, and, most likely, many (but clearly not all) signs may have arisen initially as iconic gestures. Research on historical changes in signs (Frishberg, 1975) indicates that signs develop diachronically in such a way that arbitrariness is increased and iconicity decreased. In addition, signs may be distinguished from simple iconic gestures in that there are some very definite rules for how signs may be constructed in terms of hand configuration, motion, direction, and placement in space, whereas gestures are not subject to these rules (see below). It is important, then, to stress that these rules are *linguistic* rules which govern the formation of signs, and signs may look like the objects or events they represent only so long as they obey these structure rules. That these linguistic rules themselves are arbitrary may be seen by the fact that sign structure rules in other sign languages are different from those in ASL.

The question of the iconicity of signs is very important to some people because it is the basis of their opposition to the use of signing in the classroom. Bellugi (1975) undertook an extensive study of the iconicity of ASL to see to what extent signs really did "look suspiciously similar" to the objects or events they were supposed to represent. If signs really are iconic, a person unfamiliar with American Sign Language should be able to determine the meaning of a sign by looking at it or to give a reasonable approximation to the sign when given its meaning. Bellugi conducted her tests with normal hearing people unfamiliar with ASL. She used four types of tasks. In one, she presented signs and asked the hearing people to choose from several alternatives what the meaning for each sign was. In another task, she simply presented the signs and asked the people to guess the meaning. In the third task, she gave a meaning and asked the people to choose which of several signs belonged to that meaning. In the fourth task, she gave people a meaning and asked them to produce "what the sign would look like." The subjects did much worse on the open-ended tasks than on the multiple choice tasks, and their overall performance on all tasks indicated that the supposed "iconicity" of the signs did not provide them with many helpful clues to the relationship between the signs and their meanings. That their performance on the relatively constrained multiple choice tasks was not much better than chance supports the linguistic contention that the relationship between signs and their meanings is arbitrary in the same manner as that of words and their meanings. (For further discussion on iconicity, the reader is referred to Hoemann, 1975.)

Other Criteria   As for the other criteria for *language,* it can easily be seen that reporting on the past and future, communicating about communication, forming hypotheses and lying, as well as other displacement features, are part of ASL by simply watching conversations among deaf adults or between parent and child in which various topics are discussed. This is not, however, to indicate that it is a trivial consequence. There are language situations in which speakers use a language among themselves at home which is different from the one which they use to deal with speakers of another language in working situations, for example. The communication system used at work may be a conglomeration of words and reduced syntax from several languages. Such a situation might arise when the supervising personnel do not know the workers' language, and the workers know only a small portion of the supervisors' language. The resultant communication system is referred to as a "pidgin" and is not the language used to discuss the grammaticality of Junior's description of what he had for lunch. Thus, it is important to stress that ASL does in fact function as a complete language and fully meets the communicative needs of the deaf among themselves as a linguistic and sociologic community.

It also can readily be observed that a user of ASL can be both sender and receiver. Otherwise, communication would not be possible. In addition, speakers of oral languages can learn ASL. Hearing children of deaf parents are often bilingual in ASL and English. On the other hand, the deaf generally experience difficulty in learning English. It is possible that deaf users of ASL will always experience difficulty in learning English or any other second language unless they are taught first in their native language, ASL (Charrow and Wilbur, 1975). These issues are discussed more extensively below.

Notational Conventions

In order to talk about ASL, which is a visual language, in written English, this chapter adopts the following orthographic conventions. The names of sign are written in capital letters, SIGN. The name of a sign is roughly equivalent to the name of a letter; for example, the name of "h" is different from the sound to which it refers. The meaning, concept, idea, or object to which a sign refers is in quotes, "meaning." The English word or words that are used to translate the sign are italicized, *word*. In many cases, the "meaning" of a sign and its English *words* overlap, and only one is indicated. But it is possible for a single English *word* to have many "meanings," each of which may be represented by a different SIGN.

It should be pointed out that an orthographic system for ASL has been developed by Stokoe, Casterline, and Croneberg (1965), so that it is possible to write in ASL, although this system is generally used only by linguists and in the *Dictionary of American Sign Language* (Stokoe, Casterline, and Croneberg, 1965; for other dictionaries, see Bornstein and Hamilton, 1972). Because the orthographic system developed by Stokoe, Casterline, and Croneberg is somewhat cumbersome to use, and because of the variability with which signs may be transcribed by different researchers, Hoffmeister, Moores, and Ellenberger (1975) have established a set of principles to: 1) transcribe ASL using English glosses, and 2) to count morpheme units in ASL. The ability to count morpheme units allows researchers to calculate the mean length utterance (MLU), a measure used in describing child language acquisition. The Hoffmeister, Moores, and Ellenberger guidelines for counting morphemes will allow calculation of MLU for ASL acquisition studies; this in turn will allow direct comparisons of the acquisition of ASL with other languages.

Research on Sign Language

Syntax and Semantics   Research on the syntactic structure of American Sign Language began only recently with Stokoe (1960). For several years, research focused on the "phonology" ("cherology" (Stokoe, 1960)) of ASL until McCall (1965) attempted to write a generative grammar of it. However, the fact that certain features of

ASL syntax may be conveyed simultaneously rather than sequentially like auditory languages suggested that other approaches might be more profitable. Bellugi and her associates at the Salk Institute for Biological Studies studied ASL in a variety of different ways—acquisition, memory, processing, form and structure, and use. They began by comparing various aspects of spoken English and ASL. Comparisons of the rate of speaking and signing (Bellugi, 1972; Bellugi and Fischer, 1972) revealed that, when subjects were asked to relate a story in sign and in speech separately, the amount of time needed to relate the story in sign and speech was about the same, the number of propositions and the semantic ground covered in each mode was the same, but the modality made a difference: 50% more words than signs were used in the same amount of time, since words take considerably less time to make than signs. The information conveyed was the same. The situation is comparable to the difference between the English sentence, "It is illegal to drive on the left side of the road," (which takes 12 words) and the traffic sign WRONG WAY. (The implications of this study become important in the consideration of the relative benefits and drawbacks of the sign systems discussed below.)

Space is an important part of ASL. Most signs are made in a constrained area, the "sign space" (Bellugi and Fischer 1972; Battison, 1973; Frishberg, 1975). The sign space extends from just below the waist to the top of the head on the vertical axis while horizontally and laterally it forms a "bubble" (Lacy, 1974) in front of the speaker, extending from the speaker's extreme right to the speaker's extreme left (an arc of 180 degrees). The sign space may be proportionally enlarged for signing to larger audiences ("louder") or confined for purposes of more rapid signing or to be secretive ("quieter") so as not to be "overseen." Few signs are made over the head, behind the ear, or below the waist (Lacy, 1974). Bellugi (1972) reported the observation that, in a comparison of Manual English (an unspecified variety) and ASL, when signing was intended to parallel English, the signs were produced in a more compact space in front of the signer's body, whereas when ASL was signed, the signer used a larger signing space and included eye movements and body shifts. (The eye movements, facial expressions, and body shifts ("spatialization") are probably what gives ASL the look of pantomime to the casual observer).

Significantly, when ASL is signed, locations are established in space in such a way that the intended referents of the sentence are kept clear. Bellugi suggested that the establishment of these locations in space serves an important grammatical function (rather than some esthetic visual function). Because signs move through space as they are made, the notions of "subject," "object," and other grammatical and semantic markers can be incorporated into a sign by allowing a verb sign to move from the location of the subject of the verb to the location of the object of the verb. In this way, in a single motion the subject-verb-object can be conveyed unambiguously. Locating these markers in space allows for economy of expression and takes advantage of people's reasonably good memory for locations (Norman, 1969).

   Pronouns   Lacy (1974) has made an extended study of the parameters involved in the use of the sign space for pronominal reference. Although certain pronouns in ASL may appear as random pointing gestures to those who have not learned the language, Lacy (1974, 1975) reported that each gesture establishes a particular point in space where the referent of that pronoun may be assumed to be found for the remainder of the conversation unless otherwise indicated (by a verb of motion, perhaps). Personal pronouns are placed in space according to several general rules. The center of the front of the signer is used for second person referent (*you*) for referring to the addressee. The 1st third person pronoun referent is made to the right of the signer, the 2nd third person referent is made to the left of the signer (Friedman, 1975), and the space is evenly divided if possible for greater numbers of referents (see Figure 1). Alternate linear strat-

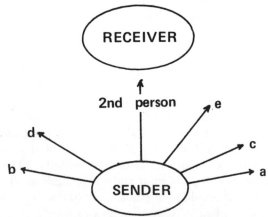

Figure 1. Approximate positioning of pronoun referents in space. *a*, first 3rd person referent; *b*, second 3rd person referent; *c*, third 3rd person referent; etc.

egies for dividing the space also have been observed (Kegl, 1976). In addition: "When the person referred to is in the vicinity, one points directly to that person rather than to an arbitrary index" (Kegl and Chinchor, 1975, p. 93).

With this strategy available, a theoretically infinite number of pronominal references can be unambiguously made. (Practically speaking, the number is constrained by memory limitations and visual perceptual limitations (Siple, 1973).) Thus, although the sentence, *Bob yelled at Bill and then he slapped him,* is ambiguous in English (and problematic for many linguistic theories), in ASL there would be no ambiguity. Bob, as the 1st third person referent, would be located in space to the signer's right, and Bill, as the 2nd third person referent, would be located to the signer's left. The direction of formation of the sign for SLAP would indicate whether *Bob slapped* Bill (right to left) or *Bill slapped Bob* (left to right) (Agent-Beneficiary Incorporation).

Furthermore, Lacy (1975) reported that the point in space which locates each pronoun referent is sufficiently well defined in three-dimensional space that, once the signer establishes the location, other members of the conversation will direct their sign so that a line extending from the end of the index finger will (more or less) pass through the point location in space of the intended referent.

Time and Space   Friedman's (1973) study also reported that there are similar possibilities and constraints on the use of space to indicate temporal and spatial relationships. A time line exists such that the space more or less parallel to the side of the body indicates present tense, the space forward of the body indicates future, and the space behind the body indicates past. When simply indicating tense, this line is placed alongside the head, roughly at the bottom of the ear. However, indications of tense can be incorporated into some signs (YEAR, MONTH, WEEK, for example) such that a motion is made in the proper direction (forward for NEXT MONTH, backward for LAST MONTH). The use of space to represent spatial relationships is not purely iconic, as some might suspect. For example, to indicate a distance far away from the signer, one does *not* simply extend the arm fully in the proper direction to indicate distance. Instead, the same type of pointing gesture used for pronominal reference is used, but rather than being directed along a line parallel to the floor, the sign is elevated several degrees; the greater the distance, the greater the angle the sign makes with the floor (up to but not including 90 degrees) (see also Frishberg and Gough, 1973b).

Juncture and Stress   In ASL, as in other languages, there are markers (junctures) that indicate the beginning and end of a conversation, sentence, phrase, or word (Covington, 1973a; Baker, 1975). These junctures are marked by certain hand movements and facial expressions. For example, Baker (1975) reported that there are several positions of the hands relevant to conversational turn-taking. When a signer is listening and not intending to take a turn, the hands remain at full rest, generally below the waist in the lap or at the sides with arms at full extension. When a signer is preparing to sign, perhaps to interrupt or simply waiting for a turn but wanting the person presently signing to acknowledge that he is waiting, the hands assume half-rest position, generally at waist level and with increased body tension (possibly a slight lean forward). Hands higher than this are in quarter-rest position, a strong indication to the current signer to yield the floor. The floor is yielded by returning hands to full-rest position or maybe to half-rest as an indication of wanting the floor back as soon as possible.

A conversation begins with direct eye contact between signer and addressee. This is necessary to ensure that the addressee is attending to the signer. During the conversation, the addressee must continue to watch the signer, but the signer need not maintain eye contact with the addressee. As in oral conversation, the sender is free to look away, for purposes of organizing thought or to maintain the floor, but must check back with the addressee every so often to be certain that the addressee is following the conversation. A signer can ignore an interruption by not establishing eye contact with the person attempting to interrupt.

In careful signing, an extremely slight pause between signs marks the end of one sign and the beginning of another. If the second sign is made in a different location than the first, the hands are moved to the new location before the second sign is made. In more rapid or casual signing, the pause (juncture) may be omitted, and the formation of the second sign may begin while the hands are still in the location of the first sign. The same slight pause may occur between two fingerspelled words or between syllables within a fingerspelled word.

A longer pause indicates the end of a sentence or clause and serves to separate sentences or clauses that otherwise might run together ambiguously (Grosjean and Lane, 1976).

A special facial expression is used to mark questions. This expression is marked by raised eyebrows and head tilted up, back, and often to one side. This facial expression is *sufficient* to mark a question; no other syntactic indication is needed, although other markers are available.

The stress on a sign is a function of meaning; it affects the "clearness" of the formation of the sign. Extremely weak stress may cause a sign, or fingerspelled letter, to be so slurred that it may be missed by a nonnative observer (Covington, 1973b). Stronger stress results in greater tension in the hands while forming the sign, with a more careful formation of the handshape, clearer and possibly longer duration of the motion, and a sharper or longer impact with the body. Moderately stressed signs may have loosely formed handshapes, only partial motion, and may not actually reach the point of contact with the body (if there is a point of contact). To indicate greater stress, the head and whole body may lean into or away from the formation of the sign. These modifications are analogous to processes that affect articulation of words in oral languages, i.e., more careful production under stressed conditions.

Stress in ASL serves the same functions as in other languages— to differentiate the topic from comments about it and to differentiate degrees of indifference, excitement, disagreement, importance, and emphasis.

Verbs   The verb system of any language forms the core of each and every utterance. Fischer (1973) and Fischer and Gough (1975) provide a detailed analysis of the verb system of ASL. Fischer (1973) reported on the use of reduplication (repetition of all or part of a form) in ASL. Verbs can be divided into Stative (*appear, seem, be, looks like,* etc.) and Non-Stative (Active), which can be further subdivided into Durative (*sleep, talk, eat*) and Non-Durative (*kill, find, win*). These divisions are semantic in nature and therefore should be appropriately differentiated in every language. In ASL, stative verbs must be reduplicated quickly while non-stative verbs can be reduplicated slowly or quickly. Slow reduplication of a non-durative verb is interpreted to mean that the action was *iterated* (*kept on Xing and Xing and Xing,* as in *eating and eating and eating*), whereas slow reduplication of a durative verb indicates that the action was *continued* (*Xed for a long time,* as in *talked for a long time*). In addition, a slowly reduplicated verb can be "rocked" ("a rhythmic movement of the body forward and back in time to the circular motion" of the reduplicated verb), in which case the sign is interpreted as meaning *too much X*. Fast reduplicated forms usually indicate a type of plural. If the reduplication is accompanied by a horizontal sweeping motion, the sign is interpreted as having either a plural subject or a plural object, each of which does *X*. Fast reduplication without horizontal movement is interpreted as *habitually does X*. In this way, the speed of reduplication, the rocking motion or absence of it, and the presence or absence of horizontal sweeping of hands can be used to indicate various semantic relationships.

Fischer and Gough (1975) investigated various linguistic properties of verbs as they are reflected in ASL. Included in their study were:

1.   Strict subcategorization: whether a verb takes an object, prepositional phrase, verbal complement, and other syntactic categories

2.   Selectional restrictions: semantic constraints on the subject, object, type of preposition, complement, etc.

3.   Directionality: whether the sign moves between subject and object—Agent-Beneficiary Incorporation

4.   Incorporation of location: whether the sign is produced closer to the place of formation of its subject or object or indirect object, if any

5.   Reversibility: whether the sign changes the orientation of the hand depending on its subject, object, etc.

6.   Incorporation of size or shape: changes in the movement or hand configuration to indicate physical features of the subject, object, etc.

7.   Incorporation of manner: whether the sign changes in speed or intensity to indicate the manner in which the action is performed

8.   Incorporation of number: fast reduplication with horizontal movement, possibly with the relevant number of fingers extended to indicate how many were involved in the action

9.   Habitual: fast reduplication, no horizontal movement

10.   Continuous: slow reduplication

11.   Reciprocal: whether the verb can (or must) take two arguments (subject and object) that perform the action on each other

12.   Reflexive: if the sign adjusts to reflect the difference between I-X-MYSELF and SOMEONE-X-ME in terms of the object of the action)

All languages have strict subcategorization and selectional restrictions. The remaining features are unique to visual languages. The acceptability of the various options that are open to each verb depends on semantic and formational constraints. For example, verbs that can be both directional and reversed are usually two-handed, symmetrical signs (HATE, BORROW, FEED), while those that can incorporate directionality and location tend to be two-handed signs in which the nondominant hand does not move. The nondominant hand serves as a base for the formation of the sign and can be placed in the proper locational area to incorporate location, while the dominant hand that moves incorporates the directionality of the sign. Signs that involve touching a portion of the body cannot generally undergo any of the possible modifications. If a verb is normally signed with a vertical movement, it cannot incorporate directionality or reversibility, but it can incorporate location. Other such constraints exist on the allowable adjustments on the formation of the signs, all of which serve to differentiate signing from hand-waving gestures (also see Frishberg and Gough, 1973a; Lacy, 1973).

Formational Constraints   Stokoe (1960) investigated the structure of sign formation, treating it as analogous to the structure of the phonologic system of oral languages. He defined three parameters that were realized simultaneously in the formation of a particular sign: TAB, DEZ, and SIG. The TAB is the place within the sign space that a sign is made. (For possible values of these parameters and the symbols used to represent them in the orthography developed for ASL, see Stokoe, Casterline, and Croneberg (1965) or Moores (1974).) Most of the TAB's are on or very near a specific place on the signer's body. DEZ refers to the hand configuration used to form the sign. These include several configurations taken from the ASL alphabet and the nine digits of the number system. The DEZ is indicated for the active hand or hands (in the case where both hands move). SIG is the parameter used to indicate motion, e.g., circular, side-to-side, sharp contact, etc. A fourth parameter, ORIENTATION, which refers to the orientation of the palm, was added later by Battison (1973; Battison, Markowicz, and Woodward, 1973).

In oral languages, parameters such as these (distinctive features) are simultaneously combined to produce consonantal and vocalic segments. Analogously, the four parameters are produced simultaneously to form signs. In oral languages, physical constraints make impossible some combinations of parameters. For example, a vowel cannot at the same time be both *high* and *low*. Other combinations are not possible on purely linguistic grounds. A number of redundancy conditions have been described for combinations of sign parameters. Adherence to these conditions defines a possible sign, whereas violations are considered impossible signs. Some of these may be attributable to constraints placed on the visual mode by perceptual mechanisms, while others may be linguistically arbitrary. Battison, Markowicz, and Woodward (1973) gave several examples. Some signs involve two sequential contacts with the body. If the body is divided into four major parts—head and neck, trunk, arm, and hand—then only the combinations summarized in Table 1 are permissible for the first and second contacts. In addition, the second contact is constrained to a centralized position in the major contact area, so that a sign may go from head to center chest, but not from head to either shoulder or to a corner or side of the trunk. A constraint such as this, not required by physical limitations, although possibly an aid to perception, distinguishes signs linguistically from pantomime.

In discussing reduplication in ASL (reduplication being the meaningful repetition of a sign two or more times), Fisher (1973) distinguished two modes of reduplication, fast and slow, and two suprasegmental features that may co-occur optionally with these, a horizontal sweeping movement and a rhythmic rocking of the body. She noted that fast reduplication cannot co-occur with rocking, and that slow reduplication cannot co-occur with the horizontal sweeping movement. Fischer wrote the following rules to account for the situation:

1. Verb $— — — \rightarrow$ [+Redup]
2. [+Redup] $— — — \rightarrow$ [±Fast]
3. [−Fast] $— — — \rightarrow$ [±Rocking]
4. [+Fast] $— — — \rightarrow$ [±Horizontal]

Rule 4, for example, says that a verb sign that is made with fast reduplication may or may not have horizontal sweeping motion, and also (by omission) implies that fast reduplication with a rocking motion is not allowed.

Battison (1974) described two further constraints, those related to signs formed with both hands. Basically, there are three types of two-handed signs: 1) both hands move independently; 2) only one hand moves but both handshapes are identical; and 3) only one hand moves (the dominant one) and the handshape of the nondominant,

Table 1. Permissible contacts with the body for double-contact signs[a]

First contact	Second contact			
	Head	Trunk	Arm	Hand
Head	+	+	+	+
Trunk	−	+	−	+
Arm	−	−	+	−
Hand	+	−	−	+

Based on Battison, Markowicz, and Woodward, 1975.

[a]+ indicates an acceptable sequence, − indicates an unacceptable sequence.

nonmoving hand is restricted to one of a limited set of the possible handshapes. For the signs where both hands move, a Symmetry Condition exists, specifying that the handshapes and movement for both hands must be identical and that the orientations and movements of both hands must be identical or polar opposites (mirror image). For two-handed signs in which the handshapes are not identical (3 above), a Dominance Condition exists, specifying that the nondominant hand must remain static while the dominant hand produces the sign. Furthermore, the nondominant hand can assume only one of the six most unmarked handshapes. The unmarked handshapes include:

1. The A-hand: a closed fist
2. The B-hand: the flat palm
3. The 5-hand: the palm with fingers spread
4. The G-hand: fist with the index finger extended
5. The C-hand: hand formed in a semicircle
6. The O-hand: fingertips meet with the thumb, forming a circle

Battison pointed out that these six handshapes are considered the least marked because they are found in all other sign languages studied to date, they are maximally distinct formationally and perceptually, and they are among the first acquired by children learning the language (Boyes, 1973). "Signs with two active hands must be symmetrical and signs which have different handshapes can only have one active hand. In these cases, a relative complexity in one part of the sign (two hands vs. one hand moving; different handshapes vs. identical ones) is counteracted by a reduction in complexity somewhere else (symmetry; one hand remains still)" (Battison 1974, p. 20) (also see Lane, Boyes-Braem, and Bellugi, in press).

Wit and Poetry   The strictures that exist on the formation of possible signs are linguistic and not physiologic. Clearly, it is possible for two hands to move along different paths simultaneously (although it is often difficult, e.g., rubbing your stomach while patting your head). The nonuse of all the possible formational combinations provides a reservoir from which puns, rhymes, and art-signs (poetry and song) may be made (Klima and Bellugi, 1975). Klima and Bellugi challenged Tervoort's (1961) claim that, "the spontaneous use of signs in an ironical or metaphorical way is rare to non-existent," and investigated the manipulation of signs for creative purposes. They pointed out that, for a pun to exist, the signers must be aware of the homonymity (or near homonymity) of two signs, and that there are many such pairs that can be used. In addition to puns, there are several types of sign-play that can be made along principles that are unique to sign language itself. Klima and Bellugi listed three basic processes that can be used: 1) the overlapping of two signs, 2) the blending of two signs, and 3) the substitution of one regular formational parameter (TAB (place), DEZ (hand configuration), SIG (motion), or ORIENTATION). Overlapping of two signs is possible because there are two hands that move independently, and, although different simultaneous motions are disallowed by the Symmetry Condition in "straight signing," for more creative purposes two signs can be produced simultaneously.

For example, to indicate mixed feelings (about taking a new job), Klima and Bellugi cited the signs for EXCITED and DE-PRESSED, produced simultaneously. Both signs are normally two-handed and are related formationally in that they differ only in the direction of motion, DEPRESSED moving down the chest, EXCITED moving up. Thus, to produce both at once, one hand moves down while the other simultaneously moves up. Another way to overlap signs is to form one with one hand and hold the hand in that position while the other hand forms another sign. A third possible way is to start with a two-handed sign, hold one hand in that position, and make another sign with the other hand. These combinations are most effective when the differences between the two signs are minimal, when they use the same handshape, or when the place of formation of the first is the starting point of the second. Blending of signs can be accomplished by combining the hand configuration of one sign with the movement and place of formation of another sign. This often occurs with name signs. Name signs are ordinarily made by using the handshape corresponding to the fingerspelled first letter of the name and then choosing some meaningful location and movement for that hand configuration. For example, the handshape S (for Shelley) is combined with the location and motion of the sign WINK to refer to Shelley Lawrence, whose eye winks frequently.

The systematic substitution of one of the parameters of a sign is a planned effort to change the meaning of the sign in a recognizable way. The results are signs that do not violate any of the constraints on signs, and thus are possible but not actual signs of the language. Klima and Bellugi illustrated several types, including change in the hand configuration (using the little finger to make the sign for UNDERSTAND instead of the normally used index finger, the little finger changing the meaning from UNDERSTAND to UNDERSTAND–a little), changes in orientation (signing NEW YORK (city) with the dominant hand underneath the nondominant hand to indicate "underhanded" NEW YORK), changes in movement (signing UNDERSTAND with the reverse motion—rather than snapping the index finger open from a closed fist, the index finger starts extended and shuts into a closed fist; to indicate DON'T UNDERSTAND, DON'T UNDERSTAND in straight signing would be indicated by NEGATIVE UNDERSTAND, two separate signs), and changes in location (to indicate a bruised eye that was swollen shut, one signer signed "My eye is deaf" by moving the sign DEAF from its normal location across the cheek to a location across the eye).

In their analysis of poetry dramatized in ASL, rather than just translated from English or "straight signed," Klima and Bellugi reported three major types of poetic structure. These are: 1) internal poetic structure, 2) external poetic structure, and 3) external kinetic structure. Internal poetic structure refers to the tendency to alliterate with the same or similar handshapes, thus modifying the actual sign to fit into the poetic line, and also to the actual choice of signs themselves. In addition, some two-handed signs are modified so that they are made single-handedly, a fact that figures into the external poetic structure. External poetic structure refers to the style of presentation of the signs, rather than their actual choice. Klima and Bellugi reported a tendency to create a balance between the two hands, by alternating hands while signing (not usually done in straight signing) and eliminating the traditional dominant hand. Because both hands can be used independently in art-sign, signs can be overlapped or blended as discussed above. The effects of this are a smoother flow of movement during the poem, with a greater continuity between signs because the transitions between signs have been softened (the nondominant hand does not drop to the side for a one-handed sign since the hands alternate in signing, both hands are active, signs are blended, etc). External kinetic structure can be seen in the greater movement through the signing space that is made during poetic signing.

This analysis of poetry and wit by Klima and Bellugi reveals that the "violations" of the Symmetry Condition, and the use of alternating hands, the lack of the traditional dominant hand, and the unrestricted use of the signing space, all combine to provide a mechanism for art-sign with the language of ASL. This art-sign is not parasitic on English or any other spoken language and represents the creative use of language that is expected in every language and culture.

Memory   In oral languages, it has been determined that the several features constituting a sound segment are a crucial part of the memory coding and recall system even when the material to be recalled is presented visually (printed word lists) (Conrad, 1962; Wickelgren, 1965). Bellugi and Siple (1971) investigated memory for signs in deaf people. They found that, whereas hearing people tend to make mistakes based on the phonologic properties of the words they hear or see, deaf people make mistakes based on the formational properties of the signs themselves. This finding held regardless of whether the deaf people were asked to sign their responses or to write the English word equivalents of the signs they were supposed to remember. For example, given the word *tea,* a hearing person might mistakenly recall it as *key* because they sound similar. A deaf person, however, might mistakenly recall the sign TEA as the sign VOTE, a sign that differs from TEA only in motion. Bellugi and Siple (1971) found that mistakes were made according to handshape, place of formation, and motion. They did not investigate orientation. Thus, at least three of the four parameters that are used to describe the formation of signs have been demonstrated to be relevant to memory in the deaf.

Other studies (Conrad and Rush, 1965; Conrad 1970, 1971, 1972, 1973; Locke, 1970; Locke and Locke, 1971) have investigated the role of phonemic, iconic visual, and dactylic (fingerspelling) coding in memory in the deaf but have not specifically attended to the possible role of sign features. Wilbur (1974a) suggested that, because hearing people convert visually presented written material to its phonologic representation for coding and storage, perhaps deaf people who know ASL utilize it in the coding and recall of written English, converting the English to a sign representation much as a compound bilingual might do. Some support for this hypothesis comes from a study by Odom, Blanton, and McIntyre (1970). They compared recall accuracy by deaf and hearing subjects on two lists of printed English words—those for which there is an exact ASL equivalent and those for which there is no exact convenient sign and thus would have to be fingerspelled. The results were as hypothesized: The deaf subjects performed significantly better on the list of signable words, while of course there was no difference between the two lists for hearing subjects. Even more interesting, however, was the fact that the performance of the deaf subjects on the list of signable words was superior to the performance of the hearing subjects on both lists (suggesting signs as an aid to learning). The data are entirely too scanty for firm conclusions to be drawn yet. However, in light of the role that sign features may play in memory coding and recall, it seems reasonable to suggest that the strict constraints on the possible combinations of parameters serve to reduce the amount of independent information conveyed to the visual perception and memory systems at any one time. (Also see Conlin, 1972.)

Historical Changes in ASL   The general linguistic constraints discussed above are also reflected in historical changes that some signs have undergone. Descriptions of signs are available from as early as 1827. Significant changes can be seen in signs in the relatively short time since Long (1918). Frishberg (1975) reported that changes in signs over time increase the symmetry of the sign (to conform with the Symmetry Condition), and the fluidity of the sign (the actual production of the sign as well as the transition from one part of a compound sign to the other). Furthermore, the place of formation of many has moved to a more central location in the area in which it is made, and the formation of signs that previously required facial expression, body or head movement has changed so that the meaning is conveyed mostly by the hands alone. The use of facial expression in modern signing is analogous to intonation in spoken languages; it conveys question, uncertainty, affirmation, negation, etc., and can be used in connection with a single sign or with an entire signed sentence. The net result of the signs becoming symmetrical, smoothed, centralized, and localized formationally in the hands is that the signs have become less iconic and more arbitrary. Frishberg (1974) reported on changes in signs that parallel language change processes in oral languages, and Fischer (1975) reported on changes in the order of signs in sentences, indicating that ASL syntax has made some adjustments to English word order.

It is important to emphasize that these changes have occurred naturally in the course of the language's history, motivated by whatever processes motivate changes in languages, not by deliberate decisions. This fact becomes important in considering the sign systems currently being used in the educational setting.

Acquisition of ASL   One of the defining characteristics of language is that it is acquired spontaneously by children who are exposed to it. Studies of the acquisition of ASL (Bellugi and Klima, 1972; Boyes-Braem, 1973; McIntire, 1974; Wilbur and Jones, 1974) indicate that children learning ASL pass through developmental stages similar to those involved in the acquisition of an oral language. Bellugi and Klima (1972) and Wilbur and Jones (1974) reported on the emergence of syntax in ASL acquisition. Both studies reported that, in the early stages, the full range of semantic relations found in children learning an oral language (Bloom, 1970) is also found in children acquiring ASL. This is not unexpected because semantic relations reflect more on the universal nature of man and his world than on the syntax in which these relations are expressed. The developmental nature of the acquisition of ASL means that the first language-processing strategies which are active in a child up until about puberty are exercised at the appropriate time in the child's development, a fact that becomes important in the later discussion of the psychoeducational considerations of choosing to use manual communication in the home or school.

Developmental stages are also seen in the acquisition of the signs themselves. That is, there are "baby" signs which occur, analogous to baby-talk. Boyes-Braem (1973) and McIntire (1974) traced the development of the hand configuration in young deaf children. McIntire (1975) reported that there are four stages. The factors which affect these stages (Boyes-Braem, 1973) are: 1) opposition of the thumb, 2) extension of one or more fingers, and 3) contact of a finger with the thumb. In the first stage, only one of the hand configurations requires a finger to make contact with the thumb. At this initial stage, the child can produce the hand configurations for the number 5, the letters S, L, A, G, and C, and what is called "baby O," in which an O is made only with the thumb and index finger rather than with all the fingers. (This does not mean that the child can fingerspell at this stage. These handshapes are involved in the formation of many signs.)

The second, third, and fourth stages include handshapes which involve touching the thumb to a finger, or more than one of the factors previously mentioned. Stage 2 includes B, F, and adult O. Stage 3 includes I, Y, D, P, 3, V, H, and W, some of which include extension of the weaker fingers. The fourth stage includes 8, 7, X, R, T, M, N, and E, some of which involve crossing fingers.

The relationship of the acquisition of spoken language to the acquisition of ASL is of considerable interest. There are three comparisons that have been made so far. One is the emergence of the first sign compared to the emergence of the first word. Although further documentation is needed, a deaf child's first sign may emerge 2 to 3 months earlier than a hearing child's first spoken word (Boyes-Braem, 1973; McIntire, 1974; Wilbur and Jones, 1974). In hearing children of deaf parents, the child's first sign may emerge several months before the same child's first spoken words (Wilbur and Jones, 1974). In addition, the child's spoken vocabulary complements his sign vocabulary, with only a small overlap of words that are both spoken and signed (Wilbur and Jones, 1974). This indicates that the child is not simply learning spoken words to correspond to signs already known, nor signs to correspond to spoken words already known. One further comparison is that of vocabulary size. McIntire (1974) reported a vocabulary of about 20 signs at age 10 months, the age at which a hearing child is likely to produce his first word. McIntire (1975) also reported two-sign utterances at 10 months (two-word utterances generally begin at 18 months in spoken language) and three-sign utterances at 18 months. The earlier emergence and growth of signs may be attributable to greater control of the hand muscles than of the oral muscles. In addition, a sign is completely visible whereas only parts of words (labial and some dental) may be seen. The early emergence also suggests that children are capable of greater linguistic capabilities than current psycholinguistic theories give them credit for. (Also see Lacy, 1972a, b.)

Dialectal Variation   As mentioned earlier, there exists a continuum ranging from ASL at one pole to (Manual) English at the other. The preceding discussions deal with ASL as though it were a single unified language; in fact, like other languages, it has several dialects of its own. These dialects have been extensively studied (Woodward 1972, 1973a, b, c, d, 1974a, b, c, d; Woodward and Erting, 1975; Woodward and Markowicz, 1975). Aside from geographic factors, it has been found that variation in lects is significantly correlated with four variables: 1) whether or not the signer is deaf, 2) whether or not the signer's parents are deaf, 3) whether or not the signer has had some college, and 4) whether or not the signer learned to sign before the age of 6 years. In a study of the occurrence of three syntactic rules— Agent-Beneficiary Incorporation, Negative Incorporation, and Verb Reduplication—Woodward found that there were lects that had none of the three rules and were thus most English-like, and that the rules were implicationally ordered such that a lect with Agent-Beneficiary Incorporation also necessarily had Negative Incorporation and Verb Reduplication, a lect with Negative Incorporation also necessarily had Verb Reduplication (but not Agent-Beneficiary Incorporation), and a lect with a Verb Reduplication did not necessarily have either of the other two rules. A lect with all three rules can be considered more ASL-like than a lect with two, which in turn is more ASL-like than a lect with only one, which again is more ASL-like than a lect with none of the three rules. Such lectal variation is also found in oral languages (Bailey, 1971) (see also Markowicz, 1972).

LINGUISTICS OF MANUAL SYSTEMS

It already has been indicated that ASL is quite different from English. It is argued below that the manual English systems are not only quite different from ASL but also quite different from English in ways which have only recently begun to attract attention (Allen, 1975; Charrow 1975b).

True simultaneous communication in ASL and spoken English is very difficult to accomplish. It is for this reason that manual systems have been created, so that signing and speech can readily parallel each other. The term *system* has been used consistently throughout to refer to several manual methods that have been developed for educational purposes but are not currently used as the home language by large groups of deaf people. A manual system is formally different in structure and function from both English and ASL, and it is the intended implication of the chapter title that the systems are not languages in the same sense that ASL is.

It also should be clear that the systems are not simply "taking the signs of ASL and putting them in English word order;" they are eliminating much of the flexibility of the signs that the users of ASL are accustomed to producing and perceiving (e.g., reduplication, Agent-Beneficiary Incorporation, etc.). The systems were not designed to parallel ASL, however; they were created on the basic assumption that, if the signs are used in an English-like manner (endings, word order), they would be more effective in teaching English than ASL would be. This basic assumption is dubious. The parallel in auditory languages would be to put Swahili words into English word order in order to better teach English to the Swahili speakers. If Swahili words in English word order were being used by the teacher, the Swahili speakers would not understand what the teacher was saying. The distortion of Swahili forms to English inflectional systems would further complicate the issue. Because ASL is not related to English historically, there is no reason to suppose that similar adjustments to ASL make it any better as a teaching medium than ASL all by itself. In addition, a child in school who learns some of the basic principles of the systems discussed below may have difficulty communicating beyond a simple level with either users of ASL or users of any of the other systems.

Probably the most important point with respect to the preceding and following discussions is that, no matter what the linguistic drawbacks of any of the systems are, there is strong evidence (Quigley, 1969; Moores, 1974; Brasel and Quigley, 1975) that manual communication in any form is itself a more effective teaching medium than straight oral approaches. For further discussion of these studies, see the latter part of this chapter on *Practical Considerations*. The point here is that there is no evidence currently to distinguish the relative benefits of any of the different systems themselves.

History

The first English-based system developed was Systematic Sign Language. The system was the result of work by Sir Richard Paget (1951), and, after his death, Grace Paget and Pierre Gorman in England. Paget was the first to delineate several basic modifications for making sign closer to spoken language. These included the following criteria: 1) each sign should represent an English word or part of an English word; 2) signs should be ordered in the same order as spoken words are; 3) signs should be inflected (endings, etc.) to reflect the inflections in spoken words; and 4) signs should be adapted to form a small, basic vocabulary for initial use (Bornstein, 1973).

The first system in the United States was developed by David Anthony (1966, 1971), who was interested in producing a simplified system to use with deaf retardates. Anthony's original system grew into Seeing Essential English, from which Linguistics of Visual English (Wampler, 1971, 1972) and Signing Exact English (Gustason, Pfetzing, and Zawolkow, 1972) were subsequently developed. Manual English was developed by the Total Communication Program at the Washington State School for the Deaf (1972), utilizing many of the principles and basic assumptions of the other systems, with differences that are noted below. Signed English includes several people's work (Fant, 1964; Bornstein et al., 1972; O'Rourke, 1973; Watson, 1973; Bornstein et al., 1975). The version of Signed English developed by Bornstein et al. (1973) is primarily aimed at meeting the communication needs of the preschool child. Bornstein et al. (1975) extends Signed English to the elementary school child.

Relationship Between Manual Systems and English

In this section, the systems are discussed with respect to the following questions: 1) What are the general principles that have been set forth for the use of the system? 2) How do these principles compare with those of English? With ASL? 3) What are the potential problems of these principles, in particular, when are they inconsistent, counter-intuitive, etc.?

The creators of each system believed that their system faithfully reflected the structure of English in a visual mode. Because English is a spoken language, many arbitrary decisions have to be made as to how to translate spoken English into signed English. It may be said of all the systems as a group that they follow English word order. But they diverge with respect to the structure of signs and the creation of new signs (sign "phonology" and morphology) (see Table 2), and the amount of permissible fingerspelling. Each system has made a different set of arbitrary decisions regarding the formation and use of signs.

The formation of past tense verbs provides an illustration of these arbitrary decisions. In English, verbs can be divided into those that form their past tense by a regular rule and those that are in some way irregular. The regular past tense rule is to add the suffix -ed to the verb (talk-talked). The irregular verbs can be subdivided into several groups. There are those for which the past tense is the same as the present, e.g., hit-hit; those that display internal vowel changes, e.g., meet-met; those that have vowel changes in both the past tense and past participle, e.g., ring-rang-rung; others that use -ought or -aught, e.g., fight-fought, catch-caught; and, of course, a few for which

Table 2. Characteristics of different manual systems

System	Author(s)	Use of ASL signs	Use of fingerspelling	Basic morphologic principle(s)
Systematic Sign	Paget (1951) Paget and Gorman (1968)	No	Only for proper names	One meaning–one sign
Seeing Essential English (SEE I)	Anthony (1966, 1971)	For the most part	Some	Two-out-of-three: sound, meaning, and spelling
Signing Exact English (SEE II)	Gustason, Pfetzing, and Zawolkow (1972)	Same as SEE I	Same as SEE I	Same as SEE I
Linguistics of Visual English	Wampler (1971, 1972)	Same as SEE I	Same as SEE I	Same as SEE I
Manual English	Washington State School for the Deaf (1972)	Yes	More than SEE	Variable: one meaning–one sign; some same as SEE I
Signed English	Bornstein et al. (1973, 1975) Fant (1964) Watson (1973) O'Rourke (1973)	Yes	Yes; variable amounts	To string together ASL signs with fingerspelling and some conjunction signs

the past tense does not resemble the present tense at all, e.g., *go-went*. The differences are all reflections of changes that occurred earlier in the history of the English language.

There are numerous possible ways in which a sign system can deal with the past tenses of English verbs. One way is to sign all of the verbs in the same way. For example: 1) sign the present tense sign followed by the ASL PAST sign (*talked* = TALK + PAST, *came* = COME + PAST), or 2) sign the present tense sign followed by another past tense marker such as fingerspelled 'D' (*talked* = TALK + D, *came* = COME + D). Another approach is to divide the verbs into regular and irregular, and use one past tense marker for the regular verbs and another for the irregular verbs. Several ways of doing this are: 3) sign the present tense sign plus the ASL PAST for the regular verbs and another marker, perhaps fingerspelled 'D' for the irregular verbs (*talked* = TALK + PAST, *came* = COME + D); 4) the opposite of 3 (*talked* = TALK + D, *came* = COME + PAST); 5) sign the present tense plus PAST marker for the regular verbs and use new signs for the irregular verbs (*talked* = TALK + PAST, *came* = CAME); 6) sign the present tense plus PAST for the regular verbs and fingerspell the irregular verbs (*talked* = TALK + PAST, *came* = C + A + M + E); 7) and 8) same as 5 or 6 but using 'D' for the regular verbs.

So far, the irregular verbs all have been treated as one class. It is of course possible to subdivide them into smaller groups, along the same lines that they are divided in English. Furthermore, all of the above possibilities can be combined in various combinations with initialized signs. Initialized signs are signs that incorporate the fingerspelling of the first letter of their English translation, such as *employment* = WORK (made with an E hand), *job* = WORK (made with a J hand), *duty* = WORK (made with a D hand).

The logical possibilities have not been exhausted, but it should be clear from the above examples that the manner in which past tenses are treated is more or less an arbitrary decision made by the creator of the system. There is nothing about the structure of English or signs that would force someone to choose any one or any combination of the above possibilities. It can be said that, because English irregular verbs are subdivided into groups, perhaps a manual system that also subdivides them would be preferable to one that does not. But the number of ways in which the verbs can be subdivided, and the way they are treated once they have been subdivided, is largely a matter of preference. Consider now how the past tenses are actually treated.

ASL   "Time . . . seems to be in sign language a sentence or utterance rather than a verb matter. Unlike an English finite verb, which must indicate tense, a sign verb will remain uninflected for time. Instead, the sentence or utterance as a whole will have whatever time reference the situation or a general or specific time sign has indicated until a change is signalled" (Stokoe, Casterline, and Croneberg, 1965, p. 282). In other words, in ASL the present and past of all verbs are signed identically and time is marked by separate markers, not necessarily one per verb or even one per sentence. In an entire conversation, it may be possible to mark the tense as past only once, after which it is assumed to be past until otherwise indicated.

Paget-Gorman Systematic Sign (PGSS)   Verbs are divided into two groups, those made with one hand and those made with two hands. The one-handed signs form their past tense by simultaneously signing the present tense form of the sign with one hand and the past tense sign PAST with the other. The two-handed signs form their past tense by sequentially signing first the present tense form of the verb and then the PAST sign. As discussed below, PGSS does not use ASL signs.

Signing Exact English   In general, the past tense is formed by signing the present tense form of the verb followed by the ASL sign PAST. The past participle is formed by signing the verb plus FINISH. Auxiliary verbs (*can-could*) do not use PAST, they use FINISH.

Manual English   All verbs form their past tense by using the sign PAST after the verb. However, verbs are divided into regular and irregular groups for purposes of forming the past participle. For regular verbs, the past participle is the same as the past tense (VERB + PAST). For irregular past participles, the sequence VERB + PAST + FINISH is used.

Signed English   Generally, the past tense form is VERB + E + D. The version used by Bornstein et al. (1973) uses two past tense markers, one for regular verbs and one for irregular verbs.

Improved Manual English   Regular verbs are all treated the same way, but irregular verbs are formed by "signing a basic verb as usual and immediately spelling out the last letter appearing in the intended tense of the word. Accordingly, 'tore' is signed-spelled TEAR (E) and 'torn,' TEAR(N). THINK(T) clearly indicates 'thought' as a verb in the context. In short, the last letter spelled out has no other function than to indicate tenses of irregular verbs" (Mossel, 1962; p. 27).

It should be clear from the above discussion and examples that each system has its own "systematic principle." Each principle is arbitrary in terms of both the structure of English and the structure of ASL. As far as the child is concerned, each system simply has its own set of signs to correspond to different concepts. Because the child does not yet know English, it makes little difference linguistically whether he learns TEAR(E) as the sign for 'torn' or TEAR + PAST, or TEAR + D, or T + O + R + E. The creators of the sign systems hoped, however, that the basic principles of their system somehow would become real and meaningful to the child, that the child would learn that all verbs signed one way have something in common. However, it remains to be seen whether the child realizes that what those signs have in common is that their English equivalents correspond to the regular rule of English past tense formation. Children are most likely to look only for generalizations about the system that they are learning, in order to organize their memory more efficiently, to make their task of comprehension and production easier. It remains to be experimentally demonstrated that these generalizations carry over into their use of English. In research on the effects of the first language on second language acquisition, Richards (1974) estimated that only 20% of all second language learning errors may be directly attributable to the structure of the first language. If this is true, and if this can be generalized to facilitation as well as interference, then the first language (here, manual systems or ASL) has little effect on the acquisition of the structure of the second language although, clearly, the first language is necessary in order to teach the second language (assuming that the second language is being taught, rather than acquired naturally as in a bilingual home).

General Comments on the Systems

Before a description of each of the systems is given, several major differences should be pointed out. In the area of sign usage and sign formation, the systems have different principles that serve as guidelines (particularly for the many words not listed in the system's dictionary or manual of usage). For example, the PGSS system utilizes a combination of basic sign + modifier sign to form most of its words.

The basic sign is a category, like PERSON or ANIMAL. The modifier sign specifies something about the nature of the particular intended referent. One hand forms the sign for PERSON and the other forms the sign for TOOTH (*dentist*), TEACH (*teacher*), FIRE (*fireman*), or STETHOSCOPE (*doctor*). For every meaning, there is a separate sign.

On the other hand, Signing Exact English (henceforth SEE, which is used as an example of Seeing Essential English and Linguistics of Visual English as well) has as a basic principle that, if two of the following three criteria are identical for two English words, the same sign is used for both of them: 1) pronunciation, 2) spelling, and 3) meaning. For example, *wind* (breeze) and *wind* (what you do to a clock or watch) are spelled the same, but they are pronounced differently and have different meanings; therefore, they have separate signs. However, *sock,* which can mean both "stocking" and "to hit," is nonetheless spelled and pronounced the same for both of its two meanings; consequently, only one sign is used for both widely divergent meanings.

Like PGSS, Manual English prefers to have one sign for each meaning, so that the English word *call* is represented by four separate ASL signs in Manual English: NAME, SUMMONS, PHONE, and SHOUT. (In SEE, one sign would be used for all four because they are pronounced and spelled the same way.) Signed English does not believe that an "altered form of the sign word will facilitate the learning of the English word form" (Bornstein, 1973, p. 462) and hence uses ASL signs for all types of English words. This is summarized in Table 2.

The systems differ also in their expressed attitude toward the use of fingerspelling. In PGSS, fingerspelling is used only for proper names. In SEE, fingerspelling is generally avoided. Manual English, on the other hand, is not opposed to the use of fingerspelling and permits it, for example, as an alternate form of the past tense formation. Signed English uses varying amounts of fingerspelling, the actual amount greatly depending on the person's fluency in English and the audience. The use of large amounts of fingerspelling by users of Signed English allows the system to be very flexible and to borrow words from English by simply spelling them. Furthermore, when learning to sign, a hearing person simply can fingerspell any word for which he does not know the sign.

Paget-Gorman Systematic Sign

PGSS was developed in England with the expressed intention that the system would be discarded by the child when it was no longer needed for communication (i.e., when the child had mastered English). Because it was developed in England, it does not use signs from ASL. The system is based on pantomimic signs that include 21 standard hand positions and 39 basic signs used in different combinations. Each basic sign serves to group together signs with a common concept. Basic signs exist for FOOD, INSECT, PERSON, ANIMAL, etc. The standard hand configurations serve to differentiate specific lexical items in each group although a basic sign is not necessary for every sign. There are also functional signs, used to form plurals, tenses, possessives, comparatives, and also to designate certain categories like parts of the body, senses, punctuation, and geometric figures. The PGSS system operates on a one meaning–one sign principle.

The PGSS pronoun system follows the pattern of English pronouns. There are separate signs for first, second, and third person singular pronouns: I, YOU, and IT. The other pronouns are variations of the main sign. For example, the pronoun *he* is signed by combining the pronoun IT in one hand with the sign MALE in the other. Reflexive pronouns are formed by signing the possessive form (formed on the nominative) and then the pronoun SELF. Thus, *myself* is MY + SELF. (Implication: the reflexive *himself* is signed as HIS + SELF, a common mistake made while learning English by young hearing children, second language learners, and deaf children.) Plurals in PGSS are formed by signing the functional sign PLURAL after the noun NOUN + PLURAL (for both regular and irregular nouns). Possessives are formed by signing the noun and then the functional sign for POSSESSIVE (NOUN + POSS). Plural possessives have the form NOUN + PLURAL + POSS.

All verbs are treated alike in PGSS except the verb *to be,* which has six distinct signs: BE, AM, IS, ARE, WAS, and WERE. The other verbs are all used unmarked in the present tense; that is, there are no endings or modifications to indicate first, second, or third person, or singular and plural, or regular versus irregular verb. The future tense is formed by using a separate sign TIME-FORWARD *before* each verb (analogous to English *will* + verb). As mentioned earlier, the past tense involves a division of verbs into one- and two-handed signs with one-handed signs stimultaneously signing the verb and TIME-BACKWARD, and two-handed signs sequentially signing the verb and then TIME-BACKWARD. The present participle is formed by a functional sign -ING, which follows the verb. The sign PAST PARTICIPLE (PAST PART) is used to form participles from the past tense, i.e., VERB + TIME-BACKWARD + PAST PART, where TIME-BACKWARD follows the rule for past tense formation.

The formation of compound and complex signs is the area in which most of the systems run into trouble. They end up being either internally inconsistent, cumbersome, or counterintuitive. The PGSS system has attempted to avoid the complexities inherent in paralleling English word formation by establishing its own morphologic rules, although a few still parallel English. The -ING functional sign can be used to derive nouns from verbs, and the -LY suffix is used to derive some adjectives and adverbs. For the most part, however, the signs are formed on productive combinations of the 39 basic signs and the 21 standard hand configurations. Examples of human signs (*dentist, fireman, doctor*) were given earlier. Others include *elephant* = ANIMAL + LONG-NOSE, *leopard* = ANIMAL + SPOTS, *lion* = ANIMAL + ROAR. Compound signs are made by combining two or more basic signs: *bedroom* = BED + SLEEP, *scent* = GOOD + SMELL, *contract* = PAPER + LAW, *breakfast* = MORNING + FOOD.

The signs of PGSS are pantomimic in some sense, but could not be taken as universal. For example, the sign for *frog* is ANIMAL + JUMP, which might be taken to refer to a kangaroo in Australia. Furthermore, PGSS violates an American cultural taboo on extended middle fingers by using this hand configuration in some of its signs (a hand configuration allowable in Chinese Sign Language).

Signing Exact English

As indicated earlier, Signing Exact English is an outgrowth of David Anthony's original work on Seeing Essential English. Signing Exact English was developed by Gustason, Pfetzing, and Zawolkow (1972), and the manual and a supplement are currently available from the National Association for the Deaf. The SEE manual includes 2,100 words and 70 affixes, with seven contractions. Words are divided into basic words, complex words, and compound words. The system uses the two-out-of-three principle described above, namely, that the same sign is used for two English words if those two words are alike in two of the three features—pronunciation, spelling, and meaning. Either one of the ASL signs is chosen to represent the two words, or a new sign is invented. The ASL sign is used if it is clear, unambiguous, and has only one English translation (Gustason, Pfetzing, and Zawolkow, 1972). The exception to the basic two-out-of-three principle is that inflected basic forms cannot be used as new basic words. For example, the past tense of *see, saw,* cannot be used as the sign for the verb *to saw.*

SEE retains some of the ASL pronoun signs—ME, MY, YOU, and YOUR. A series of initialized signs have been invented for use with the other pronouns, using for example the E hand for *he,* the M hand for *him,* and the S hand for *his.* Possessive pronouns are formed by adding -S to the possessive adjectives; for example, *yours* is signed as YOUR + S. The exception to this is the *mine* is MY + EN. The reflexives are the same as in PGSS (only using some ASL signs) with the possessive adjective (MY, YOUR, HIS, etc.) followed by SELF for the singular and SELF + S for the plural.

Regular plural nouns are formed by signing S after the noun. Irregular nouns are divided: Nouns in which the final consonant is a voiceless fricative in the singular and a voiced fricative in the plural (*leaf-leaves*) are treated like ASL plurals and reduplicated. Possessives are formed using the contraction 'S (an S hand that moves in the shape of an apostrophe), added directly to singular nouns and after the plural marker S in plural nouns (the plural marker is also an S hand, but it does not move).

Regular and irregular verbs are treated the same way in SEE. In the present tense, the third person singular is inflected with -S. The ASL sign PAST is used after the verb to indicate past tense. The future is formed with the ASL sign FUTURE, which has been initialized to stand for *will.* For the present participle, the suffix -ING is used, and for the past participle the ASL sign FINISH is used after the verb. Auxiliary verbs are differentiated, however. The past tense is formed by using the past participle sign FINISH, so that *could* = CAN + FINISH. Also, the verb *to be* has several signs associated with it. Some are derived from the ASL sign TRULY, which is initialized with A for *am,* R for *are,* I for *is,* and B for *be.* To indicate past tense, the ASL sign PAST has been initialized with S for *was* and R for *were.* Some of these signs for *to be* have worked their way back into ASL and are now being used by deaf adults in formal situations in many parts of the country.

In every language, words are created by combining one or more morphemes. For example, the word *farmers* is composed of the morphemes *farm + er + s,* where *farm* is a verb stem, *er* is an agentive suffix (one who does), and *s* is a plural marker. The PGSS system did not attempt to parallel English morphology, but the SEE system tries. It uses morphemes that are productive and have constant semantic value. (Thus, the meaning of a word composed of morphemes A + B + C is predictable from the meaning of the individual morphemes themselves. An example of an English word that does not have the meaning of its composite morphemes is *understand,* which has a meaning unrelated to either *under* or *stand*).

Again, the two-out-of-three principle holds for choice of signs. Because the affix *-ship* (as in *relationship*) has the same spelling and pronunciation as the noun *ship,* one sign is used for both, even though the meanings are radically different. Complex words, regardless of the meaning, are formed by adding an affix if there is one in English. For example, the pair *red-redden* follows an English rule for deriving verbs from adjectives (*light-lighten, white-whiten*), and an -EN suffix is used in SEE for these forms. However, the same -EN suffix is used in SEE for words where English has an *-en* ending that means something entirely different, like *chick-chicken, mitt-mitten, my-mine.* In addition, the -EN sign is actually the past participle FINISH sign, so that *chicken* is really signed as CHICK + FINISH. (The *chick-chicken* pair is particularly disturbing because it seems more appropriate for the sign to somehow indicate that *chick* is a *little chicken.*) Whether or not these system deviancies have any effect on children's learning of English remains to be seen.

Despite the fact that SEE holds to the two-out-of-three principle even in some very strange situations, as in *-ship, ship,* it nonetheless includes a number of words that are not formed along this principle at all. Some forms are actually broken down into archaic morpheme division (*height* = HIGH + T), or syllable divisions (*sorrow* = SORRY + W, *jewelry* = JEWEL + R + Y, *nursery* = NURSE + ER + Y, *any* = AN + Y). This is not done systematically, however, because *although, also,* and *already* are signed as two signs (AL + THOUGH, for example) while *almost,* which could be easily divided like the others, is nonetheless one sign.

With respect to compound signs, SEE uses two signs if the word retains the meaning of the two words of which it is composed (*babysit, shepherd*) and uses a single sign (ASL or invented) for words that have nonpredictable meanings (*carpet* has its own sign because it has nothing to do with either *cars* or *pets*). Words like *yesterday* and *today* are treated as two signs each, ignoring available ASL signs for both of them. *Hotdog* is also treated as two signs even though the relationship between its meaning and that of *hot dog* is fairly obscure. Again, it should be pointed out, first, that these are purely arbitrary decisions and, second, that most of the systems have this kind of problem with English morphology and that SEE alone cannot be faulted.

Manual English

Manual English was developed by the Total Communication Program at the Washington State School for the Deaf in order to provide a system that would parallel English sufficiently well that it could be used in conjunction with normal speech. The system is taught to adults who are in contact with a deaf child so that English structure can be reinforced through signs at all times. Again, it should be pointed out that English syntax can be reinforced this way, but that English morphology causes difficulty. Manual English uses more fingerspelling than SEE does, so that a signer has the option of forming a verb tense as VERB + TENSE or of partially spelling the word, e.g., VERB + E + D.

Manual English uses many of the ASL signs. If an English word has more than one meaning, and each of those meanings has a separate ASL sign, then the ASL signs are retained. A large number of initialized signs are used, for example, as illustrated earlier, *employ* = WORK (with the E hand), *job* = WORK (with the J hand), *duty* = WORK (with the D hand). The pronouns in Manual English are the same as those in SEE, except that *mine* = MY + E, whereas SEE uses MY + EN. The contractions, plurals, and possessives are the same as in SEE. Manual English handles the verb *to be* in the same manner as SEE but differs in its treatment of main verbs, notably in its handling of the past participle. The ASL sign for FINISH is used as a suffix marker for the past participle, but unlike SEE, Manual English divides the verbs into regular and irregular with the irregular verbs that have a distinct word for present, past, and past participle forms, as *speak-spoke-spoken,* using the past participle form VERB + PAST + FINISH. It should be borne in mind that distinctions such as this are opaque to all but the most knowledgable students, for whom this division, as most of the others, is purely an arbitrary one requiring special memorization. That is, the student must learn the list of signs that take FINISH in their past participles as exceptions to the otherwise regular rule of having simply VERB + PAST.

In compound and complex sign formation, Manual English has borrowed some signs from SEE, eliminated others, and altered others. Some nonproductive affixes like -NEATH and YESTER- have been eliminated because of their limited use, e.g., *beneath, underneath, yesterday, yesteryear.* Unlike SEE, which uses the same -ER suffix for most occurrences of the English *-er,* Manual English has three -ER signs, one for agentive *-er* (one who does) using the ASL sign PER-SON, one for the comparative *-er (bigger, smaller),* and one for everything else *(prayer, eraser, dryer).* Note that in this last category, an *eraser* is that which erases, and a *dryer* is that which dries, but a *prayer* is not that which prays, nor one who prays (one who prays would be agentive and would use PERSON), so that the third group is an arbitrary collection of leftovers.

The principles for complex word formation vary. The basic rule is supposed to be that, if no ASL sign exists for a complex word, then an affix may be used to form a sign. However, there are cases where this principle is overlooked, as seen by the use of NEAR + PERSON for *neighbor.* The same principle is supposed to hold for compound words, so that *oversight, grandmother, gentleman,* and *workshop* use the ASL signs, whereas two signs are put together when needed, for example, for *houseparent* = HOUSE + PARENT.

Signed English

Signed English is an outgrowth of the ASL-English pidginization process and reflects the work of several independent and groups (Fant, 1964; Watson, 1964; O'Rourke, 1973; Bornstein, 1973; Bornstein et al., 1973). As such, it includes a great deal of variation. Signed English uses ASL signs strung together in English word order by the use of fingerspelling and some conjunction words. The degree of English word order may vary, however, depending on the amount of finger-spelling used. Thus, the signer may use "T-h-e TWO MAN w-e-r-e-s-e-a-r-c-h-i-n-g QUIET" for "The two men were searching quietly" in a formal situation, and in a less formal situation use TWO MAN QUIET SEARCH SEARCH, using ASL reduplication to indicate the present progressive. This variability closely approximates the situation in spoken languages, where each person has several styles corresponding to the formality of the situation and the audience. Consider, for example, the difference between everyday speech and formal letter writing, or telephone calls to a friend, or to the boss, or to a client, or to a stranger. What varies is not just the content, but also the linguistic structure, the carefulness of articulation, the choice of syntactic structures, and the choice of vocabulary items. In Signed English these are reflected in the amount of fingerspelling used and the number of rules chosen from English or ASL. It provides for greater fluency because if a sign is not known, fingerspelling allows communication to continue uninterrupted.

In addition, the need for arbitrary sign formation rules is obviated because words for which no sign exists can be fingerspelled. This situation allows some new or invented signs from other systems to be tested. Some catch on (particularly some initialized signs) and are retained (for example, the different signs for the verb *to be*), and others are rejected and drop from usage. Dialects develop (a natural situation for any language) and historical changes take place. Furthermore, a teacher legitimately can insist on grammatical English in the classroom and still condone the manual communication that goes on outside the classroom as a reflection of these different linguistic styles (Nobody really talks the way English teachers would like them to, but many people expect deaf children to use classroom language outside the classroom, a highly artificial situation.) The teacher does not have to learn a new syntax (ASL) nor do the students have to learn (many) artificial or altered signs. Also, differences in sign usage, such as occur between users of SEE and users of Manual English, do not occur here.

Bornstein and his colleagues (Bornstein et al., 1973, 1975) have adapted certain portions of Signed English for use with preschool and elementary school children. The intention is to provide "a semantic approximation to the usual language environment of the hearing child" (Bornstein, 1973, p. 330). The 2500-word vocabulary is chosen for use with the young child and includes sign words and sign markers. Of these 2500 signs, 1700 are from ASL and the rest are either invented or borrowed from other systems. The 12 sign markers function for basic English structures. The plural for regular nouns is markek by fingerspelling S after the sign, and for irregular nouns it is marked by reduplication (again, an arbitrary choice of divisions). The 'S sign for possessive, which has been widely accepted into ASL, is used in Signed English. Unlike the other systems, contractions are treated as separate words, with their own signs. Thus, there is a separate sign for *don't* that is not an alteration of *do not*. The evidence from early language acquisition in hearing children supports the view that children learn contractions as separate entities. The contractions *don't* and *can't* appear in utterances in an earlier developmental stage than *can* and *do* or the other modals, suggesting that they are learned as whole units rather than as contractions of their component words.

Four sign markers are used with the verbs, one for the past tense of regular verbs, one for the past tense of irregular verbs, one for the third person singular present, and one for the past participle. The possible combinations of signs and markers are limited, so that anything not covered by these principles is fingerspelled. In all probability, the system is sufficient for the young child and many retarded individuals (see Kopchick and Lloyd, this volume).

Fingerspelling and Cued Speech

Fingerspelling and Cued Speech are separated from the other systems because their relationship with English and speech is different. They are treated individually below.

Fingerspelling   Fingerspelling (dactylology) primarily consists of 26 distinct handshapes that directly correspond to the 26 letters of the alphabet. A sign for *and* is also included in the standard fingerspelling repertoire. Because the hand configurations correspond to the letters of the alphabet, fingerspelling is a manual representation of written language and may be used for any language that uses the Roman alphabet. (For examples of fingerspelling of non-Roman alphabets, see Moores, 1974.) Fingerspelling, then, has no separate syntax, morphology, phonology, or semantics; instead, it entirely depends on the linguistic structure of the language that it represents. In this sense, it is very like Morse code, which translates each letter of the alphabet into dots and dashes. Fingerspelling combined with speech is known as the Rochester method (Scouten, 1967).

The use of fingerspelling has several advantages, but also several disadvantages. First, in its favor, anyone who can spell can learn the 26 handshape correspondences quickly, thus providing teachers, parents, and clinicians with a quick and easy way to make themselves understood to many deaf people. On the other hand, even though the average adult can learn to fingerspell in short order, learning to perceive and read fingerspelling is quite another matter. A skilled fingerspeller learns to form words as units, rather than as simple sequences of letters. Thus, the center letters of a word may be assimilated to the surrounding letters, blurring the formation of the letters and creating a perception problem. The skilled fingerspelling reader learns to rely heavily on the first and last letters of a word to help identify that word because there is often a tiny break between the last letter of one word and the first letter of the next word, making the first and last letters more distinct. In rapid fingerspelling reading, one has to make successive guesses as to what is being perceived, in which case a thorough knowledge of English grammar, which specifies what possible words can follow the words one has already deciphered, is absolutely essential. In this respect, reading fingerspelling parallels lipreading. The problem of fingerspelling reading can be mitigated if the fingerspeller slows the rate of spelling considerably. This enables the reader to follow the fingers but destroys the normal rate of conversation and interrupts the normal flow of speech and intonation.

The reading of fingerspelling is not the only problem associated with it; other problems relate to its use with very young children (below age 5). The movements of the fingers are quite small and are often quick. Fingerspelling requires a considerably greater degree of manual motor coordination than does signing. Although a child may put together two or three signs into an utterance at about 18 months, fingerspelling does not emerge until much later. Wilbur and Jones (1974) observed nearly none at age 3.5 years. In fact, the only spelling seen was the child's own name, which was not done correctly since a double consonant in the name was improperly formed by the child.

In addition to the motor problem, very young children have difficulty learning to fingerspell because, in order to be able to fingerspell, you have to be able to spell. Hearing children do not usually learn to spell until they have had considerable experience with reading and spelling practice. Spelling is one of the core subjects of the standard elementary school curriculum. Therefore, one cannot expect a very young child (an illiterate child at that, regardless of whether the child is deaf, retarded, or normal) to acquire fingerspelling without a great deal of effort (drill, patience, practice) and formal training. Language is not learned by means of formal training by hearing children, and, consequently, the learning of fingerspelling should not be viewed as a normal language learning situation.

This is not to say that children cannot learn to fingerspell. Fingerspelling has been shown to be an effective aid in educational settings. Moores (1974) reviewed several Russian studies that reported success with fingerspelling combined with speech. In a study specifically designed to assess the effectiveness of fingerspelling as an educational tool, Quigley (1969) compared two preschool programs, one using the Rochester method and the other using a traditional oral approach. He followed the two programs for 4 years. At the end of this time, he found that the Rochester method students were superior in one of two measures of speechreading, five of seven measures of reading, and in three of five measures of written language. The oral group was superior in only one measure of written language.

Quigley also compared three residential schools that used the Rochester method with three comparable schools that used simultaneous signs, fingerspelling, and speech (probably Signed English). No differences in speech or speechreading were found between the two groups. Quigley (1969, p. 87) concluded that: "1) The use of fingerspelling in combination with speech as practiced in the Rochester Method can lead to improved achievement in deaf students particularly on those variables where meaningful language is involved. 2) When good oral techniques are used in conjunction with fingerspelling there need be no detrimental effects on the acquisition of oral skills. 3) Fingerspelling is likely to produce greater benefits when used with younger rather than older children. It was used successfully in the experimental study with children as young as three and a half years of age. 4) Fingerspelling is a useful tool for instructing deaf children, but it is not a panacea."

Children of deaf parents who sign and fingerspell have considerable opportunity to observe their parents and to learn from them. But it must be kept in mind that in this situation: 1) signing is the primary language that is learned according to developmental stages and without formal instruction, and 2) the fingerspelling that is acquired emerges much later and only as an auxiliary. One should also recognize that the adult problem of perceiving and comprehending rapid fingerspelling is magnified with the very young child, both in terms of small hand movements and speed. A further caution on the use of fingerspelling is that it is difficult to see from the back of a large audience. Thus, to accommodate a larger audience, signers can enlarge their signs by increasing the space utilized in the motion, but it is not possible to enlarge one's fingers. Even though the spelling can be made more distinct by carefully forming each letter, the gain is not great, and the cost is speed. This is particularly a problem in interpreting.

Finally, fingerspelling is slow when compared to signing or speech. To get a feel for what it must be like, have someone read you the last paragraph letter by letter.

Cued Speech   Cornett (1967, 1969) described Cued Speech as a system designed "to enable the deaf child to learn language through exposure to a visible phonetic analog of speech supplied by the lip movements and supplementing hand cues." As Moores (1969) pointed out, the components ('cues') have no meaning independent of their association with those lip movements. (One cue may represent three consonants. The lip movements are required to make a decision.) Thus, the system is most appropriately viewed as an auxiliary to speech and not a separate communication channel for language. In addition to the system of Cued Speech developed by Cornett and described below, several other similar systems were developed in Europe. In the middle 19th century, a French monk, Friar Bernard of Saint Gabriel, developed a system that cued only consonants. Several years later, another Frenchman, Monsieur Fourcade, developed a similar system. Another system was developed by Dr. Georg Forchhammer of the Boarding School for Deaf and Hard-of-Hearing Children at Fredericia. Forchhammer's doctoral dissertation reported that the system had a beneficial effect on communication. His system employed hand movements to demonstrate the movement of the mouth organs that cannot be observed during normal speech (glottis, palate, etc.) (Børrild, 1972).

Cornett's system uses 36 cues for the 44 phonemes of English. The cues can be divided into vowel cues and consonant cues. Vowel cues are represented by hand position, and consonant cues are represented by hand configurations. It is possible, therefore, to represent consonant-vowel pairs by superimposing the consonant hand configuration on the vowel hand position. Diphthongs are represented by a sequence of the first vowel position followed by the second vowel position. The handshapes borrow from those of sign. The 5-hand configuration of signing is identical to the cue for /m/, /f/, and /t/. The F-hand of the fingerspelling alphabet is the cue for /h/, /s/, and /r/. The B-hand cues /n/, /b/, and /ʍ/ ('wh').[1] The L-hand cues /l/, /ʃ/('sh'), and /w/. The G-hand (upright) cues /d/, /p/, and /ʒ/.

---

[1]For readers unfamiliar with the International Phonetic Association (IPA) Alphabet, a pronunciation key is provided in Appendix B.

Vowel positions are to the right side of the face near the ear, lower on the face by the cheek, below the chin and slightly to the right, and on the right side of the lips. In other words, the cues are made near the face so that they may be easily seen in the perceptual field while the eyes are on the lips, but so that they never come in front of the lips where they would obscure the lip movement.

Like fingerspelling, Cued Speech has its advantages and disadvantages. To its credit is the fact that it can be useful for conveying fine phonetic distinctions of either standards or dialectal pronunciations to the already knowledgable speaker. Success with Cued Speech—in the form of increased accuracy in lipreading, greater vocabulary, greater relaxation among children, shortening of delay time between learning something receptively and producing expressively, increased communication among children, and increased intelligibility of children—has been reported (Rupert, 1969).

Moores (1969) has provided an extensive critical review of Cued Speech. His arguments plus comments of this author are presented in the following paragraphs.

Objections to the use of Cued Speech can be divided into: 1) those that deal with general assumptions and rationale of the system, and 2) those that deal specifically with the system's phonetic base.

1.   Assumptions: In fact, the first objection is not to an explicit assumption, but to the lack of an explicit distinction, namely, the failure of Cornett to distinguish between *language* and *speech*. As indicated above, and in the introductory paragraphs to this chapter, such distinction is crucial to understanding the nature of language and how language is acquired. Not having made this distinction leads to another assumption, quite commonly held, that language is learned by imitation. It is Cornett's belief that children copy adult cues and thus make themselves better understood by the cues even though their speech may not be accurate. This reduces frustration between adult and child and creates a better atmosphere for learning. The problem is that the considerable body of research on the acquisition of language indicates that the role of imitation is nowhere near as central to language acquisition as was previously thought. In investigating imitation, Bloom (1973) was able to sort children into those who do imitate and those who do not. Clearly, those who do not imitate stand as counterevidence to a theory of acquisition by imitation.

2.   Phonetic Problems: Moores points out that Cued Speech is intrinsically tied to the sound system and has little or no transfer

potential to reading. It is the nature of English orthography that phonemic distinctions are indicated, but predictable phonetic ones are
not indicated. For example, the English /d/ and /t/ are pronounced
as flaps when they come between two vowels. No one actually says
[raɪtɚ] /rīter/ for 'writer' and [raɪdɚ] /rīder/ for 'rider.' This flap-
ping process is a general process that holds true for all the words of
English for all the speakers. The written forms of the words do not indicate this process, yet it is a phonetic distinction. Likewise, certain
unstressed vowels are reduced to a more central, less distinct vowel.
This is also not indicated by the orthography. In addition, dialectal
pronunciation is, of course, not indicated by the orthography. One
does not write *Cuber* for the New Englanders' *Cuba,* although certainly such a major mark of New England pronunciation would have
to be cued, otherwise the child would end up missing a major feature
of the dialect.

The reason for the discrepancy between the written forms and the
types of phonetic processes just indicated is that certain phonetic distinctions do not make a difference even though they are perfectly regular. For example, every voiceless consonant is aspirated at the beginning of an English word. But if the aspiration were left out, chances
are its absence might not even be noticed. Cornett's system does not
differentiate between phonetic processes that are dialectal (the fine
distinctions mentioned earlier) and phonetic processes that are redundant, regular, not indicated in the writing systems, and, consequently,
not crucial. It is a far more serious error for the vowel in 'bat' [bæt]
to be mispronounced because it could come out as 'beat' [bit]; 'bit'
[bɪt]; 'bait' [beɪt]; 'boat' [bout]; 'bought' [bɔt]; 'but' [bʌt]; 'bet' [bɛt];
'bite' [baɪt]; 'beaut' [bjut]; etc. The system does not set guidelines for
the adult as to which phonetic distinctions are important and which are
not. In fact, one could suggest that, rather than maintain a phonetic
base, a phonemic base would be preferable, but then the benefit of
indicating fine dialectal distinctions would be lost.

This leads to the next point, namely, the competence of the average adult with respect to phonetics. Berko and Brown (1966) remarked, "The untrained adult cannot even approximate an accurate
phonetic record." From first-hand experience, this author can report
that learning phonetic transcription is tedious and boring and is a
skill that must be worked at to be developed and maintained. This
leads to the situation of an untrained adult trying to indicate phonetic
distinctions that may or may not be important, in a manner that may

or may not be accurate, to a child who may or may not imitate the cues, who may or may not produce them spontaneously on his own, and who is highly unlikely to understand what they indicate or to utilize this information in learning to read.

Børrild (1972, p. 237) reported that a cued speech system has been in use in most Danish schools for nearly 70 years and that, "it is pretty obvious that most pupils having been trained in the mouth-hand system to accompany speech are rather helpless when they have to face pure lipreading. And in spite of the past 70 years, a very small minority only of the population will be acquainted with the mouth-hand system, and a far smaller minority will really master it." It should be emphasized again that the entire system is geared toward speech and not toward language. Its utility lies in speech therapy, not in initial language learning. Børrild (1972, p. 237) concurs: "It is an indisputable fact that the mouth-hand system is an excellent medium in the articulation training, and that in many cases it is indispensable for adult persons with acquired deafness without any hearing residue but with a normal language . . ."

PRACTICAL CONSIDERATIONS
OF MANUAL COMMUNICATION

This section deals with some of the research on the feasibility and effectiveness of using manual communication. The section begins with a discussion of a small portion of the research that has been done on the general difficulty that deaf children have learning English. This is followed by a discussion of four major areas of research involving the use of manual communication in the schools and home: 1) the relationship of manual communication to the acquisition of language and the eventual acquisition of English, 2) the relationship of manual communication to the acquisition of speech, 3) the relationship of manual communication to social development and mental health, and 4) the relationship of manual communication to psychological processes such as memory. Finally, the use of manual communication with hearing nonverbal individuals such as the mentally retarded is discussed.

The acquisition of language and the subsequent acquisition of English is of primary importance in the overall education of the deaf in the United States. All subsequent academic study depends on language, including arithmetic beyond the simple nonverbal problems.

The acquisition of speech is important insofar as the need exists for deaf people to function in a hearing world. Lipreading skills can give the deaf person the ability to enjoy and profit from television, movies, lectures, and social interactions with nondeaf people. Social integration in the deaf community (which is really only possible with the knowledge of ASL) is extremely important, possibly as important as a well adjusted family situation. A deaf person who cannot speak well is almost always uncomfortable in a hearing society, and a deaf person who cannot sign is not an integrated member of the deaf community either. Finally, the development and organization of certain psychologic processes, such as memory coding, memory retrieval, and memory rehearsal, may be affected by the language learned during the child's early years.

Acquisition of Language

Learning English Syntax   The general difficulty that deaf children have learning English has been very well documented (Myklebust, 1964, 1967; Schmitt, 1968; Power, 1971; Bonvillian, Charrow, and Nelson, 1973; Quigley, Smith, and Wilbur, 1974; Quigley, Wilbur, and Montanelli, 1974, in press; Wilbur and Quigley, 1975; Wilbur, Quigley, and Montanelli, 1975; Quigley, Montanelli, and Wilbur, in press; Wilbur, Montanelli, and Quigley, in press; Wilbur, 1976).

With respect to reading, Furth (1966a) reported that less than 12% of deaf students between the ages of 15.5 and 16.5 years can read at a fourth-grade reading level or above. Traditional studies of the specific problems have focused on the number of omissions, substitutions, redundancies, and word order errors (Myklebust, 1964), but the causes for errors have remained obscure. Within the framework of transformational grammar, investigators of the syntactic problems of deaf students looked for patterns to the errors. Using a stratified random sample of 480 deaf students between the ages of 10 and 18 years old (which included students from day and residential programs, oral and manual schools, from each of the nine major geographic areas of the United States), a massive study was conducted of deaf students' difficulty with several groupings of syntactic structures. (For more information on the sample, see Quigley, Smith, and Wilbur, 1974; for a general outline of the project, see Wilbur and Quigley, 1975.)

The study indicated that, even by age 18, deaf students did not have the linguistic competence of 10-year-old hearing children in syntactic structures such as relative clauses (Quigley, Smith, and Wilbur, 1974), verbal complements (Quigley, Wilbur, and Montanelli, in press), and auxilary verbs (Quigley, Montanelli, and Wilbur, in press). In other syntactic areas, such as conjoined sentences (Wilbur, Quigley, and Montanelli, in press), pronominalization (Wilbur, Montanelli, and Quigley, in press), and certain aspects of relative clause comprehension, and in a related study of passive sentences (Power, 1971), non-English comprehension processing strategies were found to exist. In some cases, non-English rules for producing syntactic structures were found, and it was speculated that these rules may co-exist with the standard English rules in some children (also see Charrow, 1974, 1975a). It is felt that these rules arise from the child's normal process of forming hypotheses about the data and then checking the hypotheses against more data. Because of the limited amount of exposure deaf children have to English (compared to young hearing children before the age of 5), deaf children may form incorrect hypotheses with respect to English syntax, but they may not realize until they are much older that these are incorrect. Indeed, it was found that the usage of at least one deviant rule decreased significantly with age (Wilbur, Quigley, and Montanelli, in press).

It has occasionally been suggested that deaf children's difficulty in acquiring English is not limited to linguistic processing but extends to their general cognitive ability to form generalizations. Furth (1966b) has demonstrated that the general cognitive ability of deaf people is not greatly different from hearing people in nonlinguistic tasks. Given this information, it has been suggested that deaf people do not develop the ability to apply their nonlinguistic cognitive skills to linguistic tasks. This suggestion ignores the fact that the acquisition of ASL is a linguistic task which many deaf children accomplish easily. However, it is still suggested by some that the difficulty is specific to English but not specific to syntax. Wilbur (1974b) investigated nonsyntactic generalizations made by deaf students. The task required recognition of English constraints on the structure of allowable words. For example, *blick* could be a word of English, although it actually is not. However, *bnick* could not be a word of English because of the structure of the initial consonant cluster *bn*. One need not know what these words might mean in order to decide which is acceptable to English and which is not. Furthermore, these constraints,

unlike spelling rules and "proper" grammatical rules, are not specifically taught to either deaf or hearing children in school. Therefore,
any knowledge that deaf children have of these constraints must have
been extracted entirely on their own, thus giving an indication of
their processing ability relative to English. First-, third-, fifth-, and
seventh-grade deaf and third/fourth- and seventh-grade hearing children were tested on their ability to reject ill-formed words such as
bnick. Although the deaf students' scores were quantitatively below
those of the hearing children until the seventh grade, the scores were
not qualitatively different. That is, violations of English word structures constraints that were easy for the hearing children to spot were
also easy for the deaf students, and those that were hard for the hearing children were also hard for the deaf children. It was concluded
that deaf students' difficulty in learning the proper rules for the more
complex syntactic patterns is not attributable to a disturbance of general linguistic or cognitive processing (see Furth, 1966b), but rather
to difficulty in learning the specific rules for English.

The question is often raised as to the extent to which the deaf
students' difficulty with English is attributable to interference from
knowing ASL. Researchers in the area of second-language acquisition
have investigated this type of interference in a variety of ways. One
such study (Richards, 1974) reported that only about 20% of the
second-language errors may be attributed to interference from the first
language. This author admits to being unconvinced by the statistic or
the method, but nonetheless concludes that the interference from ASL
must be small. The sample used for the studies on the syntactic structures of English cited earlier included students from both manual and
nonmanual schools. The fact that nearly all of the error types were
found to some extent in all schools and at all grades strongly suggests
that the use of manual communication is not primarily responsible for
the observed errors. Many of the errors were simply the result of
"overgeneralization," a process that is found in young children acquiring any language and in all second-language acquisition. The child
hypothesizes a rule and attempts to apply it in environments where it
is not allowed. Eventually, the proper constraints are learned and the
child corrects his rule. Because of lack of feedback, however, the deaf
child displays a great delay in developing the proper constraints that
are specific to English.

A more specific study of the relationship between using manual
communication and learning English syntax recently has been com-

pleted by Brasel and Quigley (1975). They defined four groups on the basis of the educational approach of the parents with respect to the child: The parents of the first group used Manual English (ME), the parents of the second group used ASL (referred to as the Average Manual group, AM), the parents of the third group began intensive oral training with the child at an early age (IO), and the parents of the fourth group used oral communication but did not use any kind of special early training (referred to as the Average Oral group, AO). Brasel and Quigley reported that none of the parents in the ME group used any of the "morphemic types of sign language such as Seeing Essential English, Signing Exact English, or Linguistically Oriented Visual English" (p. 131) and Manual English therefore would be equivalent to what has been called Signed English here. The groups themselves each contained 18 deaf students, with a mean age for each group of 14.8 years. It should be pointed out that Brasel and Quigley's (1975) groups are confounded in the same way that many other such studies age, namely, that the parents of the deaf students in the manual groups are deaf, and the parents of the deaf students in the oral group are hearing. This entails sociologic and emotional interaction in addition to the language variable being studied (see the section *Socialization, Achievement, and Emotional Development*). An extremely detailed description of the sample group, parents, and siblings, including samples of the parents' written English, is given in Brasel and Quigley.

The groups were compared on the same tests of English syntax (the Tests of Syntactic Ability, TSA) that were used in the previously mentioned studies (Quigley et al., 1976) and on four subtests of the Stanford Achievement Test (Language, Paragraph Meaning, Word Meaning, and Spelling). The results showed, "that the two Manual groups were significantly superior to the two Oral groups on every test measure employed" (Brasel and Quigley, p. 121). Although the ME group outscored the AM group on all six major syntactic structure groupings in the TSA, only one of those differences was significant (relative clauses). Furthermore, "no differences were found between the IO and the AO group on any of the TSA sub-tests although the IO group generally did better than the AO group, and the AM group did better than the two Oral groups" (Brasel and Quigley, p. 120). On the Stanford Achievement Test sub-tests, the Manual English group "was found significantly superior to the other three groups on all four sub-tests, with the ME group being from one to nearly four grades ahead with its nearest competitor being the AM group" (p. 120). Brasel and Quigley (1975, p. 133) concluded that, "the greatest advantage appears to come when the parents are competent in Standard English and use Manual English with and around the child, as witness the marked superiority of the ME group over both Oral groups on nearly [*sic*] every test measure employed and that some advantage is found where early Manual communication exists regardless of degree of deviation from Standard English syntax."

There is a need for caution when reading and interpreting the Brasel and Quigley study. The Manual English parents are continually referred to as "language-competent" or "grammatically correct." The reader is advised to read "language-competent" as "English-competent;" "language-competent" means that someone knows a language, not necessarily English, so that someone who knows ASL is certainly language-competent, but not necessarily English-competent. "Grammatically correct" should be read as "grammatically correct with respect to English;" French and Spanish are certainly grammatically correct with respect to themselves, but not with respect to English. These findings also must be considered with caution for other reasons such as differences in age of detection between the oral and manual groups, the late age of fitting of amplication for the early intensive oral group, and the fact that many of the parents in the Manual English group were teachers.

Moores (1974) and Bonvillian, Charrow, and Nelson (1973) reviewed several studies that have been conducted on differences between groups of deaf students orally and manually trained. These studies cover a wide range of areas (social adjustment and mathematics, for example) not directly related to the topic of English syntax. These studies are reviewed below, either with respect to the relationship between manual communication and the acquisition of speech skills, or with respect to socialization and emotional development.

Early Language Learning   There is yet another aspect of the implications of manual communication for language acquisition that bears discussion. It has been well documented that the brain develops rapidly until puberty, at which time establishment of synaptic patterns ceases (see Lenneberg, 1967). At the same time, it has been observed that language acquisition before puberty happens more or less naturally, with children being able to acquire any language(s) to which they are exposed, whereas language acquisition after puberty becomes more of a process of conscious learning (as opposed to more or less spontaneous acquisition). It has been hypothesized that the high correlation between these two events, brain development and language acquisition, is in fact a causal relationship, such that the acquisition of a first language after puberty should be virtually impossible (referred to as the *Critical Age* hypothesis (Lenneberg, 1967)). Furthermore, it has been observed that the most rapid rate of brain development and organization occurs before the age of 5 or 6 years, an age that is also the time of the most rapid development of language in normal children. As the child grows toward puberty, the establishment of neural synaptic networks and language development slows. There is, then, a time in the life of a child from birth to about 6 years that is undoubtedly the most critical with respect to the proper acquisition of language.

Consider this with respect to some data from the Brasel and Quigley study. For the ME and AM groups, the children were confirmed as deaf at 7 months of age or younger. For the IO and AO groups, the children were confirmed as deaf at about 1 year, 2 months. With the exception of the IO group, the children did not begin formal schooling until they were at least 4 years old. The IO group began formal training at around 2 years (recall that the subjects were selected *because* of the early intensive training which they received). In the 4 years from birth until they began schooling, the deaf children in the ME and AM groups had an opportunity to observe the use of language in the visual mode, a mode that functions normally for them. Through this mode they were able to perceive language and use their normal linguistic processes (whatever those might be) to acquire language from their environment, utilizing the same types of early acquisition strategies as young hearing children, and passing through similar developmental stages (one-word stage, two-word stage, the several different semantic relationship stages, etc.).

The deaf child in the AO group received minimal language input (English or otherwise) until he started school at age 4, at which point nearly two-thirds of those crucial years were gone. He had missed the developmental stages that a child normally passes through in language acquisition and had to compensate for them with formal training. The deaf child in the IO group was given a partial opportunity at age 2 to begin the developmental sequence, but this was done in such a way that the child was formally presented with input, based on what the adults thought the child should be learning, in a mode that requires considerably greater effort from the child because of his auditory deficit. Furthermore, the mode and the formal presentation distract from one aspect of language acquisition, namely, the acquisition of syntax through a series of more and more refined hypotheses as to the nature of the language being learned. Even when no auditory deficit is involved, the earlier a child's linguistic processing can be set in motion, the better off he will be in the long run.

Speech Skills

If the deaf individual is to function in a hearing world, speech is clearly a useful language tool. It is a common belief that the use of manual communication necessarily hinders the development of speech. Moores (1971) summarized several studies that directly compared early oral preschool children with children who had no preschool. None of the studies cited reported any difference in oral skills (speech and speechreading) between the two groups. One of the studies (Vernon and Koh, 1970) compared deaf children of hearing parents with early intensive oral training to deaf children of deaf parents with no preschool (i.e., ASL users). Again, no differences in oral skills were found between the two groups, but the students with deaf parents were found to be superior in reading and general achievement.

Several studies have compared deaf children of deaf parents to deaf children of hearing parents. Four of those studies included results that are relevant here (Quigley and Frisina, 1961; Stevenson, 1964; Meadow, 1966; Stuckless and Birch, 1966; for a description of these, see Moores, 1971, 1974; Bonvillian, Charrow, and Nelson, 1973). The four studies reported that the deaf children of deaf parents were superior on some or all of the English skills and general measures of ability. Three of these studies reported no difference between the two groups on measures of speech production, while the fourth reported that the deaf children of hearing parents were better. One of the studies also reported that the deaf children of deaf parents were better on measures of speechreading ability, while the other three reported no difference between the two groups.

Direct studies of the effects of manual communication on speech are rare. Quigley (1969) reported no difference in speech or speechreading for students using the Rochester method (simultaneous fingerspelling) when compared with those using simultaneous signing and speech. A study of children using Swedish sign (Ahlström, 1972) reported that, "speech was not adversely affected by knowledge of signs" (quoted in Power, 1974). One study seemed to be contradictory. A group of nine children in a German school for the deaf were being taught using the Rochester method. When these children were transferred to an oral-only approach, the "quantity and quality of speech improved. Lipreading ability increased partially" (quoted in Power, 1974). Studies such as this last one are difficult to evaluate because it is not possible to determine the effects of increased age and the change in social group pressure or in numbers of opportunities to use speech.

What is striking about the studies summarized in Power (1974) and Moores (1971, 1974) is the lack of any direct evidence that the use of manual communication is in fact detrimental to the development of speech skills. If such an interference relationship existed, one would expect to see it reported in study after study. Its absence is thus noteworthy.

Socialization, Achievement, and Emotional Development

The relationship of the use of manual communication to the well-being of the deaf person interacts with the relationship of a deaf person to his parents. Several of the earlier cited studies that compared deaf students of deaf parents with deaf students of hearing parents to determine the relationship of manual communication to the acquisition of English or of speech skills are relevant here. These studies overwhelmingly reported better overall achievement for the deaf students of deaf parents, even though there were differences on some measures, and, in some cases, no differences at all. It is probable that much of this achievement directly depends on better parent-child relations, which in turn are a function of better communication channels.

Moores (1974) summarized several studies comparing deaf students of deaf parents to deaf students of hearing parents. Relevant portions are discussed here, but the reader is advised that these are only summaries. Stevenson (1964) compared 134 deaf students of deaf parents to 134 deaf students of hearing parents, and reported higher educational achievement for the deaf students of deaf parents in 90% of the comparisons, with 38% of the students with deaf parents going on to college, compared to only 9% of the students with hearing parents. Stuckless and Birch (1966) reported superior reading, speechreading, and written language for the deaf students of deaf parents, with no differences noted in speech or psychosocial development.

Meadow (1966) reported higher self-image and academic achievement for the students of deaf parents. She reported a superiority of 1.25 years in arithmetic, 2.1 years in reading, and 1.28 years overall for these students. In addition, teachers' ratings of the students were in favor of the deaf students of deaf parents on maturity, responsibility, independence, sociability, appropriate sex role, popularity, appropriate responses to situations, fingerspelling ability, written language, signing ability, absence of communicative frustration, and willingness to communicate with strangers. No difference was noted in speech or lipreading.

Vernon and Koh (1970) likewise found that deaf students of deaf parents were superior in reading, vocabulary, and written language, with an overall achievement of 1.44 years higher than the students of hearing parents (and no manual communication). No differences were found in speech, speechreading, or psychosocial adjustment. Quigley and Frisina (1961) found higher vocabulary levels for the deaf students of deaf parents, no differences in speechreading or educational achievement, and better speech for the deaf students of hearing parents. Vernon and Koh (1970) compared deaf students of deaf parents with early manual communication to deaf students of hearing parents with early intensive oral training (John Tracy Clinic program). They found that the students of deaf parents were one full grade ahead in all areas and had superior reading. No differences were found in speech or speechreading.

Comparisons of deaf students of deaf parents with deaf students of hearing parents reveal that 60% of the deaf students of deaf parents did not have preschool education, whereas only 18% of the deaf students of hearing parents have not attended preschool. The hearing parents have a significantly higher socioeconomic status than the deaf parents, and nearly 90% of the hearing parents had some contact with the John Tracy Clinic program.

Information is scarce concerning the relationship between manual communication and vocational success, psychologic problems, and other psychosocial aspects. One study (Rainer, Altshuler, and Kallmann, 1963) reported that the better the communication skills (oral or manual), the higher the probability of marriage. However, once married, the better the communication skills, the higher the incidence of marital discord. Such information, while interesting, does not directly pertain to the use of manual communication as much as to the need for communication skills. Aspects of development related to manual communication are currently being investigated by Hilde Schlesinger and Kay Meadow at the Langley Porter Institute in San Francisco. Related articles can be found in O'Rourke (1972) (see Vernon, Meadow, or Schlesinger).

Memory

With respect to the relationship between manual communication and memory, there are two questions that can be profitably asked: 1) What is the effect of signing on the organization of memory, particularly with respect to recall of English? 2) What is the effect of signing on the development of memory itself?

Organization of Memory and English   At this point, the reader should recall the earlier section dealing with research on ASL related to memory, where Bellugi and Siple's (1971) investigation of the parameters involved in recall of ASL is discussed. Their study dealt specifically with the organization of memory for ASL. It is briefly pointed out in that section that hearing people tend to make mistakes based on the phonologic properties of the words they hear or see; "phonologic" properties of signs produce similar errors in deaf persons. In order to better consider the research that has been done on memory processes of deaf individuals, the research on hearing people is now reviewed in more detail.

The recall of lists of unrelated words is heavily influenced by the sounds that constitute those words. Conrad (1962) demonstrated that hearing people have greater difficulty recalling lists of unrelated words that sound alike (phonetically similar) than lists that do not sound alike. Wickelgren (1965) investigated the contributions to memory of the major phonetic distinctive features of which sounds are composed (place of articulation: bilabial, dental, velar, etc.; and manner of articulation: voiced/voiceless, nasal/oral, aspirated/unaspirated, etc.). (The Bellugi and Siple (1971) study is entirely analogous in that it demonstrated the role in memory of the various distinctive features that constitute signs.) The use of phonologic information for memory coding was shown to be effective regardless of whether the lists were presented auditorally or visually. However, research has also demonstrated that, if at all possible, people will attempt to organize the words to be recalled according to some semantic or syntactic relationship. If a person can relate five words in a list by a sentence, or by remembering that they were all four-legged animals, this information will aid in recall.

The use of semantic information provides a greater benefit to memory than syntactic information. In fact, Sachs (1967) found that the actual syntax of a sentence is discarded very shortly after the sentence is seen or heard, probably because, once the meaning of a sentence has been extracted, the syntax is no longer useful information. Thus, for hearing people, one can expect that memory for unrelated word lists will be coded on a phonologic basis unless semantic clustering can be accomplished, and that memory for sentences will be coded on a semantic basis and not on the form (syntax) of the sentence (Bransford and Franks, 1971; Bransford, Barclay, and Franks, 1972; Crowder, 1972; Franks and Bransford, 1972; LaBerge, 1972; Norman, 1972; Paris and Carter, 1973).

To determine the role of phonologic features on deaf people's memory, Conrad and Rush (1965) investigated recall of visually presented lists of consonants (presumably the same strategies are at work with lists of letters as with lists of unrelated words). Some of the nine consonants used were phonetically similar (B, P, T, C,), others were visually similar (A, H, T, I). The recorded error patterns did not support either a phonologic or a visual encoding strategy. Locke (1970) investigated the same consonants to determine whether the fingerspelling alphabet was responsible for the errors (and would thus be a coding strategy for deaf persons) but found little support for this hypothesis.

Conrad (1970, 1971, 1972, 1973) determined that it was possible for prelingually, profoundly deaf people to use an auditory encoding strategy. In a school in which the method of instruction was predominantly oral, he compared two groups of deaf students: those for whom the phonologic properties of the consonant letters provided at least some support to coding and recall (this group was subsequently rated "above average" in speech quality by independent judges) and those for whom the auditory features seemed to be largely irrelevant (this group was subsequently rated as "average" in speech quality). Conrad inferred that the above-average group articulated while reading (not necessarily overtly) while the average group did not. He then compared the two groups on recall of visually presented material in two conditions, one where they silently read the presented material, and the other where they read out loud the presented material. Recall was not greatly improved by vocalization for the "articulating" group but was significantly hampered for the "nonarticulating" group. The inference is that the articulating group had acquired some form of a phonologic code so that actually articulating the material while reading did not either help or hinder them. But the nonarticulating group had acquired a nonphonologic coding system, and reading out loud actually interfered with their normal coding process.

A further study by Locke and Locke (1971) determined that the type of linguistic coding strategy correlated to some extent with the deaf person's articulatory skills. Unintelligible deaf subjects made more errors in recall of visually similar letter pairs that did the intelligible deaf subjects or hearing controls. Furthermore, unintelligible deaf subjects made more dactylically similar confusions (based on the fingerspelling alphabet) than did the other two groups (see Wilbur, 1974a).

The implications of the above studies are that 1) coding strategies are learned, not innate; 2) deaf people have a choice of coding language either by phonologic, visual, or manual means; 3) oral training methods do not guarantee phonologic coding strategies; 4) deaf people who do not have phonologic coding strategies, and do not use sign, do not give clear evidence of reliance on only one of the other possible strategies.

Kates (1972) compared three groups of deaf children and two groups of hearing children on several language tasks, some of which relate directly to memory for English. His groups were: oral, Rochester method, Combined (oral and signs), Hearing-Age (hearing subjects matched with the deaf subjects for age, about 14 years old), and Hearing-Achievement (hearing subjects matched with the deaf subjects for general achievement level, approximately 10 years old). On a task that investigated short-term recall memory of unconnected words, Kates found a difference between the Combined group and the Hearing-Age group, and that the other two deaf groups were not different from the two hearing groups, nor were the hearing groups significantly different from each other. At the same time, short-term recognition memory for the same words was tested (recognition being easier than recall), and no differences were found among the five groups. Kates looked only at the number of words correctly recalled or recognized and did not attempt to determine whether or not a difference existed in the types of mistakes made by the Oral, Rochester, and Combined groups.

In another study by Kates investigating noun-pair recall with the same subjects, two nouns were presented in a sentence, all the nouns being in all capital letters. Subjects were then given the first noun and were asked for the second. At the same time, subjects were asked to recall the sentence even though they had not been instructed to pay attention to the sentence (incidental recall). Kates found no differences among the five groups, presumably because the nouns and sentences were processed semantically. The last related study by Kates dealt with sentence memory, that is, memory for the exact syntax of a sentence. In this study, he found that the oral group did better than the other two deaf groups and also better than the two hearing groups. He did not find differences between the two remaining deaf groups and the two hearing groups. Kates' studies do not show consistent trends; the results may be attributable to specific instruction in the different schools.

What about the direct relationship between memory for English and ASL? Is written English converted to sign features for coding and storage? The only relevant study known to this author is Odom, Blanton, and McIntyre (1970), indicating that English words that have direct equivalents in ASL were recalled significantly better than words that did not. Further research is definitely needed. Are whole sentences converted to ASL? What is the effect of differences in syntax between the two languages? How does ASL compare with the manual systems? This author is pursuing this line of investigation.

Development of Memory   Related to the preceding discussion is the obvious question: How does learning ASL as a native language affect the eventual organization and strength of the memory process? Put another way, will someone who learns ASL as a first language have a more effective memory, and thus greater learning potential, than someone who learns ASL when he enters school at age 5? than someone who learns ASL in high school? than someone who learns ASL as an adult? than someone who never learns ASL?

The Kates (1972) study suggested that, in terms of overall amount of information to be remembered at any one time, Oral deaf students are not impaired any more than their hearing counterparts. Neither are those who use the Rochester or Combined methods. None of the deaf students in Kates' study have deaf parents, so that the comparison is between deaf students who have learned a strategy since entering school and hearing children who have acquired their strategy over normal developmental stages. (For a discussion of normal memory development, see Brown, 1975.)

Because the deaf students are not grossly deficient in their memory processing, and yet are significantly behind in their acquisition of

English, the focus should be shifted from "how much" memory to "what kind" of memory. If, as the Conrad and Locke studies indicated, many deaf people are using a variety of strategies, will early ASL usage provide a more efficient strategy, which can facilitate later learning of English? Again, the Odom, Blanton, and McIntyre (1970) study is suggestive. The deaf subjects' recall of English words with ASL equivalents is significantly better than the hearing subjects' recall of both lists of English words (those with ASL equivalents and those without). Possibly, to compensate for their deficiency with respect to English, deaf children need better memories than their hearing counterparts. Unfortunately, the central question being raised here—how does early learning of ASL affect memory?—has not been specifically studied. It is raised here for the purpose of pointing out to the reader areas related to ASL that are still unstudied.

Perception   In their comparison of signing and speech, Bellugi and Siple (1971) found that nearly 50% fewer signs than spoken words were used to relate the same number of propositions in the same amount of time. Stokes and Menyuk (1975) suggested that both ASL and English (and other natural languages) are adapted to the human central processing mechanism such that there is an optimal range of time in which linguistic processing occurs. This would include perception, attention, short-term memory, and comprehension and production processing. Because signs take longer to produce (larger muscles move more slowly), a signed language would have to be adjusted so that the semantic and syntactic content could be conveyed in fewer signs in order to keep the length of an utterance within the optimal range. Thus, the function of rules like Agent-Beneficiary Incorporation and Negative Incorporation would be to pack more information into a single sign, and fewer signs would be needed. Stokes and Menyuk reported that more recent work by Bellugi and Fischer indicated that the Signed English version takes two to two-and-a-half times longer to produce than the ASL or spoken English versions of the same sentence. Stokes and Menyuk suggested that abnormally slowed input greatly taxes storage and retrieval processes. It may be that, when difficulty is encountered in the use of sign systems in the classroom, the unusual length of a signed utterance that contains a separate sign for each English word or morpheme may be to blame. It may be that the utterance exceeds the short-term memory span and that the slow rate of input does not permit sufficient syntactic processing to aid memory coding as the input is received. As yet there are no data to support these speculations, but should they turn out to be correct, the effect would be to make the acquisition of a signed system (as opposed to ASL) a more difficult task for the young child than previously expected.

Memory and Reading   Aside from the direct implication that the Odom, Blanton, and McIntyre (1970) study has for memory, that study has another important implication for the teaching of reading. Research on hearing children indicates that children who learn letter-sound association, and then use these associations in reading (by sounding out the word), experience superior reading achievement (Chall, 1967). Consequently, reading materials intended for hearing children rely heavily on the acoustic properties of the words to serve as recognition cues to the beginning reader. Such materials would seem to be inappropriate for use with deaf children, even aside from syntactic difficulties (Quigley, Smith, and Wilbur, 1974). Instead, the study suggested that memory for English words can be strongly affected by associations with signs, and that perhaps reading materials written to reflect correspondences between English and ASL would provide a more effective teaching medium. Such an approach also might reduce the frustration involved in initial reading attempts.

Use with Other Populations

Because "other populations" includes a variety of possible problems, certain subdivisions must be made before manual communication can be considered.

1.   There are individuals who, at some point during their lives, indicate that they are capable of both sophisticated comprehension and production but who do not choose to communicate

2.   There are individuals who have excellent comprehension and are capable of good production but who suffer from performance disfluencies (consistently improper word choice, disrupted switching of stylistic level)

3.   There are individuals who have excellent comprehension but who have difficulties in production attributable to speech problems

4.   There are individuals who demonstrate comprehension on tasks not requiring verbal output but who do not speak, and make no effort to

5.   There are individuals who demonstrate generalized learning difficulties of which disturbed language is one manifestation; in such in-

dividuals there may be little or no evidence of production and possibly little or no evidence of comprehension

These five general groups are not intended to be all-inclusive, or necessarily mutually exclusive, and they do not take into account etiology, but they do represent basic variables to be considered in the remediation process. For example, the first group does not have a language disorder in the *linguistic* sense of language. In most cases of this type, some emotional disturbance is indicated, and unless the emotional problem is directly related to using speech (as in a child who refuses to talk for fear of using up his breath), it is not clear that switching to manual communication will provide any benefit.

In the second group, the disorder can be considered paralinguistic. That is, it relates to factors concerned with socially defined usage of language (conventional meanings of words, proper style for addressing friends as opposed to strangers). This type of problem has been reported with autistic adolescents (Simmons and Baltaxe, in press). It is not clear what benefit would be gained by using manual communication with this population. The probability of similar problems with ASL cannot be ruled out.

In those instances where there is an indication of aphasia of the type in which the patient finds it difficult to find the right word or where the patient substitutes semantically similar or phonologically similar words for the intended words, some benefit may be gained by switching to ASL. Markowicz (1973), Battison and Markowicz (1974), and Battison and Padden (1974), reported that evidence from brain lesions indicates that signs, fingerspelling, and speech are differentially located in the brain and are differentially impaired by lesions. It is possible, then, for speech to be lost while signs remain intact. Battison and Markowitz (1974, p. 16) suggested that: "some hearing aphasics may have an intact system capable of producing propositional gestures. That is, the language disruption of some hearing aphasics may be limited to their speech, and they may be capable of learning to sign, all problems of training aside."

Individuals with speech problems may have either nerve problems (dysarthria) or motor coordination problems (oral apraxia). In the case of dysarthria, manual communication would seem to be indicated. In the case of oral apraxia, manual communication might be a beneficial alternative, unless of course the apraxia is actually more generalized to include manual apraxia also.

Individuals who exhibit no expressive language may demonstrate a wide range of comprehension, from nearly none (a few highly frequent utterances that require simple motor responses like "stand there" or "put on your jacket") to quite sophisticated (as, for example, reported in Lenneberg, 1967). Some success in using signs with low functioning nonverbal children has been reported (see Kopchick and Lloyd, this volume; Mayberry, 1974; Fulwiler and Fouts, in press). For whatever reason, these children made no attempt to imitate auditory input and consequently produced no output. Then signs were introduced, each sign being taught with the spoken word. For each successive sign, fewer and fewer repetitions were required. The children learned both the signs and the words, and spontaneous vocalizations increased markedly. One child acquired signs so rapidly that it is difficult to consider him retarded (William Reagan, personal communication).

In the four groups discussed above, as long as some indication of comprehension was present and there was no indication of generalized learning difficulties, the focus of remediation was on providing a means for expressing language. With the retarded, particularly the severely or profoundly retarded, the establishment of receptive language becomes as important as, if not more important than, teaching means of expression.

In order to acquire a minimal receptive knowledge of a language, an individual (theoretically) must be capable of symbolic representation, in that he or she must be able to use something (not necessarily a word) to stand for (refer to, represent) something else (an object or concept). The child who can take a rattle and pretend in overt play that it is a spoon (or some similar type of representation) has indicated the ability to substitute a symbol (the rattle) for the object (the spoon). Within Piaget's (1951, 1952, 1964) theory of cognitive development, the child begins to develop such symbolic representation at Stage 6 of the sensorimotor period (roughly 18 to 24 months of age in normal children). Inherent in Piaget's theory is the notion of "readiness" to acquire language.

M. Woodward (1959) found that many profoundly retarded children and adolescents functioned at a level below Stage 6. In an explicit test of the relationship between Stage 6 functioning and the presence of meaningful language in the severely/profoundly retarded, Kahn (1975) compared a group of eight children who were able to use at least 10 words to ask for various objects, with another group of eight children who used no words at all. On four Piagetian tasks of Stage 6 functioning, Kahn found that seven of the eight children who used words functioned at the Stage 6 level on all four tasks, whereas none of the eight children who did not use words functioned at Stage 6 on all four tasks. The two best children of the nonlanguage group were able to reach Stage 6 functioning on only two of the tasks. Kahn's findings were statistically significant: the language group functioned at Stage 6, the nonlanguage group did not. Kahn (1975, p. 642) concluded that:

> . . . the implications of these findings for the training of nonlanguage profoundly retarded children to acquire language is potentially extensive. If, as these findings seem to indicate, the cognitive structures which develop during Stage 6 of Piaget's sensorimotor period are necessary for the acquisition of meaningful expressive language, then training of nonlanguage profoundly retarded children to develop language skills should begin with an assessment of their cognitive level. According to this position, those children who are at Stage 6 could then reasonably be expected to learn language skills with relative ease and operant techniques would appear appropriate. However, those children who are not functioning at Stage 6 would not be expected to learn meaningful expressive language with any reasonable degree of efficiency. These children would probably benefit more from training activities directed towards raising their cognitive level.

It should be made clear at this point that it is not the present author's intention to endorse operant techniques or for that matter any particular teaching methods. The concern here is primarily with what is being taught, rather than how it is being taught. Information about language intervention programs is covered elsewhere (e.g., Graham, this volume; Appendix D). For a general discussion of language of the mentally retarded, see Cromer (1974).

Once an individual has been deemed to be capable of acquiring language, the choice between oral language and manual language centers on matters of motor and perceptual complexity. The early emergence of signs suggests that signs are motorically simpler. Schlesinger and Meadow (1972) presented charts of the development of signs as they inter-relate with motor development. One possible advantage of using signs is their visibility. The learner is able to see the shape and movement of the modeler's hands and, crucially, of this own hands. The two sets of hands can be held together to determine the similarity, and the learner's hands can be corrected more easily than the learner's mouth. Signs also can be useful if a perceptual disorder is suspected.

That is, it might be possible to take advantage of the visual perception system if the auditory perception system seems to be disrupted (not hearing impairment, but auditory attention focusing or short-term auditory memory) (Graham and Graham, 1971).

What form of manual communication should be taught? The populations dealt with in this section represent groups that do not form their own subculture, as do the deaf. They do not have their own community organizations, social structures, and native language. In the absence of a communal language, there seems little reason to choose one form of signing over another. However, given the constraints on the structure of signs discussed earlier in this chapter and the role of signs in perception, memory, and in reducing independent movement by the two hands, those forms of manual communication that use ASL signs would be preferable to those which do not. Many of the signs created for the manual systems violate the sign constraints, which presumably are perceptually based (Siple, 1973). Thus, there are two remaining possibilities: ASL and Signed English. The use of ASL requires the teacher to learn new syntax (that of ASL), but it provides the child with the key to entering the world of the deaf. (For further discussion, see Charrow and Wilbur, 1975.) In the absence of a community with its own language, other populations (mentally retarded, autistic, schizophrenic, aphasic, etc.) can be taught Signed English, as recommended by Kopchick and Lloyd (this volume). This has the advantage of not requiring teachers to learn a new syntax. At the same time, the possibility of perceptual processing problems (raised by Stokes and Menyuk, 1975) must be kept in mind. Above all, however, it should be recalled that the weight of the evidence is in favor of any signs over no signs at all.

SUMMARY

This chapter considers the structure and function of American Sign Language and several manual systems within a linguistic framework. An attempt is made to provide extensive documentation to the claim that American Sign Language is a language. This documentation includes examples of syntactic structures and associated grammatical relations, formational constraints on possible signs that distinguish signs from nonsigns and gestures, historical changes in signs, acquisition of signs, and sociolinguistic and pragmatic aspects of signs. Perceptual processing, memory organization, and other factors are offered as reasons for the structure and function of signs and for those aspects that are restricted to visual languages.

The manual systems are considered in the same framework, and it is the contention of this chapter that the manual systems are not languages in the same sense that ASL, English, and German are. Furthermore, there is no evidence to warrant the claim that the different systems' basic principles of sign formation in any way reflect the morphology of English words. Evidence of superiority of using a manual system rather than ASL in the education of the deaf is also noticeably lacking. Fingerspelling and Cued Speech are separated from the other systems as being merely auxiliaries to written or spoken English in the same way as writing or Morse code.

The practical considerations involved in deciding to use manual communication with either a deaf or a hearing population include discussion on the relationship of manual communication to the acquisition of language in general and English in particular, to the development of speech and speechreading skills, to overall academic achievement and socioemotional development, to memory organization and functioning, and to the development of reading skills. The evidence considered does not indicate negative relationships in any of these areas and suggests that use of manual communication is beneficial in many aspects of the development and education of the deaf.

ACKNOWLEDGMENTS

The author would like to express her appreciation to those people who contributed their research papers on request, providing a massive compilation of research in the area. Special thanks go to Nancy Allen, who contributed heavily to the discussion of manual systems; to Robbin Battison, James Woodward, and Harry Markowicz for their contributions to the initial organization of the chapter and continued support throughout; to Veda Charrow, Paula Menyuk, and Judy Kegl for critical comments and suggestions; and to Lyle Lloyd for his infinite patience.

REFERENCES

Ahlström, K. G. 1972. On evaluation of the effects of schooling. *In* Proceedings of the International Congress on Education of the Deaf. Sveriges Lärarförbund, Stockholm.

Allen, N. 1975. What is said and what is signed: The relationship between English and four modes of signing English. Unpublished masters thesis, University of Southern California, Los Angeles.

Anthony, D. 1966. Signing Essential English. Unpublished master's thesis, University of Michigan, Ann Arbor.

Anthony, D. 1971. Signing Essential English. Vols. 1 and 2. Educational Services Division, Anaheim Union School District, Anaheim, Cal.

Bailey, C-J. 1971. Variation and language theory. Unpublished manuscript, University of Hawaii, Honolulu.

Baker, C. 1975. Regulators and turn-taking in American Sign Language discourse. Unpublished manuscript, University of California, Berkeley.

Battison, R. 1973. Phonology in American Sign Language: 3-D and digit-vision. Presented at the California Linguistic Association Conference, Stanford.

Battison, R. 1974. Phonological deletion in American Sign Language. Sign Lang. Stud. 5:1–19.

Battison, R., and H. Markowicz. 1974. Sign aphasia and neurolinguistic theory. Unpublished manuscript, Linguistics Research Lab, Gallaudet College, Washington, D.C.

Battison, R., H. Markowicz, and J. C. Woodward. 1975. A good rule of thumb: Variable phonology in American Sign Language. In R. Shuy and R. Fasold (eds.), Analyzing Variation in Language. Georgetown University Press, Washington, D.C.

Battison, R., and C. Padden. 1974. Sign Language aphasia: A case study. Presented at the 49th Annual Meeting, Linguistic Society of America, New York.

Bellugi, U. 1972. Studies in Sign Language. In T. O'Rourke (ed.), Psycholinguistics and Total Communication: The State of the Art. National Association of the Deaf, Silver Spring, Md.

Bellugi, U. 1975. Sign Language structure. Presented at Brown University, Providence, R.I.

Bellugi, U., and S. Fischer. 1972. A comparison of Sign Language and spoken language: Rate and grammatical mechanisms. Cognition 1:173–200.

Bellugi, U., and E. S. Klima. 1972. The roots of language in the sign talk of the deaf. Psychol. Today June: 61–64, 76.

Bellugi, U., and P. Siple. 1971. Remembering with and without words. Presented at the International Colloquium of C.N.R.S., Current Problems in Psycholinguistics.

Berko, J., and R. Brown. 1966. Psycholinguistic research methods. In P. H. Mussen (ed.), Handbook of Research Methods in Child Development. John Wiley & Sons, New York.

Bloom, L. 1970. Language Development: Form and Function in Emerging Grammar. MIT Press, Cambridge, Mass.

Bloom, L. 1973. If, when, and why children imitate in language development. Presented at the Institute for Research on Exceptional Children, University of Illinois, Urbana-Champaign.

Bonvillian, J. D., V. R. Charrow, and K. E. Nelson. 1973. Psycholinguistic and educational implications of deafness. Hum. Dev. 16:321–345.

Bornstein, H. 1973. A description of some current sign systems designed to represent English. Amer. Ann. Deaf 118:454–463.

Bornstein, H., and L. Hamilton. 1972. Some recent national dictionaries of sign language. Sign Lang. Stud. 1:42–63.

Bornstein, B. Kannapell, K. Saulnier, H., L. Hamilton, and H. Roy. 1973. Basic Pre-school Signed English Dictionary. Gallaudet College, Washington, D.C.

Bornstein, H., L. Hamilton, K. Saulnier, and H. Roy. 1975. The Signed English Dictionary for Pre-school and Elementary Levels. Gallaudet College, Washington, D.C.

Børrild, K. 1972. Cued Speech and the mouth-hand system. In G. Fant (ed.), International Symposium on Speech Communication Ability and Profound Deafness. A. G. Bell Association for the Deaf, Washington, D.C.

Boyes, P. 1973. Developmental phonology for ASL. Working paper, Salk Institute for Biological Studies, La Jolla, Cal.

Boyes-Braem, P. 1973. A study of the acquisition of the dez in American Sign Language. Working paper, Salk Institute for Biological Studies, La Jolla, Cal.

Bragg, B. 1973. Ameslish: Our national heritage. Amer. Ann. Deaf 118:672–674.

Bransford, J. D., J. R. Barclay, and J. J. Franks. 1972. Sentence memory: A constructive versus interpretive approach. Cog. Psychol. 3:193–209.

Bransford, J. D., and J. J. Franks. 1971. The abstraction of linguistic ideas. Cog. Psychol. 2:331–350.

Brasel, K., and S. P. Quigley. 1975. The influence of early language environments on the development of language in deaf children. Institute for Research on Exceptional Children, University of Illinois, Urbana-Champaign.

Brown, A. 1975. The development of memory: Knowing, knowing about knowing, knowing how to know. In H. Reese (ed.), Advances in Child Development and Behavior. Academic Press, New York.

Chall, J. 1967. Learning to Read: The Great Debate. McGraw-Hill, New York.

Charrow, V. R. 1974. Deaf English—An investigation of the written English competence of deaf adolescents. Report 236, Institute for Mathematical Studies in the Social Sciences, Stanford, Cal.

Charrow, V. R. 1975a. A psycholinguistic analysis of "Deaf English." Sign Lang. Stud. 7:139–150.

Charrow, V. R. 1975b. A linguist's view of Manual English. Presented at the World Conference on the Deaf, Washington, D.C.

Charrow, V. R., and J. D. Fletcher. 1973. English as the second language of deaf students. Report 208, Institute for Mathematical Studies in the Social Sciences, Stanford, Cal.

Charrow, V. R., and R. B. Wilbur. 1975. The deaf child as a linguistic minority. Theory into Practice 14:353–359.

Conlin, D. 1972. The effects of word imagery and signability in the paired-associate learning of the deaf. Master's thesis, University of Western Ontario, London, Ontario.

Conrad, R. 1962. An association between memory errors and errors due to acoustic masking of speech. Nature 193:1314–1315.

Conrad, R. 1970. Short-term memory processes in the deaf. Brit. J. Psychol. 61:179–195.

Conrad, R. 1971. The effect of vocalizing on comprehension in the profoundly deaf. Brit. J. Psychol. 62:147–150.

Conrad, R. 1972. Speech and reading. In J. F. Kavanagh and I. G. Mattingly (eds.), Language by Ear and by Eye: The Relationships between Speech and Reading. MIT Press, Cambridge, Mass.

Conrad, R. 1973. Some correlates of speech coding in the short-term memory of the deaf. J. Speech Hear. Res. 16:375–384.

Conrad, R., and M. L. Rush. 1965. On the nature of short-term memory encoding by the deaf. J. Speech Hear. Disord. 30:336–343.

Cornett, R. O. 1967. Cued Speech. Amer. Ann. Deaf 112:3–13.

Cornett, R. O. 1969. In answer to Dr. Moores. Amer. Ann. Deaf 114:27–33.

Covington, V. 1973a. Juncture in American Sign Language. Sign Lang. Stud. 2:29–38.

Covington, V. 1973b. Features of stress in American Sign Language. Sign Lang. Stud. 2:39–58.

Cromer, R. F. 1974. Receptive language in the mentally retarded: Processes and diagnostic distinctions. In R. L. Schiefelbusch and L. L. Lloyd (eds.), Language Perspectives—Acquisition, Intervention, and Retardation. University Park Press, Baltimore.

Crowder, R. G. 1972. Visual and auditory memory. In J. F. Kavanagh and I. G. Mattingly (eds.), Language by Ear and by Eye: The Relationships between Speech and Reading. MIT Press, Cambridge, Mass.

Fant, L. J., Jr. 1964. Say It with Hands. Gallaudet College, Washington, D.C.

Fant. L. J., Jr. 1972a. The American Sign Language. Cal. News 83(5).

Fant, L. J., Jr. 1972b. Ameslan. National Association of the Deaf, Silver Spring, Md.

Fischer, S. 1973. Two processes of reduplication in American Sign Language. Found. Lang. 9:469–480.

Fischer, S. 1975. Influences on word-order change in American Sign Language. In C. Li (ed.), Word Order and Word Order Change. University of Texas Press, Austin.

Fischer, S., and B. Gough. 1975. Verbs in American Sign Language. In U. Bellugi and E. Klima (eds.), The Signs of Language. Harvard University Press, Cambridge, Mass.

Franks, J. J., and J. D. Bransford. 1972. The acquisition of abstract ideas. J. Verb. Learn. Verb. Behav. 11:311–315.

Friedman, L. 1975. On the semantics of space, time, and person reference in the American Sign Language. Language 51:940–961.

Frishberg, N. 1974. The case of the missing length. Presented at the 49th Annual Meeting, Linguistic Society of America, New York.

Frishberg, N. 1975. Arbitrariness and iconicity: Historical change in American Sign Language. Language 51:676–719.

Frishberg, N., and B. Gough. 1973a. Morphology in American Sign Language. Working paper, Salk Institute for Biological Studies, La Jolla, Cal.

Frishberg, N., and B. Gough. 1973b. Time on our hands. Presented at the Third Annual California Linguistics Association Conference, Stanford.

Fulwiler, R., and R. Fouts. Acquisition of American Sign Language by a non-communicating autistic child. J. Autistism Child. Schizo. In press.

Furth, H. 1966a. A comparison of reading test norms of deaf and hearing children. Amer. Ann. Deaf 111:461–462.

Furth, H. 1966b. Thinking Without Language. Collier-Macmillian, London.

Graham, J. T., and L. W. Graham. 1971. Language behavior of the mentally retarded: Syntactic characteristics. Amer. J. Ment. Defic. 75:623–629.

Grosjean, F., and H. Lane. 1976. Pauses and structure in American Sign Language. Unpublished manuscript, Northeastern University, Boston.

Gustason, G., D. Pfetzing, and E. Zawolkow. 1972. Signing Exact English. Modern Signs Press, Rossmoor, Cal.

Hockett, C. F. 1958. A Course in Modern Linguistics. Macmillan, New York.

Hoemann, H. W. 1975. The transparency of meaning of sign language gestures. Sign Lang. Stud. 7:151–161.

Hoffmeister, R., D. Moores, and R. Ellenberger. 1975. The parameters of Sign language defined: Translation and definition rules. Sign Lang. Stud. 7:121–137.

Kahn, J. V. 1975. Relationship of Piaget's sensorimotor period to language acquisition of profoundly retarded children. Amer. J. Ment. Defic. 79:640–643.

Kates, S. 1972. Language development in deaf and hearing adolescents. Final report: RD-2555-S (14-P-55004). Social and Rehabilitation Service, Department of Health, Education, and Welfare, Washington, D.C.

Kegl, J. A. 1976. Pronominalization in American Sign Language. Unpublished manuscript, Massachusetts Institute of Technology, Cambridge.

Kegl, J. A., and N. Chinchor. 1975. A frame analysis of American Sign Language. In T. Diller (ed.), Proceedings of the 13th Annual Meeting, Association for Computational Linguistics. Amer. J. Comput. Ling. Microfiche 35. Sperry-Univac, St. Paul, Minn.

Klima, F., and U. Bellugi. 1975. Wit and poetry in American Sign Language. Sign Lang. Stud. 8:203–224.

Kroeber, A. L. 1958. Sign language inquiry. Int. J. Amer. Ling. 24:1–19.

LaBerge, D. 1972. Beyond auditory coding. In J. F. Kavanagh and I. G. Mattingly (eds.), Language by Ear and by Eye: The Relationships between Speech and Reading. MIT Press, Cambridge, Mass.

Lacy, R. 1972a. Development of Pola's questions. Working paper, Salk Institute for Biological Studies, La Jolla, Cal.

Lacy, R. 1972b. Development of Sonia's negations. Working paper, Salk Institute for Biological Studies, La Jolla, Cal.

Lacy, R. 1973. Directional verb marking in the American Sign Language. Presented at the Summer Linguistic Institute, Linguistic Society of America, University of California, Santa Cruz.

Lacy, R. 1974. Putting some of the syntax back into semantics. Presented at the 49th Annual Meeting, Linguistic Society of America, New York.

Lacy, R. 1975. Pronominalization in American Sign Language. Dissertation in progress, University of California, San Diego.

Lane, H., P. Boyes-Braem, and U. Bellugi. Preliminaries to a distinctive feature analysis of American Sign Language. Cog. Psychol. In press.

Lenneberg, E. 1967. Biological Foundations of Language. John Wiley & Sons, New York.

Locke, J. L. 1970. Short-term memory encoding strategies in the deaf. Psychonom. Sci. 8:233–234.

Locke, J. L., and V. L. Locke. 1971. Deaf children's phonetic, visual, and dactylic coding in a grapheme recall task. J. Exp. Psychol. 89:142–146.

Long, J. S. 1918. The Sign Language: A Manual of Signs. Athens Press, Iowa City.

McCall, E. 1965. A generative grammar of Sign. Unpublished master's thesis, University of Iowa, Iowa City.

McIntire, M. L. 1974. A modified model for the description of language acquisition in a deaf child. Unpublished master's thesis, California State University, Northridge.

McIntire, M. L. 1975. Acquisition of American Sign Language. Dissertation in progress, Department of Linguistics, University of California, Los Angeles.

Markowicz, H. 1972. Some sociolinguistic considerations of American Sign Language. Sign Lang. Stud. 1:15–41.

Markowicz, H. 1973. Aphasia and deafness. Sign Lang. Stud. 3:61–71.

Mayberry, R. 1974. Systems of manual communication and some clinical considerations for their use with normally hearing, non-communicative individuals. Unpublished manuscript. McGill University, Montreal.

Meadow, K. 1966. The effect of early manual communication and family climate on the deaf child's development. Unpublished doctoral dissertation, University of California, Berkeley.

Moores, D. 1969. Cued Speech: Some practical and theoretical considerations. Amer. Ann. Deaf 114:23–27.

Moores, D. 1971. Recent research on manual communication. Research and Demonstration Center in the Education of the Handicapped, University of Minnesota, Minneapolis.

Moores, D. 1972. Communication: Some unanswered questions and some unquestioned answers. In T. O'Rourke (ed.), Psycholinguistics and Total Communication: The State of the Art. National Association of the Deaf, Silver Spring, Md.

Moores, D. 1974. Nonvocal systems of verbal behavior. In R. L. Schiefelbusch and L. L. Lloyd (eds.), Language Perspectives—Acquisition, Retardation, and Intervention. University Park Press, Baltimore.

Mossel, M. 1962. The standard Sign Language: A useful but inadequate language training tool. Better Techniques of Communication for Severely Handicapped Deaf People Workshop, Vocational Rehabilitation Administration, Department of Health, Education, and Welfare, Washington, D.C.

Myklebust, H. 1964. The Psychology of Deafness. Grune & Stratton, New York.

Myklebust, H. 1967. Development and Disorders of Written Language. Grune & Stratton, New York.

Norman, D. 1969. Memory and Attention. John Wiley & Sons, New York.

Norman, D. 1972. The role of memory in the understanding of language. *In* J. F. Kavanagh and I. G. Mattingly (eds.), Language by Ear and by Eye: The Relationships between Speech and Reading. MIT Press, Cambridge, Mass.

Odom, P. B., R. L. Blanton, and C. K. McIntyre. 1970. Coding medium and word recall by deaf and hearing subjects. J. Speech Hear. Res. 13:54–58.

O'Rourke, T. J. 1972. Psycholinguistics and Total Communication: The State of the Art. National Association of the Deaf, Silver Spring, Md.

O'Rourke, T. J. 1973. A Basic Course in Manual Communication. National Association of the Deaf, Silver Spring, Md.

O'Rourke, T. J., T. Medina, A. Thames, and D. Sullivan. 1975. National Association of the Deaf Communicative Skills Program. Programs for the Handicapped, April:27–30.

Paget, R. 1951. The New Sign Language. The Welcome Foundation, London.

Paget, R., and P. Gorman. 1968. A Systematic Sign Language. National Institute for the Deaf, London.

Paris, S. G., and A. Y. Carter. 1973. Semantic and constructive aspects of sentence memory in children. Dev. Psychol. 9:109–113.

Piaget, J. 1951. Play, Dreams, and Imitation in Childhood. Norton, New York.

Piaget, J. 1952. The Origins of Intelligence in Children. International Universities Press, New York.

Piaget, J. 1964. Development and learning. J. Res. Sci. Tech. 2:176–186.

Power, D. J. 1971. Deaf children's acquisition of the passive voice. Unpublished doctoral dissertation, University of Illinois, Urbana-Champaign.

Power, D. J. 1974. Language development in deaf children: The use of manual supplements in oral education. Aust. Teach. Deaf 15.

Prickett, H. T., Jr. 1971. Letter to the Editor. Deaf Amer. March.

Quigley, S. P. 1969. The influence of fingerspelling on the development of language, communication, and educational achievement in deaf children. Institute for Research on Exceptional Children, University of Illinois, Urbana-Champaign.

Quigley, S. P., and R. Frisina. 1961. Institutionalization and Psychoeducational Development in Deaf Children. Council on Exceptional Children, Washington, D.C.

Quigley, S. P., D. S. Montanelli, and R. B. Wilbur. Some aspects of the verbal system in the language of deaf students. J. Speech Hear. Res. In press.

Quigley, S. P., N. L. Smith, and R. B. Wilbur. 1974. Comprehension of relativized structures by deaf students. J. Speech Hear. Res. 17:325–341.

Quigley, S. P., R. B. Wilbur, and D. S. Montanelli. 1974. Question formation in the language of deaf students. J. Speech Hear. Res. 17:699–713.

Quigley, S. P., R. B. Wilbur, and D. S. Montanelli. Complement structures in the written language of deaf students. J. Speech Hear. Res. In press.

Quigley, S. P., R. B. Wilbur, D. J. Power, D. S. Montanelli, and M. W. Steinkamp. 1976. Syntactic Structures in the Language of Deaf Children. Institute for Child Behavior and Development, University of Illinois, Urbana-Champaign.

Rainer, J., K. Altshuler, and F. Kallmann (eds.). 1963. Family and Mental Health Problems in a Deaf Population. State Psychiatric Institute, Columbia, New York.

Richards, J. 1974. Error Analysis and Second Language Learning. Longman Publishing Co., New York.

Rupert, J. 1969. Kindergarten program using Cued Speech at the Idaho State School for the Deaf. Report of the Proceedings of the 44th Meeting of the American Instructors of the Deaf, Berkeley, Cal.

Sachs, J. 1967. Recognition memory for syntactic and semantic aspects of connected discourse. Percep. Psychophys. 2:437–442.

Schlesinger, H. S., and K. Meadow. 1972. Sound and Sign: Childhood Deafness and Mental Health. University of California Press, Berkeley.

Schmitt, P. 1968. Deaf children's comprehension and production of sentence transformations and verb tenses. Unpublished doctoral dissertation, University of Illinois, Urbana-Champaign.

Scouten, E. L. 1967. The Rochester method: An oral multisensory approach for instructing prelingual deaf children. Amer. Ann. Deaf 112:50–55.

Simmons, J., and C. Baltaxe. Language patterns of adolescent autistics. J. Autism. Child. Schizo. In press.

Siple, P. 1973. Visual Constraints for Sign Language Communication. Working paper, University of Rochester, Rochester, N.Y.

Stevenson, E. 1964. A study of the educational achievement of deaf children of deaf parents. Cal. News 80:143.

Stokes, W. T., and P. Menyuk. 1975. A proposal for the investigation of the acquisition of American Sign Language and Signed English by deaf and hearing children enrolled in integrated nursery school programs. Unpublished manuscript, Boston University, Boston.

Stokoe, W. C. 1960. Sign Language structure: An outline of the visual communication system of the American deaf. Stud. Ling. Occasional Papers No. 8.

Stokoe, W. C. 1970a. The study of Sign Language. ERIC Clearinghouse for Linguistics, Center for Applied Linguistics, Washington, D.C.

Stokoe, W. C. 1970b. Sign Language diglossia. Stud. Ling. 21:27–41.

Stokoe, W. C., D. C. Casterline, and C. G. Croneberg. 1965. Dictionary of American Sign Language. Gallaudet College. Washington, D.C.

Stuckless, E., and J. Birch. 1966. The influence of early manual communication on the linguistic development of deaf children. Amer. Ann. Deaf 111:452–460, 499–504.

Tervoort, B. 1961. Esoteric symbols in the communicative behavior of young deaf children. Amer. Ann. Deaf 106:436–480.

Vernon, M., and S. D. Koh. 1970. Effects of early manual communication on achievement of deaf children. Amer. Ann. Deaf 115:527–536.

Wampler, D. 1971. Linguistics of Visual English. Early Childhood Education Department, Aurally Handicapped Program, Santa Rosa City Schools, Santa Rosa, Cal.

Wampler, D. 1972. Linguistics of Visual English (2322 Maher Drive, No. 35), Santa Rosa, Cal.

Washington State School for the Deaf. 1972. An Introduction to Manual English. The Washington State School for the Deaf, Vancouver, Wash.

Watson, D. 1973. Talk with Your Hands. George Banta, Menasha, Wisc.

Wickelgren, W. 1965. Distinctive features and errors in short-term memory for English vowels. J. Acous. Soc. Amer. 38:583–588.

Wilbur, R. B. 1974a. Reading and memory processes in deaf people who learned American Sign Language as their first language. Unpublished manuscript, Institute for Research on Exceptional Children, University of Illinois, Urbana-Champaign.

Wilbur, R. B. 1974b. Deaf and hearing children's abilities to recognize word patterns: The development of morpheme structure constraints in children. Presented at the American Speech and Hearing Association convention, Las Vegas.

Wilbur, R. B. 1976. A pragmatic explanation of deaf students' difficulty with several syntactic structures of English. Paper presented at the A. G. Bell Association Conference, Boston.

Wilbur, R. B., and M. L. Jones. 1974. Some aspects of the bilingual/bimodal acquisition of Sign and English by three hearing children of deaf parents. In M. LaGaly, R. Fox and A. Bruck (eds.), Proceedings of the Tenth Regional Meeting, Chicago Linguistic Society. Chicago Linguistic Society, Chicago.

Wilbur, R. B., D. S. Montanelli, and S. P. Quigley. Pronominalization in the language of deaf students. J. Speech Hear. Res. In press.

Wilbur, R. B., and S. P. Quigley. 1975. Syntactic structures in the written language of deaf students. Volta Rev. 77:194–203.

Wilbur, R. B., S. P. Quigley, and D. S. Montanelli. 1975. Conjoined structures in the language of deaf students. J. Speech Hear. Res. 18:311–335.

Woodward, J. C., Jr. 1972. Implications for sociolinguistic research among the deaf. Sign Lang. Stud. 1:1–17.

Woodward, J. C., Jr. 1973a. Implicational lects on the deaf diglossic continuum. Unpublished doctoral dissertation, Georgetown University, Washington, D.C.

Woodward, J. C., Jr. 1973b. Some observations on sociolinguistic variation and American Sign Language. Kan. J. Sociol. 9:191–200.

Woodward, J. C., Jr. 1973c. Interrule implication in American Sign Language. Sign Lang. Stud. 3:47–56.

Woodward, J. C., Jr. 1973d. Some characteristics of Pidgin Sign English. Sign Lang. Stud. 3:39–46.

Woodward, J. C., Jr. 1974a. Implication variation in American Sign Language: Negative incorporation. Sign Lang. Stud. 5:20–30.

Woodward, J. C., Jr. 1974b. A report on Montana-Washington implicational research. Sign Lang. Stud. 4:77–101.

Woodward, J. C., Jr. 1974c. Black Southern Signing. Presented at the 49th Annual Meeting, Linguistic Society of America, New York.

Woodward, J. C., Jr. 1974d. Variety is the spice of life. Presented at the First Annual Conference on Sign Language, Gallaudet College, Washington, D.C.

Woodward, J. C. Jr. and C. Erting. 1975. Variation and historical change in American Sign Language. Lang. Sci. 37.

Woodward, J. C., Jr., and H. Markowicz. 1975. Some handy new ideas on pidgins and creoles: Pidgin sign languages. Presented at the International Conference on Pidgin and Creole Languages, Honolulu.

Woodward, M. 1959. The behavior of idiots interpreted by Piaget's theory of sensori-motor development. Brit. J. Educ. Psychol. 29:60–71.

12

TOTAL COMMUNICATION PROGRAMMING FOR THE SEVERELY LANGUAGE IMPAIRED: A 24-HOUR APPROACH

George A. Kopchick, Jr., and Lyle L. Lloyd

CONTENTS

Importance of Total Communication _____ 504

The 24-hour Approach _____ 505

    Gaining administrative support/506
    Administrative considerations/507
    Special roles of the audiologist/507
    Selection of clients/508
    Selection of staff/509
    Staff training/510
    Living area/511
    Selection of sign language system/512
    Selection of teaching method/513
    Residential activities/514
    Schedule for Client A.G./515

Conclusion _____ 518

References _____ 518

This chapter presents a rationale and methodology for a total communication program instituted on a 24-hour basis for severely language-impaired individuals who live in private or public residential centers.

Within a residential setting, the operational definition of total communication has two aspects. The first is the traditional, which suggests utilization of all available language modes for the purpose of achieving communication, such as gestures, postures, facial expressions, tones of voice, formal speech and nonspeech systems, and simultaneous communication. The second aspect is a broader one, which suggests a communication program that is available throughout the client's total environment—in short, a program that does not cease at the end of the school day. In this chapter, the significance of this second meaning is stressed.

The use of nonspeech communication systems, especially total communication, with the severely language impaired is attracting increasing interest (e.g., Berger, 1972a; Bricker, 1972; Eliott and Nirje, 1972; Creedon, 1973; Imaoka, 1974; Kent, 1974; Schiefelbusch and Lloyd, 1974; Shaffer and Goehl, 1974; Fristoe, 1975; Kopchick, Rombach, and Smilowitz, 1975; Vanderheiden et al., 1975; Wilson, Goodman, and Wood, 1975). Several reports indicate that mentally retarded individuals who have not developed the ability to talk despite years of training can be taught to communicate with signs from American Sign Language (ASL) or with other nonspeech systems (e.g., Sutherland and Becket, 1969; Hall and Talkington, 1970; Berger, 1972a, b; Stohr and VanHook, 1973a; Coggins, Eng, and Gill, 1974; Brookner and Murphy, 1975).

Several nonspeech systems are presented in this volume (see chapters by Carrier, Vanderheiden and Harris-Vanderheiden, and Wilbur). This chapter deals with the specific application of one such system—total communication as defined above. In contrast to systems that depend on some type of device involving manipulation of equipment and/or nonspeech symbols, most modes of total communication employ only the tools that are always available to trainer or client—hands, fingers, mouth, etc. In this ready availability lies the main power of the system: It has the potential to be used during all aspects of the client's daily living routine. The consistent utilization of total communication on a 24-hour basis provides the ample repetition required by many slow learners and promotes immediate functional application of each appropriate response. When a client makes an appropriate response, the immediate functionality also can serve as a reinforcer that is likely to generate additional spontaneous communication.

Utilization of a combination of visual/motor and aural/oral expression is often called "simultaneous communication" and is considered an important segment of any total communication program. However, as Lloyd (1973) cautioned, the term *simultaneous communication* can become only a euphemism for a completely manual approach. In dealing with the severely language impaired, the oral/aural stimuli (words) and motor/visual stimuli (signs) always must be presented together. Anything less than this truly simultaneous communication can cause confusion and impair effectiveness, resulting in failure to achieve the maximal benefit offered by a total communication approach.

IMPORTANCE OF TOTAL COMMUNICATION

Because higher functioning clients generally have a better prognosis for developing speech, and, in the past, few successful language training programs have been available for the severely retarded, the work of the speech pathologist in mental retardation facilities usually has been concentrated on clients classified as mildly to moderately retarded. Although it would be unwise to state that verbal skills can never be taught to severely language-impaired clients, it seems safe to say that, for many, the goal of intelligible speech production will be difficult to obtain.

Now that the thinking of the field has broadened to the point where speech is viewed as only one of several possible expressive modes, professionals are realizing that language often can be taught to even profoundly retarded clients through other methods (Stohr and VanHook, 1973a; Kent, 1974; Fristoe, 1975; Wilson, Goodman, and Wood, 1975). Consequently, responsibilities of speech pathologists in residential settings have been enlarged to include teaching language to severely language-impaired clients. Most now feel a professional and sometimes even a legal obligation to give each individual the opportunity to develop to the limits of his or her potential. For some the final goal will be communication through speech; for others the final goal will be communication through some other means. Whatever the end goal, a total communication approach may best meet the severely language-impaired client's communication needs because it will both be useful at the client's present level of functioning and will allow progression at an individual rate until that person's maximum level is reached.

THE 24-HOUR APPROACH

The importance of functional language has been emphasized (e.g., Miller and Yoder, 1972; McLean, Yoder, and Schiefelbusch, 1972; Brown, 1973; Guess, Sailor, and Baer, 1974; Schiefelbusch and Lloyd, 1974). To be functional, language must have the power to permit manipulation and modification of one's environment. Burrows and Lloyd (1972) have stated that it is difficult to build functionality into a total communication program unless the environment in which the client's personal and physical needs are met can enhance and reinforce the use of this total communication. In a recent survey, Brannan, Sigelman, and Bensberg (1975) found that institutions for the retarded provide less than 1 to more than 6 hours of language instruction daily; but, regardless of amount of time spent, this training is usually confined to a classroom or clinic. Administrators of language programs frequently bemoan the lack of skill generalization outside the clinical area when in fact there is an almost total lack of communication exchanges available to the severely language-impaired client anywhere else in the environment.

Kopchick, Rombach, and Smilowitz (1975) have reported that stressing total communication only in the classroom does not result in a change of communication behaviors in the living environment. Although severely language-impaired clients could recognize and produce signs in the classroom, once outside they reverted to their old behaviors of withdrawal and esoteric gesturing. Clients involved in only a daytime classroom approach did not comprehend the true communicative potential of what they were learning.

The living environment of severely language-impaired clients is not limited to the classroom or clinic. Their environment also consists of their dining, living, and recreation areas. With a lack of adequate language stimulation in the living area, the communication interactions and opportunities presented in the classroom or clinic can have little impact on clients' lives. With limited opportunity for functional implementation, generalization from the clinic is unlikely to occur. Language cannot become functional if it is not used everywhere that clients live, or if it is used only during a small proportion of their waking hours.

In order to meet these environmental language stimulation needs, the environment must be considered to include all other persons who interact with the client. Certainly, direct-care staff at the living area who do not recognize or comprehend the developing expressive skills of a client will not help this language to become functional. Ideally, simultaneous communication training should be provided for the entire staff of the residential center. A more realistic approach, which would meet the Accreditation Council for Facilities for the Mentally Retarded standard requiring that, "the grouping of program and residence units shall be based upon a rational plan to meet the needs of the residents. . . ," would be to group a segment of clients according to language needs and then provide simultaneous communication training to those personnel who would staff this area. The enivronment in that living area then would be one in which all staff and clients could share the same simultaneous communication methods.

Gaining Administrative Support

A prerequisite to the establishment of a 24-hour total communication program is gaining the support of the facility administrator, who will need considerable information in order to judge the feasibility of such a program. A well written, comprehensive proposal justifying the program, designating environmental and staff needs, and specifying management and training procedures is essential. In addition to the general considerations presented in this chapter, the plan should include the following:

1.   Reasons for the proposal, including a list of client's needs that are not currently being met
2.   Total number and names of all clients that the program will serve
3.   Equipment and space needed, including an environmental living area and modifications that should be made to the area
4.   Number of staff needed on each shift, classified by working title
5.   Description of how the administration of the program fits into the facility's table of organization
6.   Objectives of the program that go beyond increasing language and communication skills, such as developing personal hygiene, self-care skills, etc.

Numbers 2, 3, and 4 may be presented in the proposal in the form of several alternatives, with two or three different sized groups and areas being described. These alternatives provide the administrator with an option of selection. An administrator who may not accept a large request may approve a small project involving only a dozen or so clients and perhaps seven or eight staff members. Twelve or 18 months after beginning the pilot project, it should not be difficult to gain additional support if the project has shown positive results.

Administrative Considerations

The administrative supervision of the 24-hour total communication program is naturally a critical factor in its success. There must be an appropriate emphasis on communication throughout every client's daily activities. As a communication specialist, the speech pathologist, audiologist, or educator of the hearing impaired should have major responsibility for the administration and supervision of this program, which is designed to maximize development of communication skills. This responsibility includes authority over and responsibility for all direct-care staff assigned to the program. In facilities operating under a unit system, this communication specialist would act as unit director, with the total communication program functioning as a small unit. This would allow some administrative autonomy and would result in the communication specialist assisting in the selection of the clients to be assigned and then coordinating the entire program of each of these clients.

Some of the problems which would exist in a program that is developed and instituted by a communication specialist and then subsequently administered by medical or nursing staff are obvious. By having direct-care staff report directly to the communication specialist, the vital need for close coordination between the communication training that occurs in the clinic and that which occurs at the living area will be obtainable. Close contact between these training areas will ensure adequate reinforcement of the communication concepts being taught.

Special Roles of the Audiologist

The audiologist can play an important role in the total communication program. A relatively high prevalence of hearing problems is found in a population of severely language-impaired individuals

(Bensburg and Sigelman, this volume; Lloyd, 1970). Systematic hearing screening and rescreening programs (Cox and Lloyd, this volume; Lloyd and Cox, 1972) provide the audiologist with the opportunity to identify and refer many clients to the program through acquaintance with the entire institutional population. Because most of the language-impaired clients with a hearing impairment must have consistent use of quality amplification, the audiologist plays a critical role in monitoring hearing aids and in training staff and clients in hearing aid maintenance (McCoy and Lloyd, 1967; Moore, Miltenberger, and Barber, 1969; Hanners and Sitton, 1974).

Ross (this volume) discusses the major aspects of providing amplification and the difficulties of hearing aid maintenance experienced in schools for the deaf. Similar difficulties can be expected in a mental retardation or other type facility; thus, it is recommended that the audiologist make at least weekly visits to the living area to spot-check the aids and perform simple preventive maintenance. This weekly hearing aid check should be a regularly scheduled activity and should be made a mandatory part of the schedule of all hearing aid users until they show that they can consistently care for their own aids. Staff training should include instructions in the maintenance of hearing aids, and daily hearing aid checks should be made part of the direct-care staff routine. If the supervisor of the program also makes periodic hearing aid checks, maximal benefit can be derived from their use. The importance of these daily and weekly checks to ensure proper functioning of the clients' aids cannot be overemphasized. With clients who have such severe communication handicaps, the risk of eliminating input through a major sensory channel cannot be tolerated.

Selection of Clients

Prime candidates for a 24-hour total communication program are those individuals who are nonverbal, noncommunicative, unintelligible, and nonresponsive to oral modification, or those who demonstrate high receptive skills but very limited expressive skills. However, the candidates also may have hearing impairments compounding their problems, or they may have been diagnosed as autistic, schizophrenic, brain damaged, mentally retarded, aphasic, or any combination of these. Diagnosis or etiology should not be the determining factor for selection. The determination should be based on the assessment of language skills and the conclusion that these clients may derive more benefit from nonspeech language training than from more traditional communication training. A rule of thumb that is often used for selecting clients for a total communication program is simply the failure to imitate speech.

Because of the difficulties of determining the intelligence level of severely language-impaired persons, any intelligence test scores must be considered highly tentative (Vernon, this volume). The lack of adaptive behaviors often noted in these clients may be attributable to an inability to relate to their environment, sometimes resulting in attempts either to destroy it or to withdraw from it. For the most part, these clients may not indicate personal needs or respond to gesture or contact with adults. For these reasons, it is also difficult to estimate reliably their potential for development (Berger, 1974). Developmentally, they may need first to achieve basic attending and gross motor imitation skills before they can profit from more specific communication training.

Because there is no evidence at present that using a nonspeech communication method deters eventual development of oral communication, there is no reason to think that putting clients into such a program is committing them to a perpetual nonspeech state. They may or may not eventually develop oral communication, but regardless of their eventual accomplishments they will have an interim method available to them to take care of their current communication needs.

The best method for selecting clients for the program is to conduct an interdisciplinary team staffing to determine the needs of each client with a language problem. The speech and hearing specialist always must be prepared, however, to provide major input into the recommendations for these language-impaired individuals. When an interdisciplinary team staffing is not possible, the speech and hearing specialists should determine which clients are most appropriate for the program, based on the criteria mentioned above.

Selection of Staff

The most critical aspects of developing a 24-hour total communication program may be staff selection, training, and supervision. Any attempt to rush the selection or in-service training process would be unwise. It is essential to attract staff members who have a real interest in working with language-impaired clients. An advertisement in the facility's newsletter or bulletin is a good way to reach all direct-care employees. The application should be worded to discourage applicants who are primarily interested in getting away from disliked assignments. Indicating the necessity of having to develop sign language fluency on one's own time may serve to eliminate those who are inappropriately motivated.

Personal interviews with all applicants may give information regarding the applicants' appreciation of the effects of language handicaps, their willingness to learn, and their openness to new procedures. Talks with their supervisors and a review of their personnel files may give additional information about their flexibility, special skills in interacting with clients, dependability, attitudes, and work habits. Knowledge of what in-service training or other courses they have taken may indicate their past interest in gaining new skills and techniques.

Select the number of staff needed on each shift, plus at least two alternates on each shift. The alternates or relief personnel will ensure adequate coverage and continuity of services should any of the original selections resign.

The importance of selecting capable and enthusiastic direct-care staff cannot be overemphasized. These people will be spending much more time with the clients than will any speech pathologist, audiologist, or educator. If the program is successful, it will be primarily because of their input (Sigelman and Bensberg, this volume; Bensburg, 1965).

Staff Training

The staff must be afforded the best possible training in simultaneous communication and in behavior management principles and techniques. Behavior management has been discussed in other chapters of this volume (Baker; Spradlin, Karlan, and Weatherby; Sigelman and Bensberg). An understanding of the principles of behavior modification and skill in devising management strategies is essential to the handling of clients who have limited communicative abilities. Simultaneous communication training should be provided to direct-care and other interested staff by a consultant or someone skilled in the specific system selected (e.g., Signed English). Experience indicates that the signing fluency necessary to initiate a 24-hour total communication program cannot be readily acquired in less than a month of daily classes. These classes should be scheduled twice daily in order to reach staff from all three shifts.

The staff of the 24-hour total communication unit should develop their skill in simultaneous communication until it becomes easy for them to communicate in this way. Simultaneous communication should be required among trained staff at all times and should be encouraged even when communication takes place with other ancillary staff. Such use will create increased awareness of its importance, and at least some incidental learning may occur among untrained staff members. This constant use of simultaneous communication provides a model for clients who observe the communication interaction, and it demonstrates to them that this interaction is a productive functional tool that causes environmental changes. In effect, the functionality of communication in a 24-hour total communication program is taught by example.

Living Area

Haviland (1972) has presented a view of most residential environments that demonstrate their negative influence on communication development. One must be cognizant of these factors in selecting a living area for a 24-hour total communication program. Most living areas in residential centers were built for convenience of staff and not for programming needs of the clients living there. Most facilities do not have living areas that stimulate clients to realize their communicative potential. The Accreditation Council for Facilities for the Mentally Retarded (1975) *Standards for Residential Facilities for the Mentally Retarded* may be used as a guide for selecting the living space. These standards specify a maximum of four clients per bedroom area and a minimum of 60 square feet per client in multiple sleeping quarters. The large dormitory areas that are so common in many facilities are not appropriate because of their poor acoustics, which lessens the positive impact of aural stimulation and all but destroys the effectiveness of hearing aids.

Furthermore, smaller bedroom areas contribute to the development of independent living skills and self-management. A homelike living environment adds to the ease with which staff and clients can interrelate and mingle, resulting in more communication exchanges taking place between them. The living area must be one that *fosters* communication. If such an area is not present, the initial proposal must delineate the environmental changes that will be necessary to provide such a suitable and stimulating living area.

Selection of Sign Language System

The director of a total communication program should study carefully all sign language systems in order to select one that will provide maximal benefits, with particular regard to consistency within the program (see Wilbur, this volume). Although there have been reports of methods utilizing esoteric or modified sign language systems for teaching communication skills to a specific severely language-impaired group (Wilson, 1974b; Topper, 1975), development of a special manual system, while interesting, is not usually necessary. Most reports indicate that many severely language-impaired individuals can learn manual communication symbols such as those used in American Sign Language (Grecco, 1972; Hall and Talkington, 1972; Hoffmeister and Farmer, 1972; Kent, 1974; Fristoe, 1975; Kopchick, Rombach, and Smilowitz, 1975). These authors stated that their major reason for choosing root signs from ASL was to make communication as functional and as broad-based as possible, having use in many different environments. There is another practical side: Videotapes, 8mm films, and a number of good illustrated booklets are available to aid in staff training (Riekehof, 1963; Saunders, 1968; Fant, 1972; O'Rourke, 1973; Bornstein et al., 1975; Christopher, 1976).

Publication of the Babbidge Report of Health, Education, and Welfare's Committee on Education of the Deaf in 1965 made apparent the need for use of manual systems other than ASL. This report indicated that the average graduate of a public residential school for the deaf had only an eighth grade education, largely the consequence of low language and reading attainment rather than low intelligence. Also, ASL does not lend itself well to true simultaneous communication because its morphology and syntax differ from that of spoken English. Other systems—Signed English, Systematic Sign Language (Paget-Gorman system), Seeing Essential English, Signing Exact English, and Linguistics of Visual English— have been designed to parallel more closely the morphology and syntax of spoken English (see Wilbur, this volume).

Whatever successes these other systems achieve in residential schools for the deaf, it is doubtful whether the strict application of any of these systems is useful with the severely language-impaired, such as the mentally retarded deaf or the profoundly retarded. The complexities of these systems increase the difficulty of mastery by those with severe multiple handicaps.

A reasonable alternative is a modification of Signed English, as described by Bornstein (1973) and Bornstein et al. (1973, 1975), *without* the initial use of inflectional markers. Thus, as particular clients become skilled in its use, tense and plurality may be added through signed markers when such complexities can be handled. Therefore, the authors recommend this modification and simplification of Signed English as the system that is best suited for severely impaired individuals. It can be made as complex or as simple as the needs of the individual require, and it can present exactly the same message to the receiver through both visual and auditory channels, hence permitting a true simultaneous presentation. Bornstein and his group at Gallaudet College have developed a number of storybooks, posters, and a dictionary for use with preschool deaf parents. Many of these materials are also quite appropriate for severely retarded individuals.

Selection of Teaching Method

Consistent stimulation from a 24-hour total communication environment will not solve all communication problems. These clients, except for those with severe to profound hearing impairments, have heard speech all their lives without learning spoken language. It is doubtful that mere exposure to sign language will result in its being learned. A language (or communication) teaching approach based solely on environmental stimulation lacks the intensity and consistency needed to ensure success. A specific approach, based on functional goals and procedural structure, must be chosen and followed by all staff members. Berger (1972a, b) has presented a systematic approach to teaching the various expressive modes according to an empirically determined scale of increasing complexity, from gross motor responding (sitting, walking, standing), to specific motor responding (pointing, selecting matching), and then to manual signing, fingerspelling, writing, and speaking. Following is her own brief description of the method (Berger, 1972b, pp. 119–120):

> Prerequisite to response development of any communication mode is an ability to discriminate the salient features of that mode. Therefore, the following sequence of discriminative stimuli was arranged, again according to increasing complexity: gestures (gross and specific), manual signing, alphabet symbols (printed and signed), graphemes, finger spelling, visual-kinesthetic-auditory features of spoken language.

Procedurally, a continuing interchange between discriminative responding and response development takes place, with stimulus discrimination always preceding modal response development. Utilizing a paired-association procedure, new stimuli are matched with previously learned ones; the first-learned stimuli are faded so that independent discriminative responding to the new stimulus can be elicited. Through imitation and successive approximation the new response modes are developed.

Because some clients will not be able to use even simple signs at the beginning of their training, Berger included the use of gross motor responses and gestures as an available mode for primary training. Some clients must begin with work at this level with additional work on developing attending skills. These very gross motor responses can consist of imitating the teacher's gross motor action (e.g., standing, sitting, bending from the waist, raising hands over head). Initially the client's body may have to be physically shaped to imitate the movement. However, this one-to-one personal contact plus a tangible reinforcer for completion of the movement almost always results in some successful imitation at this very basic level. Eventually, the client will produce gestures with merely a cue from the teacher.

After determining the appropriate level and mode of responding, taking small steps of increasing complexity eliminates the possibility of stifling potential that can be caused either by trying to advance in increments of too great a magnitude or by failing to utilize learned stimuli to achieve a higher level of response. Signed English used in simultaneous communication encourages staff members and clients to strive consistently for a higher level. One of the valuable features of Berger's hierarchy is that it can provide poorly discriminating, noncommunicating clients with the skills necessary to indicate their discriminations at least in gestural form. However, clients who progress beyond this level will develop a more sophisticated awareness of the communication process. For some, the development of manual language, fingerspelling, or even speech may become viable goals.

Residential Activities

While stressing the importance of communication skills, several clinicians emphasize the importance of training the severely language-impaired in other adaptive behaviors, including self-help, education, socialization, and vocational skills (e.g., Hall and Talkington, 1970;

Hall and Conn, 1972; Burrows and Lloyd, 1972; Brannan, Sigelman, and Bensberg, 1975). In developing an individualized program to enhance adaptive behaviors, the residential living segment should be different for each individual according to needs for adaptive behavior training.

The following is an example of a daily schedule of a 50-year-old client with a profound hearing loss who was involved in a 24-hour total communication program. The schedule was arranged after an interdisciplinary team staffing was held to set up an individualized program for this man.

Schedule for Client A.G.

Monday through Friday:
 6:00 Self-care skills (showering, dressing, toothbrushing, hair combing, etc.)
 7:00 Breakfast (mealtime training program)
 8:00 Grooming (wash up and shave)
 8:30 Vocational training
 9:00 Vocational training
10:00 Vocational training
11:00 Grooming (wash up, comb hair)
11:30 Lunch
12:30 Free time (Wednesday—Speech and Hearing Clinic, hearing aid preventive maintenance)
 1:00 Community orientation class (sight vocabulary, community signs, etc.)
 2:00 Sign Language class (signs of daily living)
 3:00 Education class (number concepts, identity, time, etc.)
 4:00 Grooming (wash up and comb hair)
 4:30 Dinner
 5:30 Free time
 6:00 Recreation and socialization (movies, dances, sports, games)
 7:30 Free time
 8:00 Communication skills (second shift staff reviews first shift classroom lessons)
 9:00 Self-care skills (shower and prepare for bed)
 9:30 TV time
10:00 Lights out

Client A.G. had been institutionalized for over 40 years. At the beginning of the program, he had a very complex system of esoteric signs that only he could understand. The staff had learned to smile when he gestured, nod their heads, and pat him on the back. This of course pleased him. On the Leiter International Performance Test, he scored an IQ of 45, but the staff did not believe it. They thought he was more capable and more alert than an IQ of 45 would indicate, There is no way of ascertaining the adverse effects of over 40 years of institutional living, but there is no doubt that it could cause a certain amount of cultural retardation.

This client had been able to exist for all those years with a complete lack of expressive and receptive language. His records showed a history of violent temper tantrums and behavioral outbursts along with a history of stealing and fighting. Staff and clients learned to leave him alone. A speechreading and auditory training program proved to be of little value to him. When a classroom total communication program was started, he quickly learned to imitate and produce the signs that were taught. These signs were never carried over to his living environment, however.

When a 24-hour total communication program was initiated (Kopchick, Rombach, and Smilowitz, 1975), the first month was spent teaching A.G. and 10 other nonverbal clients the signs for the clothes they wore and the food and drink they consumed as listed in Appendix F at the back of this book.[1] At all times the direct-care staff provided a model for the clients by engaging in simultaneous communication according to Van Riper's (1972) parallel talking format. That is, the staff provided a simultaneous communication model for all that was happening in the environment, especially during times of dressing, eating, and bathing. The clients learned to imitate what the staff did. At the end of this month, the clients were then expected to use signs to ask for what they wanted, rather than having everything provided automatically.

At this point, A.G. was deliberately sent to the shower without his soap, towel, or toothbrush. At first he reverted to his old behavior and became angry, grunted, and pointed at the closet where the soap was kept. The aide who worked during bathing time looked at him inquisitively and asked, "You want soap?" in simultaneous communication. A.G. responded with the sign for "soap" and the aide

---

[1]A listing such as the one provided in Appendix F is designed to assist clinicians and teachers in developing functional vocabularies for their clients. In developing this basic or functional vocabulary, it should be noted that some terms vary from setting to setting, and the vocabulary of the individual must be used rather than a printed list that someone else has developed for another environment. There are a number of limited vocabulary sign language booklets designed especially for the retarded (Owens and Harper, 1970; Talkington and Hall, 1970; Stohr and VanHook, 1973b; Andreas et al., 1974; Topper, 1974; Vail and Spas, 1974; Wilson, 1974a).

opened the door and gave it to him. He and the other clients became somewhat perturbed when their clothes were not in the usual place after their shower. The first day resulted in some confusion and tears, but eventually the clients learned that by using the hand and arm configurations that they had learned during the past month, they could manipulate people around them to do what they wanted.

Within a week, communication had increased dramatically. Some of the clients enjoyed asking staff members for things just to see them active. It was as if they had found a power that they never had before. They learned that it was easier to manipulate people through specific and structured gestures than to scream and pound tables.

To make residential programming for the clients' adaptive behavior effective, direct-care staff members trained in simultaneous communication were scheduled to participate with the clients in most daily living activities. That is, staff members were assigned to accompany clients periodically to the workshop or the school where additional services were received. The direct-care staff member then explained to the clients in simultaneous communication what was expected of them. When A.G. attended a recreational program or participated in leisure time activities, a direct-care staff member, through simultaneous communication, would make these programs as meaningful as possible. The staff member also attempted to have A.G. and the other clients communicate at their highest level during these activities.

During these times, the direct-care staff also acted as "sign language teachers" to the staff members who provided ancillary services. Each department at the facility that provided support services to these clients was encouraged to have one or more members of its staff assigned the responsibility of learning sign language to a degree adequate for them to assume responsibility for providing their specialty to the severely language-impaired population. This involvement of other staff members increased the effectiveness of all residential activities for the clients and ensured acceptance and success of the program. Even in areas where this training of ancillary staff members had been done, however, the total communication program direct-care staff still assisted in carrying out all aspects of residential programming.

The success of any residential program necessarily depends on the training and supervision that the direct-care staff members receive

(Sigelman and Bensburg, this volume). In-service training sessions in sign language must be continually scheduled to provide refresher courses to the total communication staff as well as to offer ancillary staff members the rudiments of the system.

CONCLUSION

This chapter is written to provide information primarily for persons interested in developing or currently operating a 24-hour total communication program.

As more professionals concerned with the welfare of the institutionalized severely language impaired become aware of the benefits to be obtained from a 24-hour program, the number of such programs should increase. Presently, according to the results of a survey of state institutions for the retarded by Brannan, Sigelman, and Bensberg (1975), there are only seven total communication programs that operate on a 24-hour basis. So-called total communication programs that are not operating on a 24-hour basis are failing to realize their fullest potential. It is the consistency and continuity provided by the type of model program described in this chapter that provides maximal opportunity for the development of communication skills in the severely language impaired.

REFERENCES

Accreditation Council for Facilities for the Mentally Retarded. 1975. Standards for Residential Facilities for the Mentally Retarded. Joint Commission on Accreditation of Hospitals, Chicago.

Andreas, J., D. Bell, J. Bentley, G. Buck, and D. Klee. circa 1974. Let Your Fingers Do Your Talking: A Teaching Manual for Use with Non-Verbal Retardates. Department of Communication Disorders and Education and Training, Craig Developmental Center, Sonyea, N.Y.

Bensburg, G. 1965. Teaching the Mentally Retarded, Handbook for Ward Personnel. Southern Regional Educational Board, Atlanta, Ga.

Berger, S. L. 1972a. A clinical program for developing multimodal language responses with atypical deaf children. In J. E. McLean, D. E. Yoder, and R. L. Schiefelbusch (eds.), Language Intervention with the Retarded. University Park Press, Baltimore.

Berger, S. L. 1972b. Systematic development of communication modes: Establishment of a multiple-response repertoire for non-communicating deaf children. Report of the Proceedings of the 45th Meeting of the Convention of American Instructors of the Deaf, Little Rock, Ark., Arkansas School for the Deaf, June, 1971, pp. 118–122. U.S. Government Printing Office, Washington, D.C.

Berger, S. L. 1974. Establishing and developing initial communication for the non-communicating deaf child. Paper presented at the Council for Exceptional Children Convention, New York.

Bornstein, H. A. 1973. A description of some current syntax systems designed to represent English. Amer. Ann. Deaf 118:454–463.

Bornstein, H., L. B. Hamilton, K. L. Saulnier, and H. L. Roy. 1975. The Signed English Dictionary for Pre-School and Elementary Levels. Galladdet College Press, Washington, D.C.

Bornstein, H. A., B. M. Kannapel, K. L. Saulnier, L. B. Hamilton, and H. L. Roy. 1973. Basic Pre-School Signed English Dictionary. Gallaudet College Press, Washington, D.C.

Brannan, A. C., C. K. Sigelman, and G. J. Bensberg. 1975. The Hearing Impaired Mentally Retarded: A Survey of State Institutions for the Retarded, Research and Training Center in Mental Retardation Monograph 4, Texas Tech University, Lubbock.

Bricker, D. D. 1972. Imitative sign language as a facilitator of word-object association with low functioning children. Amer. J. Ment. Defic. 76:509–516.

Brookner, S. P., and N. O. Murphy. 1975. The use of a total communication approach with a non-deaf child: A case study. Lang. Speech Hear. Serv. Schools 6:131–139.

Brown, R. 1973. A First Language: The Early Stages. Harvard University Press, Cambridge, Mass.

Burrows, N., and L. L. Lloyd. 1972. Programming considerations for the deaf retarded. Report of the Proceedings of the 46th Meeting of the Convention of American Instructors of the Deaf, Little Rock, Ark., 1971. U.S. Government Printing Office, Washington, D.C.

Carrier, J. K., Jr., and T. Peak. 1975. Program Manual for Non-SLIP (Non-Speech Language Initiation Program). H & H Enterprises, Lawrence, Kan.

Christopher, D. A. 1976. Manual Communication: A Basic Text and Workbook with Practical Exercises. University Park Press, Baltimore.

Coggins, K., D. Eng., and M. Gill. 1974. A proposed program for teaching signs as a means of functional communication to non-verbal retarded individuals. Unpublished manuscript, University of Wisconsin, Madison.

Creedon, M. P. (ed.). 1973. Appropriate Behavior Through Communication: A New Program in Simultaneous Language for Non-Verbal Children. Dysfunctioning Child Center, Michael Reese Medical Center, Chicago.

Eliott, L. S., and B. Nirje. 1972. The deaf mentally retarded in Ontario mental retardation facilities: A program proposal. Unpublished manuscript, Prince Edward Heights, Ontario, Canada.

Fant, L. 1972. Ameslan: An Introduction to American Sign Language. National Association of the Deaf, Silver Spring, Md.

Fristoe, M. 1975. Language Intervention Systems for the Retarded: A Catalogue of Original Structured Language Programs in Use in the U.S. State of Alabama Department of Education, Montgomery, Ala.

Grecco, R. 1972. Manual Language Programs. Unpublished manuscript, Mansfield Training School, Mansfield Depot, Conn.

Guess, D., W. Sailor, and D. M. Baer. 1974. To teach language to retarded children. In R. L. Schiefelbusch and L. L. Lloyd (eds.), Language Perspectives—Acquisition, Retardation, and Intervention. University Park Press, Baltimore.

Hall, S. M., and T. F. Conn. 1972. Current trends in services for the deaf retarded in schools for the deaf and residential facilities for the mentally retarded. Report of the Proceedings of the 45th Meeting of the Convention of American Instructors of the Deaf, Little Rock, Ark., 1971. U.S. Government Printing Office, Washington, D.C.

Hall, S. M., and L. W. Talkington. 1970. Evaluation of a manual approach to programming for deaf retarded. Amer. J. Ment. Defic. 75:378–380.

Hall, S. M., and L. W. Talkington. 1972. The redwood project. Train. School Bull. 69:10–12.

Hanners, B. A., and A. B. Sitton. 1974. Ears to hear: A daily hearing aid monitor program. Volta Rev. 76:530–536.

Haviland, R. T. 1972. A stimulus to language development: The institutional environment. Ment. Retard. 10:19–21.

Hoffmeister, R. J., and A. Farmer. 1972. The development of manual sign language in mentally retarded deaf individuals. J. Rehab. Deaf 6:19–26.

Imaoka, N. 1974. Development of Communication Skills. Paper presented at American Association on Mental Deficiency Convention, Toronto.

Kent, L. R. 1974. Language Acquisition Program for the Severely Retarded. Research Press, Champaign, Ill.

Kopchick, G. A., D. W. Rombach, and R. Smilowitz. 1975. A total communication environment in an institution. Ment. Retard. 13:22–23.

Lloyd, L. L. 1970. Audiologic aspects of mental retardation. In N. R. Ellis (ed.), International Review of Research in Mental Retardation, pp., 311–374. Vol. 4. Academic Press, New York.

Lloyd, L. L. 1973. Mental Retardation and Hearing Impairment. PRWAD (Professional Rehabilitation Workers with the Adult Deaf) Deafness Annual, Vol. 3. Washington, D.C.

Lloyd, L. L., and B. P. Cox. 1972. Programming for the audiologic aspects of mental retardation. Ment. Retard. 10:22–26.

McCoy, D. F., and L. L. Lloyd. 1967. A hearing aid orientation program for mentally retarded children. Train. School Bull. 64:21–30.

McLean, J. E., D. E. Yoder, and R. L. Schiefelbusch. 1972. Language Intervention with the Retarded. University Park Press, Baltimore.

Miller, J., and D. E. Yoder. 1972. On developing the content for a language teaching program. Ment. Retard. 10:9–11.

Moore, E. J., G. E. Miltenberger, and P. S. Barber. 1969. Hearing aid orientation in a state school for the mentally retarded. J. Speech Hear. Disord. 34:142–145.

O'Rourke, T. J. 1973. A Basic Course in Manual Communication. National Association of the Deaf, Silver Spring, Md.

Owens, M., and B. Harper. 1970. Sign Language: A Teaching Manual for Cottage Parents of Non-Verbal Retardates. Pinecrest State School, Pineville, La.

Riekehof, L. 1963. Talk to the Deaf. Gospel Publishing House, Springfield, Mo.

Saunders, J. I. (ed.). 1968. The ABC's of Sign Language. Manca Press, Tulsa, Okla.

Schiefelbusch, R. L., and L. L. Lloyd. 1974. Language Perspectives—Acquisition, Retardation, and Intervention. University Park Press, Baltimore.

Shaffer, T. R., and H. Goehl. 1974. The alinguistic child. Ment. Retard. 12:3–6.

Stohr, P. G., and K. E. VanHook. 1973a. The development of manual communication in the severely and profoundly retarded. Paper presented at American Speech and Hearing Association Convention, San Francisco.

Stohr, P. G., and K. E. VanHook. 1973b. Have Hands—Will Sign: A Manual Communication Program for the Severely and Profoundly Retarded. Ranier School, Buckley, Wash.

Sutherland, G. F., and J. W. Becket. 1969. Teaching the mentally retarded sign language. J. Rehab. Deaf.

Talkington, L. W., and S. M. Hall. circa 1970. A Manual Communication System for Deaf Retarded. Austin State School, Austin, Tex.

Topper, S. 1975. Gesture language. Ment. Retard. 13:30–31.

Topper, S. circa 1974. Gesture Language for the Severely and Profoundly Mentally Retarded. Denton State School, Denton, Tex.

Vail, J., and D. L. Spas. circa 1974. A Manual Communication Program for Non-Verbal Retardates. NWSEARCH—Title I, DeKalb, Ill.

Vanderheiden, D. H., W. P. Brown, P. MacKenzie, S. Reinen, and C. Schiebel. 1975. Symbol communication for the mentally handicapped. Ment. Retard. 13:34–37.

VanRiper, C. 1972. Speech Correction Principles—Methods. Prentice-Hall, Englewood Cliffs, N.J.

Wilson, P. S. 1974a. Manual Language Dictionary: Functional Vocabulary for the Retarded. Office of Mental Retardation Developmental Team, Hartford, Conn.

Wilson, P. S. 1974b. Sign language as a means of communication for the mentally retarded. Paper presented at Eastern Psychological Association, New York.

Wilson, P. S., L. Goodman, and R. Wood. 1975. Manual Language for the Child without Language. Paula Starks Wilson, Hartford, Conn.

13

APPLICATION OF A NONSPEECH LANGUAGE SYSTEM WITH THE SEVERELY LANGUAGE HANDICAPPED

Joseph K. Carrier, Jr.

CONTENTS

Background and Rationale for a Nonspeech Language System _____ 525
  Premack's work with a nonspeech language system/525
  Pilot work with Premack's training procedures/527
  Development of a child-oriented training program/528

Description of the Child-Oriented Training Program _____ 529
  Sequencing training/530
  Labeling training/531
  Subject noun training/533
  Verb training/533
  Object of preposition training/534
  Preposition training/534

Current Application of Program _____ 538
  Subjects with whom Non-SLIP has been used/538
  General progress in Non-SLIP/539

Current Status of Non-SLIP _____ 541
  Recommended use of programs/541
  Areas in need of additional study/543

Summary _____ 544
References _____ 545

During recent years, trends in clinical management of communication disorders have resulted in reasonably optimistic potentials for nearly anyone with a specific problem. The point has not been reached where it is possible to guarantee success for any one individual, but it is possible, in most cases, to provide viable treatment and to be reasonably certain that the treatment will benefit the individual. Children with articulation disorders now have the benefit of highly programmed and highly efficient training procedures (e.g., Mowrer, Baker, and Schutz, 1968; Carrier, 1970; McLean, this volume, 1970). Children with language disorders, but without severe confounding problems, usually can be treated successfully with available programs (McGinnis, 1963; Berieter and Engelmann, 1966; Gray and Ryan, 1971; Bricker and Bricker, 1972; Kent, 1972; Miller and Yoder, 1972; Stremel, 1972).

The population of severely and profoundly mentally retarded is one for which such optimism is not currently possible. Speech and language training procedures that are generally effective with higher functioning children are seldom successful with children in this group. Speech and hearing clinics in residential institutions most often focus on the higher level children and resort to treatment of severe and profound retardates only when necessary. Procedures used with those children are usually termed *prelanguage*, usually consist of concept building or direction following, and seldom lead to a child's learning much—if any—functional communication. Some research has been done in attempting to teach spoken communication to such children (Baer, Peterson, and Sherman, 1967; Garcia, Baer, and Firestone, 1971), and, although results show that precisely defined training procedures can be effective, the time requirement for teaching small numbers of single spoken word responses are clearly prohibitive in most current clinical budgets.

BACKGROUND AND RATIONALE
FOR A NONSPEECH LANGUAGE SYSTEM

Premack's Work with a Nonspeech Language System

The recently published work of Premack (1970, 1971; Premack and Premack, 1972, 1974), although not initially intended as a means of treating severely and profoundly retarded children, suggested a perspective that seemed to have potential implication. Premack's principle concern seemed to be to demonstrate that a chimpanzee was capable of learning "language." Defying the history of past failures to teach chimps verbal language (e.g., Kellogg, 1931) and arguments that language is uniquely human (Hockett and Ascher, 1964; Bolinger, 1968; Campbell, 1970), Premack devised a system based on current behavioral technology and logic. He began by suggesting that one of the reasons chimps had not learned spoken language may have been the lack of a physiologic capability to produce the sounds requisite to speech. If speech is behavior that produces communicative symbols and if language[1] is a set of rules for using those symbols, it is clear that an organism with no symbols hardly can be expected to learn or to demonstrate usage of language. The chimp or any organism could be totally capable of learning language, the rules for using symbols, but could not demonstrate this capacity without a viable set of symbols.

Premack attempted to circumvent the physiologic limitations of the chimp by devising another symbol set to function as an alternative to speech. He prepared a series of different plastic shapes, each to represent a "word" or to function as a symbol. His hypothesis was essentially that, if a chimp had the potential for learning language, even though it might not be able to learn speech, it might be able to learn to use the plastic shapes as words and might be able to learn to manipulate them in accord with the linguistic rules more commonly associated with spoken symbols.

A second major outcome of Premack's work was the analytical manner in which he approached defining the training goals for the chimps—how he went about determining those behaviors that he would accept as governed by "linguistic" rules. Premack (1970, p. 108) stated:

> The functions an organism carries out when engaged in language need to be separated from the form these functions take in man. Not only human phonology but quite possibly human syntax may be unique to man; both may encompass mechanisms not found in any other species (Chomsky, 1965; Lenneberg, 1968 [sic]). But if this is so, it does not commit the mechanisms of logic and semantics to the same status. The latter may be more widely distributed and it may be them, not the human form of syntax and phonology, upon which the basic functions of language depend.

---

[1]More complete definition and discussions of language are presented by Siegel and Broen (this volume) and Wilbur (this volume).

From this basic premise, Premack went on to define classes of behavior that had the logical and semantic characteristics of human language, but that conceivably could be emitted without precise duplication of human utterances. Using the plastic symbols and this analytical system, he was able to teach his chimpanzee to communicate in a linguistic fashion.

The implications of Premack's work for clinical management of children with severe language handicaps may well have been one of the major contributions ever made to solving that problem. He demonstrated quite clearly that spoken symbols, although basic to most human communication and basic to most training goals, are little more than one of numerous symbol sets that can be used to teach communication. In the same sense, he demonstrated that certain constraints generally placed upon language training, because of the defined nature of human language, are not necessary for an organism to learn a functional language. The point Premack made so nicely was that functional linguistic "communication" can exist independent of many of the characteristics traditionally considered basic to its existence.

Besides this shedding of traditional views, Premack's work had even further implications for work with severely impaired humans. One of the most critical maxims in any educational programming is to begin training at a level that is simple enough to ensure success. (Mathematics students do not enroll in calculus until they have had more basic, prerequisite courses.) Those working with low functioning nonverbal children have been aware of this maxim but have not been successful at finding ways to implement it with such cases. The lowest levels of behavior were still far beyond most of these children. Premack's approach to communication training, however, was a new lower-level task and offered the potential of reaching some children.

Pilot Work with Premack's Training Procedures

Immediately after the publication of Premack's work with the chimpanzee, an attempt was made to replicate the same basic procedures with three severely retarded children (8, 12, and 14 years old) and with seven 2- to 3-year-old Down's syndrome children (Parsons and Carrier, 1971; Schmidt, Carrier, and Parsons, 1971). The purpose of this work included the study of two general questions:

1.   Can severely impaired, nonverbal children with either a history of failure or a low probability of success in conventional communication therapy learn the Premack system?

2.   Can linguistic rules, learned using the geometric shape symbols like those used by Premack, be used to facilitate learning of spoken language with children in the target population?

The answers to these questions were clearly affirmative. All subjects learned part or all of the system described by Premack and all showed some transfer to spoken responses. The most remarkable subject was a 14-year-old child who had received over 5 years of speech and language therapy before this pilot work. At the onset of the pilot work, he had no spoken responses, but within 6 months he was generating seven- to eight-word grammatically correct spoken sentences. Furthermore, he was communicating with individuals in several different environments. This case was exceptional but did illustrate the potential of such a system.

Development of a Child-Oriented Training Program

The success of the pilot work with Premack's procedures was encouraging enough to stimulate development of a set of training programs using the same basic principles but geared more directly toward meeting the needs of the human child with a severe communication handicap. Much of the rationale is discussed in depth elsewhere (Carrier, 1974a; Carrier and Peak, 1975) and is not repeated here. However, the primary efforts in preparing the training program included:

1.   Developing a language model from which specific response classes to be taught could be derived

2.   Determining, from the model, specific classes of linguistic behavior to be taught (i.e., establishing and sequencing the subgoals of training)

3.   Preparing formal training procedures, based on the experimental analysis of behavior models, to teach each of the goal behaviors

4.   Testing these programs on a small group of children

5.   Revising procedures as indicated in the data

6.   Retesting and revising procedures until viable programs were developed

7.   Revalidating the final set of procedures with other subjects and with other trainers in a variety of different clinical settings (field testing) (LaCroix and Carrier, 1973)

DESCRIPTION OF THE
CHILD-ORIENTED TRAINING PROGRAM

The program evolving out of the four years of research activities listed above is referred to as the *Non-Speech Language Initiation Program (Non-SLIP)*. The term *nonspeech* refers to the fact that the programmed training uses pieces of masonite cut in various shapes, rather than spoken words. The term *language* refers to the proper use of linguistic rules and to communication in general. The term *initiation* is included to emphasize that the program is not intended as a total language training program but rather as a means of getting children started in the process of learning linguistic communication skills. It is viewed as a program for training children who are not viable candidates for learning through other more conventional speech and language training procedures. In essence, it is viewed as a starting point for children who are not able to meet entry requirements for other more advanced programs. Finally, the term *program* refers to the fact that all training procedures are very explicitly defined and sequenced in a finely graded fashion, beginning with very basic, easy tasks and proceeding on toward terminal goals.

There is one additional aspect of Non-SLIP that should be clarified. This training program is designed to teach a child a set of conceptual skills necessary to the acquisition of functional linguistic communication. Thus, it focuses on teaching a child tactics for learning language rather than teaching a circumscribed set of "functional" communicative responses. As a result, the vocabulary, the grammar, and the specific sentences trained are quite unlike those traditionally viewed as appropriate for such children. Some specifically taught responses might be viewed as surrealistic on the surface (e.g., *The cow is sitting on the car*), but these same responses serve to teach the child critical tactics for rule acquisition and thus serve an invaluable long-term function. The role of Non-SLIP is not so much one of teaching functional communication responses as it is one of teaching tactics for acquiring those responses.

The materials necessary to administer Non-SLIP include:

1.   A set of symbols of varying shapes; these are to be the child's vocabulary and can be used to express words or sentences: a square, for example, represents the noun *boy,* a circle represents *lady,* etc.
2.   A response tray, similar to the tray of a chalkboard but divided by vertical painted lines into seven 4-inch wide slots
3.   A set of pictures to be used as stimuli for the child
4.   An instruction set
5.   Record-keeping sheets
6.   Reinforcers

The specific reinforcers used in this training vary from child to child. Some respond best to edibles, others to verbal praise, others to physical contact, etc. The most crucial aspects of reinforcement are to find a reinforcer that is appropriate to the child, to use it consistently, and to deliver it with immediacy. More complete discussions of the processes of selecting and delivering reinforcers is presented by Spradlin, Karlan, and Wetherby (this volume), and by Carrier and Peak (1975).

Sequencing Training

The first phase of training is designed to teach a child to respond in a sequential fashion, a behavior he must be able to perform if he is ever to produce grammatical utterances in which two or more words must be arranged in proper order. The basis for this behavior in Non-SLIP is a rote sequence of seven units. The terminal behavior requires the child, when presented with seven appropriately cued symbols, to place the symbol with one red marker in the slot at the left of the response tray, then place the symbol with one orange marker in the second slot of the tray, the symbol with a green marker in the third slot, the symbol with a blue marker in the fourth slot, the symbol with a black marker in the fifth slot, the symbol with two red markers in the sixth slot, and the symbol with two orange markers in the seventh slot. In order to accomplish this, the child must be able to discriminate between symbols with one marker and those with two markers and to discriminate among the five different colors—red, orange, green, blue, and black.

After a child has been taught to sit in his chair and to place symbols (from the table in front of him) on the response tray, formal discrimination training commences (Peak and Carrier, 1973).

The "Number Matching Program" (NMP) is designed to teach the child a simple match-to-sample task in which the number of color markers on a symbol are the salient characteristics. Two symbols, one with one marker and another with two markers, are placed on the table in front of the child. The child is then shown another symbol with either one or two markers (varies randomly from trial to trial) and required to place the matching symbol, the one with the same number of markers, on the response tray. When the child is consistently matching symbols on the basis of number of markers, he is moved to the next program.

The "Color Matching Program" (CMP) uses the same basic procedures as the NMP, but the stimuli are the colors of the markers on the symbols. In step 1 of training, the child has two colors in front of him from which to select. When he is matching them a third is added, then a fourth, and finally a fifth. When he is matching all five colors, it is concluded that the child is capable of the necessary color discriminations and is ready to move on to the next program.

The "Rote Sequencing Program" (RSP) teaches the child to use the color and number cues to arrange symbols in a seven-symbol left-to-right sequence. The child's behavior is carefully shaped, beginning with teaching him to place one symbol in the appropriate slot of the tray, then two symbols in their slots, etc., until all seven symbols are being properly placed. The terminal behavior for the RSP requires the child to place the symbols by color/number cues as shown in Table 1.

Labeling Training

When the seven-symbol sequence based on color and number cues has been established, training shifts to teaching the use of symbols as words. The first 10 symbols to be taught are subject nouns—man, lady, horse, cow, etc. The child's task is to select, when shown a picture of one of those nouns, the correct symbol from the 10 symbols on the table in front of him and to place it on the response tray. Labeling training is preceded with match-to-sample training on the 10 symbols and the 10 pictures to be used. In the "Symbol Matching Program" (SMP) the child is taught to select, from symbols in front of him on the table, the one matching another shown to him by the trainer. In the "Picture Matching Program" (PMP) the child is taught in the same manner to match the 10 picture sitmuli.

Table 1. Arrangement of symbols in sequence training

	Slots on response tray						
	1	2	3	4	5	6	7
Cues on symbols indicating which slot to use	1 red marker	1 orange marker	1 green marker	1 blue marker	1 black marker	2 red markers	2 orange markers
Sentence constituent represented	Subject; noun phrase article	Subject; noun	Verb; auxiliary	Verb	Preposition	Prepositional phrase; article	Prepositional phrase; noun
Sample sentence	The	boy	is	sitting	on	the	bed

When this training (SMP and PMP) is complete, it can be concluded that the child is able to discriminate among the symbols and pictures. The child is then ready to be taught to match symbols to pictures— to label the pictures by selecting the appropriate symbol. The "Labeling Program" (LP) is identical to the match-to-sample programs (SMP, PMP, etc.) except that, rather than matching identical colors, numbers, symbols, or pictures, the child must match symbols to pictures. The symbols are placed on the table in front of the child, and he is taught to select them in response to stimulus pictures. The specific procedures and child performance in this program are presented in detail in Carrier (1974b; Carrier and Peak, 1975).

Subject Noun Training

When a child has completed LP, he has two classes of behavior that can be combined to move him a step closer to using language to communicate. He has learned a seven-unit response with the sequential characteristics of a seven-word sentence, and he has learned to use 10 symbols as nouns to label 10 different pictures. The program for combining these behaviors is called the "Constituent Selection Program" for subject nouns (CSP_{sn}). The program has a large number of finely graded stages (detailed in Carrier and Peak, 1975), but the basic constructs of the program are quite simple. The child has in front of him on the table a set of symbols. These include all 10 subject nouns learned in the LP and six other symbols, color and number cued, so that there is one symbol for each of the other slots in the tray. In a given trial, the child is shown a picture of one of the subject nouns engaged in some action. His response begins by placing the symbol with one red marker in the first slot of the tray. He then selects from the 10 symbols with one orange marker, the one that matches the stimulus picture. After he places that symbol— the correct subject noun—in the second slot of the tray, he completes the sequence with the remaining color/number cued symbols. He is responding with the symbols—one red + correct subject noun (one orange) + one green + one blue + one black + two red + two orange. The subject noun is now being used meaningfully in the context of the seven-symbol sequence.

Verb Training

The next phase of training teaches the child to use verbs (symbols with blue markers) meaningfully in the sequence. The "Constituent

Selection Program" for verbs (CSP_v) is designed to teach verbs in context. Training begins with two verbs, *sit* and *stand*. The child has symbols for the 10 subject nouns, for the two verbs, and color/ number cued symbol each for the remaining five slots in the sequence. He begins, when shown a picture, by placing the symbol with one red marker in the first slot, selecting the correct subject noun and placing it in the second slot, and then placing the symbol with the green marker in the third slot. He must then choose the verb appropriate to the picture, from the two symbols with blue markers— *sit* and *stand*. If he does this, he can then complete the sequence by color and number cues. When two verbs have been learned, others are then added one at a time to increase the vocabulary that the child uses meaningfully.

In some cases, teaching verbs in context is quite difficult, probably because the children have not learned the concept of verb usage. A branch program is designed to focus the child's attention on the parameters of the pictures that cue verb usage. He is thus taught to "label" pictures of people sitting and standing with the appropriate verb symbols. Finally, he is taken back to the CSP_v to learn to use the verbs in context.

Object of Preposition Training

The next phase of training teaches meaningful use of the object of preposition nouns. Ten new nouns, appropriate to the last slot of sentences of the sequential structure, are taught using the previously discussed LP procedures. Then these nouns are fit into the seven-unit sequence in the object of preposition slot (two orange markers). Procedures for this program, the "Constituent Selection Program" for object of preposition (CSP_{op}), are essentially identical to those used for teaching subject nouns and verbs in context (CSP_{sn} and CSP_v). When a child finishes this training, he is responding: symbol with one red marker + correct subject noun + symbol with green marker + correct verb + symbol with black marker + symbol with two red markers + correct object of preposition noun. He is filling three of the slots in the seven-word sentence in a meaningful fashion.

Preposition Training

The final major phase of training with the nonspeech symbols is to teach children to select and to use prepositions appropriately in the context of the sequence. The "Constituent Selection Program" for prepositions (CSP_p) is essentially like the one for verbs (CSP_v). Prepositions are trained in context until the child can select and place them in an appropriate, meaningful fashion.

Summary and Comments

Table 2 summarizes the major subprograms of nonspeech training and identifies the function of each. At the end of the nonspeech training, children are able to produce grammatically correct, seven-word sentences of the form: article + noun + verb auxiliary + verb + preposition + article + object of preposition + noun. Furthermore, they are able to produce these responses in response to various picture stimuli. Generalization tests throughout training are used to further ensure that the responses are not just to specifically trained pictures, but rather that the children can respond to new

Table 2. Subprograms in Non-SLIP[a]

1. Number Matching Program (NMP)—teaches discrimination between symbols with one colored strip on their faces and those with two strips
2. Color Matching Program (CMP)—teaches discrimination among five colors
3. Rote Sequencing Program (RSP)—teaches child to sequence seven symbols on the basis of color (CMP) and number (NMP) cues
4. Symbol Matching Program (SMP)—teaches discrimination among 10 symbols on the basis of shape
5. Picture Matching Program (PMP)—teaches discrimination among 10 pictures of 10 different nouns (man, lady, dog, etc.)
6. Labeling Program (LP)—teaches discriminative use of symbols (from SMP) to label pictures of 10 nouns (from PMP)
7. Constituent Selection Program for subject nouns (CSP_{sn})—teaches use of 10 nouns (from LP) in seven-unit sequence (from RSP)
8. Constituent Selection Program for verbs (CSP_v)—teaches discriminative use of verbs in seven-unit sequence (from RSP and CSP_{sn})
9. Verb Branch Program (VB)—teaches discriminative use of first two verbs if CSP_v is not adequate
10. Labeling Program A (LP_A)—teaches discriminative use of 10 more noun symbols (same procedures as LP above)
11. Constituent Selection Program for object of preposition (CSP_{op})—teaches discriminative use of 10 LP_A nouns in context of seven-unit sequence
12. Constituent Selection Program for prepositions (CSP_p)—teaches discriminative use of prepositions in seven-unit sequence

[a]Presented in the order in which they are used.

pictures and can generate new appropriate sentences or combinations of symbols. By the completion of the nonspeech training, the children are actually generating appropriate seven-word sentences. They have further demonstrated the ability to learn a variety of behaviors that are absolutely necessary if they are ever to use language to communicate (Bosley and Carrier, 1973). They are able to:

1.   Discriminate among members of at least one set of symbols— the shapes
2.   Discriminate among picture stimuli that call for different linguistic responses
3.   Use symbols to represent picture stimuli
4.   Respond symbolically to parameters of a stimulus that cue verb selection
5.   Respond symbolically to parameters of a stimulus that cue preposition selection
6.   Use symbols taught in response to one or more stimuli of a class to respond to other stimuli of the same class
7.   Sequence symbols in appropriate grammatical order
8.   Combine all these skills to produce complete, correct communication responses
9.   Use the combination of all these skills to generate new untaught syntactically and semantically correct sentence responses

It might be noted that the early research with Non-SLIP went much further in the grammar and the vocabulary that were taught than does the current form of the program. Children have been taught, using the nonspeech symbol set to:

1.   Produce declarative sentences with direct objects rather than prepositional phrases (e.g., *The boy is hitting the ball*)
2.   Produce a variety of interrogative sentences including "wh" questions (who, what, where, etc.) (e.g., *Who is hitting the ball? What is the boy hitting? Where is the boy sitting?*)
3.   Use plurals (e.g., *The boys are playing on the sidewalk*)
4.   Change verb tense (e.g., *The boy was sitting on the floor*)
5.   Use adjectives (e.g., *The big girl is sitting on the black horse*)
6.   Use compound forms such as compound subject nouns, compound objects, compound verbs, compound adjectives, and compound sentences (e.g., *The boy and the dog are running and playing*, etc.)

7. Use all of these skills discriminatively—i.e., to select, from all alternatives, the one appropriate to the current available stimulus

Training on these additional structures is no longer being done, primarily because most children were ready, after learning the first sentence structure, to make the transition to speech and to conventional speech and language training programs. In essence, it was concluded that training on additional structures was feasible but not maximally profitable to the child.

After the early research had indicated that children could learn communication skills using the nonspeech symbols and training procedures, an attempt was made to study the transition of children from nonspeech to spoken responses. It was discovered that all but a few children could at least partially make such a transition by the time they had finished training on prepositions (CSP_p) (Carrier, LaCroix, and Critcher, 1973; Critcher, Carrier, and LaCroix, 1973). Some with severe motor problems or severely deformed articulatory mechanisms were not able to make such a transition and were placed in manual communication training; but the others were able to produce, with some training, enough speech to emit intelligible phrases and short sentences. They were able, at the same time, to retain the linguistic rules they had learned in Non-SLIP and thus had enough language to generate such utterances appropriately. It was thus concluded that children at this stage of skill acquisition were ready to move into more conventional training. They were now able to succeed in learning speech responses and various linguistic rules.

The speech training that is included in Non-SLIP is described in the program manual (Carrier and Peak, 1975) but is not highly programmed. In essence, the speech training, a form of paired associate training, is conducted concurrently with the nonspeech work but at the pace of the child. Every time a child places a symbol on the tray, the trainer says the word represented by the symbol. If the child attempts to vocalize or imitate the trainer's speech, the trainer begins to encourage and reinforce spoken responses as well as those responses with the nonspeech symbols. The child's speech is then gradually shaped from that base. If the child never shows any inclination toward speech, no speech is required until CSP_p (preposition training) is completed. Then speech becomes the central focus of training and is worked on until the child is emitting intelligible spoken sentence responses or has demonstrated that he is not a viable candidate for speech training because of some organic or physiologic problem.

Table 2 presents a list of the subprograms in Non-SLIP, the order in which they are presented, and the general purpose of each subprogram. Detail beyond that presented in this chapter is available in the Non-SLIP clinical management package (Carrier and Peak, 1975), which includes a detailed manual and step-by-step instructions for using the programs.

CURRENT APPLICATION OF PROGRAM

Subjects with Whom Non-SLIP Has Been Used

Non-SLIP was originally designed for training severely and profoundly retarded nonverbal children. However, because of problems with clear etiologic classification and because of the need for similar procedures with other diagnostic groups, it has been used with several other populations. Most of the 180 children who have gone through or are currently progressing through Non-SLIP are children with a primary diagnosis of severe or profound mental retardation. Nearly all such children were nonverbal at the onset of training, and many have had a history of failure in speech and language therapy. The 180 children have also included a large number of children who had been diagnosed as autistic, psychotic, or in some way emotionally disturbed. In some cases, retardation was not considered a significant part of their diagnosis, and in other cases retardation and emotional disturbance could not be clearly delineated. Still other children had mild to moderate motor problems (cerebral palsy), and others had defective sensory channels.

Non-SLIP has been used in one center as part of the training for deaf-blind children and has been particularly helpful in teaching such children some of the syntactic components of language. With these children, it should be noted that sitmuli had to be made appropriate, according to the child's ability to perceive, and that the tactile sense was used for discriminating and arranging the masonite symbols. In all cases, regardless of etiology, subjects had shown severely retarded behavior, particularly with communication skills. Most children did not use even one-word responses when they began, but some did have single-word responses or a few short phrases. Some of the emotionally disturbed children emitted echolalic responses before training but did not use them for communication purposes.

It also should be pointed out that, although there was little if any observable pretraining language behavior in any of these children, the results of posttraining generalization tests have indicated that over 90% of the children did have some preestablished concepts. For example, after teaching children to respond on the LP by labeling 10 pictures, one of each of 10 nouns, most children were able to generalize immediately to correct labeling of a different set of pictures of the same nouns. Unless it is possible to establish a concept by teaching only one exemplar, it is necessary to conclude that these children had learned the concepts or at least some of the concepts before training on Non-SLIP. At this writing, it is not clear why or how such concepts have been learned, but it seems quite clear that they were in the repertoires of most children.

General Progress in Non-SLIP

At this writing, part or all of the Non-SLIP has been used with 180 children, some in the research laboratory and some in field-test clinics. Of these, only three children have not been able to complete the early phases of training. Some children have been discontinued because they were no longer available for training or because of prolonged illness, and the others have either completed or are currently progressing through training. Speech has been included in the training of 57 children, and of these, 56 have moved on to successful training in conventional speech and language therapy. At least 21 children are known to be using speech in environments outside of the training room and are, at this time, learning language in their everyday environment. Non-SLIP does seem to be a means of reaching many of the children for whom it was intended.

In general, it can be concluded that, as children progress through Non-SLIP, they learn new skills at an increasing rate. Non-SLIP requires, for example, an average of 2 hours, 11 minutes to learn the first set of 10 nouns, but only 48 minutes to learn the second set of 10 nouns. The first two verbs take the longest time to teach, and each successive verb requires less and less training time.

The first two verbs and the first two prepositions are the most difficult parts of Non-SLIP to teach. This may be because children do not generally have verb and preposition use concepts in their repertoires before training. The children who show difficulty learning the first verbs and prepositions are also children who do not show generalization of a concept after teaching of the verbs or prepositions to the first pictures. Rather, they require training with several pictures before generalizing and thus showing that they have learned the concepts.

The amount of time required to complete Non-SLIP varies from child to child and depends on a number of factors. Most children are scheduled for one session per day, 5 days a week. Children with fewer sessions per week require more calendar time to complete training. Some children work well in 20- to 30-minute sessions, and other children cannot work for more than a few minutes at a time. This also affects calendar time required. Some children are ill much of the time and thus progress more slowly. Finally, although the clock time for training (hours and minutes actually in training) is a more meaningful indication of time requirements than is calendar time, the children vary somewhat in that measure as well. In fact, of the children who have been on Non-SLIP, there seems to be a bimodal distribution with about 90% falling into one normal distribution around 11 hours and about 10% falling into another around 35 hours (see Carrier, 1974a, for a sample distribution).

Table 3 presents mean training times to complete the various phases of training and to complete all of Non-SLIP. It also presents the training times for the slowest child on each subprogram and on the total program. These times represent the times actually spent in training the children and do not include time for preparing materials, setting up the training room, or recording data after a session. It

Table 3. Training times for subprograms of Non-SLIP[a]

Subprogram	Mean training time	Slowest child
RSP	2 hr, 10 min	10 hr, 15 min
LP	2 hr, 11 min	12 hr, 30 min
CSP_{sn}	1 hr, 10 min	4 hr, 18 min
CSP_v[b]	5 hr, 11 min	14 hr, 30 min
LP_A	48 min	2 hr, 45 min
CSP_{op}	45 min	3 hr, 35 min
CSP_p	2 hr, 44 min	11 hr, 30 min
Total	14 hr, 53 min	59 hr, 23 min

[a]NMP, CMP, SMP, and PMP times are not included because of the small number of subjects who have required complete training in those programs (i.e., most met criterion without going through all of the programs).

[b]Includes data for Verb Branch Program where it was used.

should be further mentioned that these training times are not directly related to calendar times. Some children have completed training on Non-SLIP in 2 to 3 months, and other children have taken as much as 2 years. Some of the children at the outer end of this sample have session times that are at or below the means of the entire group for subprograms and for the entire program. Previously mentioned variables such as illness, length of session, and attendance seem to be responsible for this lack of correlation.

Table 4 presents error rates in terms of means for the entire group; it also presents the rate for the child with the most errors. Error rate data have been used, along with session time data, to identify various phases of programming that have been in need of improvement.

CURRENT STATUS OF NON-SLIP

Recommended Use of Programs

At this writing, Non-SLIP has been field tested in several different clinics with several different trainers. The data have been carefully monitored to determine whether they are consistent with the laboratory data generated during earlier phases of program development and consistent from trainer to trainer and center to center. The data have been consistent, with two exceptions. The laboratory work, including speech, was conducted by research assistants with no experience with speech training, and the field work has been primarily

Table 4. Error rates for subprograms of Non-SLIP[a]

Subprogram	Mean errors (%)	Highest error rate (%)
RSP	10.5	22
LP	13	21
CSP_{sn}	15	30
CSP_v[b]	NA[c]	NA[c]
LP_A	2.5	18
CSP_{op}	1	16
CSP_p	13.7	44.7

[a]NMP, CMP, SMP, and PMP times are not included because of the small number of subjects who have required complete training in those programs (i.e., most met criterion without going through all of the programs).

[b]Includes data for Verb Branch Program where it was used.

[c]A straightforward percentage of errors is not possible because of the nature of the program.

conducted by professional speech pathologists. The speech pathologists have been more successful in training speech production, i.e., have accomplished speech training in less time. The other exception was the data from one center in which the trainers did not follow the program instructions. These deviations from the specified training routines increased training times, increased error rates, and frequently required that the child be taken back and repeat portions of the program.

In essence, it is reasonable to conclude at this time that Non-SLIP is ready for general clinical application. It is a tool that is an effective means of getting a large percentage (over 90% in available data) of children, with previously low likelihood of success, started in the process of learning communication skills.

These conclusions are further validated by the work of Hodges and Deich (1975) in which similar procedures were used successfully. Their data were quite similar to those generated by Non-SLIP.

Non-SLIP has been tested with a variety of individuals with different etiologies and with different behavioral symptoms. It seems, from reliable data, that most children with primary emotional problems do quite well in Non-SLIP. In fact, some of the most remarkable success cases have been children who had been diagnosed as autistic. McLean and McLean (1974) reported success using a similar approach with autistic children. Only a small number of children with a primary diagnosis of hearing impairment have been run through Non-SLIP, but these children have been quite successful and indicate that this program is appropriate for them as well.

Similar procedures used by Maison (1975) also strongly suggest that deaf children are viable candidates for such training. The reported success with hearing-impaired children is no great surprise because many of the concepts basic to Non-SLIP are similar to those used in education of the hearing impaired for many years (e.g., the Fitzgerald key, discussed in Davis and Silverman, 1965, pp. 446–447). Concurrent training on Non-SLIP and on manual communication has resulted in very rapid learning of syntax by a small number of deaf children. Children with a primary diagnosis of retardation (measured intelligence levels of IV and V, and adaptive behavior levels of IV—Heber, 1961) also have been quite successful on Non-SLIP, and degree of success has not been related to measured degree of retardation. The programs have been conducted with individuals in nearly every age group ranging from 2- to 3-year-olds to retarded adults in their 50's. The data on children under 8 years of age are not comprehensive enough at this time to conclude much about the rate of learning, but such children have been able to complete Non-SLIP successfully. The data on adults, although also somewhat limited, seem to indicate that they learn much more slowly than children.

The present author has used Non-SLIP successfully with a small number of adult aphasics. Others (Velletri-Glass, Gazzaniga, and Premack, 1973; Gardner et al, 1975) also have found the nonspeech symbol system to be a viable approach for teaching adult aphasics.

The children with whom Non-SLIP is least successful fall into three groups. Children with motor problems that interfere with the required responses have learned very slowly and in some cases have not been able to go beyond training of motor responses. This problem may be reduced by using some of the techniques and devices described by Vanderheiden and Harris-Vanderheiden (this volume). Children with frequent and severe seizures have been a problem as far as retaining behavior learned before a seizure, but a set of specially developed procedures called the Retention Program (Carrier and Peak, 1975) has largely eliminated this problem. The most problematic group of children has been a few subjects with primary diagnosis of severe or profound retardation and with clear emotional overlay. At least two such subjects have shown what seem to be a form of resistance to learning. One was on the Labeling Program at a step where criterion levels were 15 consecutive correct responses. He began running 14 consecutive correct responses, then missing one, running 14 more, missing one, etc. The other child was working on the SMP and was supposed to select from two symbols the one matching the one on the tray. She would perform correctly to the preset criterion on some days but would never repeat the behavior for the next session, even if it were only a few minutes later. These two children gave continued indications of being able to learn the necessary tasks but unwilling to cooperate long enough to meet criterion and move from step to step. It would seem that children showing such patterns over a large number of sessions have very low likelihood of succeeding in Non-SLIP.

Areas in Need of Additional Study

Although Non-SLIP is currently ready for clinical applications, it is still in need of further research. As mentioned earlier, the teaching of the first two verbs and the first two prepositions is particularly difficult. These programs and the actual processes of teaching verbs and prepositions might be further studied and improved. Speech training is another major area in need of additional work. The procedures for speech training are not currently specified in a carefully programmed fashion nor are the most effective procedures really known. The entire training process would be greatly improved if more study were done on the speech issues.

The dynamics of this approach are quite similar to those involved in reading and writing. Kuntz (1974) studied the transfer of this training to printed words and reported a high degree of success with severely retarded children. More attention to this matter and the ultimate adaptation of research data to reading programs might be a profitable undertaking.

Another general area in which Non-SLIP might be further studied is in training children with severe motor problems and/or children with severe sensory problems. In some cases, alternative stimuli should be developed. In others, alternative symbol sets should be studied. The basic procedures used in Non-SLIP could function as a starting point in such work and could possibly expedite development of effective procedures for such special children.

In addition to the clinically oriented issues mentioned above, there remain a variety of research questions about why children are as successful as they are with Non-SLIP. It might be profitable, for example, to compare processing of auditory versus visual stimuli. The results of such research might lead to further improvement in training and to ways to deal more effectively with some of the children who have difficulty with Non-SLIP as it currently exists.

SUMMARY

This chapter reviews the development and use of the Non-Speech Language Initiation Program (Non-SLIP). Premack's (1970, 1971; Premack and Premack, 1972) use of an analytical system and plastic symbols to teach his chimpanzee to communicate in a linguistic fashion is reviewed as the basis of the program. Non-SLIP is described from selection of reinforcers through initial matching and sequencing tasks to the production of grammatically correct seven-word sentences of the form: article + noun + verb auxiliary + verb + preposition + article + object of preposition + noun with the generalization of responses to various picture stimuli. The use of this nonspeech system to initiate language and subsequently speech is discussed. Although the program was designed for use with severely and profoundly retarded children, it has been applied successfully to other populations. The current status of Non-SLIP and areas needing additional study are also considered.

REFERENCES

Baer, D., R. Peterson, and J. Sherman. 1967. The development of imitation by reinforcing behavioral similarity to a model. J. Exp. Anal. Behav. 10:405–416.

Berieter, C., and S. Engelmann. 1966. Teaching Disadvantaged Children in Preschool. Prentice-Hall, Englewood Cliffs, N.J.

Bolinger, D. 1968. Aspects of Language. Harcourt, Brace & World, New York.

Bosley, S., and J. Carrier. 1973. Establishing linguistic behavior in severely retarded children. Presented at the Region V American Association on Mental Deficiency Convention, October, Wichita, Kan.

Bricker, W. A., and D. B. Bricker. 1972. The use of programmed language training as a means for differential diagnosis and educational remediation among severely retarded children. Final Report, George Peabody College, Contract OEG 2-7-070218-1629, U.S. Office of Education.

Campbell, B. 1970. The roots of language. In J. Morton (ed.), Biological and Social Factors in Psycholinguistics. University of Illinois Press, Urbana.

Carrier, J. K., Jr. 1970. A program of articulation therapy administered by mothers. J. Speech Hear. Disord. 35:344–353.

Carrier, J. K., Jr. 1974a. Application of functional analysis and a nonspeech response mode to teaching language. In L. V. McReynolds (ed.), Developing Systematic Procedures for Training Children's Language. Asha monogr. 18.

Carrier, J. K., Jr. 1974b. Nonspeech noun usage training with severely and profoundly retarded children. J. Speech Hear. Res. 17:510–517.

Carrier, J., Z. LaCroix, and C. Critcher. 1973. Use of nonspeech training to facilitate learning of spoken communication skills. Presented at the spring conference of the Oklahoma Speech and Hearing Association, April, Oklahoma City.

Carrier, J. K., Jr., and T. Peak. 1975. Non-Speech Language Initiation Program. H & H Enterprises, Lawrence, Kan.

Chomsky, N. 1965. Aspects of the Theory of Syntax. MIT Press, Cambridge, Mass.

Critcher, C., J. K. Carrier, Jr., and Z. LaCroix. 1973. Speech and language training using a nonspeech response mode. Presented at the Annual Meeting of the American Speech and Hearing Association, October, Detroit.

Davis, H., and S. R. Silverman. 1965. Hearing and Deafness. Holt, Rinehart and Winston, New York.

Garcia, E., D. Baer, and I. Firestone. 1971. The development of generalized imitation within topographically determined boundaries. J. Appl. Behav. Anal. 4:101–112.

Gardner, H., E. Zurif, T. Berry, and E. Baker. 1975. Visual communication in aphasia. Unpublished manuscript, Aphasia Research Center, Boston University School of Medicine and Psychology Service, Boston Veterans Administration Hospital, Boston.

Gray, B. B., and B. P. Ryan. 1971. Programmed Conditioning for Language. Accelerated Achievement Association, Monterey, Cal.

Heber, R. 1961. Adaptive behavior: A manual on terminology and classification in mental retardation. Amer. J. Ment. Defic. monogr. suppl. 2nd Ed.

Hockett, C. F., and R. Ascher. 1964. The human revolution. Amer. Scientist 52:71–92.

Hodges, P., and R. Deich. 1975. Teaching an artificial language to nonverbal retardates. Unpublished manuscript, California State College, Los Angeles, and California Department of Mental Hygiene, Pacific State Hospital, Los Angeles.

Kellogg, W. N. 1931. Humanizing the ape. Psychol. Rev. 38:106–176.

Kent, L. 1972. A language acquisition program for the retarded. In J. E. McLean, D. Yoder, and R. Schiefelbusch (eds.), Language Intervention with the Retarded. University Park Press, Baltimore.

Kuntz, J. B. 1974. A nonvocal communication development program for severely retarded children. Unpublished doctoral dissertation, Kansas State University, Manhattan, Kan.

LaCroix, Z., and J. K. Carrier, Jr. 1973. Clinical application of experimental language programs for severely and profoundly retarded children. Presented at the American Association on Mental Deficiency Convention, June, Atlanta.

Lenneberg, E. 1967. Biological Foundations of Language. John Wiley & Sons, New York.

McGinnis, M. A. 1963. Aphasic Children. The Volta Bureau, Washington, D.C.

McLean, J. E. 1970. Extending stimulus control of phoneme articulation by operant techniques. Asha monogr. 14.

McLean, L., and J. McLean. 1974. A language training program for nonverbal autistic children. J. Speech Hear. Dis. 39:186–193.

Maison, E. P. 1975. Teaching pre-school deaf children to use written language: A pilot study of a new approach. Unpublished manuscript, Oral Education Center of Southern California, Los Angeles.

Miller, J., and D. Yoder. 1972. A syntax teaching program. In J. E. McLean, D. Yoder, and R. Schiefelbusch (eds.), Language Intervention with the Retarded. University Park Press, Baltimore.

Mowrer, D. E., R. L. Baker, and R. E. Schutz. 1968. Modification of the Frontal Lisp, Programmed Articulation Control Kit. Educational Psychological Research Associates, Tempe, Ariz.

Parsons, S., and J. K. Carrier, Jr. 1971. A proposed language program based on David Premack's program for Sarah, a chimpanzee. Presented at the spring Meeting of the Oklahoma Speech and Hearing Association, April, Oklahoma City.

Peak, T., and J. K. Carrier, Jr. 1973. Establishing prelinguistic responses in severely retarded children. Presented at the Region V American Association on Mental Deficiency Convention, October, Wichita, Kan.

Premack, D. 1970. A functional analysis of language. J. Exp. Anal. Behav. 14:107–125.

Premack, D. 1971. Language in chimpanzee? Science 172:808–822.

Premack, A. J., and D. Premack. 1972. Teaching language to an ape. Scient. Amer. 277:92–99.

Premack, D., and A. J. Premack. 1974. Teaching visual language to apes and language-deficient persons. In R. L. Schiefelbusch and L. L. Lloyd (eds.), Language Perspectives—Acquisition, Retardation, and Intervention. University Park Press, Baltmore.

Schmidt, M. J., J. K. Carrier, Jr., and S. Parsons. 1971. Use of a nonspeech mode for teaching language. Presented at the American Speech and Hearing Association Convention, Chicago.

Stremel, K. 1972. Language training: A program for retarded children. Ment. Retard. 10:47–49.

Velletri-Glass, A., M. Gazzaniga, and D. Premack. 1973. Artificial language training in global aphasics. Neuropsychologia 11:95–104.

14

GRAPHIC SYSTEMS OF COMMUNICATION

*Charlotte R. Clark and
Richard W. Woodcock*

CONTENTS

Graphic Systems _____ 552
    Model/552
    History/554

Alphabetic Systems _____ 556
    Traditional orthography/557
    Phonemic alphabets/567

Nonalphabetic Systems _____ 579
    Syllabic systems/579
    Logographic systems/582

Summary _____ 599
References _____ 600

"In order to communicate thoughts and feelings there must be a conventional system of signs or symbols which, when used by some persons, are understood by other persons receiving them" (Gelb, 1963, p. 1). As early man's world expanded geographically and intellectually, he needed some form of graphic communication to provide permanence and accuracy. Prehistoric attempts at graphic communication are found in many parts of the world. For example, the Altamira cave paintings of northern Spain, done over 20,000 years ago, graphically portray aspects of early life. It is not known, however, whether cave painters and those who carved pictures in rocks were engaging in simple aesthetic expression or were attempting to communicate messages.

True written language did not emerge until around 3100 B.C. (Falk, 1973). Most of the drawings and carvings before that time, though the forerunners of writing, were not symbols systematically arranged according to a formal set of rules. Thus, they were difficult if not impossible to interpret. One did not know where to begin a message, if indeed there was a message, or if there was a sequence to follow. With time, however, graphic systems evolved and became increasingly more systematized.

In spite of the utility of systematized written languages, they usually present a complex task for the learner. To some children, the acquisition of language in graphic form may be formidable and unrewarding.

English orthography or *traditional orthography* (T.O.), which is employed as the graphic system in English-speaking countries, is considered relatively difficult to master. This difficulty is experienced by many children, but particularly by certain populations of handicapped individuals. To lessen problems in types of learning that require the use of a graphic system, or in learning to read T.O., alternative graphic systems as well as methods for control or for elaboration of T.O. have been devised. Such devices include a variety of modified alphabets, nonalphabetic symbol systems, colored symbols, or diacritical markings used as aids to decoding (converting to intelligible language) in beginning reading.

Presented in this chapter are descriptions of several of the graphic systems which have been suggested as modifications or as alternatives to T.O. and descriptions of various schemes which have as their intent the control of spelling pattern variance in beginning reading programs. Examples of instructional programs and materials utilizing these systems are also included.

GRAPHIC SYSTEMS

Model

For the purposes of this chapter, a *graphic system* is defined as a *system comprised of a rule-governed set of visible marks that provide a means of linguistic intercommunication.* Graphic systems may be divided into two major categories. The first is the *alphabetic* category consisting of *traditional orthography* and *phonemic alphabets.* Traditional orthography divides into: 1) systems which control the introduction of spelling patterns of T.O. (*controlled T.O.*), and 2) systems which elaborate on T.O. in the form of colors, diacritical marks, or other accentuations (*elaborated T.O.*). In alphabetic systems the symbols represent phonologic (sound) units of a language. For example, in written English the alphabetic symbol "d" usually represents the phoneme /d/,[1] while the symbol "c" usually represents the phonemes /k/ or /s/.

The second major category of graphic systems is the *nonalphabetic* one which consists of *syllabic systems* and *logographic systems.* A characteristic of both syllabic and logographic systems is that they contain symbols which represent language in units larger than individual phonologic units. The symbols of a syllabary, or syllabic system (syllables) usually stand for two or more phonemes in combination, whereas a logograph (the symbol unit of a logography, or logographic system) represents one or more words. The syllabic systems divide into: 1) *pictographic syllabaries,* and 2) *nonpictographic syllabaries.* Similarly, the logographic systems divide into: 1) logographies which employ primarily *pictographic logographs,* and 2) logographies which employ primarily *nonpictographic logographs.*

Figure 1 portrays the model described above. Also included in the figure are examples of some instructional programs or materials which have utilized the various graphic systems. Some of the programs and materials listed in Figure 1 have borrowed types of symbols from early writing systems. These systems tended to evolve through the centuries from logographs to syllables to alphabets. A brief reach into the history of writing will clarify this evolution and suggest why borrowing from early systems might have advantages for certain instructional situations.

---

[1]For readers unfamiliar with the International Phonetic Association (IPA) Alphabet, a pronunciation key is provided in Appendix B.

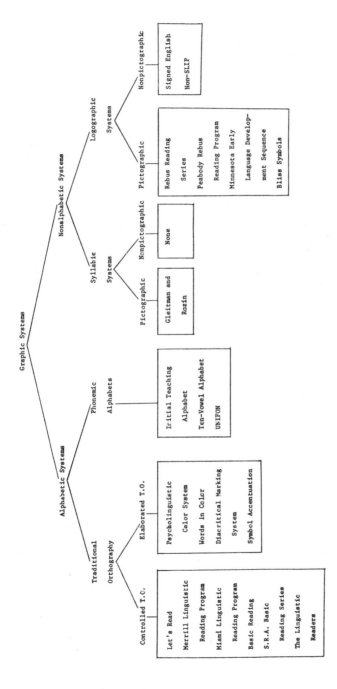

Figure 1. A model of graphic systems and related instructional materials.

History

Although pictures such as petroglyphs (rock carvings) and petrograms (rock painting or drawings) were the precursors of writing systems and were, perhaps, essential to their development, they did not represent language (Diringer, 1962). Their influence, nevertheless, is seen in Figure 2, which shows the evolution of modern graphic systems from pictographs.

In the first nonalphabetic systems the pictographic symbols were primarily logographic. These symbols were not pictures but rather were highly stylized drawings. The word *wife,* for instance, might be a stick figure holding a broom; *foot* a simplified drawing of a foot. Most of the symbols were easily decipherable, especially those words which could be depicted simply. The reader could relate the symbol directly to meaning. Some words, however, could not be represented concretely with a pictograph. The English words *be, would,* or *belief,* for example, would be difficult to portray. Frequently, words of this nature were represented by employing what is known as the *rebus principle* (Diringer, 1962; Gelb, 1963; Langacker, 1968; Antilla, 1972). This principle capitalizes on homophones (words which sound alike such as *rose* and *rows* but which have different meanings). With the rebus principle a pictograph is used to represent several words which sound the same, or different pictographs are employed to represent each syllable of a word. The English word *would* might be represented by:

or the word *belief* by:

Instead of going directly from symbol to first-order meaning, as would be possible with a pictograph representing *foot,* the reader decoding words represented by the rebus principle is required to transfer the meaning of the pictographic symbols into sound chunks, then process the sound chunks into a new or second-order meaning. Thus, early logographic systems were not purely comprised of iconic representations. Furthermore, several authorities on written language (Gelb, 1963; Langacker, 1968) believe that a pure word-writing system never existed but rather that logographic systems incorporated

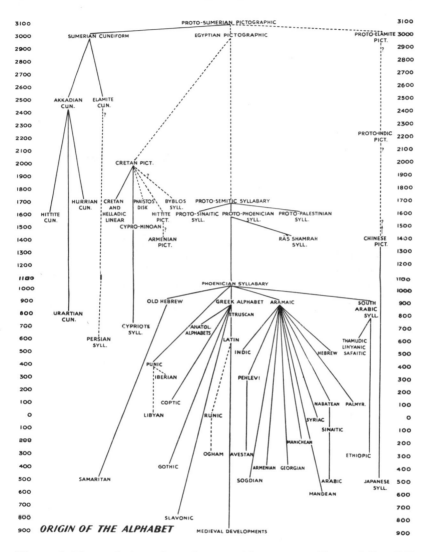

Figure 2. The evolution of modern graphic systems. (From Gelb, 1963; reprinted by permission of The University of Chicago Press.

syllabic representation along with logographs. Because of problems in representing words and because vast amounts of symbols had to be learned and remembered, most logographic systems gradually evolved to complete syllabic representation.

With the development of syllabaries, certain efficiency in writing not afforded by logographies was achieved. Fewer symbols were now required because of the combinatorial quality of syllables to form words. Hence, the load on memory was reduced for those learning and using the system. On the other hand, decoding of the symbols involved extra steps beyond that of the word-writing systems. No longer could a symbol be converted directly into meaning as with many logographic symbols.

In time, pictographs used in both syllabic and logographic systems frequently became stylized to the point of being difficult to recognize. This was the case with Chinese symbols, which have evolved into increasingly more abstract characters. This abstractness, naturally, added to the difficulty of learning such systems. The Chinese reader of today must know at least 1500 basic symbols and many combinations of these in order to form words or ideas (Ullman, 1963).

The Greek alphabet evolved from syllabaries about 900 B.C. Similar alphabets emerged shortly thereafter, including the Roman alphabet, which is used in nearly all of Western Europe and the new world. Most languages today employ an alphabet as their graphic system. With the emergence of alphabets, a new level of efficiency in writing was achieved. Because symbols in such systems represent phonologic units, the language can be written using fewer different symbols than would be required by a syllabary or logographic system. Hence, alphabets are the most efficacious of known symbol systems (Diringer, 1942; Falk, 1973). For the beginning reader, however, they are probably the most difficult to learn to decode. Thus, as symbol systems evolved, from logographies to syllabaries to alphabets, they tended to increase in efficiency but decrease in ease of decodability for the novice reader.

ALPHABETIC SYSTEMS

Alphabetic systems are efficient because a few symbols are used in combinations to form thousands of different words. In some languages, there is a close correspondence of grapheme (letter) to phoneme (sound). Once these correspondences have been learned, they can be applied generally to all situations. Thus, such alphabets are intended to be more or less phonemic, that is, one letter for each phoneme and one phoneme for each letter. In written English, however, there are many irregularities in phoneme-grapheme correspondence. These irregularities, which are vestiges from many centuries of use and change, increase the difficulty of learning written English.

Traditional Orthography

Gleason (1961) noted that writing systems change much more slowly than spoken forms of languages. English orthography has many so-called silent letters. However, at one time, a great number of these letters actually did represent sound segments such as the "gh" in the word *fight,* pronounced as the gutteral sound segment [x] ('kh') in Old English. Through the centuries, the pronunciation of certain grapheme combinations changed or ceased to be used completely. The spelling patterns, though, were retained in the written language and came to be referred to as "irregularities." Other irregularities have been added as a result of "borrowing" from other languages. For example, in the early part of the Middle English period of history, literate people of the English court usually spoke French rather than English. In the 13th century, when English was restored as the national language of Britain, many new words had been added as carryovers from French.

Well meaning scholars also have been responsible for some of the borrowing, particularly from the Latin and Greek languages, which experienced a revival during the Renaissance (MacLeish, 1970). The spelling of Latin-based English words was frequently changed to show the origin of the words. The word *doubt,* for example, was borrowed originally from the French language as *doute.* The Latin form of this word was *dubitum.* Because *dubitum* contained a "b," some scholars felt that the English form should too—hence the word *doubt* with a "b" that no one has ever pronounced (Falk, 1973). Similar tampering with spelling resulted in the insertion of an "s," which is not pronounced in words such as *aisle* and *island* (MacLeish, 1970). Because spellings have frequently occurred indiscriminately and often do not reflect the current pronunciation in spoken English, it is not difficult to understand the desire of educators and others to pursue the possibility of a simplified orthography for the beginning reader.

Controlled T.O.

Leonard Bloomfield, a distinguished linguist, might be called the "father" of the "linguistic" approach to reading instruction, an approach that controls spelling patterns of T.O. Bloomfield, who bitterly criticized phonic and meaning-emphasis approaches to reading, argued that the child's first task in reading is to learn the code; as the code is broken, meaning will come naturally but should not be stressed (Bloomfield, 1942).

One of the basic tenets of the linguistic approach is that children will learn to read easier and faster when presented words with minimal contrasts in spelling. For this reason, linguistic reading series and programs tend to control the introduction of irregularly spelled words until children have learned to read a great number of words that primarily are spelled as they sound.

Control of vocabulary in early materials is accomplished by utilizing mostly phonemically regular words taught as whole units in consonant-vowel-consonant (CVC) monosyllables. The words are presented in word "families" or spelling patterns such as *bat, cat, fat, hat,* and so on. Letter sounds are not taught in isolation; rather, phoneme-grapheme correspondences are learned through the repetition of words of certain patterns. The "linguistic" emphasis is on whole-word learning and inference of sound-letter patterns, and not on syntactic patterns or on phonics.

Spache and Spache (1973, p. 219) stated: "This group of materials offering a linguistic theory is proving to be somewhat confusing to the average classroom teacher." They further suggested that the confusion may stem in part from the differences in approaches among the materials. Some materials are purposely devoid of pictures so that readers will concentrate only on the print. Other materials are profusely illustrated. Some programs initially present only lists of isolated words; other programs present words in complete sentences. Differences exist in the emphasis or deemphasis on meaning and in the use of regularly spelled words versus an early inclusion of irregularly spelled words. Various "linguistic" programs began to appear in the 1960's and were hailed as new and innovative when, in fact, they often resembled reading materials from the 1800's.

Several reading authorities have voiced concern about the soundness of the theoretical bases of linguistic programs. Spache and Spache (1973, p. 218) asserted that many linguists have done a disservice to the field of reading by ". . . propounding conflicting and naive theories of the reading process . . . and by refusing to accept that much of current reading instruction is based on psychological and physiological principles unfamiliar to them . . ." Goodman (1964, p. 355) stated that the linguist ". . . is not on firm ground when he produces reading programs that are based solely on linguistic criteria."

One program that is a "true" linguistic approach is entitled *Let's Read* and is discussed somewhat in detail. Others that have a modified linguistic orientation are discussed only briefly.

Let's Read Leonard Bloomfield is credited by many linguists with identifying the basic phonemes of English. It is this research on phonemes which was the basis for *Let's Read: A Linguistic Approach* (Bloomfield and Barnhart, 1961). Bloomfield tried to popularize his approach to reading before his death in 1949 but was generally ignored by educators.

His instructional materials and notes on reading were willed to his protégé, Clarence Barnhart, who compiled them into a large volume and published them in 1961. Later Barnhart formed his own company, divided the volume into smaller units, and republished the materials (Bloomfield and Barnhart, 1966).

Let's Read consists of nine small books with workbooks for classroom use and mimeographed teacher's manuals. No illustrations are present in any of the materials, and very little reading of connected discourse occurs. There is heavy emphasis initially on learning names of the capital and small letters. In the first three books, words are presented in isolation and taught in lists in the same way as Bloomfield's earlier materials (Figure 3). The lists are arranged in nine different patterns that allow children to compare monosyllables for similarity and contrast. Spelling is stressed as a key to unlocking the code. In later materials, irregular words are presented along with phrases such as *a bat, a cat, a hat*. Then meaningless sentences of the nature, *a fat cat ran at a fat cat,* are presented, followed by stories illustrating certain sounds.

Only a few studies in which the Bloomfield-Barnhart materials were used have been reported. Sister Mary Edward Dolan (1966) compared *Let's Read* to a more traditional basal reader program but confounded the resultant superiority of the linguistic approach by incorporating into it some basal materials and phonic training. Another study that compared three reading approaches in first grade was continued into second and third grades (Sheldon, Nichols, and Lashinger, 1967; Sheldon, Stinson, and Peebles, 1969). The three approaches—basal, modified linguistic (Stern's *Structural Reading*), and true linguistic (*Let's Read*)—produced different results at each grade level. Basal pupils were superior in accuracy of oral reading and in rate of reading at the end of first grade. The two linguistic approaches produced better results in word meaning, spelling, and

1

can Dan fan man Nan pan ran tan an
ban van

a can a fan a pan a man a van
a tan van a tan fan

Dan ran.　Nan ran.
Van ran.　A man ran.

Nan can fan Dan.
Can Dan fan Nan?
Dan can fan Nan.
Nan, fan Dan.
Dan, fan Nan.

Dan ran a van.
Dan ran a tan van.
A man ran a tan van.

Figure 3. The first lesson from *Let's Read: A Linguistic Approach*. (Reprinted by special permission of Clarence L. Barnhart, Inc., from *Let's Read: A Linguistic Approach* by Leonard Bloomfield and Clarence L. Barnhart, 1961, page 60.)

oral comprehension at the end of second grade. However, at the end of third grade there were no differences among the three approaches.

　　Merrill Linguistic Reading Program　Charles C. Fries, a linguist who has agreed almost wholeheartedly with Bloomfield's theory, set forth his philosophy of an approach to reading in *Linguistics and Reading* (Fries, 1963). Like Bloomfield's approach, the *Merrill Linguistic Reading Program* (Fries, Wilson, and Rudolph, 1966) was unillustrated, had a heavy initial emphasis on alphabet learning, and presented words first in isolation and then in sentences. Unlike *Let's Read,* however, Fries' materials used storybooks for practice in reading the words just learned in isolation. Materials consisted of an alphabet book and six readers with annotated teacher's manuals. Three major spelling patterns were stressed: those of the CVC pattern (*pig, bat*), those of the CVCe pattern (*take, line*), and those of the CVVC pattern (*boat, rain, meat*). The program since has been revised and expanded into 11 readers and supplementary materials. The present authors (Otto et al., 1975) have added illustrations to the advanced readers.

Schneyer (1969), extending a first-grade study into third grade, compared the Fries materials to a basal reader series (Scott, Foresman & Co., Glenview, Ill.). In first grade, the basal series produced superior results in word meaning, spelling, and phonic skills. However, by third grade the only difference that occurred was in phonic skills and was in favor of the basal reader group.

A program similar to Bloomfield's and Fries' is *Sounds and Letters* by Frances A. Hall (1964). It is presented in basically the same way as Bloomfield's program with no illustrations and no story plot.

Miami Linguistic Readers   Designed for Cuban-American children, *The Miami Linguistic Readers* (Robinett, 1966) are used as a language arts program as well as a reading program to teach English to Spanish-speaking children. The 2-year program consists of 21 small illustrated paperback books and 16 workbooks plus teacher's manual. A whole-word approach is used, and much emphasis is placed on intonation and stress. This linguistically oriented program probably departs more from Bloomfieldian theory than most "linguistic" programs.

Other linguistic based series include the *SRA Basic Reading Series* (Goldberg and Rasmussen, 1970), which is illustrated and presents irregularly spelled words early in the materials; *The Linguistic Readers* (Smith and Stratemeyer, 1970), which utilizes meaningful content from the beginning; and *Basic Reading* (McCracken and Walcutt, 1971).

As mentioned earlier, proponents of the "linguistic" approaches believe that children learn to read easier and faster when presented words with minimal contrasts in spelling. Levin and Watson (1963) have shown this to be the case in learning lists of words but found that, once the learning set or pattern was established, it was even more difficult to learn irregularly spelled words. Related findings from a laboratory study on the acquisition of sight words were reported by Samuels and Jeffrey (1966). They concluded that training on a list of words with maximal contrasts in spelling forced attention on all the letters. Consequently, the child adopted a strategy that resulted in a better basis for learning new words.

The value of learning to read words in isolation with a deemphasis on reading for meaning has been questioned, and the practice has not been favorably received by many. The significance of contextual clues as valuable aids in reading has been discussed by Goodman (1970), Kolers (1970), Weber (1970), and many others.

Elaborated T.O.

Several graphic systems have been devised for facilitating decoding of T.O. through the elaboration of symbols but without changing T.O. spelling patterns. Systems using color, diacritics, and other forms of elaboration are discussed in this section. Most of the reading programs utilizing these systems begin with a phonic approach rather than a whole-word approach.

Psycholinguistic Color System   According to Bannatyne (1971), the developer of the Psycholinguistic Color System (PCS) (Bannatyne, 1968), the program evolved out of research and clinical practice over two decades. Bannatyne recommended the system for beginning readers, for the learning disabled (particularly "dyslexic" children), and as a preventive program. PCS includes sequencing of phonemes, graphemes, and words in meaningful context.

Bannatyne (197) noted that dyslexic children have difficulty primarily in phoneme-grapheme association of vowels. Color coding in PCS involves 17 vowel phonemes only. Words are coded ". . . in such a way that the name of the color itself indicates the sound of the vowel phoneme" (Bannatyne, 1971, p. 646). For example, the color *green* is used with the long "e" sound $(/i/)$[2] in words such as *field, receipt, bean*. The color *lime* is used in words with a long "i" sound $(/aɪ/)$, for example, *light, tie, eye*.

---

[2]Although IPA is employed throughout this volume to represent phonemes or words when they are presented as examples, the present chapter is an exception to this convention. Instead, in representing examples, this chapter employs T.O., as is customary in the field of reading.

A series of programmed workbooks, teacher's guides, wall charts in color, and flash cards comprise most of the materials. Colored pencils are used by children to trace over vowels in the workbooks, thereby giving a teacher immediate feedback on a child's knowledge. The material is taught in four stages. At the end of stage 4, children discard color for standard black-on-white reading.

Words in Color   The beginning reading program by Caleb Gattegno (1962, 1969), *Words in Color,* is an outgrowth of the author's work with illiterate adults in several countries including the United States. Fifty-two colors and shades of colors are used to differentiate what Gattegno considers to be the 52 sounds of American English.

Materials include 29 colored wall charts of letter sounds and spelling patterns, a book on background and principles, a teacher's guide, and word cards. Four books in black-and-white print and worksheets in black and white are offered for pupils. Basic learning in the 8-week program is accomplished through: 1) work with wall charts, 2) considerable oral drill on each letter sound, and 3) copying onto paper in cursive script what has been printed on the chalkboard by the teacher in manuscript.

In a study of first-grade subjects, Hill (1967) found no differences when comparing *Words in Color* with another phonic approach. Hinds and Dodds (1968) found no differences among a small number of first- and second-grade students except on vocabulary and spelling, which favored *Words in Color.* In a longitudinal study from kindergarten to third grade, Dodds (1966) compared *Words in Color* with a traditional reading approach. At the end of third grade, there were no differences in comprehension, spelling, or word recognition even though Gattegno's system had produced better results in word recognition in the early stages of the study.

Other color systems are available. For example, *Colour Story Reading,* (Jones, 1965), printed in Great Britain, uses only three colors, red, blue, and green. Colors are printed in round, square, or triangular backgrounds with black letters.

Studies on color elaboration methods versus other methods of reading instruction are sparse. However, some research on the effect of color cues in learning words has shown that color does aid initial learning but interferes with transfer to black and white (Samuels, 1968).

Diacritical Marking System   The use of diacritical marks to simplify the learning of written English dates from at least 1580 A.D. (Pitman and St. John, 1969). The Diacritical Marking System (DMS) devised by Edward Fry (1964) is used for elaborating T.O. and is thus intended for the simplification of decoding during the beginning reading stage. The marks, which are those found on any standard typewriter keyboard, are gradually phased out after initial reading ability has been established.

Fry's basic rules for using the system follow (Fry, 1964, p. 527):

1.   Regular consonants and short vowels are unchanged.
2.   Silent letters have a slash mark. (writé right)
3.   Long vowels have a bar over mark. (mādé mājd)
4.   Schwa vowels have a dot over mark. (àgo lemòn)
5.   Other consistent sounds than those above are indicated by the bar under. (is̲ a̲u̲tō)
6.   Digraphs have a bar under both letters. (s̲h̲ut c̲h̲at)
7.   Exceptions to the above stated basic rules have an asterisk above the letter. (ȯf ŏncé)

A DMS specimen is given below (Fry, 1964, p. 529):

Thė Littlé Red Hen

Ŏncé upon à tīmé Littlé Red Hen livéd in à ba̲rn wit̲h̲ hér fīvé chiéks. À pig, à cat, and à duék mādé thèįr hōmé in t̲h̲é sāmé ba̲rn. Éach dāy t̲h̲é littlé red hen led hér chiéks o̲u̲t to l̲o̲o̲k fo̲r fōod. But t̲h̲é pig, t̲h̲é cat, and t̲h̲é duék wŏu̲ld not l̲o̲o̲k fo̲r fōod.

As a part of the "First Grade Reading Studies" (27 first grade reading projects (Bond and Dykstra, 1967)), DMS marks were applied to the Allyn & Bacon series and compared to the regular Allyn & Bacon series and to Initial Teaching Alphabet materials in several first-grade classes (Fry, 1966). Results at the end of the first grade showed no significant differences in reading among groups nor any relationship of method to IQ, age, or sex. Fry (1969) extended the study to third grade and found similar results.

Symbol Accentuation   A "perceptual-discrimination" approach to beginning reading, *Symbol Accentuation,* was designed by Arnold Miller (1968a) originally for use with severely retarded people. It since has been utilized with adult aphasics (Miller, 1968); educable mentally retarded children, deaf children, and "high-risk" first-grade children (Brown, 1971); and other populations.

Initially, the program used only flash cards with the word on one side distorted in shape, or accentuated, to reflect the word's meaning. The word *cold,* for example, has icicles on the letters. The word *dry* is hanging by clothespins from a line. *Symbol Accentuation* evolved from a total flash card format to flash cards plus animated motion pictures, which gradually phase out the accentuation. Figure 4 presents an example of accentuated words.

The materials, thirty 8mm film cartridges, workbooks, flashcards, and a teacher's manual, are divided into three phases. In phase 1, a 51-word sight vocabulary is presented by animated filmed sequences that gradually transform each accentuated word into the letters of normal T.O. The learner watches the transformation, says the word, and uses body actions to mimic meaningful aspects of the word. For example, the child would mimic a bird's flying motion as *bird* ap-

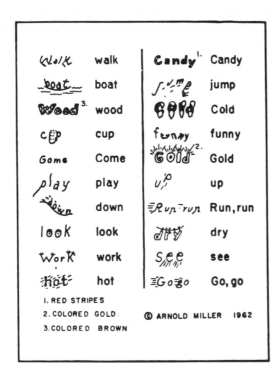

Figure 4. A sample of "accentuated" words. (From Miller and Miller, 1968, p. 204; reprinted by permission of the authors.)

peared on the screen and changed into the T.O. form. Phase 2 is a transition from the sight-word vocabulary to a partial phonic breakdown of the previously learned words such as *b-ird*, or *c-up*. Phase 3 utilizes motion pictures to teach individual sounds. As a sound is formed by the movement of a filmed mouth, the mouth phases into the printed letter. Learners are then taught how to blend the letters into meaningful units.

Two studies, using retarded persons ranging in age from 9 to 27 years with an IQ range of 25 to 75, indicated significantly better results in learning T.O. words with accentuation than learning T.O. words without accentuation (Miller and Miller, 1968). Similar results were found in a later study by Miller and Miller (1971). Three- and four-year-old normal children, as well as retarded adolescents (mean IQ 44) were reported by Miller (1968b) to have performed significantly better on a word-learning task when words were accentuated rather than simply paired with an illustration of the word's meaning. Miller further reported that normal 5- and 6-year-old children learned significantly more letter-sound relationships under accentuated conditions than under nonaccentuated conditions.

Messier (1970) studied disadvantaged 5-year-old children who received reading instruction by *Symbol Accentuation*. At the conclusion of instruction, subjects scored significantly higher on the Metropolitan Reading Readiness Test than control groups of children who had not had such training.

There may be limitations on types of words that can be presented by accentuation; however, it is possible that the method enhances formation of visual images, thus aiding memory. In addition, the uses of body movement and hand gestures, a vital aspect of the program, has been found to enhance acquisition and retention of printed words.

Several schemes have been devised for elaborating on T.O. in such a way that irregularities in spelling are accommodated for while the spellings themselves remain unchanged. Theoretically, this provides the beginning reader with a system that is easier to learn than T.O. alone.

Summary   Research on systems of elaborated T.O. is meager, and the results are inconsistent from system to system. It does seem, however, that reading ability is enhanced while the system is being used, but generally this enhancement tends to diminish once the system is removed.

Phonemic Alphabets

Persistent criticisms of T.O. have stemmed from the belief that the English language in print has a shortage of symbols. The rationale for this shortage theory is based on the claim that there exist approximately 44 phonemes in English, yet there are only 26 letters in the Roman alphabet to represent these phonemes.

As a consequence of the symbol shortage notion, numerous *phonemic alphabets* have been devised. Such graphic systems provide a close sound-to-symbol relationship by increasing the number of alphabetic symbols (beyond that of 26) so that they more nearly match the number of English phonemes. With the use of a phonemic alphabet, a sound usually has only one spelling. Table 1 illustrates this point by comparing some of the various spellings of the long "i"

Table 1. Comparison of T.O. and i.t.a. spellings for the long "i" sound (/aɪ/)

T.O.	i.t.a.
I	ie
aye	ie
eye	ie
lie	lie
high	hie
by	bie
buy	bie
ride	ried
rye	rie

sound (/aɪ/) in T.O. and in the Initial Teaching Alphabet (i.t.a.), one of the most widely used phonemic alphabets.

There have been two purposes for phonemic alphabets: 1) as alphabets underlying proposed spelling reforms of the English language, and 2) as symbol systems to be used temporarily during the early stages of reading instruction. To date none of the efforts at reform has been successful although such notables as George Bernard Shaw and President Theodore Roosevelt strongly advocated alphabet and spelling reform. The use of phonemic alphabets for beginning reading instruction, however, has been more accepted. After a child learns to read materials using the phonemic alphabet, these symbols are phased out and replaced by T.O. spellings.

Phonemic alphabets should not be confused with phonetic alphabets. A phonemic alphabet is used to represent the sounds of a particular language, such as English, when the reader knows the language. The alphabets used in reading instruction, for example, are phonemic, not phonetic. A phonetic alphabet such as the alphabet of the International Phonetic Association (IPA) presented in Figure 5 was not designed to teach reading. It is a system employed primarily by audiologists, speech pathologists, linguists, and other scholars to represent the sounds used in speaking. A person who is familiar with IPA notation can pronounce a passage from an unfamiliar language without knowing anything about the contents or meaning of what is being said. Some singers learn songs in foreign languages in this way. Transcription using the IPA alphabet can be either broad or narrow. Broad transcription, using the symbols shown in Appendix B, presents the recognized sound categories or speech sounds of a given language. Narrow transcription uses modifying notations to represent variations within sound categories, for example, the exact pronunciation of speech sounds by a specific speaker or in a given context or sound environment, and is very detailed. Thus, broad transcription can be thought of as approximating the phonemic aspects of a spoken language while narrow transcription represents the phonetic aspects. Examples of T.O. and i.t.a. representations are compared with broad and narrow IPA representations in Table 2. Although IPA was not designed for reading instruction, if it were used as a symbol system it actually would be a phonemic system in its application.

Initial Teaching Alphabet   In 1844, Sir Isaac Pitman developed a 42-character phonemic alphabet called "Phonotypy." Pitman was not interested in using the alphabet for spelling reform but rather

	Bi-labial	Labio-dental	Dental and Alveolar	Retroflex	Palato-alveolar	Alveolo-palatal	Palatal	Velar	Uvular	Pharyngal	Glottal
Plosive	p b		t d	ʈ ɖ			c ɟ	k g	q ɢ		ʔ
Nasal	m	ɱ	n	ɳ			ɲ	ŋ	N		
Lateral Fricative			ɬ ɮ								
Lateral Non-fricative			l	l			ʎ				
Rolled			r						R		
Flapped			ɾ	ɽ					R		
Fricative	ɸ β	f v	θ ð s z ɹ	ʂ ʐ	ʃ ʒ	ɕ ʑ	ç ʝ	x ɣ	χ ʁ	ħ ʕ	h ɦ
Frictionless Continuants and Semi-vowels	w ɥ	ʋ	ɹ				j (ɥ)	(w)	ʁ		

CONSONANTS

	Front	Central	Back
Close	i y	ɨ ʉ	ɯ u
Half-close	e ø	ə	ɤ o
Half-open	ɛ œ	æ	ʌ ɔ
Open	a	ɑ	ɑ ɒ

(y ʉ u) (ø o) (œ ɔ) (ɒ)

VOWELS

Figure 5. The alphabet of the International Phonetic Association (IPA) presented according to place and manner of articulation. (Reprinted by permission of the International Phonetic Association.) A pronunciation key to the IPA symbols used in American English is provided in Appendix B.

Table 2. English words represented by T.O., by a phonemic alphabet (i.t.a.), and by broad and narrow IPA transcription

T.O.	i.t.a.	Broad IPA[a]	Narrow IPA[a]
tan	tan	tæn	t^{h}æ̃n
pot	pot	pɑt	p^{h}ɑt
spot	spot	spɑt	spɑt
coat	cœt	kot	k^{h}o^{w}t

[a]A pronouncing key for IPA is provided in Appendix B.
[b]The ^{h} refers to aspiration; ~ refers to a nasalized vowel; and ^{w} refers to the rounding of /o/.

as a means of providing temporarily the advantages of a spelling reform at the time a child first learned to read and write. Pitman strongly believed that learners would have no problem in converting from Phonotypy to T.O. Phonotypy was widely acclaimed in schools in the middle and late 19th century in Great Britain and the United States (Mathews, 1966). Several other phonemic alphabets appeared and were tested in the latter part of the 1800's. In spite of their reported success, these graphic systems declined in use by the end of the century. Competition among the phonemic systems themselves and from the more traditionally oriented McGuffey readers and Webster's Blue-back spellers was probably the cause (Mathews, 1966).

Approximately 100 years after the introduction of Phonotypy, Sir James Pitman, grandson of Isaac Pitman, became interested in the alphabet, revised it, and presented the 44-character system, now known as i.t.a., in a May 1959 edition of the *London Times*. Pitman's i.t.a. (Figure 6) was originally called the "Augmented Roman" alphabet because it retained 24 characters from the Roman alphabet, dropping the redundant letters "q" (kw) and "x" (ks), and added 20 new characters similar in form to Roman letters or combinations of them. Only lower-case letters are used. If capital letters are needed, the size of the symbol is simply increased by about one-third to one-half.

Ostensibly, each i.t.a. character represents only one sound and each sound is represented by only one character. However, i.t.a. was not intended to be a perfectly regular code for the phonemes of English. The character ꝡh, for example, represents the "ch" sound in the words *church* and *chair* but not in *nature* and *question*. The

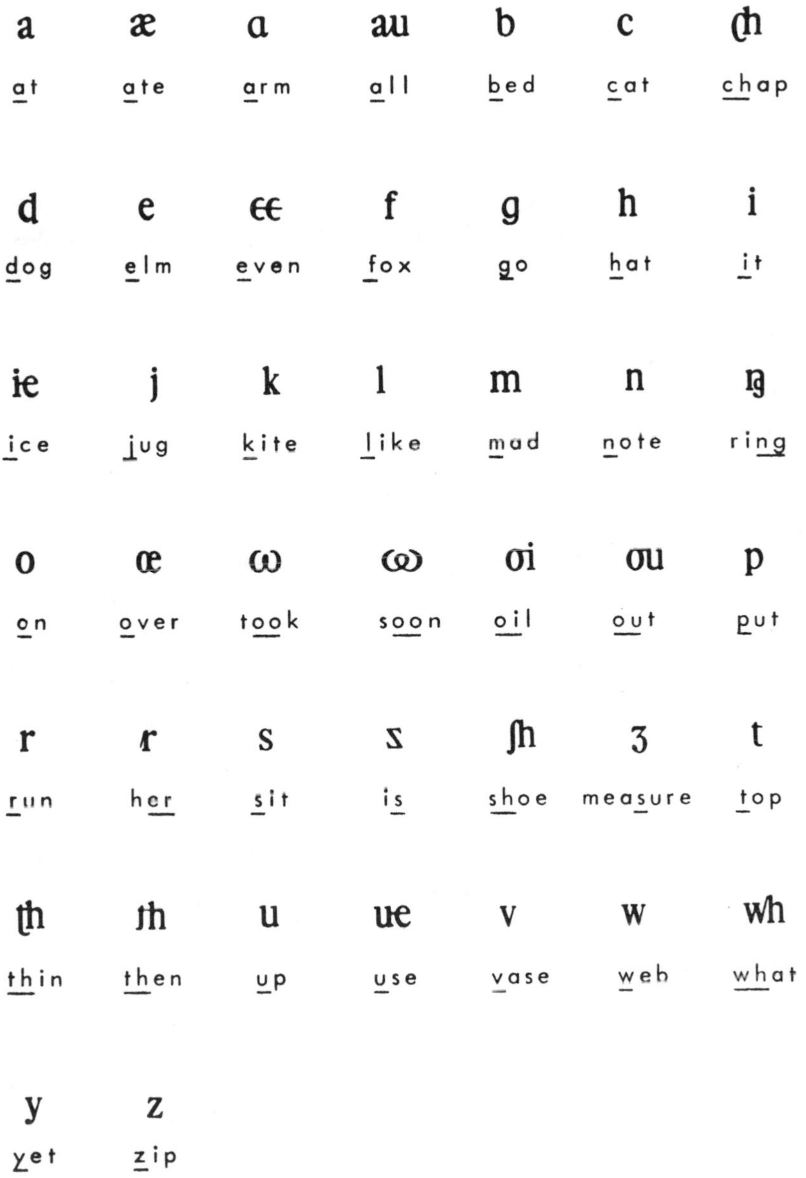

a	æ	ɑ	au	b	c	ʧh
at	ate	arm	all	bed	cat	chap

d	e	ɛɛ	f	g	h	i
dog	elm	even	fox	go	hat	it

ie	j	k	l	m	n	ŋ
ice	jug	kite	like	mad	note	ring

o	œ	ω	ꙍ	ɔi	ou	p
on	over	took	soon	oil	out	put

r	ɾ	s	ʒ	ʃh	3	t
run	her	sit	is	shoe	measure	top

ʧh	ʃh	u	ue	v	w	wh
thin	then	up	use	vase	web	what

y	z
yet	zip

Figure 6. The Initial Teaching Alphabet.

phoneme is written /t/, as it would be in T.O., so that the words appear as *kwestion and nætuer*. These exceptions are intended to help alleviate problems in transition to T.O.

Pitman was instrumental in launching the first i.t.a. reading experiment in Great Britain. This study involved over 1700 pupils and 158 teachers.

In 1962, John Downing, the British study's chief spokesman, introduced i.t.a. into the United States (Downing, 1967). Impetus was added to the i.t.a. movement in this country by Harold Tanyzer and Albert Mazurkiewicz, who met in England while observing the British. experiment. They returned to the United States and prepared the *Early-to-Read i/t/a Program* (Tanyzer and Mazurkiewicz, 1963). These materials were first used in Bethlehem, Pennsylvania, in a major study that began in the fall of 1964. i.t.a. became widely used during the 1960's in the United States, Great Britain, and other English-speaking countries and was heralded as a possible panacea for the prevention of early reading difficulties.

The *Early-to-Read* materials have an early phonic emphasis that is employed systematically throughout the series. The series is divided into three phases and approximates the format of typical basal reading series used in the United States. The materials include basal readers, supplementary reading materials, and teacher guides. By the end of phase 1, children are reading and writing i.t.a. Phase 2 is designed to reinforce the skills taught in phase 1. Phase 3 provides a gradual transition to T.O. This transition usually occurs during the first year of reading instruction but may be postponed until the second year if necessary.

The earlier i.t.a. materials such as *The Downing Readers* (Downing, 1963), published in Great Britain, differ from the American series primarily in their deemphasis on early phonic skill training. Considerable emphasis is placed on language experience activities and creative writing, with no emphasis on spelling and the mechanics of writing until the second year of instruction (Downing, 1967). In Britain complete transition to T.O. may not occur until the third year.

Extensive research in both Britain and the United States has attempted to assess the efficacy of i.t.a. as a medium for beginning reading instruction. Spache and Spache (1973) stated that American research in the area frequently has been contradictory or inconclusive and has received severe criticism from competent reviewers. Downing (1970) asserted that researchers in the United States have confounded the results of their studies by employing different instructional materials and different teaching methods in the comparison of i.t.a. to T.O.

British researchers, however, have exercised more stringent controls and have not produced such contradictory results. The British studies for the most part have employed parallel translations of T.O. materials in i.t.a. Unlike most American studies, this procedure allows for evaluation of the graphic systems themselves.

Although much of the i.t.a. research must be interpreted cautiously, the results suggest these answers to the following important questions:

1. When tested in the graphic system of instruction, are i.t.a.-trained children superior readers to children trained in T.O.?
Nearly all of the investigations, British and American, lend support to the notion that i.t.a.-trained children were superior in their medium of instruction compared to T.O.-trained children in their medium. i.t.a. readers had larger reading vocabularies (Mazurkiewicz, 1966), were well above the T.O. median on tests administered (Mazurkiewicz, 1965; Tanyzer, Alpert, and Sandel, 1965), and read more difficult materials (Harrison, 1964; Downing and Jones, 1966; Downing, 1967).

2. Are i.t.a.-trained children better readers in T.O. after the transition?
In the U.S. Office of Education First Grade Reading Studies (Bond and Dykstra, 1967), four of the five investigators who compared i.t.a. with T.O. approaches found no significant differences among groups at the end of first grade. The only exception occurred in measures of word recognition that favored i.t.a. subjects (Fry, 1966; Hayes, 1966; Mazurkiewicz, 1966; Tanyzer and Alpert, 1966). These studies, in which many of the children had undergone transition, employed the *Early-to-Read i/t/a Program*, which has a strong phonic emphasis. The fifth investigator (Hahn, 1966) used *The Downing Readers* and found significant differences in every area favoring i.t.a. However, Fry (1969) noted that, in a later replication of this study, Hahn found no differences. In a 3-year extension of his first-grade studies, Fry (1969) still found no differences, while Hayes and Wuest (1969) found first-grade i.t.a. superiority only in word recognition and found the third-grade group, initially

trained with i.t.a., to be significantly superior to others in silent reading. These third-grade i.t.a. subjects were at that time reading in T.O. in the *Merrill Linguistic Readers;* therefore, it is difficult to know whether the superiority was attributable to the initial i.t.a. instruction, to the Merrill materials, or to both.

In a review of several substantive American and British studies, Warburton and Southgate (1969) concluded that children tend to read easier, earlier, and faster using an i.t.a. approach, but after about 3 years of schooling the reading achievement of T.O.-trained and i.t.a.-trained children is approximately equal.

3. Does instruction in i.t.a. foster poor spelling later in T.O.? Block (1972) reviewed 47 studies that measured the spelling of children who had been taught initially by i.t.a. versus those taught by T.O. in first, second, and third grades. At the end of first grade, approximately one-third of 21 studies reported i.t.a. students as poorer spellers than T.O. students, one-third found no differences, and one-third found i.t.a. spellers significantly superior to T.O. spellers. At the end of second grade, i.t.a. students were found to be superior spellers in 11 out of 18 studies. The remainder of the 18 studies found no differences. The eight studies with third- and fourth-grade children generally found no differences in spelling.

4. Is i.t.a. better suited for one group of children than another? There has been some evidence that bright students fare better with i.t.a. than do slower students (Downing, 1967). Slower students do just as well with T.O. as with i.t.a. The Initial Teaching Alphabet has been reported to be helpful with learning-disabled children (Rampp and Covington, 1972; Lane, 1974), primarily in remedial instruction.

In a study of six different approaches to reading with 120 classes of primary educable mentally retarded students, Woodcock (1968a) found no differences in achievement after 2 years. Two of these approaches were i.t.a.

The initial teaching alphabet enjoyed great popularity in the 1960's. However, when studies failed to show i.t.a.'s long range superiority over T.O., its use declined.

Fōnetic English   A graphic system called Fōnetic English (Rohner, 1966) was devised not merely as a transitional orthographic system but as a permanent system to simplify the spelling of English. No materials are available; only a compilation of the phonemic elements of the language exists, with many suggestions for spelling reform based upon the compilation. The suggested alphabet presented in Figure 7 provides a one-to-one relationship of symbol to sound by using 29 letters instead of 26. The five long vowel sounds

Letter	Its Name	Word Example
ā	ā	āt (ate)
a	a(t)	at
b	bē	best
c	cē (hard c)	cat
d	dē	dog
ē	ē	ēt (eat)
e	e(t)	eg (egg)
f	ef	fat
g	gā (hard g)	get
h	hā	had
ī	ī	īs (ice)
i	i(t)	it
j	jā	jet
k *	kā	Karl
l	el	let
m	em	man
n	en	not
ō	ō	ōld
o	o(t)	hot or father
p	pē	pen
q *	cyū	Quebec
r	or (är)	rat
s	es	sat
t	tē	top
ū **	ū (also yū)	fūd (food)
u	u(t)	up
v	vē	veri (very)
w	wā	wish
x	ecs	fix
y	yā	yes
z	zē	zērō

* Used only in proper nouns.

** Within a word, ū is pronounced without the y (as in *food*); for starting a word and for the pronoun *you* it is pronounced yū. See p. 13.

Figure 7. The 29-letter Fōnetic English Alphabet. (Reprinted with permission of the Fōnetic English Spelling Association.)

are inserted as new letters with the macron (long vowel mark) over them. The "k" and "q" are eliminated except as capital letters in proper names. Numerous spelling changes are suggested such as contracting words to simplify them, for example, using *th* for *the,* and *r* for *are.*

The Fōnetic English Spelling Association, publisher of the alphabet, makes the system available without charge to anyone who will use it. The aims of the association are: to eliminate adult illiteracy, to provide a superior method for teaching reading to children, and, eventually to encourage everyone in the English-speaking world to write and print in Fōnetic English (Rohner, 1966). A sample of the "Star Spangled Banner" written in the alphabet follows (from Spache and Spache, 1969, p. 494):

> O sa! can U se, bi th dawn'z irli lit
> whot so proudli we hald at th twilit's
>   last gleming
> Huz brawd strips and brit storz,
>   thru the perulus fit . . .

Ten-Vowel Alphabet   Many hours have been spent each year by Leo G. Davis, a retired teacher, in his quest for orthographic reform. The 31-letter "fonetik alfabet" (Davis, 1965) retains Roman letters but has a 10-vowel arrangement in which small capital letters are used for long vowels and the usual lower-case letters for short vowels. Silent and double letters are eliminated, and simplicity is increased by substituting spellings such as "k" for hard "c," "f" for "ph," or "j" for soft "g."

Spache and Spache (1969) remarked that Davis' approach to reading is a spelling approach. This is delineated in "the davis speller" (Davis, 1965), a guide for teachers on transliterating materials into 10-vowel orthography. A small reader, "k-a-t spelz cat," (Davis, 1963) is available for use with children.

UNIFON   John Malone, a former inventor, economist, and newspaperman, developed UNIFON, or the Single-Sound Alphabet, in the late 1950's. Malone's keen interest in spelling reform for all reading matter prompted him to devise the alphabet to match the sounds of English and of other major European languages (Malone, 1962). He was also interested in UNIFON's adaptability to language-using machines (Durr, 1967). A few small experiments with UNI-FON led to the establishment of "The Foundation for a Compatible and Consistent Alphabet," an organization directed by Malone for the promotion of phonemic alphabets and for the eventual adoption of a universal phonemic alphabet.

Malone's original 40-character UNIFON alphabet has been revised slightly by Margaret Ratz, the developer of the reading system employing UNIFON. The revised symbol system, as well as the original system, is always presented in block capitals as shown in Figure 8. There are 16 vowels and vowel diphthongs, and 24 consonants. Using the alphabet, one spells ". . . each word as it sounds: i.e., 'alfubet, kat, kup, met, etc.' " (Malone, 1962, p. 441). UNIFON uses neither silent nor double letters.

Materials for children were published by the Western Publishing Company of Racine, Wisconsin, in 1966. These readers are now out of print. Other materials, however, since have been developed. Medcalf and Ratz (1973) have described briefly a set of five basic English-UNIFON books in preparation. These have now been completed, and other materials have been developed (Ratz, 1975).

Only a few studies have dealt with the effectiveness of UNIFON. Nold (1968) compared one UNIFON class to one control class and found no significant differences. McClintick (1973) compared i.t.a., Distar, UNIFON, Diacritical Marking System, and Simplified Signaling System (a beginning reading alphabet devised by McClintick) in the transition to T.O. Transition was said to be quite workable when using the author's system compared with the other methods.

In 1971, a Title III project was initiated in Hammond, Indiana, comparing 10 first-grade UNIFON classes to 10 T.O. classes. At the end of first grade there were significant differences favoring the UNIFON classes in word recognition skills and comprehension of T.O. (Ratz, 1975).

Summary   Research on phonemic alphabets used for beginning reading shows that their use, like elaborative systems, seems to accelerate *initial* reading achievement beyond that of T.O. readers. This advantage, however, tends to fade after complete transition to T.O. Very few studies have been conducted with handicapped individuals; therefore, any special advantages of phonemic alphabets with this population is not completely known.

THE NEW SINGLE-SOUND ALPHABET

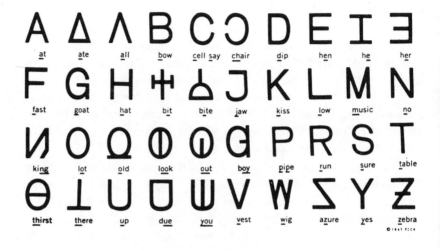

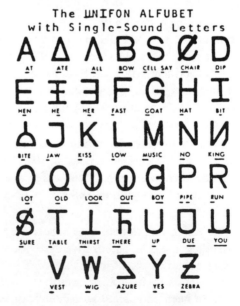

Figure 8. Malone's original UNIFON alphabet (*top*) and Ratz's revision (*bottom*).

NONALPHABETIC SYSTEMS

Although alphabets are the most widely used of all graphic systems, some cultures including those of Japan and China still employ syllabaries, logographies, or combinations of the two. Syllabic and logographic systems have had special application in instructional situations for the purpose of providing a code that initially is easier to learn and use than an alphabetic system.

Syllabic Systems

In the early 19th century, Sequoyah, for whom the giant trees of the Pacific Coast were named, devised for his people what is believed to be the first graphic system of the American Indians (Gelb, 1963). This system was an 85-character nonpictographic syllabary designed for the Cherokee language. The writing system (Figure 9) was of great usefulness to the Cherokee nation for many years. With the system, ". . . there is nearly one-to-one correspondence between the pronunciation and the writing" (Gleason, 1961, p. 415).

Other syllabaries were created for North American Indian languages later in the 19th century. Most of these, however, were developed by missionaries rather than tribal members themselves. Some of the systems form the core of syllabaries currently used by many Alaskan and Canadian Eskimo tribes.

Syllabic systems are also utilized by the highly literate country of Japan. Writing is accomplished with two kana syllabaries, hiragana and katakana (presented in Figure 10), plus a logographic system of some 1850 characters called kanji. The kanas are used mainly for affixes, names, and foreign words (Gleason, 1961; Gelb, 1963); the kanji usually represent nouns, adjectives, and verbs (Makita, 1968; Gibson and Levin, 1975).

Makita (1968) has claimed that Japan has less than a 1% rate of reading disability because of the ease of learning the logographic-syllabic system. This claim is contrary to earlier findings (Gray, 1956), but, nevertheless, has focused some attention on the possibility of using syllabaries for teaching reading in the United States.

Recently, Gleitman and Rozin (1973) suggested using a small pictographic syllabary (60 characters) to teach beginning readers that the writing system "tracks the sound stream" of English. Figure 11 shows a sample of writing from the Gleitman and Rozin syllabary, which employs the "rebus principle" (discussed pp. 554, 584) in con-

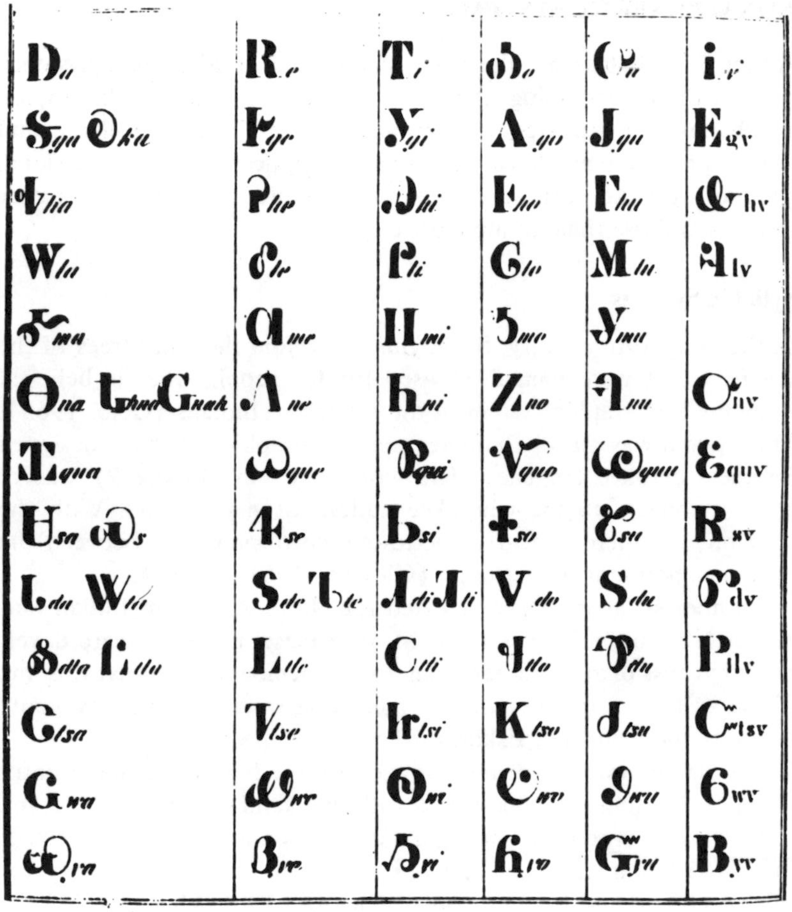

Figure 9. The Cherokee syllabary. (Photograph no. 1474 in the Phillips Collection in the Western History Collections, University of Oklahoma Library. Reprinted by permission.)

junction with spelled words. The method was tested with kindergarten and first-grade classes in Philadelphia. Reportedly, children learned very rapidly. Whether or not the method enhances transfer to phonemic analysis of T.O. is not known.

Syllabaries are not used currently in the United States to teach reading. English, with some 4000 or more syllables, might be extremely difficult to learn in a syllabic system.

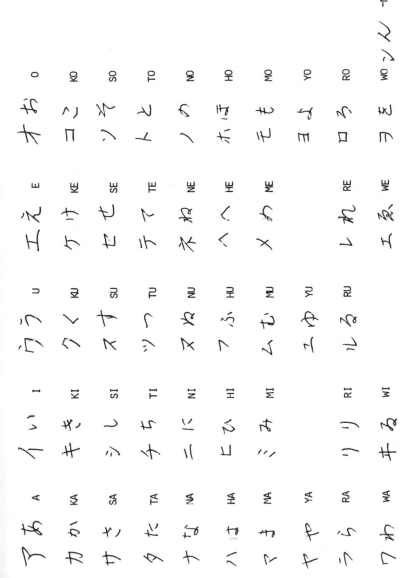

Figure 10. The katakana and hiragana syllabaries.

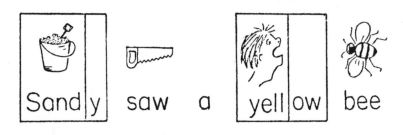

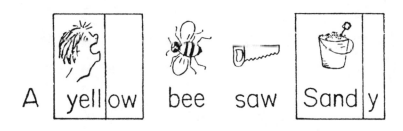

Figure 11. A sample passage using the Gleitman and Rozin rebus syllabary. (From Rozin, P., and L. R. Gleitman, "The Syllabary Curriculum: Pilot Materials," Curriculum Development Associates, Inc., Washington, D.C., 1973.) Reprinted with permission of the authors.

Logographic Systems

Logographic systems, albeit not as efficient for total language representation as syllabaries or alphabets, have some advantages over other systems. One such advantage is that logographs represent word units or ideas, and, therefore, are probably easier to learn and use initially than systems that represent units smaller than words. A second advantage lies in the fact that some logographic systems and many symbols within systems can be understood in almost any language. This occurs even though logographs range in character from pictographic (concrete) to nonpictographic (abstract). The abstract logographs of a mathematical language, for example, know few language boundaries. $1 + 1 = 2$ can be read by speakers of French, English, Greek, Russian, Chinese, and many other languages. A concrete pictograph of a cow represents that animal in any language whereas the alphabetically written word *cow* is decipherable only to readers of English.

The simplicity of a picture-type system, which allowed man to set his thoughts into writing, has been recaptured many times for use with individuals who do not read well in a particular language. Huey (1908, p. 326) believed that such a system represents ". . . a stage of reading and writing that is a natural one for the child, and he will make much use of it if encouraged a little."

Pictographic Logographs

Pictographs are often referred to as *rebuses*. Many 19th century reading texts used pictures and rebuses for words not yet in the reading vocabularies of their users. The practice has continued into the 20th century. *The Harper and Row Basic Reading Program* (O'Donnell, 1966), for example, uses pictures in some of the pre-primers (Figure 12).

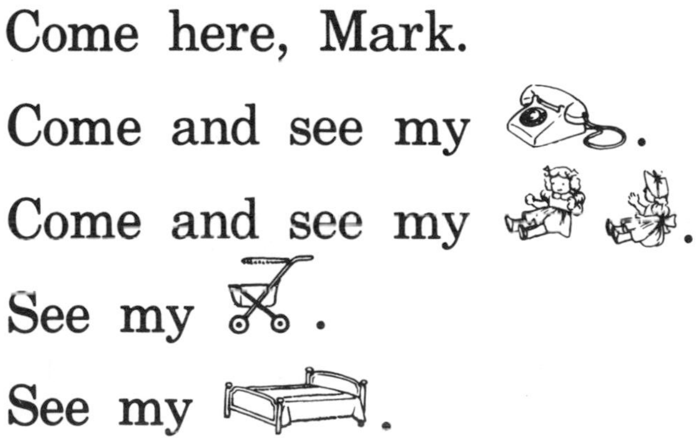

Come here, Mark.

Come and see my .

Come and see my .

See my .

See my .

Figure 12. A page from *Janet and Mark,* the first preprimer of *The Harper and Row Basic Reading Program.* (From JANET AND MARK by Mabel O'Donnell. Copyright © 1966, Harper & Row, Publishers, Incorporated. Reprinted with permission.)

Rebuses are used widely as international symbols for equipment controls and road signs. In these capacities, logographs usually represent more than one word. Dreyfuss (1972) has compiled a number of such symbols in his *Symbol Sourcebook*.

Anyone can design rebus symbols. The rebus symbols described in this section, however, are taken from a published set of rebuses known as the *Standard Rebus Glossary* (Clark, Davies, and Woodcock, 1974). This glossary contains 818 different rebuses plus over 1200 combinations of rebuses or rebuses with letters.

Rebus symbols in general may be classified into three types: concrete, relational, or abstract. Rebuses can be combined with other rebuses or with letters to form new words. Figure 13 presents an example of types of rebuses and some possible combinations. A passage written completely with rebuses is illustrated in Figure 14.

Although the use of rebuses to represent the complete or virtually complete text of reading material has been limited, this use has been applied in several situations such as testing, beginning reading instruction, early language development, teaching English as a second language, and as the symbol system for communication boards used with individuals with neuromuscular involvement (see Vanderheiden and Harris-Vanderheiden, this volume). Woodcock (1958) developed a test to predict success in remedial reading; the test required the child to learn a vocabulary of 72 rebuses (mostly relational and abstract) and then to read test passages written in this vocabulary. The procedure for teaching the rebuses and administering the test passages took from 30 to 45 minutes per subject. The number of oral reading errors made on the test passages was used as a relative index for predicting success in subsequent remedial reading instruction. O'Connor (1964), in describing the symbol system in Woodcock's test, suggested that it might serve as an aid to the "coding problems" in the severely retarded and "make the reading of simple material that much easier for them."

The Rebus Reading Series In 1965 an experimental rebus approach was developed for teaching reading to young mentally retarded children. *The Rebus Reading Series* (Woodcock, 1965) was a basal reader program in which children learned to read using a vocabulary of rebuses that were gradually transliterated into T.O. The program was designed to replace the readiness, preprimer, and primer levels of a traditional T.O. basal reading program. The materials were part

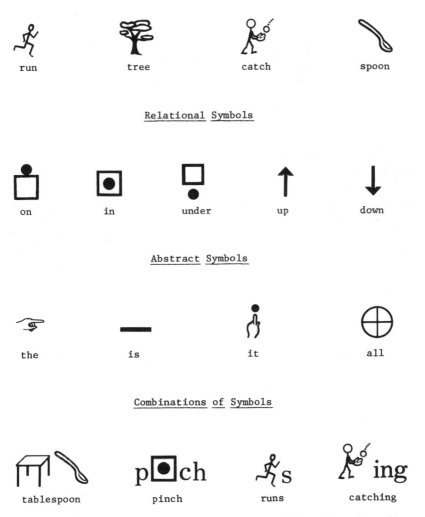

Figure 13. Examples of the three types of rebus symbols, and word combinations utilizing rebuses with letters. (Rebuses from Clark, Davies, and Woodcock, 1974.)

of the Peabody-Chicago-Detroit Reading Project (Woodcock, 1968a), which compared six different approaches to beginning reading with young retardates in Chicago and Detroit.

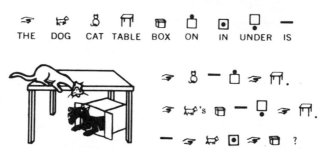

Figure 14. Illustrative rebus vocabulary and passage (one-half actual size).

Peabody Rebus Reading Program The *Peabody Rebus Reading Program* (Woodcock, Clark, and Davies, 1968) is an outgrowth of *The Rebus Reading Series.* The instructional goals of the program approximate the readiness and preprimer objectives of traditional reading programs. Two characteristics which particularly set the *Peabody Rebus Reading Program* apart from traditional beginning reading programs are the incorporation of a programmed text format with an emphasis on developing comprehension skills, and the use of logographs (rebuses) as a link between spoken language and the discrete patterns of language in print. Figure 15 presents two frames from the first workbook. The vertical lines beneath the answer choices are printed with a special water-sensitive ink. The pupil wipes a moist eraser across the lines. If the choice is correct, the ink turns green and the pupil moves to the next frame. If the choice in incorrect, the ink turns red, which is a signal for the pupil to stop and work that frame again.

With the exception of two words, *airplane* and *into,* each rebus in the program represents a morpheme (the smallest linguistic unit of meaning). Inflectional morphemes "s," "'s," and "ing" are presented in T.O. as part of the rebus word, as illustrated in Figure 13.

The instructional materials include three programmed workbooks, two readers, and supplementary materials. In the third workbook, which is correlated with the two readers, words in T.O. are gradually introduced so that at the end of the Transition Level the reader has a vocabulary of 122 "spelled words" (T.O.) and 172 rebuses (Figure 16). The method is primarily a whole-word approach, but the latter portion introduces phonic skills through a "semiphonic" presentation, that is, rebus families preceded by T.O. letters. For

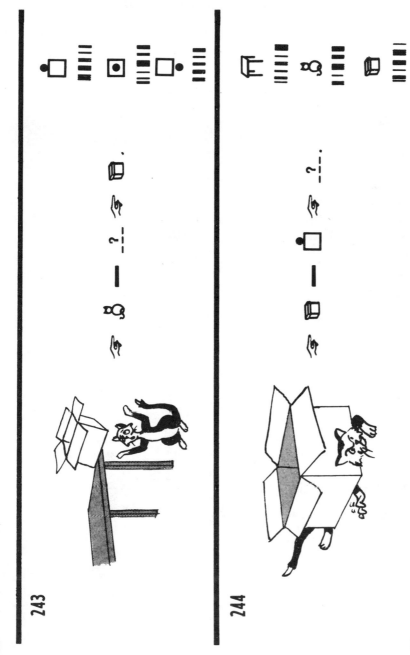

Figure 15. Sample frames from *Introducing Reading: Book One of the Peabody Rebus Reading Program.* [The cat is—the box (on, in, under). The box is on the—(table, cat, box).] (Reprinted with permission of American Guidance Service, Circle Pines, Minn.)

REBUS VOCABULARY—BOOK THREE

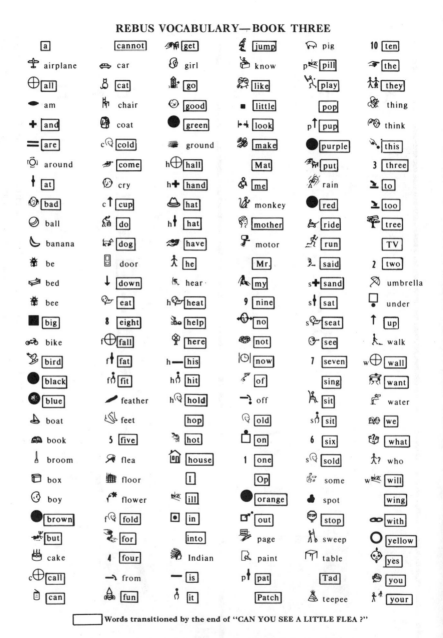

Words transitioned by the end of "CAN YOU SEE A LITTLE FLEA ?"

Figure 16. The vocabulary of the *Peabody Rebus Reading Program.* (Reprinted with permission of American Guidance Service, Inc., Circle Pines, Minn.)

example, the rebus *and* presented early in the program later would be preceded by the letter "h" to produce *hand*:

$$h \; \textbf{+}$$

Minnesota Early Language Development Sequence   The *Minnesota Early Language Development Sequence* (MELDS) (Clark, Moores, and Woodcock, 1975) was developed in response to the need for a receptive language program for young hearing-impaired children who had little or no language. Using a multimodality approach, the program combines with the speech mode, two visual language systems—rebuses (from the *Standard Rebus Glossary* and the vocabulary of American Sign Language[3]—presented in a planned sequence of English syntactic patterns. MELDS contains 120 structured classroom lessons that correlate with 120 parent lessons. This correlated design provides continuity in the child's language environment. The materials may be employed with children as young as 2.5 years or with older children who need further receptive language training to enhance their expressive language. In addition to its use with the hearing impaired, MELDS has been used with severely mentally retarded individuals and with children having developmental language deficits.

MELDS' instructional materials include the teacher's manual of lessons and a parent's manual of lessons. Both classroom and parent materials include rebus cards, picture cards, sentence cards, and pupil workbooks. A supplementary publication, *MELDS Glossary of Rebuses and Signs* (Clark and Greco, 1973), presents the 393 pairs of rebuses and signs utilized in MELDS. This publication may serve as a reference source for anyone wishing to use rebuses jointly with signing.

The MELDS teaching procedure follows a basic sequence in which rebus words, phrases, or sentences are put into a pocket chart. The teacher or parent points to, says, and signs each word and demonstrates the meaning physically or with objects or pictures. The

---

[3]American Sign Language (ASL or Ameslan) is discussed by Wilbur (this volume). Also, the vocabulary of ASL is the primary vocabulary of the total communication program presented by Kopchick and Lloyd (this volume).

lessons are designed for constant and active involvement of the child in the teaching-learning process. A great variety of sentence patterns are presented using the 393-word vocabulary. Although MELDS is primarily a receptive language program, the lessons contain optional expressive language activities.

The use of a logographic system such as rebus symbols for partial presentation of language has several advantages: 1) the constructed language patterns may be left on display for review and rehearsal; 2) written language, in the form of rebuses, may be manipulated manually long before a child is able to read and write in T.O.; 3) the use of a pictographic based symbol system (rebuses) reinforces the meaning of the transitory and nongraphic systems of sign language and speech. In most cases rebuses and signs represent morphemes and, as in the *Peabody Rebus Reading Program,* inflectional endings such as "-s," "'s," "-ed," "-ing," "-er," and "-est" are presented in T.O. Concomitantly, the signing component of MELDS utilizes separate signs for inflections.

Research Using Rebuses   The Peabody-Chicago-Detroit Reading Project (Woodcock, 1968a), which extended over a 2-year period, was a large study (over 600 subjects) on beginning reading conducted with retarded children. Subjects were the nonreading children in 120 primary classrooms for educable mentally handicapped in Chicago and Detroit. Twenty classrooms were randomly assigned to each of the six treatments. Woodcock compared the experimental program, *The Rebus Reading Series,* with five other reading approaches. Two of these were i.t.a. approaches, one a language experience approach and the other a basal reader approach using the *Early-to-Read i/t/a Program.* The other three approaches in traditional orthography were: 1) the Sullivan *Programmed Reading* materials (Buchanan, 1964); 2) a language experience program; and 3) the basal reader program, *The Macmillan Reading Program* (Harris and Clark, 1965).

There were no significant differences among the six approaches at the end of the second year. During the early months of the project, however, it was apparent that learning to read passages and stories written with rebuses was much easier for those children instructed in the "rebus" approach than passage reading was for children in the other approaches. It was hypothesized that preschool nonreaders might display equal ease in learning to read rebus passages, thus implying that children could acquire a great deal of knowledge about the reading process and the structure of symbolic written language long before they were presented the more difficult task of decoding T.O.

To test this hypothesis, Woodcock (Woodcock, 1968b; Clark, Davies, and Woodcock, 1974) conducted a study with 10 culturally disadvantaged preschool nonreaders in which he compared the subjects' oral reading performances on a learning-to-read task. For one group of five subjects the task utilized passages composed of a 20-word rebus vocabulary (mostly concrete and relational). The task for the second group of five subjects utilized parallel passages with the same 20-word vocabulary but in T.O. A significant difference at the 0.001 level was found favoring the rebus group. Hence, Woodcock's hypothesis that preschool nonreaders could learn easily a simple logographic system comprised of rebuses was supported. Unlike the T.O. words that were mostly unlearned, the 20 rebus words were learned and read in passages in only 15 to 20 minutes. The comparable learning time of the first 20 words in a basal reader program would be approximately 10 to 15 reading periods of at least one-half hour each (usually following a "readiness" program).

The ease of a rebus-type approach to communication for a population of severely and profoundly retarded individuals was noted by Kuntz (1974). She reported that rebus symbols (mostly concrete) were learned much faster than abstract symbols of the type employed by Carrier (this volume). However, the six subjects in the abstract symbols treatment group made a more rapid transition to T.O. than the six subjects in the rebus treatment group.

Wolf and McAlonie (in press) reported on a study of language acquisition using some of the lessons from the *Minnesota Early Language Development Sequence* with severely retarded preschoolers ranging in age from 26 to 37 months at the beginning of the study. The materials were used three sessions per week for 7 months. Subjects, who initially had a pattern of nonverbal behavior but the ability and willingness to vocalize, all made substantial gains in receptive language, and four of the eight subjects gained in expressive language skills.

Fifteen severely hearing-impaired preschool students were followed for 1 year as they progressed daily through the *Minnesota Early Language Development Sequence*. All but one child made substantial gains on a receptive language measure (Clark, Moores, and Woodcock, 1975).

Bliss Symbols   Charles Bliss, a former Austrian engineer, designed an international symbol system while in China during 1942. The system of Bliss symbols, patterned after written Chinese, was formerly called "semantography" because, according to Bliss, it was based on symbolic logic, semantics, and ethics. The symbol combinations frequently represent more than one word, making the system logographic in the same way as Chinese characters, which are ideational combinations of 1500 or so basic symbols.

Bliss symbols were not utilized with children until a teacher, in Canada, Shirley McNaughton, happened upon them in the early 1970's while searching for something simpler than T.O. to use on language boards for cerebral palsied individuals. The symbols since have been employed in Canada and the United States.

There are approximately 100 basic symbols in the system; the symbols are used singly at times, but more often they are used in combination to represent a given word or idea. Although a few of the Bliss symbols are pictographic, most are relational or abstract. Figure 17 presents some of the basic symbols and their combinations.

The system has been used primarily as a means for expressive communication by children who have some language but who are unable to employ functional oral or gestural expression. This includes individuals with neuromuscular impairment or severe intellectual retardation.

A Teaching Guide has been prepared by the Ontario Crippled Children's Centre (1974) in which approximately 450 symbols, including some of the basic symbols and combinations of these, are presented. The Guide is devoted to procedures for teaching the symbols, implementing them on language boards, and to lists and matrices of symbols. Rather than first teaching the basic symbols and then the logic for their combinations, the instructor presents words or ideas as wholes with the semantics of the combinations to be inferred and generalized by the learner as vocabulary is acquired. The T.O. counterpart of the Bliss word is always printed beneath the symbol so that those unfamiliar with the system can communicate with Bliss users. Currently, there are no materials for use with children other than the language board implementations. For further information on this use of Bliss symbols, the reader is referred to the chapter by Vanderheiden and Harris-Vanderheiden (this volume).

BASIC SYMBOLS

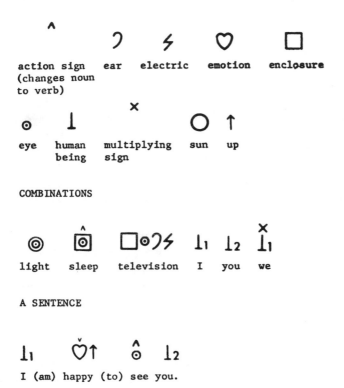

A SENTENCE

I (am) happy (to) see you.

Figure 17. Selected examples of Bliss symbols.

Nonpictographic Logographs

Although abstract or nonpictographic logographs may be more difficult to learn and to remember than concrete or relational logographs, they do tend to be easier to learn and use than alphabets in
certain situations. Such a situation was reported by Rozin, Poritsky,
and Sotsky (1971). Chinese logographs were used with eight second-
grade, inner-city students who had failed to learn to read with an
alphabet (T.O.). The subjects learned 30 abstract Chinese characters
and read with fair to good comprehension after 3 to 6 hours of
tutoring.

Recently, the abstract logographic system of printed sign language has been popularized. Such a system is particularly bene-

ficial to the deaf, who have used manual signs for thousands of years (Moores, 1971, 1974) but not in printed form.

Other types of abstract logographs have been employed with animals as well as humans. In attempts to foster linguistic communication between man and chimpanzee, several researchers have utilized nonpictographic logographs in chimp-training procedures. The chimpanzee, Lana, at the Yerkes Regional Primate Research Center in Atlanta, Georgia (Rumbaugh, Gill, and von Glasersfeld, 1973), learned to communicate with humans by means of abstract logographic symbols printed on a keyboard that was connected to a computer. Lana typed a sequence of "sentences," or received a sequence on a TV-type screen from her trainer.

Premack (1971) and Premack and Premack (1974) used movable abstract symbols in "language" training exercises with the chimpanzee named Sarah, who was trained to place the plastic logographs in sequential orders to form sentences.

The Premack symbols and training procedures, sometimes referred to as "Premackese," were employed by Hughes (1974/75) with four aphasic children who were seriously language deficient. The subjects, ranging in age from 9.5 to 12 years, learned to express several of the "language" functions. Hughes, however, questioned the linguistic status of "Premackese" and suggested it might be viewed more appropriately as nonlinguistic communication. Carrier (this volume) describes the development and use of a nonspeech language initiation program (Non-SLIP) based on Premack's plastic logograph system (also see Hollis, Carrier, and Spradlin, this volume).

Two very different applications of nonpictographic systems are explored in the following sections. The application of printed sign language is discussed in detail, while a nonprinted movable system is touched on only briefly.

Signed English Bornstein (1974), the innovator of Signed English, stated that Signed English is a manual parallel to spoken English and is made up of two kinds of gestures. The first kind of gesture, ". . . called a 'sign word,' represents the meaning of a target word as it is used in the syntax of the target language" (p. 331). The second class of gestures is "sign markers." These represent inflectional endings, the past tense for irregular verbs, irregular nouns, and an agent (person or thing). For example, in the sentence, *He saw the teacher looking at him,* the following are "sign words": HE SEE THE TEACH LOOK AT HIM. The sign markers in the sentence are: 1) a sign marker denoting the irregular past tense of *see,* which would follow the sign for SEE; 2) a sign marker after the sign for TEACH to denote *person* (TEACH PERSON); and 3) a sign marker for "-ing" after the sign LOOK. Figure 18 illustrates the various sign markers.

The present "teaching-aid" materials (Bornstein et al., 1972–1976) consist of more than 21 colored paperback books of stories and poems, several posters, and two dictionaries. The most recent dictionary contains 2200 signs or words (Bornstein et al., 1975). A total of 50 teaching aids, using the total vocabulary of 2500 words, is planned. Each of the teaching aids is self-contained and is usable without reference to any others.

Although Bornstein did not develop these materials to teach reading specifically, they can be read and signed to children or read by the children themselves. The materials illustrate the story action, present a printed word and its sign or signs, and illustrate for each sign word ". . . the most distinctive shape of the first visible lip movement" (Bornstein, 1974, p. 340). This is shown on the character (whether human or animal) making the signs. A page from *Happy Birthday Carol* (Bornstein et al., 1973) is presented in Figure 19. The Signed English materials began a formal 3-year evaluation program in the fall of 1974.

For unsophisticated signers, including young children, there may be a problem in the placement of "sign markers" in the illustrations of Signed English materials. The T.O. words read from left to right. The sign words are represented above the T.O. words, and they, too, read from left to right. Nearly all of the sign markers, however, are placed to the left of their sign words, as seen in Figure 19. This causes them to be read in an incorrect reading sequence as the reader moves across the line from left to right. The obvious reason for their being placed where they are is that they are signed on that particular side of the body. Nevertheless, they are sequentially misplaced and, in some instances, seem to belong to the preceding sign because nothing directs the reader from the sign word to the sign marker. The materials perhaps would be more readable to those learning signs if these markers were represented in another manner (for example, a dotted figure signing to the anatomical left of the sign word character) so as to synchronize the spatial sequencing of T.O. words and signs with the temporal sequence experienced by the reader who signs along while reading the story. The linguistic

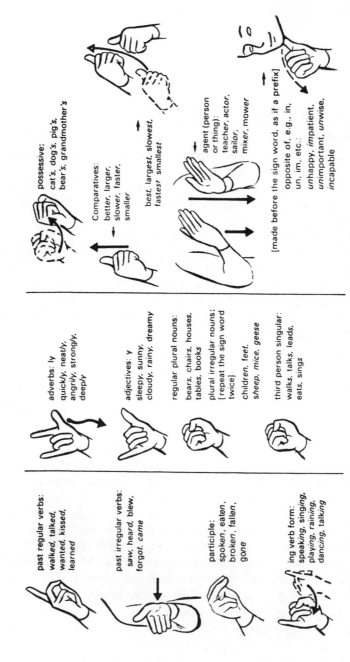

Figure 18. Sign markers used in Signed English. (From *The Ugly Duckling;* reprinted by permission of Gallaudet College.)

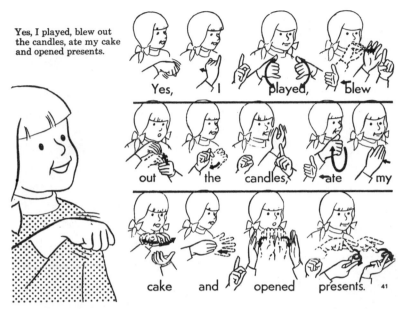

Figure 19. A page from *Happy Birthday Carol*. (From Bornstein et al., 1973, p. 41; reprinted with permission of Gallaudet College.)

aspects of Signed English are discussed in detail by Wilbur (this volume).

Non-Speech Language Initiation Program (Non-SLIP)   The same type of symbol and behavioristic approach as that used by the Premacks with chimpanzees has been employed by Carrier and Peak (1975) to train severely retarded individuals in a nonspeech communication system. The program is designed as an initiation into language for those with whom auditory input alone has been unsuccessful. Figure 20 shows a sample of the Non-SLIP symbols, which consist of 20 nouns, five verbs, three prepositions, and the functors *the* and *is*. Non-SLIP is presented in Carrier's chapter (this volume); therefore, it is not discussed in detail here except to note that it is a system utilizing movable abstract plastic shapes as symbols for communication in a manner similar to the way that one might use written words on cards. Because the program is nonoral, muscles for verbalization are not needed; only those for moving the plastic shapes are necessary.

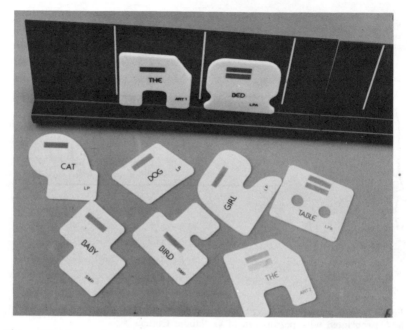

Figure 20. A sample of the Non-SLIP plastic symbols. (Courtesy of H & H Enterprises, Inc., Lawrence, Kan.)

Summary   In summary, logographic systems may have several advantages over alphabetic systems for certain purposes and with certain populations of handicapped individuals. Pictographic logographs are easily and quickly learned, even by very young children or by severely retarded persons. Although relational and abstract logographs are somewhat more difficult to learn, they, like pictographic symbols, can be used singly to represent a word or a morpheme whereas alphabets require combinations of symbols for the same purpose.

If an instructional objective is one of language enhancement, and not specifically the reading of T.O., then it seems logical to employ the most easily learned symbol system. In such a case, the graphic system is merely a means to an end and eventually may be unnecessary in language training.

If the purpose is to introduce a child to the language flow as it appears when converted to printed words, then the logographic unit may be ideal. This permits the child to develop a set for language patterns in print without having to employ initially the fine decoding required for T.O. Finally, logographs themselves can be functional as communication systems for the nonverbal individual.

SUMMARY

Mastering the traditional orthographic representation of the English language has proved to be a difficult learning task for many individuals and for many centuries. Consequently, various graphic systems have been devised to alleviate some of the problems of traditional orthographic representation, particularly at the beginning stages of reading instruction. Some systems designed for early reading control the spelling patterns of T.O. or elaborate on T.O. in the form of color cues, diacritical marks, or accentuation of words. Phonemic alphabets, syllabaries, and logographies completely replace T.O. in the early stages of learning and gradually may phase in traditional orthography later. A few graphic systems are intended not as precursors to T.O. but as means of communication, language enhancement, or alphabet reform.

The majority of research on graphic systems and their program utilization is ambiguous at best. In most instances, the value of such systems over T.O. has neither been proved nor disproved. This is particularly true in relation to handicapped individuals on whom graphic-system research has been sparse. One large study that supports the equivocalness of much of the research is the Peabody-Chicago-Detroit Reading Project, cited previously. This study, which involved over 600 mentally retarded children, is important in that it compared several graphic systems and varied uses of the systems, yet found no significant differences among the six treatments in the reading of T.O. after 2 years of instruction.

At present, the research that has evaluated the effectiveness of various graphic systems as compared to T.O. must be deemed inconclusive. There is, however, a consonance among research results. Many of the graphic systems are easily learned by individuals for whom literacy in T.O. is impossible. Furthermore, it seems that, while most of the graphic systems are being used, initial reading achievement is accelerated beyond that of T.O. readers. The types of learning that might occur during this acceleration are unresearched, yet they may be significantly important, particularly to the handicapped. It is possible that, while using graphic systems that are alternatives to regular T.O., children more readily develop various learning sets, such as a set for printed language patterns, a set for the discrete units of language, a set for interpreting printed symbols, a set for decoding and stringing symbols together. A great deal more research needs to be conducted with handicapped individuals utilizing various graphic systems for various purposes in order to determine their full impact on learning.

REFERENCES

Antilla, R. 1972. An Introduction to Historical and Comparative Linguistics. Macmillan, New York.

Bannatyne, A. D. 1968. Psycholinguistic Color System: A Reading, Writing, Spelling and Language Program. Learning Systems Press, Urbana, Ill.

Bannatyne, A. 1971. Language, Reading and Learning Disabilities. Charles C Thomas, Springfield, Ill.

Block, J. R. 1972. But will they ever lern to spel korectly? Educ. Rev. 14:171–176.

Bloomfield, L. 1942. Linguistics and reading. Elem. Eng. Rev. 19: 125–130.

Bloomfield, L., and C. L. Barnhart. 1961. Let's Read: A Linguistic Approach. Wayne State University Press, Detroit.

Bloomfield, L., and C. L. Barnhart. 1966. Let's Read. Clarence L. Barnhart, Bronxville, N.Y.

Bond, G. L., and R. Dykstra. 1967. The cooperative research program in first-grade reading instruction. Read. Res. Q. 2:5–142.

Bornstein, H. 1974. Signed English: A manual approach to English language development. J. Speech Hear. Disord. 39:330–343.

Bornstein, H., B. M. Kannapell, K. L. Saulnier, L. B. Hamilton, and H. H. Roy. 1973. Happy Birthday Carol. Signed English Series, Gallaudet College Press, Washington, D.C.

Bornstein, H., B. M. Kannapell, K. L. Saulnier, L. B. Hamilton, and H. H. Roy. 1972–1976. Signed English Series. Gallaudet College Press, Washington, D.C.

Bornstein, H., K. L. Saulnier, L. B. Hamilton, and H. L. Roy. 1975. The Signed English Dictionary for Pre-School and Elementary Levels. Gallaudet College Press, Washington, D.C.

Brown, M. 1971. SEIMC's Evaluation of the Symbol Accentuation (SA) Program. Regional Special Education Instructional Materials Center, State University College at Buffalo, Buffalo.

Buchanan, C. D. 1964. Programmed Reading. Webster Division, McGraw-Hill, New York.

Carrier, J. K., and T. Peak. 1975. Non-Speech Language Initiation Program. H & H Enterprises. Lawrence, Kan.

Clark, C. R., C. O. Davies, and R. W. Woodcock. 1974. Standard Rebus Glossary. American Guidance Service, Circle Pines, Minn.

Clark, C. R., and J. A. Greco. 1973. MELDS Glossary of Rebuses and Signs. Research, Development and Demonstration Center in Education of Handicapped Children, University of Minnesota, Minneapolis.

Clark, C. R., D. F. Moores, and R. W. Woodcock. 1975. The Minnesota Early Language Development Sequence. Research, Development and Demonstration Center in Education of Handicapped Children, University of Minnesota, Minneapolis.

Davis, L. G. 1963. k-a-t spelz cat. Carlton Press, New York.

Davis, L. G. 1965. the davis speller. Carlton Press, New York.

Diringer, D. 1942. The Alphabet, A Key to the History of Mankind. Philosophical Library, New York.

Diringer, D. 1962. Writing. Thames and Hudson, London.

Dodds, W. G. 1966. A longitudinal study of two beginning reading programs: Words in color and a traditional reader. Diss. Abst. 27:1084B.

Dolan, M. E. 1966. Effects of a modified linguistics word recognition program on fourth grade reading achievement. Read. Res. Q. 1:37–66.

Downing, J. A. 1963. The Downing Readers. Initial Teaching Publishing Co., London. (With teachers' manual, 1965.)

Downing, J.A., and B. Jones. 1966. Some problems of evaluating i.t.a.: A second experiment. Educ. Res. 8:100–114.

Downing, J. 1967. Evaluating the Initial Teaching Alphabet. Cassell, London.

Downing, J. 1970. Cautionary comments on some American i.t.a. reports. Educ. Res. 13:70–72.

Dreyfuss, H. 1972. Symbol Sourcebook. McGraw-Hill, New York.

Durr, W. K. (ed.). 1967. Reading Instruction: Dimensions and Issues. Houghton Mifflin, Boston.

Falk, J. S. 1973. Linguistics and Language. Xerox Corp., Lexington, Mass.

Fries, C. C. 1963. Linguistics and Reading. Holt, Rinehart and Winston, New York.

Fries, C. C., R. G. Wilson, and M. K. Rudolph. 1966. Merrill Linguistic Reading Program. Charles E. Merrill, Columbus, Ohio.

Fry, E. B. 1964. A diacritical marking system to aid beginning reading instruction. Elem. Eng. 41:526–529.

Fry, E. B. 1966. First grade reading instruction using Diacritical Marking System, Initial Teaching Alphabet and basal reading system. Read. Teach. 19:666–669.

Fry, E. 1969. Comparison of beginning reading with i.t.a., DMS, and T.O. after three years. Read. Teach. 22:357–362.

Gattegno, C. 1962. Background and Principles: On Words in Color. Educational Solutions, New York.

Gattegno, C. 1969. Reading with Words in Colour: A Scientific Study of the Problems of Reading. Educational Explorers, Reading, England.

Gelb, I. J. 1963. A Study of Writing. Rev. Ed. University of Chicago Press, Chicago.

Gibson, E. J., and II. Levin. 1975. The Psychology of Reading. MIT Press, Cambridge, Mass.

Gleason, H. A. 1961. An Introduction to Descriptive Linguistics. Holt, Rinehart and Winston, New York.

Gleitman, L. R., and P. Rozin. 1973. Teaching reading by use of a syllabary. Read. Res. Q. 8:447–483.

Goldberg, L., and D. E. Rasmussen. 1970. SRA Basic Reading Series. Science Research Associates, Chicago.

Goodman, K. S. 1964. The linguistics of reading. Elem. School J. 64: 355–361.

Goodman, K. S. 1970. Reading: A psycholinguistic guessing game. In H. Singer and R. B. Ruddell (eds.), Theoretical Models and Processes of Reading, pp. 259–271. International Reading Association, Newark, Del.

Gray, W. 1956. The Teaching of Reading and Writing. Scott, Foresman, Glenview, Ill.

Hahn, H. I. 1966. Three approaches to beginning reading instruction— ITA, language arts and basic readers. Read. Teach. 19:590–594.

Hall, F. A. 1964. Sounds and Letters. Linguistica, Ithaca N.Y.

Harris, A. J., and M. K. Clark. 1965. The Macmillan Reading Program. Macmillan, New York.

Harrison, M. 1964. Instant Reading. Pitman & Sons, London.

Hayes, R. B. 1966. ITA and three other approaches to reading in first grade. Read. Teach. 19:627–630.

Hayes, R. B., and R. C. Wuest. 1969. A three year look at i.t.a., Lippincott, phonics and word power, and Scott, Foresman. Read. Teach. 22:363–370.

Hill, F. G. 1967. A comparsion of the effectiveness of words in color with the basic readiness program used in the Washington Elementary School District. Diss. Abst. 27:3619A.

Hinds, L. R., and W. G. Dodds. 1968. Words in color: Two experimental studies. J. Typogr. Res. 2:43–52.

Huey, E. B. 1908. The Psychology and Pedagogy of Reading, Macmillan, New York. (Paperback reprint: MIT Press, Cambridge, Mass., 1968.)

Hughes, J. 1974/75. Acquisition of a non-vocal "language" by aphasic children. Cognition 3:41–55.

International Phonetic Association. 1949. The Principles of the International Phonetic Association. Department of Phonetics, University College, London.

Jones, J. K. 1965. Research report on phonetic color. New Educ. 1: 28–30.

Kolers, P. A. 1970. Three stages of reading. In H. Levin and J. P. Williams (eds.), Basic Studies on Reading, pp. 90–118. Basic Books, New York.

Kuntz, J. B. 1974. A nonvocal communication development program for severely retarded children. Unpublished doctoral dissertation. Kansas State University, Manhattan, Kan.

Lane, A. 1974. Severe reading disability and the initial teaching alphabet. J. Learn. Disabil. 7:479–483.

Langacker, R. W. 1968. Language and Its Structure: Some Fundamental Linguistic Concepts. Harcourt, Brace and World, New York.

Levin, H., and J. Watson. 1963. The learning of variable grapheme-to-phoneme correspondences: Variations in the initial consonant position. *In* A Basic Research Program on Reading. Final report, U.S. Office of Education Cooperative Research Project 639, Cornell University, Ithaca, N.Y.

McClintick, O. F. 1973. Simplified Signaling System: A Beginning Reading Orthography. Unpublished doctoral dissertation, St. Louis University, St. Louis.

McCracken, G., and C. C. Walcutt. 1971. Basic Reading. J. B. Lippincott, Philadelphia.

MacLeish, A. 1970. Do you pronounce it as it's spelled? *In* W. L. Anderson and N. C. Stageberg (eds.), Introductory Readings on Language, pp. 303–314. Holt, Rinehart and Winston, New York.

Makita, K. 1968. The rarity of reading disability in Japanese children. Amer. J. Orthopsychiatr. 38:599–614.

Malone, J. R. 1962. The larger aspects of spelling reform. Elem. Eng. 39:435–445.

Mathews, M. M. 1966. Teaching to Read, Historically Considered. University of Chicago Press, Chicago.

Mazurkiewicz, A. J. 1965. First Grade Reading Using Modified Co-basal Versus the Initial Teaching Alphabet. Lehigh University Office of Education Co-operative Research Project 2676, Bethlehem, Pa.

Mazurkiewicz, A. J. 1966. ITA and TO reading achievement when methodology is controlled. Read. Teach. 19:606–610.

Medcalf, R. L., and M. Ratz. 1973. A coding system that makes sense. Elem. Eng. 50:44–48.

Messier, L. P. 1970. Effects of reading instruction by Symbol Accentuation on disadvantaged five-year-old children. Diss. Abst. 70-22,460.

Miller, A. 1968a. Symbol Accentuation—A New Approach to Reading. Doubleday Multimedia, Santa Ana, Cal.

Miller, A. 1968b. Symbol accentuation: Outgrowth of theory and experiment. *In* E. Meshorer (ed.), Symbol Accentuation: A New Approach to Language Development with Retardates. First International Congress for the Scientific Study of Mental Deficiency, Montpellier, France.

Miller, A., and E. E. Miller. 1968. Symbol Accentuation: The perceptual transfer of meaning from spoken to printed words. Amer. J. Ment. Defic. 73:202–208.

Miller, A., and E. E. Miller. 1971. Symbol accentuation, single track functioning and early reading. Amer. J. Ment. Defic. 76:110–117.

Miller, E. E. 1968. Symbol accentuation: Application to special language problems. *In* E. Meshorer (ed.), Symbol Accentuation: A New Approach to Language Development with Retardates. First International Congress for the Scientific Study of Mental Deficiency, Montpellier, France.

Moores, D. 1971. Recent Research on Manual Communication. Occasional Paper 7. Research, Development and Demonstration Center in Education of Handicapped Children, University of Minnesota, Minneapolis.

Moores, D. F. 1974. Nonvocal systems of verbal behavior. In R. L. Schiefelbusch and L. L. Lloyd (eds.), Language Perspectives—Acquisition, Retardation, and Intervention, pp. 377–417. University Park Press, Baltimore.

Nold, J. T. 1968. The effect of UNIFON on teaching beginning reading: A pilot study. Ill. School Res. 4:38-40.

O'Connor, N. 1964. Educating the ineducable. New Soc. 4:18–19.

O'Donnell, M. 1966. The Harper and Row Basic Reading Program. Harper & Row, New York.

Ontario Crippled Children's Centre. 1974. Teaching Guide. Symbol Communication Research Project, Toronto.

Otto, W., M. Rudolph, R. J. Smith, R. G. Wilson, et al., 1975. Merrill Linguistic Reading Program. Charles E. Merrill, Columbus, Ohio.

Pitman, J., and J. St. John. 1969. Alphabets and Reading: The Initial Teaching Alphabet. Pitman, New York.

Premack, D. 1971. Language in chimpanzee? Science 172:808–822.

Premack, D., and A. J. Premack. 1974. Teaching Visual Language to apes and language-deficient persons. In R. L. Schiefelbusch and L. L. Lloyd (eds.), Language Perspectives—Acquisition, Retardation, and Intervention, pp. 347–376. University Park Press, Baltimore.

Rampp, D. L., and J. R. Covington. 1972. Auditory perception, reading and the initial teaching alphabet. J. Learn. Disabil. 5:497–500.

Ratz, M. 1975. Personal communication.

Robinett, R. F. 1966. Miami Linguistic Readers. D. C. Heath, Lexington, Mass.

Rohner, T. 1966. Fōnetic English Spelling. Fōnetic English Spelling Association, Evanston, Ill.

Rozin, P., S. Poritsky, and R. Sotsky. 1971. American children with reading problems can easily learn to read English represented by Chinese characters. Science 171:1264–1267.

Rumbaugh, D. M., T. V. Gill, E. C. von Glaserfeld. 1973. Reading and sentence completion by a chimpanzee (Pan). Science 182:731–733.

Samuels, S. J. 1968. Relationship between formal intralist similarity and the von Restorff effect. J. Educ. Psychol. 59:432–437.

Samuels, S. J., and W. D. Jeffrey. 1966. Discriminability of words and letter cues used in learning to read. J. Educ. Psychol. 57:337–340.

Schneyer, J. W. 1969. Reading achievement of first grade children taught by a linguistic approach and a basal reader approach—Extended into third grade. Read. Teach. 22:315–319.

Sheldon, W. D., N. J. Nichols, and D. R. Lashinger. 1967. Effect of first grade instruction using basal readers, modified linguistic materials and linguistic readers—Extended into second grade. Read. Teach. 20: 720–725.

Sheldon, W. D., F. Stinson, and J. D. Peebles. 1969. Comparison of three methods of reading: A continuation study in the third grade. Read. Teach. 22:539–546.

Smith, H. L., and C. Stratemeyer. 1970. The Linguistic Readers. Benziger, Beverly Hills.

Spache, G. D., and E. B. Spache. 1969. Reading in the Elementary School. Allyn & Bacon, Boston.

Spache, G. D., and E. B. Spache. 1973. Reading in the Elementary School. Allyn & Bacon, Boston.

Tanyzer, H. J., and H. Alpert. 1966. Three different basal reading systems and first grade reading achievement. Read. Teach. 19:636–642.

Tanyzer, H. J., H. Alpert, and L. Sandel. 1965. Beginning Reading: Effectiveness of Different Media. Nassau School Development Council, Mineola, N.Y.

Tanyzer, H. J., and A. J. Mazurkiewicz. 1963. (Revised 1966.) Early-to-Read i/t/a Program. Initial Teaching Alphabet Publications, Inc., New York.

Ullman, B. L. 1963. Ancient Writing and its Influence. Cooper Square, New York.

Warburton, F. W., and V. Southgate. 1969. i.t.a.: An Independent Evaluation. John Murray, London.

Weber, R. M. 1970. First-graders' use of grammatical context in reading. In H. Levin and J. P. Williams (eds.), Basic Studies on Reading, pp. 147–163. Basic Books, New York.

Wolf, J. M., and M. L. McAlonie. A Multi-Modality language program for retarded preschoolers. Educ. Train. Ment. Retard. In press.

Woodcock, R. W. 1958. An experimental test for remedial readers. J. Educ. Psychol. 49:23–27.

Woodcock, R. W. (ed.). 1965. The Rebus Reading Series. Institute on Mental Retardation and Intellectual Development, George Peabody College, Nashville.

Woodcock, R. W. 1968a. The Peabody-Chicago-Detroit reading project— A report of the second year results. In J. R. Block (ed.), i.t.a. as a Language Arts Medium, pp. 186–196. The i.t.a. Foundation, Hofstra University, Hempstead, N.Y.

Woodcock, R. W. 1968b. Rebuses as a Medium in Beginning Reading Instruction. IMRID Papers and Reports 5:(4). (Available from American Guidance Service, Circle Pines, Minn.)

Woodcock, R. W., C. R. Clark, and C. O. Davies. 1968. Peabody Rebus Reading Program. American Guidance Service, Circle Pines, Minn.

15

COMMUNICATION TECHNIQUES AND AIDS FOR THE NONVOCAL SEVERELY HANDICAPPED

*Gregg C. Vanderheiden and
Deberah Harris-Vanderheiden*

CONTENTS

Simple Model for Expressive Communication Channel _____ 611

Selecting/Developing a Physical Mechanism for Indicating
    Message Elements _____ 614

Three Basic Approaches to Providing a Physical Mechanism for
    Nonvocal Communication _____ 615
    Scanning/615
    Encoding/619
    Direct selection/621
    Combination techniques/623
    Levels of implementation/624
    Comparison of approaches/630

Selecting/Developing a Symbol System and Vocabulary _____ 632
    Basic considerations for selecting a symbol system/632
    Symbol systems for use with nonvocal communication
        techniques and aids/633
    Summary of symbol systems/637

Applications of Nonvocal Communication Techniques and Aids _____ 639
    Symbol communication for mentally retarded children/639
    Preliminary evaluation of an independent aid/642

Summary and Conclusions _____ 646

References _____ 647

Suggested Readings _____ 648

The ability to communicate is basic to human development and interaction and, therefore, fundamental to any educational process. It is through communicative interaction that persons are able to relate and exchange thoughts, ideas, feelings, needs, and desires to learn and to share experiences of others. For many severely handicapped children, however, effective communication is not possible through traditional channels. These nonvocal (nonoral) motorically impaired children (many of whom have normal or above normal intelligence) are unable to speak or write and are left with only undifferentiated guttural sounds and gross gestures to relay their thoughts and ideas to others.

Educational opportunities are now being provided to many severely handicapped children through statewide enactment of federal legislation that specifies that every child must be provided with educational programming no matter what the type or degree of handicap. However, if these educational programs are to be meaningful and productive, the children must be provided with an effective means of communicating. Without effective communication channels, these children have no means of interacting with their teachers or peers. They have no means of asking questions when tasks presented are unclear, nor can they respond to questions from the teacher. They also are unable to do productive independent work, do homework, or take tests without the constant, undivided attention of a second person.

Teachers often have extreme difficulty integrating the nonvocal, nonwriting child into their classroom because no effective program exists for successfully integrating the child into a group. The education of nonvocal, severely handicapped children is greatly limited by their need for one-to-one tutorial attention, their inability to work independently, and their reliance on others' interpretation of their thoughts, unless they can be provided with an effective means of communicating and writing.

Information contained in this chapter has been cumulated from research projects sponsored by the National Science Foundation (EC 40316) and the Bureau for the Handicapped, U.S. Office of Education (OEGO-74-7461 and OEC 0-74-9057).

The field test of the Auto-Com was made possible through grants by the National Science Foundation (EC-40316) and the Bureau for the Education of the Handicapped (OEG-0-74-7461). The Bliss symbol research program is being carried out as a cooperative effort with Central Wisconsin Colony, Madison, Wisconsin.

Techniques and aids that can help these children overcome their severe communication deficit are now available, and new aids are appearing frequently. These techniques and aids can serve to augment the communication abilities of these children and provide them with more effective systems of communication. *It is important to note that these techniques and aids should be thought of as augmentative channels of communication and not substitute channels of communication.* They are not meant to replace the existing communication abilities of the child, but to act as additional channels of communication for the child in much the same manner as writing and gesturing are additional means of communication for a speaking child. There has been some fear that introducing augmentative nonvocal communication channels might decrease vocalization or discourage speech development. However, studies to date have shown that introduction of nonvocal communication techniques has not decreased functional vocalization or speech development in these children but has, in many cases, increased both their attempts at vocalization and their intelligibility (McDonald and Schultz, 1973; McNaughton and Kates, 1974; Vicker, 1974; Harris-Vanderheiden et al., 1975).

Although augmentative techniques and aids are now becoming available, applying the techniques and choosing the appropriate one(s) for a particular child are not simple tasks. Augmentative systems range from very basic techniques, such as gesturing and yes-no guessing, to highly sophisticated and often expensive communication aids. Just as there is a great diversity in the form and degree of a child's handicap, there is also tremendous diversification in the types of aids and in their sophistication, benefits, and costs. Moreover, the benefits of a particular aid for a particular child or adult depend on a great many factors including the person's:

1. Type and degree of physical handicap
2. Cognitive abilities and potential
3. Social and physical environment
4. Other functional or partially functional communication channels
5. Communication function to be fulfilled by the aid

There is not one ideal or most appropriate communication aid for any particular type of handicap. Neither are cost, sophistication, or number of features necessarily indicators of a better aid. In many cases, a simpler, less sophisticated aid may be a more appropriate choice for a particular child than a more advanced aid.

Moreover, it is very important to note that the communication aid itself is only one component of the child's communication system and perhaps the easiest one to identify and provide for the child. A better perspective on what is involved in providing an augmentative communication system or channel for a child can be obtained by examining a simple model for an expressive communication system.

SIMPLE MODEL FOR EXPRESSIVE COMMUNICATION CHANNEL

Many models can be drawn depicting an expressive communication system (see Sanders, this volume; Hollis, Carrier, and Spradlin, this volume). This chapter, however, deals only with the external or physical aspects of a child's communication system; those aspects that could be affected by a strictly physical impairment. The model used is a simple three-component model of an expressive communication system. The three components of this model are:

1. A *physical mechanism* or means of indicating or transmitting the elements of a message to a receiver
2. An *ideo-symbol system and vocabulary* to provide the child with a set of symbols that can be used to represent things and ideas for communication to a receiver
3. *Rules and procedures* for combining and presenting the ideo-symbols so that they will be most easily interpretable by a receiver

To better understand these components, one needs to examine how they relate to the communication system of a normal vocal child (see Table 1).

The *physical mechanism* that the normal vocal child uses to present or transmit the elements of his message is his oral speech mechanism. With this mechanism, the child is able to transmit specific sound patterns that represent different ideas or concepts. These sound patterns, or spoken words, form the child's *ideo-symbol system*. The child uses these sound patterns (spoken words) to transmit his ideas to a receiver. In presenting these words to a receiver, however, the child must follow certain *guidelines* concerning their combination and order of presentation if the message is to be easily and correctly interpreted by the receiver (see Sanders, this volume).

Table 1. A simple model of expressive communication components for normal and nonvocal motor-impaired children

Component	Function	Component as represented in the normal speaking child	Component as represented in a child using a communication board
Physical mechanism	To provide the child with a means of specifying or transmitting the elements of his message to a receiver	Oral speech mechanism	Pointing board
Ideo-symbol system and vocabulary	To provide the child with a set of symbols that he can use to represent things or ideas for communication	Spoken words	Pictures, printed words, other symbols
Rules for combining and presenting symbols	To provide the rules and procedures for presenting the ideo-symbols so that the message will be most easily understood by the receiver	Syntax, grammar, etc.	Syntax, grammar, etc.

Fortunately for the vocal child, the potential to develop these three components is present in infancy.

Given normal stimulation, these components develop early in the child's life and provide an effective means of communication and interaction during most of the child's growth and development.

For the nonvocal severely physically handicapped child, physical and sometimes cognitive impairments often prevent the development of one or more of the components of the child's communication system. In the case of the physically handicapped child who is unable to communicate through his oral speech mechanism, at least two of the three components are missing or unavailable. To supply an augmentative communication channel for the nonvocal child, alternative mechanisms for providing these basic components must be developed.

Table 1 shows an example of what these components might be in a nonvocal communication system involving the use of a communication board. The *physical mechanism* for such a child would be a pointing board. Using this board, the child would be able to indicate the various *ideo-symbols* displayed on it that make up his message. These ideo-symbols may be in the form of pictures, printed words, or other symbols, such as Bliss symbols. Again, as with the vocal child, there are certain *rules* for combining and presenting symbols (words, pictures, Bliss symbols, etc.) so that they can be easily understood by a receiver.

The overall procedure for developing a nonvocal communication system for a severely handicapped child therefore consists of:

1. Selecting/developing a technique or aid to provide the child with an effective means of indicating the elements of his message
2. Selecting/developing a symbol set and vocabulary system that can meet and fulfill the child's communicative needs
3. Developing in the child the necessary communication skills that will permit him to use his symbol set in such a way that he can be clearly understood by the message receiver

A detailed discussion on any of these topics easily could fill several books. The remainder of this chapter briefly explores some of the options and considerations of the first two topics. Basic approaches and techniques for providing a nonvocal child with a means of communication are described along with a brief description of some of the aids and techniques that are presently available or under development. For further information on these topics and for advice on vocabulary selection and communication skills development, the reader is referred to other chapters in this volume (e.g., Clark and Woodcock; Graham; Kopchick and Lloyd) and the readings cited at the end of this chapter. Worthy of particular note in this regard are the publications by McDonald and Schultz (1973), McNaughton and Kates (1974), Vicker (1974), and Vanderheiden and Luster (1975).

SELECTING/DEVELOPING A PHYSICAL
MECHANISM FOR INDICATING MESSAGE ELEMENTS

A basic step in developing a communication system for a child is the selection/development of a mechanism to provide the child with a means of indicating or specifying the elements of his message for a receiver. For a child who uses a nonvocal communication technique, this step usually means developing some means for the child to indicate which visual symbols on a display make up the message he is trying to transmit. Pointing to symbols himself or nodding when someone else points to the desired symbols are just two examples of techniques for indicating message elements.

Many different nonvocal communication techniques have been developed by teachers, clinicians, and researchers over the years. Each technique has advantages and disadvantages and is more applicable to some types of disability than to others. Some require minimal muscular control while others use more refined movements. In general, the greater the number and complexity of a child's controlled movements, the faster his speed of communication can be. To achieve optimal speed, however, a child must be matched with the technique that best utilizes his particular type and degree of control.

The child's age and cognitive abilities also influence the applicability of a technique or aid. Both the complexity of the technique and the types of symbols that can be used with the technique or aid must be examined in relation to the child's present and future capabilities. A technique that requires the use of a complex code or an aid that requires spelling skills may be inappropriate for a very young child or a child with severe mental handicaps.

The various operational aspects of different techniques and aids must be understood if the most appropriate and efficient system is to be selected/developed for a child. There is no "one system" for a particular child; usually a child is physically capable of using any one of several different techniques. The objective is to find the technique that is most effective for the child, given his environment and communication needs, as well as his cognitive and physical abilities. As a child develops, his environment, his communication needs, and his cognitive and physical abilities will change. In all likelihood, the technique or aid that is most appropriate for him also will change. Aids that are more flexible are therefore usually more desirable.

THREE BASIC APPROACHES TO PROVIDING A PHYSICAL MECHANISM FOR NONVOCAL COMMUNICATION

Although there are a great many different techniques for providing a child with a means for indicating message elements or symbols, these techniques are all essentially variations or combinations of three basic approaches: *scanning, encoding,* and *direct selection.* Because understanding the theory, advantages, and disadvantages of each approach is important in selecting an appropriate aid for a child, each of these approaches is described, and several examples of specific techniques utilizing each approach are provided. A summary section reviews and compares the three approaches.

Scanning

Scanning techniques are techniques where the message elements are presented to the child in a sequential manner and where the child specifies his choice by responding to the person or display presenting the elements.

Basically, any technique would be considered a scanning technique if it involves a person or aid that presents the various symbols or words to a child, who essentially remains passive until the correct item is presented. At this point, the child makes some kind of signal indicating that the correct item or category had been selected. In other words, the person or aid scans over the various choices until the child responds, indicating a correct choice has been reached, thus the term *scanning* approach.

The simplest example of a scanning technique is the "yes/no" guessing game. Here the person trying to communicate with the child presents the child with choices, one at a time, and the child nods "yes" when (and if) the second person reaches the desired message (Figure 1A). Another example of a scanning technique (Figure 1B) is a second person pointing individually to pictures, words, or letters on a communication board. Here again the child

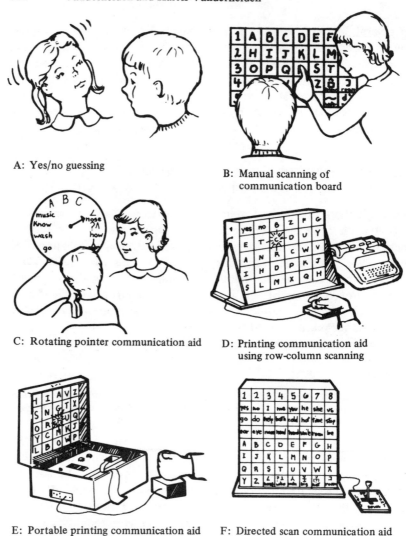

A: Yes/no guessing

B: Manual scanning of
   communication board

C: Rotating pointer communication aid

D: Printing communication aid
   using row-column scanning

E: Portable printing communication aid

F: Directed scan communication aid

Figure 1. Scanning techniques and aids.

responds to the second person by nodding or making some movement
to signal "yes" when the person points to the correct element of the
child's message.

   To help make this process easier for the second person, aids
are available that can do the sequencing automatically. One example

is the rotating arrow aid shown in Figure 1C. Here the child controls the pointer by using a switch specially designed to respond to some movement over which the child has good control. With this aid the child is able to start and stop and the pointer to indicate the various elements of his message. The second person still must be present but is relieved of the task of pointing to each element and watching for a response from the child.

For the more advanced child, scanning aids have been developed that can provide the child with a completely independent means of communication and writing. These aids not only do the sequencing or scanning automatically but also print out or display the letter or word finally chosen by the child (Figure 1D). With these aids the child does not require the constant attention and presence of a second person to watch his movements or assemble his message, and he can work completely independently. The second person need only take the time to read the completed message. Such aids also allow the child to do independent work, assignments, etc., especially if they can be used to control typewriters or television displays (similar to those used in airports to present flight information).

Scanning Techniques and Aids   The aid pictured in Figure 1B uses a linear scanning technique. In linear scanning aids, each and every letter, picture, word, etc., is presented until the child signals that the correct message element is being presented. Because this method can be very slow, several other scanning techniques have been developed that significantly decrease the time it takes for a child to reach his desired message element on the display. One method for doing this is to use a two-speed scan. With this technique the child can push a button, causing the aid to begin scanning rapidly. The child then waits until the scan gets close to the desired element, at which time he releases the button, causing the aid to scan more slowly so that he can stop it easily on the correct element of the display.

Another technique is the row-column scanning technique (Figure 1D and E). Here the aid (or person) points to each row in turn and the child responds when the row containing the desired element is indicated. The aid (or person) then points to the elements in that row until the child indicates that the desired element has been reached. This method can reduce to less than a third the average time required to reach a given square on the display. When the alphabet is used, the speed can be increased even further by positioning the most used letters close to the upper lefthand corner of the display (where the scanning process begins) as in Figure 1D.

Another type of commonly used scanning is directed scanning. Here the child can control the *direction* of the scan (up, down, left, right) as well as being able to stop it when it reaches the proper position of the display. A joystick (Figure 1F) would be one way of controlling such a display.

Finally, a technique that has been developed recently to increase further the speed of scanning aids using the alphabet is the "predictive scanning" technique (also called "anticipatory" or "computeraided scanning"). With this technique the aid uses the last two letters that the child has indicated to try to predict which letter the child will want next. It then presents those letters to the child first before scanning over the other letters of the alphabet. For example, if the first two letters of the child's message were T and H, the aid would indicate that the six letters most likely to occur in the next space after letters in this sequence would be (in order of probability) E, SPACE, A, I, O, and S. Using this system and looking only at the last two letters printed, the probability is 81.3% that the next letter the child wants will be one of the first six letters presented by a predictive scanning aid. This technique, of course, only works for the alphabet and cannot be easily applied to aids utilizing pictures, symbols, whole words, or phrases.

Scanning Overview   The scanning approach is a particularly powerful approach because it can be used by any child no matter how severe his physical handicap. This is possible because all that is necessary to use these techniques is that the child have some movement or signal that can be detected by a second person or by an aid. To allow children to use scanning aids, a great number of different switches have been developed that can take advantage of most any movement or signal the child can make. Some of them are: touch switches, impact switches, knee switches, proximity switches, eyebrow switches, breath switches, whistle switches, joysticks, eye switches, muscle potential switches, and even brain wave sensors.

The major advantages of techniques and aids that use the scanning approach are that they:

Can be very simple to operate for low cognitive level children
Require little effort to operate
Can be used by almost anyone, no matter how severe the physical
    disability

The major disadvantage of the scanning approach is its relatively slow speed. With these techniques the child must wait while the indicator steps over many unwanted positions before it reaches the desired message element. The rate of scanning must remain quite slow for many children because the indicator must rest at *each* location long enough for the child to be able to respond and select it without error. The slowness of these techniques as compared to the other approaches also increases as the number of pictures, symbols, or words on the display increases.

Encoding

Encoding techniques are techniques where the desired message elements are indicated by multiple signals from the child which are presented in a pattern that must be memorized or looked up on a chart.

In the encoding approach, any number of switches or movements may be used. The code may involve activating switches or making movements sequentially, simultaneously, or in a specific time pattern (as in Morse code).

Encoding Techniques and Aids   A very simple example of an encoding technique is one in which the letters of the alphabet are arranged in a 5 $\times$ 5 matrix (Z excluded) (Figure 2A). With this system a child can indicate that he wants the letter L, for instance, by holding up two fingers indicating the second column and then three fingers indicating the third letter down. Another encoding technique is shown in Figure 2B. Here pictures, words, or other symbols are presented on a vocabulary chart with a number pair beside each symbol. The child specifies the symbols that make up his message by pointing to the two numbers that are next to the appropriate symbols. For the child who cannot point with his hand, arm, head-stick, etc., an eye gaze chart similar to the one shown can be used. This clear plastic chart (called an ETRAN chart) allows effective communication for children who have control over only their eyes. For the child who is not ready for two-number pairing, colors can be used in conjunction with the numbers so that the child specifies a color and a single number to indicate the appropriate element on his vocabulary chart.

Another encoding technique involves the use of Morse codes and other two-switch, multiple movement encoding techniques. In

A: Unaided encoding technique

B: Two-movement encoding techniques

C: Morse code decoder
display communication aid

D: Sip and puff encoding communication aid

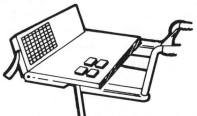

E: Portable printing encoding communication aid

Figure 2. Encoding techniques and aids.

general, if these techniques are to be used for communication with the general public, an aid similar to the one pictured in Figure 2C, which can decode and display the encoded character, is usually necessary. Encoding aids are also available that use any of these techniques (except eye gaze, which is currently being researched) to control a typewriter or other output form. There are also systems that use varying degrees of puff and sip on a mouthpiece to control a typewriter as shown in Figure 2D, and portable techniques that can use any of the above techniques (Figure 2E).

The number of switches or encoding elements and the number of movements in the various schemes vary widely. In general, the greater the number of switches, the simpler the code. An increased number of switches, though, means that a greater range of motion is required on the part of the child. Thus, a compromise between the two factors—simplicity of code and number of encoding elements—must be worked out. The specific abilities of the child determine which of the techniques is best suited for him.

Encoding Overview   The basic advantage of encoding techniques over the scanning approach is the potential for greater speed, a most important factor. These encoding techniques, however, do require a greater degree of control on the part of the child. More complex movements and more responses per message element are also required. In addition, the encoding scheme must be learned before the child can use the aid or technique. Clinicians who are using encoding techniques with their children, however, have indicated that the process of learning an encoding system was much faster and easier for their children than they had first thought.

Another advantage of the encoding system is that it permits access to large vocabularies for a child with very limited abilities. Using only the numbers from 1 to 10 and a three-movement encoding scheme, a child can retrieve any one element out of a 700-element vocabulary in just a few seconds. Accomplishing this by direct pointing would require very fine motor control, and it would be very slow using scanning techniques.

In summary, encoding techniques provide a faster means of communication and a means of accessing relatively large vocabularies with limited movements. However, they do require greater physical control than the scanning aids and higher cognitive abilities than either scanning or direct selection.

Direct Selection

Direct selection techniques are any techniques where the child directly selects the elements of his message.

The simplest example of a direct selection technique is the gesture. Here the child points directly to the object to express his message—a faucet for a drink of water, the bathroom when he wants to go to the toilet, or the door if he wants to go outside (Figure 3A).

Direct Selection Techniques and Aids   A very familiar direct selection technique is the use of the pointing board or communication board (Figure 3B). With this aid the child points directly to the various pictures, symbols, words, or letters that make up his message.

All types of expanded, guarded, and otherwise modified keyboards (Figure 3C) are also examples of direct selection aids. These specially modified keyboards have provided many moderately involved children with a means of producing written communication. The keyboards, however, do require a greater range of motion than either the scanning or encoding aids and also require more control than the letterboards.

To provide a means of communication for the child who can use a letterboard but who could not use a modified keyboard, a technique called the "automonitoring" technique was developed. Incorporated into a communication board, it forms an "automonitoring

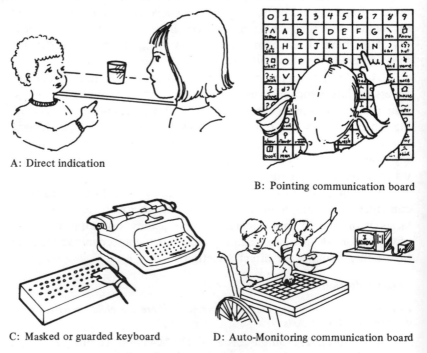

A: Direct indication

B: Pointing communication board

C: Masked or guarded keyboard   D: Auto-Monitoring communication board

Figure 3. Direct selection techniques and aids.

communication board" that can interpret the erratic pointing motions of a letterboard user and automatically print out the letters or words as the child tries to point to them (Figure 3D).

Direct Selection Overview   The major advantages of the direct selection approach are that it is straightforward and that no learning of the technique is required. This approach also provides very good direct feedback and can be used with very low cognitive level children. The potential speed of this approach is also quite high and is limited only by the pointing speed of the child.

The major limitation of these aids is that they require a greater range of motion on the part of the child. Thus, the direct selection approach provides a comparatively fast, simple, and straightforward means of communication for the child who can develop the range of motion and control to use a letterboard or keyboard.

Combination Techniques

Different approaches often can be combined to take advantage of some of the characteristics or advantages of each approach to provide a solution for a particular child. For example, the scanning and encoding techniques can be combined to form the scan-encode system shown in Figure 4A. This system provides very simple one-switch control for a severely physically impaired individual and also allows for quick access to a vocabulary that could be as large as 1000 words.

Another example of a combination of approaches is shown in Figure 4B. It was devised for a child who had moderate communication board pointing ability (about 40 squares) and a vocabulary considerably larger than 40 items. The direct selection and encoding approaches were combined to form a "direct selection and encoding system." The child uses the number line at the bottom to encode whole words, phrases, and sentences from his vocabulary chart. He then uses the faster and simpler direct selection technique to spell out additional words to complete his messages. This same combination technique could be implemented in an independent aid that would print out either individual letters as the child points to them or full words, phrases, or sentences as the child encoded them.

A third combination technique combines direct selection with the scanning approach. This technique provides a moderate or large vocabulary for an individual who has only limited pointing skills. With this technique, the handicapped individual uses a standard pointing board (communication board) but is able to point only to the general

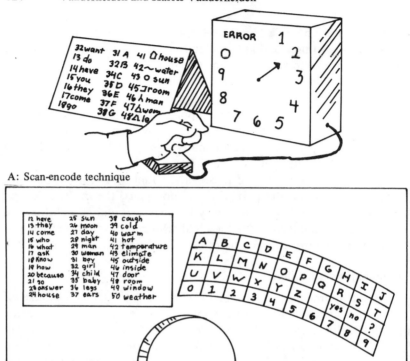

A: Scan-encode technique

B: Combination of direct selection and encoding

Figure 4. Combination techniques.

area where the desired symbol is located. The second person then scans that area, pointing to the individual symbols until the handicapped individual indicates that the correct symbol has been reached. This system can provide fairly quick access to a large number of vocabulary elements while still only requiring minimal skill on the part of the user. A second benefit of this approach is that it provides good training for the development of more accurate pointing skills. As the user improves his pointing, the speed of communication increases because scan time decreases. Eventually, some children develop sufficient pointing skills to enable them to indicate directly the desired symbols. If the child cannot point with an arm, headstick, etc., then eye gaze may be used, but it is usually not as effective.

Levels of Implementation

As can be seen from the previous examples, existing techniques and aids cover a wide range of complexity, from techniques that involve no aid at all, to electronic aids that can provide a child with a completely independent means of communicating and writing. This range can be broken down into five levels of implementation, each with its own basic characteristics. These five levels are:

1. Unaided techniques
2. Fundamental aids
3. Simple electronic and mechanical aids
4. Nonportable fully independent aids
5. Portable fully independent aids

Figure 5 illustrates the three approaches and the five levels of implementation. This figure is a composite of Figures 1, 2, and 3 and classifies the techniques described above. Each successive level represents an increase in the function and also in the cost of the associated aids. It also represents an increase in the independence of communication for the handicapped child as well as a decrease in the amount of effort on the part of a second person who is needed to interpret and record the child's message.

Unaided Techniques   Unaided techniques are communication techniques that do not involve any physical communication aid. They tend to be very personal communication systems between the handicapped child and a small number of people who frequently interact with the child. As such, they can fulfill only very few of the child's communication needs.

Fundamental Communication Aids   Fundamental communication aids have no electronic or moving parts. Most aids in this category can be easily constructed in the classroom or by a person who is handy with simple tools. These aids provide the child with a means of indicating his message more directly and generally expand the number of individuals with whom the handicapped child can communicate. With aids of this level, a second person is required to determine which message element the child is trying to indicate, to write down or remember each element as it is chosen, and to assemble the complete message. This takes considerable time and concentration on the part of the second person. For this reason, these aids, although very flexible and effective, are seldom used to their full potential and usually do not fulfill many of the communication needs of the handicapped child. Fundamental aids generally cost from $10 to $100 depending on the materials used and labor involved in constructing the aid.

CLASSIFICATION TYPE / DEGREE OF SOPHISTICATION	SCANNING	ENCODING	DIRECT SELECTION
Unaided techniques	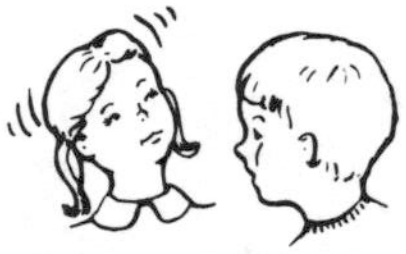	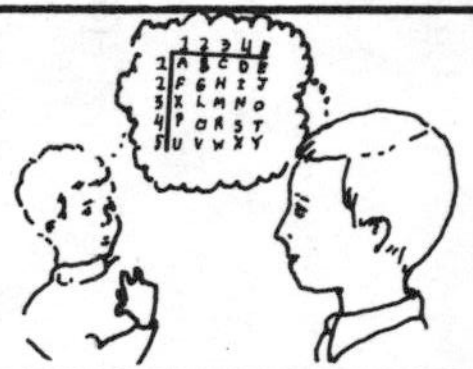	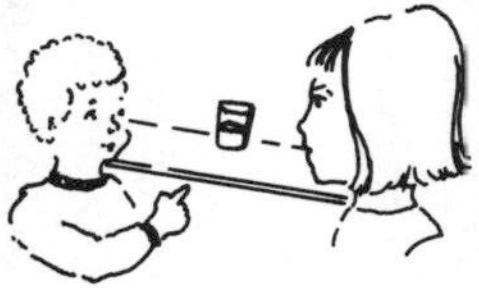
Fundamental aids	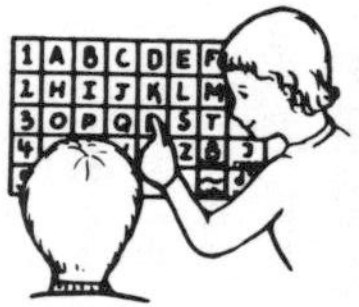	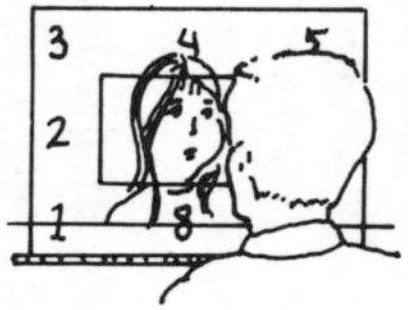	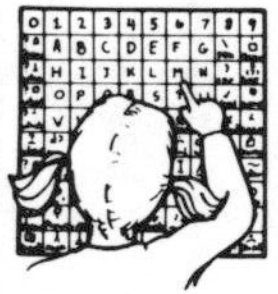

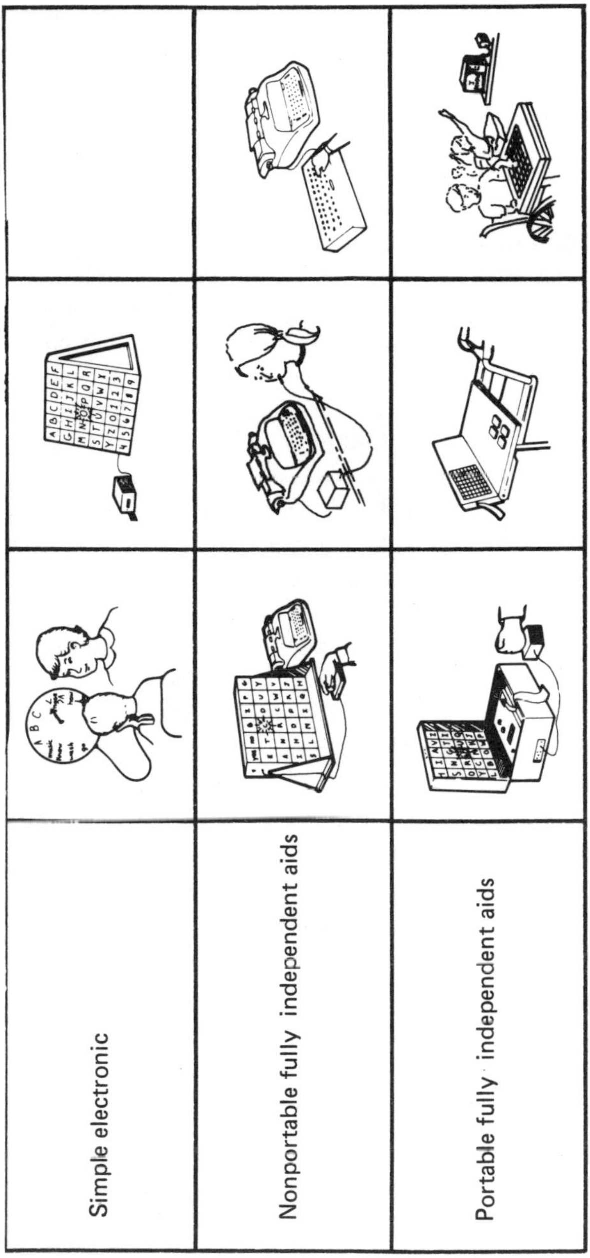

Figure 5. Basic approaches to providing nonvocal communication and major levels of implementation for each.

Simple Electronic and Mechanical Aids   Simple electronic and/
or mechanical aids also require help from a second person. With
these aids the child is able to indicate directly the elements (pictures,
words, etc.) that make up his message, but a second person is still
required to write down or remember the various elements indicated
by the child and to assemble the child's message. Because the elements of the message are directly specified by the child, very little
knowledge of the system is required on the part of the message receiver. Thus, the child generally can communicate with almost anyone who will take the time to work with him and assemble his
messages as he indicates the elements. Because of the slow nature of
spelling or using some of the techniques, this process is still usually
quite time consuming for the second person. For this reason, aids in
this category are also not usually utilized to their full potential.

The cost of these simple electronic and mechanical aids generally ranges from $100 to $1000.

Independent Communication Aids   An independent aid allows
the child to produce entire messages in a correctly assembled form
without assistance. A second person need only read or listen to the
completed message. Most independent aids either produce printed
copy of the message or are able to store and play back a completed
message. Many of these aids incorporate a typewriter or printing
device that enables the child to print out entire messages and do
papers, letters, homework, or creative writing.

These aids also enable the child to participate more easily in
group discussion or group conversations. In these situations, the
child's ability to assemble his own messages independently allows
him to have much more opportunity to communicate. Without an
independent aid, the child would require the assistance of another
person to work with him for a significant amount of time each time he
wanted to say something. This is often quite inconvenient for the second person. The handicapped child often has little opportunity to participate in conversation or discussion.

Although independent aids can be a definite advantage in group
conversations, they are often no faster in one-to-one conversation
than most of the aids from the two lower levels. In fact, many times
the independent aids are slower when used for one-to-one conversations because they do not allow the second person to fill in obvious
words for the child as the message is assembled. In these cases, how-

ever, many of the aids can be operated with their printers turned off so that they function in the same manner as the lower level aids.

Portable versus Nonportable Independent Aids   Independent communication aids can be broken down into two categories, nonportable and portable. Portable communication aids are given their own classification because they can move with the handicapped person, thus providing him with a means of communication in a great variety of settings. As a result, portable independent communication aids can function as a mobile "voice" for the nonvocal individual. A "fully portable" independent aid is an aid that requires no external power source for operation and weighs less than 20 pounds. The cost of nonportable and portable communication aids is approximately the same and ranges from $1000 to $7000. The nonportable systems usually have a typewriter as the standard output mechanism, while typewriter output would have to be an option or an accessory with the portable communication aids.

Implications and Advantages of Various Levels of Implementation   Although the highest level of implementation (portable fully independent communication aid) seems to provide the most benefits for the handicapped child, it is not necessarily the best solution for every child. Many factors may make one of the lower level aids more appropriate for a given individual. Some of these are: cost, age and cognitive level of the child, the mobility of the child, the communication functions to be fulfilled by the aid, and the symbol form (picture, symbol, word, or letter) to be used with the aid.

Cost is currently a much greater consideration than it should be or than it has to be in the future. Because of the newness of the field, relatively few aids are currently available, and these aids are not yet widely known or applied. As a result, the aids cost more now than they will when they are in more widespread use. In addition, as communication aids become more widely recognized, they will probably come under the coverage of medical insurance plans as have other special services and aids for the severely handicapped.

For very young children, the fundamental aids are generally preferable to the more complex aids. For these children, or children with lower cognitive abilities, aids that can be used with pictures, symbols, and other forms of pictographic representation are probably more appropriate than the more advanced aids with letter or word options only. Aids that can be used developmentally (first with pictures, then symbols, and finally with words and the alphabet) may be the most effective because they allow the child's communication abilities to expand and develop as his abilities grow.

The mobility of the child or individual also must be considered in the selection of a communication aid. If the child is completely bedridden, a stationary communication aid may fulfill most of his communication needs. If he is mobile but wheelchair bound, a portable communication aid may be more appropriate. If he is partially ambulatory (i.e., uses a walker or crutches), he may have to use one of the simple electronic or fundamental aids because only very few independent aids are currently available for the partially ambulatory child.

The communication function to be fulfilled by the aid is another point to consider in selecting the appropriate aid. If the handicapped person is vocal but needs a means of writing, then the stationary communication systems may be most appropriate. If the person is partially vocal and only needs a communication aid as a backup when his speech is unintelligible, a simple electronic or fundamental communication aid might be the best choice, depending on how often and for how long these aids are needed. If the aid is meant only to facilitate the communication of basic needs, or for very short (one to three word) communication, a simple electronic or fundamental aid may again be most appropriate.

Handicapped persons who are of normal intelligence but who are unable to speak or write generally can benefit most from a portable independent communication aid. If the individuals are to be enrolled in an educational program, then this type of aid would be necessary for them to participate effectively in the programs. Only these higher level aids can provide them with the independent means of communication and writing necessary for them to respond in class, complete written assignments and homework, take tests, and do the independent work required of them.

Comparison of Approaches

From these discussions it becomes apparent that there are a large number of different techniques, each with its own advantages and disadvantages. There are no valid "general rules" for sorting out the techniques or for trying to select an appropriate aid for a particular child. The only valid procedure is to try different approaches that seem appropriate and see whether the child has or can develop the skills necessary to use them.

Remembering that there are no rules that are valid in all cases, the following general statements are offered to help in formulating a plan for trying different techniques with a particular child. It should be stressed that these are general categorical statements and that they do not hold for all techniques with each category:

1.   Scanning techniques generally are slower but can be used with the most severely physically handicapped children; any child should be able to be fitted with a scanning aid of some sort
2.   Ways exist for making basic scanning techniques faster if the child can handle a little more complexity
3.   Encoding systems are best for large vocabulary systems
4.   Encoding is not very difficult for many children and may be most appropriate if direct selection is not possible
5.   Direct selection techniques are the simplest and potentially the fastest if the child has the ability to use them; they can be used with very low cognitive level children but do require more range of motion than scanning or encoding techniques
6.   Specific shortcomings of a particular approach or technique often can be overcome by using a combination of techniques

Other considerations to keep in mind when developing a communication system for an individual are:

1.   Speed of communication is a very important factor if a technique is to be used to communicate with others. The child's communication opportunities are directly limited by the time it takes for him to express himself. A 2- to 3-minute message seems to be much faster than a 5- to 6-minute message even though they only differ by a factor of two. Thus, techniques that are only twice as fast as others will seem to be much faster in a conversational situation
2.   Because it is important to provide the child with an effective communication system as early as possible, it is sometimes appropriate to provide a child with a slower technique that he can begin to use immediately, while at the same time working on the development of skills necessary to use a more efficient technique
3.   If a technique or aid is to be used as the child's primary means of conversation and communication interaction, then the aid must be very portable, convenient, and require little or no setup. Preferably the aid should be accessible to the child at all times without requiring the aid of another person

4.   If an aid is to be used in an educational setting, then some form of page display, either a video display or printed page, is desired if the individual is to do independent work effectively. Visibility, correctability, and printed copy are all important features for an output form to be used with a severely handicapped child, even though all three features are only available at a high cost with presently available technology

5.   Finally, the selection/development of a technique or aid for a given child is an ongoing process taking much time and patience. An appropriate selection requires not only an understanding of the different approaches and their relative advantages, but a very good understanding of the child, his abilities, his environment, and those with whom he will be communicating

SELECTING/DEVELOPING A
SYMBOL SYSTEM AND VOCABULARY

The preceding section considers various approaches and techniques for providing the child with a means of *indicating* or *transmitting* his message elements to a second person. This section discusses various symbol systems that the child might use with these techniques. The purpose of these symbol systems is to provide the child with a means of representing his thoughts in a form that can be physically transmitted or presented to those with whom he will be communicating.

Basic Considerations for Selecting a Symbol System

For young cognitively impaired children, the selection/development of the child's symbol system(s) and vocabulary is usually more important to the effectiveness of the child's overall communication system than is the particular *mechanism* (techniques or aid) that is used. Careful study and selection of this component, therefore, is very important to the success of the communication system for the child. In the selection of a symbol system, the particular approach first chosen may not be the most appropriate approach. As with selection of a physical communication aid, the most effective system for a child may change as the child develops and acquires additional skills. The selection/development process, therefore, is not a one-time decision; it is a continual process. Often, no best system exists for a child in all environments, and more than one system in fact may be appropriate for a child (e.g., using one system for general communication and interaction and another for educational purposes).

This section is designed only to introduce the symbol 'systems commonly used with communication aids for nonvocal physically handicapped children. Each symbol system is defined and briefly described, followed by examples and illustrations of its use with different techniques or aids. A more detailed description of these and other symbol systems is presented by Clark and Woodcock (this volume).

The following factors should be considered both when selecting a symbol system for use with a particular aid or technique and when selecting the most appropriate symbol system for the child who is to communicate with the aid or technique. The symbol system chosen should be:

1. Compatible with the aid or technique with which it is used
2. As nonrestrictive of the child's communication as possible
3. Appropriate to the child's current level of receptive and expressive ability
4. Developmental and flexible to allow for the child's changing communication needs
5. Adaptable to current therapy and educational procedures and approaches
6. Acceptable to the child, his parents and teachers, and those with whom he will communicate

Symbol Systems for Use with Nonvocal Communication Techniques and Aids

Traditional Orthography   The basic elements in the system of traditional orthography (T.O.) are the letters of the alphabet, A to Z. All symbols (words) in the T.O. system are formed by combinations of these 26 basic elements. Therefore, T.O. can be implemented in two ways. First, the symbols (words) themselves can be placed on the communication aid and used by the child to communicate. As mentioned before, however, this usually results in problems related to vocabulary size because only a very limited number of words (10 to 500) usually can be placed effectively on a communication aid, thus severely limiting the expressive power of the child. The second means of implementing the T.O. system (which is often used in conjunction with the first) is to provide the child with the 26 elements (letters of the alphabet) from which all of the symbols (words) in the system are formed. In this manner, the child's vocabulary potential is unbounded.

This second approach, however, does require that the child develop more advanced skills, both cognitively (additional levels of abstraction) and academically (acquisition of spelling skills). It also can be a much slower process because the child would have to specify an average of five to six elements for each symbol or idea he was trying to convey.

Because T.O. is the principal *augmentative* communication system of the normal vocal individual, there is great incentive to implement this system as the primary *augmentative* system for the nonvocal child as well. This system does require reading and/or spelling skills before it can be effectively implemented, however, so that it poses for the nonvocal child a communication difficulty that is not present with the vocal child.

The nonvocal child for whom T.O. is the first and only system of communication, is placed in the position of having to learn to read and/or spell before he can communicate effectively. For the normal child, acquisition of these skills is not attempted until long after effective communication has been established and used by the child. The exact implications of this situation have not been determined and additional research in this area is needed. Some researchers and clinicians believe that effective and versatile communication is necessary before the child's acquisition of reading and spelling skills; this belief has led such individuals to develop or explore other symbol systems. These systems are being studied both as initial systems (systems that are used until reading/spelling skills are acquired) and as primary systems (systems that always will be used by a child in addition to the traditional orthography system). In either case, however, T.O. is a very important communication system that should be learned eventually by every child who is capable of learning to read and spell.

The T.O. system can be applied to aids and techniques at all levels of implementation. It is the easiest system to implement at the *independent* level because of the ready availability of typewriters, teletypes, television displays, strip printers, and other alphanumeric printers and displays.

Picture Vocabularies   One alternative symbol system involves the use of pictures. Pictures as a symbol system for communication are here defined as the use of illustrations or pictographs to represent thoughts, feelings, or ideas. Typically, a child using a picture vocabulary system sequentially points to pictures that represent objects or ideas in order to communicate his thoughts to another person. Very often, the child who is communicating through pictures communicates on a holophrastic or "one picture" level to express his thoughts. He points to a picture of food to represent thoughts such as *I am hungry, I want to eat,* or *I have eaten,* or points to a picture of a glass of liquid to express *I am thirsty, I want a drink,* or *I had juice for lunch.*

When the child is communicating with a picture vocabulary system, the message receiver is almost always required to make use of contextual clues in order to interpret the child's message. Because the child cannot spell out his thought or idea very specifically using pictures, he must rely on the message receiver to interpret the picture in the same manner that he does, so that the desired message is effectively relayed. This can lead to confusion and misinterpreted messages. However, this same ability to interpret a picture in more than one way can be advantageous in that it allows the child to communicate a larger number of different ideas with a limited set of symbols. The effectiveness of this latter technique largely depends on the skill of the second person and his familiarity with the child. Picture systems, therefore, are limited in their versatility and generally are not very functional with strangers except on a very fundamental basis. They are, however, the easiest systems to implement with the very young or severely mentally retarded child.

Pictures are applicable to nearly all of the basic techniques and can be applied at most levels of implementation except for higher level independent aids that have some form of printouts. Because pictures most probably will serve as the symbol system for the child who is just learning to communicate through a nonoral means, or for the child who may not be capable of communicating with a more traditional orthographic symbol system, they are most applicable at the more fundamental or basic levels of a nonoral system.

Bliss Symbols   Bliss symbols are unique, ideographic symbols that represent concepts (as opposed to words only) through simple line drawings. Bliss symbols were originally designed and developed as a universal language system by Charles K. Bliss. A complete description of the development of the Bliss symbols is covered in Bliss (1965), and application of the symbols as a communication mode for nonvocal physically handicapped children has been documented by McNaughton and Kates (1974), Harris-Vanderheiden et al. (1975), and the published reports of the Ontario Crippled Children's Centre. A more detailed description of Bliss symbols as a communication system is presented in Clark and Woodcock (this volume). This section focuses on implementing and applying Bliss symbols as another type of symbol system that may be utilized with nonoral communication techniques and aids.

Bliss symbols are both ideographic and pictographic. By ideographic, it is meant that a Bliss symbol represents an idea or a concept that may be expressed by the child. Pictographic implies that the symbol is also "picture-like." Consider the following examples:

want   like   happy   sad

The above samples all have one similar component, the heart, and all have similar meanings: They have to do with emotion of some sort. The heart symbol, then, is representative of the concept *emotion* and consistent throughout the system wherever an emotion is expressed.

From the next set of examples, it is seen that Bliss symbols are also pictographic:

man   lady   father   mother

Bliss symbols often visually resemble the concept or ideas that they are portraying. It is important to note that the Bliss symbols always appear with a word describing the basic meaning of the symbol printed directly beneath them. Thus, the system can be used with total strangers, and there is no need to "learn" the system to be able to communicate with someone who uses Bliss symbols.

Like picture systems, Bliss symbols can be used with young prereading and mentally retarded children. Although they may not be useful with the profoundly mentally retarded, the Bliss symbols have been found successful with very severely mentally retarded cerebral palsied children (Harris-Vanderheiden et al., 1975). Also, like picture systems, the Bliss symbol system uses generalization to allow more diversified communication with a limited symbol set. Because the symbols are idea based instead of object based, as picture systems are, the Bliss system is able to use generalization even more effectively than picture systems do. It also contains many concepts and abstractions that could not be easily depicted with pictures.

Bliss symbols may be used at all "levels" of implementation although their use with independent aids may require the use of special printers or displays. They can serve as a communication mode for the child who cannot read or spell, as a transition symbol system for the prereading child who eventually will communicate using traditional orthographic systems, or as a conversational communication system for the child who already can read and "write."

Other Symbol Systems   Clark and Woodcock (this volume) present in detail a number of different symbol systems, including systems such as the rebus and the Initial Teaching Alphabet (i.t.a.). Most of these symbol systems can be implemented with the communication aids and techniques discussed in this chapter. In addition, pictures of the manual alphabet, American Sign Language (ASL), or other manual systems used with deaf children can be used also (see Kopchick and Lloyd, this volume; Wilbur, this volume). These are not specifically discussed in this chapter inasmuch as the focus here is on symbol systems that are currently in widespread use with nonvocal communication aids.

Summary of Symbol Systems

The basic considerations for applying symbol systems to communication aids and techniques, introduced at the beginning of this section, are again presented with further elaboration:

1. *The symbol system chosen for use should be compatible with the aid or technique with which it is used.* When selecting a symbol system for use with a particular communication aid, it is important to consider the functions that the aid will serve. Pictures or symbols such as Bliss symbols are compatible with the fundamental or even the simple electromechanical aids. These aids do not involve printed copy of any sort. The "independent" or "independent and fully portable" aids and techniques most often utilize printed copy of some sort, however, and pictures or special symbols may not be appropriate symbol system selection. T.O. can be easily implemented at all levels.

2. *The symbol system chosen should place the least possible amount of restriction on the child's communication.* There is no way of getting around the fact that any vocabulary system provided to a child using a nonoral communication aid or technique will be limited. If

the vocabulary system has to be displayed for the child through a communication board, an eye chart, or whatever, there is a finite amount of space. Therefore, symbol systems should be chosen to allow the child to express as much as possible with the least number of symbols (words, pictures, etc.). With this in mind, Bliss symbols (which cover a wider range of meaning and concepts with a fewer number of actual symbols) may be chosen instead of pictures. Or, a wordboard with an alphabet that allows the child to spell words not appearing on the display may be chosen over a word-board alone.

3. *The symbol system chosen should be appropriate to the child's current level of expressive ability.* If a communication aid is to be effective for a child, the symbol system chosen for use with the aid should be one that is commensurate with the child's present expressive ability. If a child is not yet able to spell or recognize sight words, then pictures, Bliss symbols, or other alternate symbol systems should be considered, even if a strictly traditional orthographic system is the final goal. It is important both to the developmental and educational processes of the child that he be provided with an effective communication system at as early an age as possible.

4. *The symbol system chosen should be developmental.* The child's communication needs are not static; they are dynamic and will change and grow, just as his ability to utilize the symbols for expressive communication will change and grow. Therefore, the symbol system chosen for use with a particular aid or technique should be flexible enough to allow for the child's growing communication needs. As the child grows it may become necessary to change symbol systems as with the young child who moves from pictures to Bliss symbols or words.

5. *The symbol system must be adaptable to current therapy and educational techniques and approaches.* This consideration concerns the environment and circumstances in which the symbol system and communication aid is to function. If the child is going to be able to participate successfully in educational programs planned for him, then he must be able to communicate effectively with those who will implement the programs. Whatever symbol system is chosen as the child's communication system, it should be compatible with the educational and communication programs in which he is currently enrolled.

6. *The symbol system must be acceptable to the child, his parents, and those with whom the child will communicate.* This is one of the

most important considerations in the selection of a symbol system. The system chosen, above all, must be acceptable to the child as a means of communication. If he is not happy with the system, then he will not communicate with it. Likewise, the system must be acceptable to those who will be communicating with the child. If not, communication attempts generated by the child may not be given adequate attention and response so that, after a period of frustration, the child's attempts may be reduced to conveying only basic wants and needs, or else the child may not use the system at all.

Developing an appropriate symbol system and vocabulary for a child who will communicate through a nonoral means is not an easy task, and many times involves much trial and error. Many other considerations also will be necessary once the symbol system has been selected (i.e., content and arrangement of content on the display). For a discussion of these and other considerations the reader is referred to McDonald and Schultz (1973) and Vicker (1974).

APPLICATIONS OF NONVOCAL COMMUNICATION TECHNIQUES AND AIDS

As an example of the application of the previously discussed techniques in developing nonvocal communication programs for handicapped children, two such programs are briefly discussed.

The first application describes a symbol communication program for nonvocal severely mentally retarded cerebral palsied children, and the second describes use of a communication aid in orthopedic classroom settings with nonvocal severely physically handicapped children.

Symbol Communication for Mentally Retarded Children

Bliss symbols, a unique system of communication, have been adapted as an alternate mode of communication for both retarded and nonretarded nonvocal cerebral palsied children at the Ontario Crippled Children's Centre and at other centers and clinics throughout the United States and Canada.

Results of a variety of programs have indicated that Bliss symbols can be effectively implemented as an augmentative means of communication for the child with average or near average cognitive ability and for the child with severe mental retardation and motoric involvement (McNaughton and Kates, 1974; Harris-Vanderheiden et al., 1975). Bliss symbols have provided many children with their first adequate and effective means for expressing themselves to peers, parents, teachers, and residential institution personnel. Mentally retarded adolescents with a chronological age of 10 to 16 years and a mental age equivalent of two to five years, have demonstrated an ability to use Bliss symbols effectively for both responsive and spontaneous communication. (Responsive communication is defined here as the child's use of the symbols to answer questions and respond to statements posed to him. Spontaneous communication refers to communication that is "child initiated." Here, the child uses symbols to initiate conversation in addition to using them to respond to conversation.)

For a detailed description of the system and its application as a communication system for handicapped children, the reader is referred to publications by Bliss (1965), Ontario Crippled Children's Centre Project Reports (1971–1974), and McNaughton and Kates (1974). The film about Bliss and his symbols, *Mr. Symbol Man,* distributed by the Canadian Film Board, is also very highly recommended (Lynes, 1974).

Pilot Symbol Communication Program with Mentally Retarded Children   A pilot Bliss symbol communication program was implemented at Central Wisconsin Colony and Training School, a residential institution for retarded persons. Five nonvocal, cerebral palsied children with severe mental retardation were enrolled in the program. Before initiation of the program, the children's communication consisted of yes/no gestures, undifferentiated vocalizations, or a very limited number of intelligible utterances (yes, no, hello, goodbye, etc.). Other approaches to communication either had been implemented without much success in the past or were not considered feasible communication systems for these children. Fingerspelling, ASL, and typing were not implemented because of the children's motoric involvement, and pictureboards and wordboards had not been successful as communication systems for those children with whom they had been tried. Bliss symbols were chosen as a communication alternative for the children because:

1.   The symbols were easily generalizable and more universal than pictures
2.   They could be understood by almost anyone with whom the child would communicate because the word representing the symbol is always written directly below the symbol
3.   They could be easily adapted as vocabulary elements on a

pointing board, an aid that all of the children were able to use

4. The system allowed for presentation of the vocabulary elements in a left to right, modified Fitzgerald key arrangement, and contained parts of speech that allowed the child to construct correct grammatical symbol sentences (when and if the child achieved this level)

Ward personnel, teachers, and other support staff were integrated into the program from its inception and were encouraged to use the Bliss symbols with the children and reinforce the the children's attempts to communicate with the symbols. Support, encouragement, and cooperation from the institution staff were among the prime factors in the success of the program. Although initially skeptical, the staff became enthused about the Bliss symbols and began to interact and communicate with the children once the children had learned the symbols and begun communicating.

Results of Pilot Program   In the initial pilot program (total teaching time of 20 hours) the five severely retarded children enrolled learned from seven to 50 symbols each and had begun to use symbols both to respond to questions and to initiate simple symbol sentences spontaneously. Over a 3-month summer period, during which there was no formal program, these five children were taught new symbols by ward aides, foster grandparents, parents, and teachers, and two additional children were brought into the program. When formal programming was reinitiated in September, it was discovered that the children had retained the symbols over the summer and were still using them for communicative purposes.

Most of the children in the program were able to use pointing boards, but some modifications were made for children whose pointing responses were erratic and ambiguous. A series of "flip card packets" (Figure 6) were arranged for one child. To use this system, the child would indicate through gross pointing which packet contained the symbol she wanted to communicate. The teacher would then flip the cards until she got to the card displaying the desired symbol, at which point the child again would make some movement of confirmation. Then the teacher would slowly scan the symbols on the card by pointing to them one at a time. When she pointed to the desired symbol, the child again would confirm the movement. Although effective, this method was slow and frustrating for the child, and she has been diligently working on her pointing response so that she can communicate her thoughts via direct selection of the Bliss symbols.

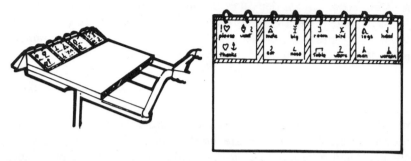

Figure 6. Flip card communication system. Flip cards on tray: *left,* side view; *right,* top view.

Presently, the original five children have greatly expanded their symbol repertoire (some have gone from 10 to 15 symbols to 30 and 60 symbols), and some are able to communicate in sentences up to four symbols in length. As a direct result of their increased communication ability, these children have been viewed by the staff as appearing to be "more normal," and teachers have related that they feel that the children know and are capable of learning much more than they had previously thought they could. Many people are surprised and delighted that the children can "talk" with them and express their needs, thoughts, emotions, and humor. Bliss symbols have provided both the children and staff with a means of interacting and communicating.

This pilot program now has been expanded to include over 20 children, with greater diversities of physical and cognitive handicaps. Results from the pilot study and initial results from the expanded study are extremely encouraging and support continued implementation of nonvocal communication techniques and aids with the severely mentally and physically handicapped child.

Preliminary Evaluation of an Independent Aid

In this study, the use of a portable independent communication aid was evaluated in order to determine its effect on the educational progress and communication development of seven nonvocal cerebral palsied children. Before using the independent communication aids, these nonvocal severely motorically impaired children found effective participation and interaction in their educational environments to be very difficult, if not nearly impossible. Unable to speak or write to communicate, the children were unable to ask questions or participate in class discussions without interrupting the class while the teacher worked out their message through guessing or using a manual communication board. These children were also unable to do any type of independent work or homework without the constant and undivided attention of a second person. As a result, much of their time was relegated to passive observation in classroom activities.

The objective in giving them an independent communication aid was to provide them both with a means to communicate spontaneously in individual and group situations and to provide them with a means of doing independent work and homework and of taking tests. The communication aid that was used in the program was the "auto-monitoring communication board" (Auto-Com), developed at the University of Wisconsin.

Description of Auto-Com   The Auto-Com (Figure 7) is a direct selection, "self-monitoring" communication board designed for

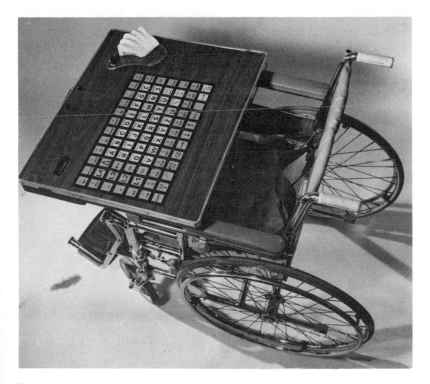

Figure 7. Auto-Com.

physically handicapped persons who have had to rely on manual communication boards as a primary expressive mode of communication. It is a completely independent communication aid that is built into a special wheelchair laptray. The Auto-Com is operated in the same manner as a traditional communication board except that a magnet is used, instead of a finger, knuckle, fist, or headstick, to point to the letters or words. Designed especially for use by nonvocal cerebral palsied children, the Auto-Com requires only minimal pointing skills to operate. The child may use the aid by operating it with his head, hand, finger, wrist, foot, or any other part of the body with which he can point.

In actual operation, the child "points" with a magnet to the desired letters or words that make up the message. Through an electronic sensing system, the child's pointing movements are interpreted, and letters or whole words are printed out on a small strip printer mounted inside the Auto-Com. Because of the special automonitoring system in the Auto-Com, the aid is able to decipher even the very erratic pointing motions of the athetoid cerebral palsied children in the program.

Because the aid is fully portable and battery operated, it can accompany the child wherever he goes, enabling him to communicate at any time without the need for a second person to interpret his pointing and put together his message for him. In addition, the Auto-Com also controls a television display that allows the child to print out messages up to 512 characters long and display them on an ordinary television screen. This television output gives the child a highly visible and completely correctable display of his work.

Results of Evaluation Program   Although the following results were obtained through the use of a particular communication aid, the Auto-Com, these same results can be expected from the implementation of any portable independent communication aid that has the same basic features and fulfills the same functions for a child.

Before using the Auto-Com, the children in this field test were communicating through gestures, pointing, limited vocalizations, or letter wordboards; none were able to use guarded keyboard typewriters. Although effective for relaying messages to persons familiar with them, these communication attempts were not effective overall communication systems for the children. Classroom participation was limited to those small amounts of time that teachers could spare in order to work with them on a one-to-one basis. After using the

Auto-Coms on a regular basis as their primary mode of communication, however, these children were able to spend productive hours doing schoolwork independent of their teacher and were also able to communicate more effectively with their parents, families, and peers.

The Auto-Com had a significant effect on the children's acquisition and development of skills in basic educational areas, especially mathematics and language skills. The aid's most direct effect on the children's acquisition of and progress in the mathematics skills was that it enabled the children to write out their arithmetic problems on a visual display and to correct their mistakes.

In the language skills area, the aid provided the children with the ability to see their letters forming words and the words forming sentences. Through this, many of the children began to communicate in full thought patterns and sentences for the first time.

Teachers found that, with the Auto-Com, the children completed their work more slowly but were able to do the same amount of work with much less teacher time. This enabled the students to move at a faster rate than when they were strictly dependent on one-to-one attention from the teacher. One instructor estimated that she could now teach the child in less than 2 years what would have taken 3 or more years without the aid. The work of the children was also judged to be more comprehensive and of a better quality.

In addition to increasing the ability of the children to participate in educational programs, the Auto-Com was also viewed as an invaluable skill assessment tool by the teachers. The Auto-Com allowed the children to produce a reliable and consistent response that could be visually displayed. Utilizing this display teachers were able to diagnose more accurately problems and deficiencies in learning that the children were experiencing. In some cases, it was found that the children knew much more than the teachers had thought, but many times the teachers discovered that the children had not learned basics that had been assumed to be a part of their repertoire.

The use of the independent communication aid also affected the social and personal development of the children. Academically, they were more eager to learn and took great pride in their accomplishments. The ability to do something completely independently for the first time seemed to have a great effect on their self-concept. Teachers and parents of some of the children also remarked about a "deeper" personality developing in the children. The children started expressing themselves spontaneously and on a larger variety of topics. They were forming their own opinions and, for the first time, argued with and contradicted their teachers and parents. The personal identity and aspirations of the children were heightened and others' attitudes toward them also changed markedly.

In summary, this field testing has demonstrated that the application of an independent communication aid can significantly affect the educational progress of nonvocal motorically involved children. Furthermore, it has shown that such an aid also can enhance the communication skills and the personal and social development of the child. Results discussed here are not considered to be specific to the children's use of the Auto-Com but rather to be the result of providing the children with an effective and independent mode of communication.

SUMMARY AND CONCLUSIONS

This chapter provides a basic framework for looking at the development of augmentative communication systems for the nonvocal severely handicapped child, along with some information concerning recent research and development in this area. The information presented is far from complete, and supplemental reading is advised. As a means of summarizing and integrating the information presented in this chapter, the following points are reemphasized.

1. Many communication aids and techniques are currently available. Some of these aids and techniques are fundamental and can be easily constructed in the classroom or at home. Others are more advanced and may involve electromechanics or electronics. The people working with the child should select the most appropriate aid or technique; each aid or technique considered should be carefully evaluated in terms of the current benefit to the child and the child's future needs. The most effective communication aid or technique is the one that is most beneficial to the child and not necessarily the one that is most advanced or most costly

2. Selecting and implementing a symbol/vocabulary system for use with a particular aid or technique is not an easy task. The development of an appropriate system should be approached with the previously mentioned considerations in mind, and it must be remembered

that the vocabulary system provided most likely will influence the entire communication ability of the child. Alternative symbol/vocabulary systems can be effective communication systems for nearly any child, including the severely cognitively and physically impaired child
3.   In order to provide the child with an effective means of communication as soon as possible, it is most appropriate to find a technique and symbol system that can be used immediately, and then work toward developing skills that will allow the child to communicate more swiftly or effectively
4.   Studies to date have shown that introduction of nonvocal communication techniques does not decrease functional vocalization or speech development but has, in many cases, increased the attempts at and intelligibility of vocalization

Finally, it should be remembered that providing communication alternatives for the nonvocal physically handicapped child does not fall within the realm of any one particular profession. It must be a cooperative interdisciplinary effort involving educators, speech clinicians, parents, occupational and physical therapists, engineers, and medical personnel. Only through the combined, co-ordinated efforts of these and other professions can the full potential of severely communicatively impaired individuals be realized.

With recent rapid advances in both technology and the social sciences, knowledge and tools are now becoming available for providing nonvocal, nonwriting individuals with effective and efficient communication systems. Even today the potential exists to provide meaningful and productive employment for nonvocal, nonambulatory, nonwriting individuals who have the appropriate language and technical skills. By providing children with effective communication systems at an early age, there is little reason why many of them could not achieve the level of competency necessary to secure and hold such jobs.

REFERENCES

Bliss, C. K. 1965. Semantography. Semantography Publications, Sydney, Australia.
Harris-Vanderheiden, D., W. P. Brown, P. MacKenzie, S. Reinen, and C. Scheibel. 1975. Symbol communication for the mentally handicapped: An application of Bliss symbols as an alternate communica-

tion mode for nonvocal mentally retarded children with motoric impairment. Ment. Retard. 13(1).

Harris-Vanderheiden, D. The Auto-Com as an aid to the nonvocal physically handicapped child's education and communication skill. In preparation.

Lynes, G. 1974. Mr. Symbol Man (film of Charles Bliss and the use of Bliss Symbols). National Film Board of Canada, Montreal.

McDonald, E. T., and A. R. Schultz. 1973. Communication boards for cerebral palsied children. J. Speech Hear. Disord. 38:73–88.

McNaughton, S., and B. Kates. 1974. Visual symbols: Communication system for the pre-reading physically handicapped child. Paper presented at the American Association on Mental Deficiency Annual Meeting, June, Toronto.

Ontario Crippled Children's Centre Bliss Project Team. 1973. Ontario Crippled Children's Centre Symbol Communication Research Project 1972–1973. Ontario Crippled Children's Centre, Toronto.

Vanderheiden, G. C., and M. J. Luster. 1975. Nonvocal communication techniques and aids as aids to the education of the severely physically handicapped: A state of the art review. Trace Center, University of Wisconsin, Madison.

Vicker, B. 1974. Nonoral communication system project 1964–73. Campus Stores Publishers, University of Iowa, Iowa City.

SUGGESTED READINGS

Because communication aids for the nonvocal severely handicapped are a rapidly growing area of communication disorders, the following bibliography is presented. The list is arranged categorically.

Summary Information

Copeland, K. 1974. Aids for the Severely Handicapped. Spector Publishing Co., Ltd., London.

Kafafian, H. 1971–1973. A Study of Man-Machine Communication Systems for the Handicapped. 3 Vols. (1970–1973). Cybernetics Research Institute, Washington, D.C.

Luster, M. 1974. Preliminary Selected Bibliography of Articles, Brochures and Books Related to Communication Techniques and Aids for the Severely Handicapped. Trace Center, University of Wisconsin, Madison.

Luster, M., and G. C. Vanderheiden. 1974. Preliminary Annotated Bibliography of Researchers and Institutions. Trace Center, University of Wisconsin, Madison.

Luster, M., and G. C. Vanderheiden. 1974. Preliminary Annotated Bibliography of Communication Aids. Trace Center, University of Wisconsin, Madison.

Vanderheiden, G.C., and M. J. Luster. 1975. Nonvocal Communication Techniques and Aids as Aids to the Education of the Severely Physically Handicapped: A state of the art review. Trace Center, University of Wisconsin, Madison.

Vicker, B. 1974. Nonoral Communication System Project 1964–73. Campus Stores Publishers, University of Iowa, Iowa City.

Communication Boards

Davis, G. A. 1973. Linguistics and language therapy: The sentence construction board. J. Speech Hear. Disord. 38:205–214.

Dixon, C. 1965. Some thoughts on communication boards. C. P. J. 26:12–13.

Dixon, C. C., and B. Curry. 1973. Some thoughts on the communication board. J. Speech Hear. Disord. 38:73–88.

Feallock, B. 1958. Communication for the non-verbal individual. Amer. J. Occup. Ther. 12:60–63.

Goldberg, H. R., and J. Fenton. 1960. Aphonic Communication for Those with Cerebral Palsy: Guide for the Development and Use of a Conversation Board. United Cerebral Palsy of New York State, New York.

McDonald, E. T., and A. R. Schultz. 1973. Communication Boards for Cerebral Palsied Children. J. Speech Hear. Disord. 38:73–88.

Miller, K. 1964. Electronics for communication. Amer. J. Occup. Ther. 18:20–23.

Picken, S. R. 1974. Development, use and application of a communication board with a cerebral palsy child. Marquette, Mich.

Remis, A. The Cerebral Palsied Child and the Development of a Conversation Device. New York State College of Teachers, Buffalo.

Robenault, I. P. 1973. Functional Aids for the Multiply Handicapped. Harper & Row, New York.

Roe, H. The Hall Roe Conversation Board. Distributed by Ghora Khan Grotto, St. Paul, Minn.

Sklar, M., and D. N. Bennett. 1956. Initial communication chart for aphasics. J. Assoc. Phys. Ment. Rehab. 10:43–53.

United Cerebral Palsy Association. (circa 1969). Aphonic Communication for Those with Cerebral Palsy. United Cerebral Palsy Association, New York.

Communication and the Cerebral Palsied Child

Bosley, E. 1954. Normal language in its application to the cerebral palsied child. C. P. Rev. June/July.

Christman, D. 1956. Problems of communication of individuals with cerebral palsy. C. P. Rev. September/October, vol. 17.

Mecham, M. 1954. Complexities in the communication of the cerebral palsied. C. P. Rev. February, vol. 15.

Nicol, F. 1972. Breakthrough to communication. Spec. Educ. December.

Scanning Communication Aids

Charbonneau, J. R., C. Cote, and O. Z. Roy. 1974. NRC's "Comhandi" communication system technical description and application at the

Ottawa Crippled Children's Treatment Center. Paper presented at the seminar, Electronic Controls for the Severely Physically Handicapped, Vancouver, B.C.

Foulds, R., G. Balesta, and W. Crochetiere. 1975. Effectiveness of language redundancy in nonvocal communication. *In* Proceedings from the Conference on Systems and Devices for the Disabled. Krusen Center for Research on Engineering, Temple University, Philadelphia.

Foulds, R., and E. Gaddis. 1975. A practical application of an electronic aid in the special needs classroom. *In* Proceedings from the Conference on Systems and Devices for the Disabled. Krusen Center for Research on Engineering, Temple University, Philadelphia.

"Physically handicapped children learn to communicate." 1973. Sci. Dimen. April:8–13.

Sampson, D. 1970. A communication device for patients unable to speak. Med. Biol. Eng. January:99–101.

Encoding Communication Aids

"Jack H. Eichler: Builds communication device." 1973. Case Alumnus 211:2. Case Institute of Technology Alumni Association, Cleveland.

Hagen, C., W. Porter, and J. Brink. 1973. Nonverbal communication: An alternate mode of communication for the child with severe cerebral palsy. J. Speech Hear. Disord. 38:448–455.

"Handicapped youth 'talks' with eyes." 1974. News J. (22 October 1974), Mansfield, Ohio.

Direct Selection Communication Aids

Bullock, A., G. F. Dalrymple, and J. M. Danca. The Auto-Com at Kennedy Memorial Hospital: Rapid and accurate communication by a multi-handicapped student. Amer. J. Occup. Ther. In press.

"Handicapped aid (PILOT) is demonstrated." 1972. Winnipeg Free Press (16 February 1972). Winnipeg, Canada.

Harris-Vanderheiden, D., C. D. Geisler, M. Spielman, V. Valley, and R. Schultz. Evaluating the Auto-Com as an aid to the nonvocal physically handicapped child's education and communication skill. In preparation.

Harris-Vanderheiden, D., and R. Schutz. Providing independence through communication: A case study of the use of the Auto-Com. In preparation.

Hill, S. D., J. Campagna, D. Long, J. Munch, and S. Naecher. 1968. An explanation of the use of two response keyboards as a means of communication for the severely handicapped child. Percep. Mot. Skills 26: 699–704.

Soede, M., and H. G. Stassen. 1973. A light spot operated typewriter for severely disabled patients. Med. Biol. Eng. 1973:641–644.

Stassen, H. G., M. J. Soede, and W. J. Luitse. 1974. The light spot operated typewriter: The evaluation of a prototype. *In* 5th International Seminar on Rehabilitation, pp. 1–21. London.

Vanderheiden, G. C., D. F. Lamers, A. M. Volk, and C. D. Geisler. A portable nonvocal communication prosthesis for the severely physically handicapped. In preparation.

Vanderheiden, G. C., G. A. Raitzer, D. P. Kelso, and C. D. Geisler. 1974. An automated technique for the interpretation of erratic pointing motions of severely cerebral palsied individuals. Cerebral Palsy Communication Group, Madison, Wis.

Vanderheiden, G. C., C. D. Geisler, and A. M. Volk. 1973. The auto-monitoring technique and its application in the auto-monitoring communication board: A new communication device for the severely handicapped. In Proceedings of the 1973 Carnahan Conference on Electronic Prosthetics, pp. 47–51. Lexington, Ky.

Wendt, E. 1975. Habilitation: A team approach to communication. Teach. Exc. Child. 8(1).

Special Language Systems/Techniques

Bliss, C. K. 1965. Semantography. Semantography Publications, Sydney, Australia.

Harris-Vanderheiden, D., W. P. Brown, P. MacKenzie, S. Reinen, and C. Scheibel. 1975. Symbol communication for the mentally handicapped: An application of Bliss symbols as an alternate communication mode for nonvocal mentally retarded children with motoric impairment. Ment. Retard. 13(1).

Levett, L. M. 1972. A method of communication for non-speaking severely subnormal children—trial results. Brit. J. Disord. Commun. October:125–128.

Lynes, G. 1974. Mr. Symbol Man (film of Charles Bliss and the use of Bliss symbols). National Film Board of Canada, Montreal.

McNaughton, S., and B. Kates. 1974. Visual symbols: Communication system for the pre-reading physically handicapped child. Paper presented at the American Association on Mental Deficiency Annual Meeting, June, Toronto.

Moore, M. V. 1972. Binary communication for the severely handicapped. Arch. Phys. Med. Rehab. 53:532–533.

Ontario Crippled Children's Centre Bliss Project Team. 1973. Ontario Crippled Children's Center.

Symbol Communication Research Project 1972–1973. Ontario Crippled Children's Centre, Toronto.

Other Aids and General Information

Ehrlich, M. D. 1974. The Votrax voice synthesizer as an aid for the blind. In 1974 Proceedings on Engineering Devices in Rehabilitation, Boston.

Goodwin, M., and T. C. Goodwin. 1969. In a dark mirror. Ment. Hyg. October.

Israel, B. L. 1969. Responsive environmental program, Brooklyn, New

York. Institute for Applied Technology, U.S. Department of Commerce, Springfield, Va.

Martin, J. H. 1969. Kaleidoscope for learning. Sat. Rev. June 21.

Rahimi, M. A., and J. B. Eylenberg. 1973. A computer terminal with synthetic speech output. Paper presented at the National Conference on the Use of On-Line Computers in Psychology, October, St. Louis.

Rahimi, M. A., and J. B. Eylenberg. 1974. A computing environment for the blind. In AFIPS Conference Proceedings of the 1974 National Computer Conference. Vol. 43.

"The responsive environment corporation follow through model." 1970. Division of Compensatory Education, U.S. Office of Education, Washington, D.C.

Rueter, D. B. 1974. Speech Synthesis Under APL. In Proceedings of the Sixth International APL Users Conference, pp. 585–596.

Sachs, R. M. 1973. Technology comes to telecommunications for the hearing impaired. Q. Bull. N.Y. League for the Hard of Hearing 52:(2).

Smith, N. B., and R. Strickland. 1969. Some approaches to reading. Association for Childhood Education International, Washington, D.C.

Steg, D. (undated). The oralographic learning system. The Language Arts Center of the New Jersey Association for Children with Learning Disabilities, Convent Station, N.J.

Steg, D. 1971. The limitations of learning machines and some aspects of learning. Focus on Learning (A Journal of the School of Education, Indiana University of Pennsylvania), Vol. 1.

Steg, D., and A. D'Annunzio. 1969. Some theoretical and experimental considerations of cybernetics, responsive environments, learning and social development. Paper presented at the International Congress of Cybernetics, London.

Steg, D., and A. D'Annunzio. 1972. Helping problem learners during the early childhood years. Paper presented at the American Educational Research Association, Chicago.

Steg, D., and A. D'Annunzio. 1974. A learning print approach toward perceptual training and reading in kindergartens. Paper presented at the International Reading Association, May, New Orleans.

Steg, D., and R. Schulman. 1974. Remarks on the possible economic significance of "pre-school" education technology. Drexel University, Philadelphia.

Zaslov, S. S., and R. I. Frazier. 1969. A comparison of the Edison responsive environment learning system with an alternative system for teaching reading. A report sponsored by the Division of Research and Development of the Maryland State Department of Education.

16

SUPPORTIVE PERSONNEL FOR THE DEVELOPMENTALLY DISABLED

Carol K. Sigelman and Gerard J. Bensberg

CONTENTS

Supportive Roles _____ 655

Supportive Personnel within a Service System _____ 658
    Need for coordination/658
    Administrative concerns/660

Characteristics of Supportive Personnel _____ 661
    Background characteristics/661
    Attitudes/663
    Actual patterns of functioning/665

Effective Uses of Supportive Personnel _____ 667
    Proved potential/667
    Special concerns in programs for the hearing-impaired retarded/671

Training and Supervising Supportive Personnel _____ 674
    Training priorities and practices/675
    Supervising and motivating supportive staff/679

Conclusions and Future Prospects _____ 681

References _____ 684

Most of this volume focuses on the professional's role in communication assessment and intervention. However, it is a simple fact that professionals need help in their work, as has been noted in several other chapters of this volume (Baker; Cox and Lloyd; Graham; Kopchick and Lloyd). There are simply not enough professionals, particularly those trained to work with the multiply handicapped, to go around. But even if there were, it would be uneconomical and inefficient to rely on professionals in every phase of service delivery.

Supportive personnel are service deliverers who extend the impact of professionals. Some classes of supportive personnel—for example, aides or attendants in institutions—have been functioning for years, although, recently, increasing emphasis has been placed on expanding their roles to include more direct training activities. Other supportive roles—for example, those of audiometric technicians or aides—are only beginning to emerge as gaps in service are recognized.

The best organized plans of professionals cannot be translated into effective service on a broad scale without the efforts of supportive personnel. Moreover, it is often up to the professional to recruit, train, and motivate supportive staff. Consequently, this chapter is devoted to supportive staff and, more specifically, to the ways in which professionals can channel the energies of supportive staff for the good of handicapped persons.

SUPPORTIVE ROLES

Today, supportive personnel are found in almost any setting where communication programming takes place—residential schools for the deaf or mentally retarded, speech and hearing clinics, and public school classrooms—but their titles and functions are varied.

Direct-care staff (or attendants, cottage parents, child-care technicians, or resident counselors, as they are variously termed) are critical in staffing residential facilities. In many ways, the term *supportive personnel* is a misnomer, because attendants are typically primary care personnel who have more contact with, and presumably more influence on, residents than most professional staff members in an institution (Fleming, 1962). Yet they are supportive in the sense that professionals must depend on them if new treatment and training programs are to be implemented and reinforced in daily living activities. Direct-care staff, who traditionally have spent most of their time maintaining dorm or ward environments, managing residents, and providing basic care, can become central in communication training efforts.

More recently, a new role has emerged that is much like the attendant's role. As the trend toward deinstitutionalization has taken hold, community residences have been developed, either in the form of small foster homes for children or larger group homes and halfway houses for adults. In such programs, the foster parents or "houseparents," as they are often called, take primary responsibility for the care and maintenance of residents. If trained and supervised by professionals, however, they also can play an important role in training activities and function as more than parent surrogates. In residential institutions, as well as in smaller community residences, coordination between professionals and supportive personnel who supervise residents during the bulk of the day is critical.

Teacher aides—another type of supportive personnel—are fast becoming an integral part of American education (Brighton, 1972). Under the guidance of a certified teacher, aides can manage many clerical tasks that formerly fell on the teacher's shoulders and, if trained and used wisely, work directly with students to provide the individual instruction so often essential with the multiply handicapped. In the field of mental retardation, professional manpower shortages almost necessitate the use of assistants to provide instruction in classes for the educable and trainable and of behavior-shaping technicians to teach self-help in day care or residential settings. Other supportive positions similar to that of the teacher aide are being created in speech and hearing clinics and departments. For example, audiometric technicians without professional degrees can assume some of the duties of an audiologist, by conducting screening and fuller audiometric tests and handling many reporting and recording tasks. Similarly, aides to speech and hearing clinicians have been used to conduct specific therapy programs under professional direction (Alpiner, Ogden, and Wiggins, 1970).

These types of aides are representative of a larger corps of supportive personnel spawned by the "new careers" concept. First spelled out in the Economic Opportunity Act of 1966, this concept includes plans to develop entry-level jobs in human service fields for unemployed and low-income persons, and to create prospects of advancement in meaningful vocations (Gartner, 1971). The new careers concept soon spread to other areas of legislation (Gartner, 1971), so that opportunities for paraprofessionals were included in amendments to acts such as the Elementary and Secondary Education Act (Public Law 90-247, January 2, 1968), the Vocational Rehabilitation Act (Public Law 90-391, July 7, 1968), and the Mental Retardation Facilities and Community Health Centers Construction Act (Public Law 91-517, October 30, 1970, renamed the Developmental Disabilities Services and Facilities Construction Amendments of 1970). In addition to aide roles in institutions, schools, and clinics, many supportive positions were created to bridge the gap between service agencies and the communities they serve. Indigenous paraprofessionals, acting as home visitors, might detect needs, help citizens obtain the services to which they are entitled, and even train handicapped persons or their parents in the home. In a well developed community program, a referral clinic worker can aid in arranging and coordinating services for the developmentally disabled, and a homemaker service worker can relieve parents of responsibilities in times of family crisis (Bensberg, 1966).

While paraprofessionals are paid, volunteers typically are not. Of course, volunteer services have existed for centuries, but now there are formal programs with financial backing that channel volunteer efforts. The Domestic Volunteer Service Act of 1973 (Public Law 93-113) consolidates several existing programs—including VISTA (Volunteers in Service to America), University Year in ACTION,[1] and the Retired Service Volunteer Program—under a single legislative authority. The 1973 Act specifically authorizes the Director of ACTION to support volunteer work with developmentally disabled and other handicapped adults, in order to supplement the focus of earlier programs on handicapped children. VISTA workers can be assigned to work in care and rehabilitation programs for the handicapped, particularly the severely handicapped. Many different volunteer programs already have been used successfully in work with the mentally retarded. The Foster Grandparent program, for example, often provides individual attention and stimulation for the institutionalized retarded in return for meaningful activity and a salary. The SWEAT (Student Work Experience and Training) program has been successful in supplementing institutional programs while at the same time attracting talented youth to the field of mental retardation (Allen and Foshee, 1966). Volunteers also have been used in speech clinics (Boone, 1964). Finally, as community services for the development-

---

[1]Originally, ACTION was an acronym for American Council to Improve Our Neighborhoods, but it now includes other groups such as The Peace Corps.

ally disabled have expanded, a new volunteer role has emerged—
that of the citizen advocate (Wolfensberger, 1972). The citizen
advocate serves as a friend to the handicapped child or adult in the
community and aids the handicapped person in carrying out daily
activities and meeting crises.

Although the list of roles that supportive personnel can and do
play is by no means exhaustive, the breadth of their involvement has
been indicated. It is important to note that professionals are often considered to be supportive personnel, depending on whose viewpoint is
considered. For example, the audiologist in a residential facility may
need the help of other professionals such as vocational counselors,
social workers, and nurses in order to carry out a full habilitative
strategy. In many ways, working with supportive professionals poses
the same problems as working with nonprofessional supportive personnel because, in both cases, the people involved do not have thorough training in developmental disabilities, hearing impairment, or
communication programming. This chapter emphasizes direct-care
staff, teacher aides, and volunteers because they have been studied
more thoroughly by researchers and because they are often overlooked in total programming.

SUPPORTIVE PERSONNEL WITHIN A SERVICE SYSTEM

Before discussing specific characteristics and potentials of supportive
personnel, it is useful to view them within a total service system. This
is particularly true in regard to programs for the severely and multiply
handicapped in residential facilities, but the administrative concerns
raised here are relevant in schools and clinics as well.

Need for Coordination

Effective programming for the multiply handicapped with communication disorders must be coordinated horizontally, so that various
daily training activities fit together, and vertically, so that an orderly
progression of services is provided.

Rarely do handicapped persons interact with only one type of
professional; they are more likely to interact with an entire staff
during the course of a day. This point is well exemplified by Watson
and Nicholas (1973), who described a typical day in the life of a
deaf-blind, low cognitive functioning child in a residential school for
the blind (p. 1):

He has one housemother who wakes him and is with him from 6:30 a.m. until 8:00 a.m. From 8:00 a.m. until 3:00 p.m., he is under the direct supervision of his teacher and aides. During his school day, he may leave the classroom for work with the speech pathologist, physical therapist, occupational therapist, gym instructor, and swimming instructor. A different aide may help him to dress in the morning or work with him at lunch. After school, he may have supervised play with one or two part-time employees and/or volunteers and supper with another staff member. From Friday through Sunday, he follows his home routine, living and playing with family and friends.

In this situation, four different types of personnel—houseparents, teacher aides, volunteers, and a host of professionals—form the child's environment. Their efforts must be coordinated in a consistent 24-hour program as outlined by Kopchick and Lloyd (this volume). Just as the progress of students learning French is likely to be greater in France, where almost every daily activity becomes a learning experience, the progress of handicapped children will be greater if they are in an environment where all staff can act consistently and reinforce one another's efforts. A communication program almost certainly will fail to have a strong impact if it affects the learner for only a few hours a day; therefore, the cooperation of other staff members, particularly those in the child's living quarters, is essential. The gap between class and afterclass activities has been recognized as a critical problem in residential schools for the deaf (Naiman and Mashikian, 1973), as well as in institutions for the mentally retarded (Kopchick and Lloyd, this volume; Kopchick, Rombach, and Smilowitz, 1975).

No less important than horizontal coordination is vertical coordination. Although the concept of the mentally retarded as developing persons is fully embraced today, a full developmental continuum of programs is difficult to establish, and decisions regarding movement along such a continuum are difficult to make. For example, the hearing-impaired, mentally retarded in an institutional setting first must acquire self-help, social, and communication skills; then, as they mature, educational and sheltered workshop programs aimed toward vocational development should be made available to them (Mitra, 1971). In many cases, attendants or cottage parents are useful sources of information about a resident's progress through a developmental continuum because they have a continuing relationship with the resident.

Furlough and discharge from the institution also must be orderly, starting with a campus job placement, trial off-campus competitive employment, and movement to the community when vocational competence has been demonstrated. As movement to the community is planned, a volunteer citizen advocate might play a central role in smoothing the transition.

Administrative Concerns

For 24-hour, consistent programming and movement along a developmental continuum to occur, staff organization must be conducive to coordination (see Kopchick and Lloyd, this volume). Many older residential institutions and other treatment facilities have been organized in a hierarchical structure or medical model. In this model, distinctions among different types of professionals and between professionals and nonprofessionals are rigid. Because information must pass up and down a long chain of command, as well as between departments horizontally, communications are often lost or distorted along the way. Most critically, the innovative plans of professionals may not be translated into action at the front line. This model is also associated with a structured and authoritarian administrative style that may inhibit free communication among all levels of the hierarchy.

A newer administrative model, the "team" model, attempts to reduce barriers among various disciplines and between professionals and various supportive personnel, including direct-care staff, by fostering interdepartmental planning, diagnosis, and treatment. In the team model, the audiologist, teacher, speech pathologist, psychologist, social worker, and attendant work together to see that a total program for each individual is designed and implemented. Lloyd and Cox (1972) advocated such a team approach—headed by the audiologist and involving supportive personnel and other professionals—in programming for the audiologic aspects of mental retardation. The team model, favored in the Accreditation Council for Facilities for the Mentally Retarded *Standards for Residential Facilities for the Mentally Retarded* (1975), represents a more participative organizational style. Many residential facilities have adopted the team model, which is sometimes referred to as the "unit system."

There are several reasons for suspecting that this model facilitates both horizontal and vertical coordination of programming. Scheerenberger (1971), using a scale tapping staff members' perceptions of the organizational structure of a facility for the mentally retarded, considered four different management systems—autocratic, benevolent autocratic, consultative, and participative. Although most attendants saw their organization as consultative, they desired a more important role in decision-making, one that would be more characteristic of the participative or team model. As Naiman and Mashikan (1973, p. 39) said of afterclass staff in facilities for the deaf: they ". . . know that their position is pivotal in the program but that their salaries, their training and their inclusion in the decision-making apparatus are inconsistent with their alleged importance." A study of management practices in vocational rehabilitation offices (Viaille and Hills, 1973) suggested that a participative model is indeed more effective than a more authoritarian model. The styles of supervisors were highly related to the morale, efficiency, and effectiveness of the counselors working under them.

It is not enough to train supportive personnel to execute plans handed to them by professionals; professionals must be trained to use effective supervisory styles in their interactions with supportive personnel, styles that promote effective teamwork.

CHARACTERISTICS OF SUPPORTIVE PERSONNEL

Effective working relationships with supportive personnel are predicated on knowledge of: 1) their backgrounds and general levels of competency; 2) their attitudes toward their job, the handicapped they serve, and their supervising professionals; and 3) their typical patterns of operation. This section considers several characteristics of direct-care staff and other supportive personnel that have implications for programming.

Background Characteristics

In residential institutions for the mentally retarded, attendants typically constitute a majority of institutional employees. Their very ubiquity makes them an important factor in communication programming.

Yet the qualifications for the job of attendant are less clear than those for almost any other role in the institution. In a survey of residential facilities in the United States and Canada, it was found that requirements ranged from none to a high school diploma, but fewer than 20% of the institutions required a diploma and almost none required previous experience (Parnicky and Ziegler, 1964).

In a review of the literature, Butterfield (1967a) concluded that the attendant typically has no prior experience, has less than a complete high school education, falls in the lower part of the normal IQ range, and often comes from a rural or small-town background. If not employed in an institution, most direct-care staff might be found in unskilled or semi-skilled jobs in the community. The turnover rate among attendants is high, particularly in the first months of employment (Tarjan, Shotwell, and Dingman, 1955; Fleming, 1962). But this seems to be less a function of working conditions within the institution than of the general employment picture in the area (Butterfield, Barnett, and Bensberg, 1966). Quite simply, the turnover rate is lower when the unemployment rate is high, suggesting that if the persons who take attendant positions have access to other jobs, including those with more competitive salaries, they are likely to leave the institution for greener pastures.

This profile of attendants is not drastically different from profiles of other types of supportive personnel, although the trend recently has been to upgrade qualifications and salaries. For example, residential programs in the community, although they sometimes recruit well trained, college-level houseparents, often draw from less educated, less experienced groups. Mamula and Newman (1973), drawing on information from small family care homes for the mentally retarded in California, described the typical care-provider as middle-aged, married, lower middle-class, and conservative, with a high school education. Their description closely parallels one of foster parents in Pennsylvania (Guerney, 1974). Teacher aides and other paraprofessional workers, particularly if they are part of a "new careers" program, are typically recruited from the unemployed and unskilled of the local area. For example, recruits for an instructional aide program at the Houston Speech and Hearing Center were generally black women with a high school education or less who performed on academic achievement tests at approximately the seventh- or eighth-grade level (Rister, 1974). Volunteers often enter a program with more education (e.g., Rich, Gilmore, and Williams, 1964), but in programs such as the Foster Grandparent program, many volunteers do not have relevant experience or education.

These basic descriptive characteristics have implications for mobilization of supportive personnel. The paucity of education and relevant experience suggests that the kinds of formal instruction used in training professionals may not be successful with supportive personnel. The fact that salaries and other incentives for supportive personnel are often low suggests that the possibility of high turnover rates must be reckoned with, perhaps by arranging for continuous training and attempting to equip supportive personnel with basic skills in a very short period of time.

Attitudes

The problems in utilizing supportive personnel become even clearer when one considers some of the attitudinal factors that often create a barrier between supportive personnel and the professional and administrative staff. One very basic disagreement often arises with respect to the proper function of supportive personnel, particularly direct-care staff in institutions. Shotwell, Dingman, and Tarjan (1960), for example, had attendants, their immediate supervisors, and professional personnel at an institution rate statements about the role of an attendant according to their importance. Professional personnel stressed the attendant's interaction with residents, emphasizing roles such as playing games with residents and being friendly toward them. Attendants and their immediate supervisors (typically experienced attendants) attached more importance to activities such as being neat, being punctual, following instructions, and keeping the ward clean. Schmidmayr and Weld (1971) also reported that, although professionals emphasized the resident-oriented responsibilities of attendants, attendants ranked "object-oriented" statements higher in importance, although specially trained aides in an intensive care unit deviated from the general pattern and valued resident-oriented responsibilities. Several studies converge to indicate that, although professionals view attendants as trainers and stimulators, attendants see their roles primarily as custodial.

Attendants also tend to emphasize managing large groups of residents; psychologists, on the other hand, place greater value on individual residents and their progress (Rettig, 1956). This suggests that attendants, fearing that they will seem to have favorites if they do not treat all residents the same, may resist attempts by professionals to launch programs for individuals in need of special attention or training. More generally, the professional cannot simply assume that attendants will operate special training programs because of their inherent interest in developing residents' potentials. In fact, in one study supervisory attendants at an institution tended to believe that society should be protected from the mentally retarded, an attitude that is totally contradictory to habilitative programming (Overbeck, 1971).

The implications of attendant attitudes for innovative programming were spelled out in some detail by Bogdan et al. (1974) on the basis of 3 years of observation of attendants in three wards. Attendants' attitudes toward professionals and supervisors were summarized in one sentence: "They don't know what it's really like." In other words, attendants felt that professionals were ignorant of residents' needs and attendants' roles, and they questioned the competence of professionals, expressing skepticism about the value of test scores and professional jargon. To most attendants, their job was just a job, valued for its salary and fringe benefits rather than for any intrinsically satisfying properties. As for the residents, most attendants tended to define them in terms of their deficits and capacities for making trouble and saw little hope that they would progress. Attendants defined their job as custodial to the extent that one was quoted as saying, "We sometimes have to tie people up so that we can carry on with the work."

As a natural consequence of these perspectives, programs introduced in these three wards by professionals were typically aborted. Failing to appreciate the value of such programs and seeing involvement in training as something "outside" their job requirements, attendants simply stopped conducting training programs. The most successful program was a token economy to reward appropriate behavior in a ward for adolescent girls, but attendants continued its use primarily because they saw it as a way to punish girls for inappropriate behavior—namely, by threatening them with loss of points and privileges. In other words, attendants either failed to conduct an innovative program, or they subverted the intended goals of the program to make the program consistent with their own priorities.

Attendants' attitudes are not always as starkly different from professionals' attitudes as the study by Bogdan et al. (1974) suggests. Nonetheless, the possibility of attitudinal barriers must be considered, whether it is between teacher aides and teachers or between volunteers and the professionals supervising them. The attitudes of professionals toward supportive personnel are as important as the attitudes of supportive personnel toward professionals, residents, and their roles. Just as many professionals in institutions adopt a condescending attitude toward direct-care staff, teachers and other professionals sometimes have difficulty accepting the presence of supportive personnel, particularly when they fear that their own job security and status is threatened (Alpiner, Ogden, and Wiggins, 1970; Gartner, 1971; Rister, 1974).

Actual Patterns of Functioning

In view of the attitudinal barriers discussed above and the characteristics of supportive personnel, particularly direct-care staff in residential facilities, it is hardly surprising that there is often a large gap between roles officially espoused by administrators and actual daily activities of attendants. If attendants are first and foremost parent surrogates and trainers, one would never know it from their daily activity patterns. Bensberg and Barnett (1966) had graduate students observe attendant behavior in four institutions for the mentally retarded. Eleven categories of attendant behavior were used in classifying observations. In all, supervision (watching, checking, and giving orders) and leisure (activities, such as reading and watching television, which had nothing to do with work assignments) were the two most prevalent activities, each accounting for approximately 30% of attendants' time. Only 8% of their time was spent providing personal care, and less than 5% was devoted to teaching residents skills. Moreover, it was noted that, on the relatively rare occasions when they interacted with residents by supervising them or attending to their needs, attendants rarely took advantage of the opportunity to interact verbally with the children.

Similarly, Warren and Mondy (1971) reported that attendants rarely respond to either the appropriate or inappropriate behaviors of retarded children in their care. For example, of a total of 493 appropriate behaviors displayed by 49 children, 82% were not responded to at all by attendants. In a study of one cottage for profoundly to moderately retarded children, Dailey et al. (1973) found that the average resident engaged in positive or social-play interactions with caretakers in fewer than 1% of the intervals during which he was observed. Dailey et al. (1973) aptly termed attendants' ignoring of residents "an inadvertent extinction program."

Research suggests that this commonly observed lack of involvement of attendants in stimulating and training residents has detrimental effects. Klaber (1969) was able to relate attendant behavior to "effective" institutional care, as defined by resident happiness and level of adaptive functioning. In one "effective" institution, a high percentage of resident behavior involved interaction with attendants, and residents spent relatively more time interacting with attendants and other nonretarded adults than with retarded peers. This pattern contrasted with that found in less effective institutions. In reviewing research on the effects of institutionalization, Butterfield (1967b) hypothesized that the diminished intellectual, verbal, and personality functioning often found among the institutionalized retarded is in part attributable to a lack of verbal stimulation from adults.

It is tempting to attribute this lack of stimulation by attendants to excessive demands on their time caused by staff shortages, but as Bensberg and Barnett (1966) reported, attendants spend much of their time on the job pursuing leisure activities rather than caring for the cottage or its residents and do not effectively use the time available to them to stimulate residents. Moreover, there is evidence that increasing staff size does not necessarily increase the amount of interaction between residents and caretakers (Thormahlen, 1965; Wills, 1973; Harris et al., 1974). For example, Thormahlen (1965) reported that the attendants he observed spent only 2% of their time training self-help skills, while they used 36% of their time to foster dependency by doing things for residents. A larger number of attendants simply meant more time doing things for residents, and as the staff became more stratified, staff members became more heavily involved in administrative and maintenance tasks rather than resident interaction. Wills (1973) reported that, when extra staff help was available, attendants spent more time socializing with one another, assuming duties of working residents, and improving the ward physically. The point is not that institutions should be deliberately understaffed; rather, attendants' understanding of their roles and behavioral interactions with residents must be modified so that they contribute more powerfully to the habilitative goals of the institution. The challenge is to train direct-care staff to provide verbal stimulation, reinforce appropriate behavior, and in a broader sense, to enrich the environment through the types of visual, tactile-kinesthetic, and auditory stimulation outlined by Haviland (1972).

Although the problem is not as great, teacher aides in public schools, like attendants, have not always functioned as effectively as they might. Certainly, goals of teacher aide programs include providing more individual attention to students. However, in most settings, teacher aides devote most of their time to what can be called "secretarial" or clerical duties (Gartner, 1971). However, this pattern seems to be attributable not to the aides' perceptions of their roles, but to the teachers' perceptions of an aide's functions. A National Education Association survey cited by Gartner (1971) indicated that over 90% of the teachers surveyed thought aides were helpful, but, whereas 73% favored their use in clerical work, only 44% favored their involvement in certain types of classroom instruction. As research reviewed in the next section suggests, supportive personnel have been and can be used effectively in innovative programming, but their promise will not be realized unless role perceptions of both supportive personnel and professionals are altered.

EFFECTIVE USES OF SUPPORTIVE PERSONNEL

Whereas the previous section stresses obstacles to effective programming by supportive personnel, this section turns to evidence of the successful use of supportive personnel in a variety of settings. Unfortunately, it is difficult to assess the independent effects of supportive staff on programs, and as a result, relatively little evidence is available. The evidence falls in four categories: acceptance of supportive personnel by professionals, benefits to professionals, benefits to supportive personnel, and benefits to handicapped persons.

Proved Potential

Although evidence that supportive personnel are accepted by professionals is not sufficient grounds for proclaiming their effectiveness, a comfortable working relationship between supportive personnel and professionals is requisite for a successful program. Several studies report initial skepticism by professionals, later replaced by acceptance and appreciation. For example, Alpiner, Ogden, and Wiggins (1970) found that speech clinicians in public schools initially feared being replaced by aides, but most came to accept the program, and 11 of 14 wanted the aide program continued. In a survey of large state, day, and private schools for the deaf, 96.8% of the administrators returning surveys indicated that aides were of "great value" (Butler and Hanks, undated). In a National Education Association survey in 1968 (cited by Gartner, 1971), 90% of the teachers surveyed found teacher aides helpful, and over half said that they were of great assistance.

This acceptance of supportive personnel by professionals is no doubt related to the benefits that accrue to professionals. Alpiner, Ogden, and Wiggins (1970) reported that speech clinicians felt that they had more time for preparation and contact with children as a result of the aide program. According to school teachers in the Minneapolis Public Schools, aides saved them, on the average, 14 hours per week to do planning and 3 hours to work directly with students (Bennett and Falk, 1970). Not only are supportive personnel often time-savers; they also may spawn new role perceptions among professionals. Bowman and Klopf (1968) detected evidence that, with paraprofessional aides as the catalysts, professionals developed higher levels of professionalism, placing more emphasis on diagnosis, planning, and coordination of eductional activities. Similarly, the introduction of high school and college students in institutions for the mentally retarded led many staff members to comment on the positive effects of the students on their own work (Allen and Foshee, 1966).

Benefits to the professional are complemented by benefits to the paraprofessional. Beyond the obvious benefits of employment and salary, paraprofessionals, particularly those in new careers programs with incentives and vehicles for advancement, often gain in the long run by becoming motivated to pursue a career. For example, many of the student workers in SWEAT programs made verbal or written commitments to pursue a career in mental retardation (Allen and Foshee, 1966), and of the 209 paraprofessionals in schools for the deaf surveyed by Butler and Hanks (undated), 28% planned to become certified as teachers of the deaf, even though 48% came to the job with only a high school diploma.

Of course, neither potential benefits to professionals nor to supportive personnel themselves are as important as benefits to the handicapped children and adults with whom supportive personnel work. Research suggests that supportive personnel in a variety of settings have positive effects on program outcomes, although rigorous evaluative studies are rare.

Several studies point to the value of one-to-one training through the use of volunteers. Cytryn and Uihlein (1965) noted anecdotal and case history evidence of gains in the social adjustment, speech, and reading of mentally retarded children who had volunteers working with them. In another project for mentally retarded children (Freeman and Thompson, 1973), both student teachers and mothers contributed to gains. Eight young children received 1 hour of one-to-one tutoring from a student teacher while the mothers participated in group counseling. During the second hour, each mother worked with a child on behavior control and language development. Although there was no control group, the 8-week program produced an average growth in mental age of over 5 months and improvements in functional skills. High school and college volunteers have been used effectively to improve reading comprehension in severely retarded students (Barrett and McCormack, 1973). Largely through use of behavior modification principles in one-to-one relationships, academic gains were achieved. Volunteers quickly learned to execute the structured program with very few errors.

Attendants or cottage parents have been effective in improving cottage behavior, typically in behavior modification or token economy programs. For example, Bath and Smith (1974) instituted a token economy to change the social skills and volunteering behavior of retarded women. Gains were significant, although performance dropped off when the illness of a ward charge attendant precipitated the introduction of new, untrained staff to the system. In fact, behavior modification, as described in another chapter (Spradlin, Karlan, and Wetherby, this volume), is a tool that can be successfully employed by direct-care staff as well as other supportive staff under supervision. For example, Craig (1970) demonstrated the efficacy of token reinforcement in improving visual attending among deaf students. Osborne (1970) designed a behavior change program for a deaf student; the program demanded the participation of the student's teacher and dormitory counselors in observing and reinforcing behavior. Eveslage and Buchmann (1973) reported that deaf 10-year-old children orally read word cards in a manner more intelligible to their teacher when they were given feedback on performance and reinforced for intelligible responses (i.e., responses that the teacher could write down, not knowing which word card the child had). And finally, Tharp and Wetzel (1969) demonstrated the potential of paraprofessional "behavior analysts" in instituting behavior change programs within the public schools. Under the direction of supervising psychologists, the behavior analysts taught teachers and parents to dispense rewards appropriately. Such a role might serve to extend the influence of the psychologist within a residential facility or to achieve consistency between training programs and afterclass activities.

Recent developments in the mental health field have immediate application to work with the developmentally disabled. Supportive personnel can help prepare persons to leave residential facilities. For example, Beck, Kantor, and Gelineau (1965) reported significant improvements in the social behavior of chronic psychotic patients who had continued contact with volunteer college students, but not among control subjects without such one-to-one relationships. Moreover, the volunteer program permitted a relatively high proportion of patients to be discharged from the hospital (Beck, Kantor, and Gelineau, 1963). Once mental health patients are discharged, volunteers can serve as effective aftercare workers. In one program, volunteers checked to see that clients kept appointments and took medicines, evaluated their progress, assisted them in finding housing and jobs, and offered supportive counseling (Katkin et al., 1974). The result was a recidivism rate of 10%, which compared extremely favorably with a rate of 35% for patients offered traditional follow-up services. In another aftercare program, trained paraprofessionals evaluated the functioning of and provided supportive services to physically handicapped persons released from a rehabilitative hospital, maintaining high levels of functioning in these released clients (Thornhill et al., 1974).

Volunteers or supportive personnel, therefore, might serve two important roles in the deinstitutionalization of developmentally disabled persons: preparing residents for furlough or discharge, and supporting them once they are placed in the community. Already, college students have been used as tutors in community training programs, and volunteer citizen advocates have eased the transition process for mentally retarded adults leaving institutions, although such programs have not been formally evaluated.

Even more impressive and provocative are demonstrations that volunteers or supportive personnel are at least as effective as professionals in providing therapeutic counseling and, most importantly, in producing positive changes in clients (Carkhuff, 1968). In one study, patients at the Hot Springs (Arkansas) Rehabilitation Center were assigned to professional, experienced counselors with masters' degrees, to professional counselors helped by a closely supervised aide, and to aides working with minimal supervision—generally former secretaries with little or no college work (Truax and Lister, 1970). All clients had behavioral problems and a good number of them had speech and hearing defects or were mentally retarded. In terms of client performance in the vocational training program, the best results were obtained by aides working alone with minimal supervision from a professional counselor. One explanation for the finding that supportive personnel are sometimes more effective counselors than professionals is their potential for achieving rapport and reducing social distance (Pope et al., 1974). This interpretation is supported by evidence that doctoral training in the helping professions is associated with lower levels of empathy, warmtn, and genuineness (Carkhuff, Kratochvil, and Friel, 1968). Although this evidence does not support wholesale abandonment of professionals, it certainly suggests that trained supportive personnel can take on more complex responsibilities than is generally assumed.

Special Concerns in Programs for the Hearing-Impaired Retarded

In programming for the hearing-impaired retarded and other multiply disabled groups, supportive personnel can be mobilized to meet specific critical needs, including the need for training in the use and care of hearing aids, the need for consistent approaches to communication, and the need for structured programming in all areas of life functioning.

Brannan, Sigelman, and Bensberg (1975) reported that individual hearing aids are not available to most hearing-impaired residents of state institutions for the mentally retarded. Two-thirds of the respondents to a mail survey indicated that hearing-impaired residents have difficulty caring for hearing aids, a factor that partially may account for the scarcity of hearing aids. Funding problems aside, the critical problem seems to be one of training residents to wear and care for aids and supervising their use (McCoy and Lloyd, 1967; Moore, Miltenberger, and Barber, 1969). The first step is to convince all staff members of the value of aids, not just in the classroom but throughout the day. The attendant's involvement is pivotal if hearing aids are to become a fact of life. McCoy and Lloyd (1967) described a step-by-step hearing aid orientation program that involves repeated contacts with cottage parents, the key to effective follow-up. As the resident is introduced to the hearing aid, the cottage parents are acquainted with aids and their functions, informed of the resident's progress, and trained to monitor adjustment as the resident gradually works toward full-time use of the hearing aid. For a more extensive discussion of hearing aid care and use the reader is referred to the chapters by Cox and Lloyd (this volume) and by Ross (this volume).

A second critical area of programming for the hearing-impaired retarded is a coordinated approach to communication, which, in some cases, may include manual communication (e.g., Kopchick and Lloyd, this volume). Data reported by Brannan, Sigelman, and Bensberg (1975) indicated that manual communication systems are not heavily used in state facilities for the mentally retarded. In large part, this can be traced to the fact that only a handful of institutions group hearing-impaired and deaf residents in special living quarters. With hearing-impaired residents dispersed across campus, it is impractical to train all staff to use manual communication methods. If hearing-impaired residents were more often grouped or clustered, residents would be able to communicate manually with one another and intensive training of attendant personnel in total communication would be feasible. There have been numerous reports of the value of manual communication, particularly early in the life of the hearing-impaired child (e.g., Vernon, 1970; Moores, 1974). Furthermore, it is clear that mentally retarded children with communication difficulties can learn sign language (e.g., Kopchick and Lloyd, this volume; Wilbur, this volume; Sutherland and Beckett, 1969; Wilson, 1974).

Some practitioners have developed special or adapted sign languages and designed structured programs for teaching communication. For example the Pinecrest State School in Pineville, Louisiana, has developed a sign language manual for cottage parents that has promise (Owens and Harper, 1970). It includes diagrams of approximately 300 functional signs, guides on how to express signs, and a simple training procedure for use with residents. Using a behavior modification approach, attendants are instructed to reinforce correct signing by residents with praise and with the use of signs for *good* and *thank you*. Praise expressed through signs is paired with social and edible rewards. The steps in training a resident to use signs are as follows: 1) gain the child's attention; 2) have the child match colors, objects, and so on; 3) give a sign; 4) ask for an item using the sign; 5) help the child make the sign; 6) point to the item and have the child sign it; 7) ask for the item using signs; and 8) have the child ask for the item using signs.

In one institution, the feasibility of teaching a simplified esoteric sign language to severely and profoundly retarded nonverbal children was demonstrated, but the program specialists were unable to induce the rest of the staff to adopt the system (Wilson, 1974). Attendant participation is essential if sign language or any approach to communication is to permeate the lives of institutionalized persons. Kopchick and Lloyd (this volume) argue that the use of signs by supportive personnel is facilitated by homogenous grouping and by use of more standard signs rather than an esoteric system.

Other kinds of communication programming can be conducted by supportive personnel if the procedures are simple. In fact, higher functioning residents in an institution for the mentally retarded can contribute to language programming. Hall and Talkington (1970), recognizing the need for individualized programming, multiplied staff through the use of paid resident aides. The mentally retarded aides were trained to answer the telephone, then to cut and paste pictures for language training, and later to make transparencies. Five aides, themselves severely retarded, were trained to serve as models for other residents learing to follow commands and to reinforce their students for correct responses. Working under the supervision of ward staff and using the Peabody Language Development Program (Dunn, Smith, and Horton, 1968), these resident aides contributed to significant language age increases among 26 severely and profoundly retarded residents. Hall and Talkington (1970) also used resident aides trained in manual communication in a classroom for the deaf retarded.

Glovsky and Rigrodsky (1963) placed strong emphasis on cottage parents in generalizing language training to everyday life. The words being learned by six language-delayed, hearing-impaired retarded children were distributed to other staff members, particularly to cottage parents, who were encouraged to use them as frequently as possible in daily activities. In another communication program for the hearing-impaired retarded, a teacher aide working with the teacher helped to conduct academic training which relied on sign language, fingerspelling, and speech (Mitra, 1974). The results were significant increases in vocabulary, sentence structure, and reading comprehension.

The potential of volunteers in working with the hearing-impaired mentally retarded should not be overlooked. Ludtke and Elliott (1969), noting that volunteers in residential facilities are often restricted to the role of friendly visitor, mobilized volunteers as trainers of children, involving them in manual language and social skill training for deaf-retarded residents and as speech aides, among other things. Although they offered no evaluative data, they observed that volunteers are motivated when given clear expectations and challenging assignments.

One of the authors had success using a modification of the Wisconsin General Test Apparatus (Zeaman and House, 1963) to structure a variety of training activities. In a cubicle with side doors, the instructor sits behind a curtain across a table or "stage" from the child and presents tasks. An object or card is held over one of three holes in the stage and a reinforcer is placed in the correct hole. For example, the instructor might say, "Show me the car," and then let the child grab a peanut from the hole if he or she reaches for the car. The professional prepares a developmental program, which can deal with language concepts, reading, color discrimination, or any variety of subjects, and the attendant, aide, or volunteer executes it. The apparatus makes learning a game for the child, and if side walls are used, cuts down on distractions. At the same time, it provides trainers with simple step-by-step procedures and often motivates them as much as it motivates the learner.

Finally, the "model home" approach to training hearing-impaired children is a promising model that can be readily adapted for use by supportive personnel (Simmons, 1967; Horton, 1974). For example, in the Home Teaching Program for Parents of Very Young Deaf Children, the basic strategy, a highly effective one according to research reports, is to train parents to make use of everyday activities in the home as the context for auditory stimulation and training (Horton, 1974). The needs of the hearing-impaired retarded are such that communication training must be incorporated into a broader habilitative program. For example, Vockell, Vockell, and Mattick (1973), in describing Project LIFE, emphasized the need for perceptual and cognitive training accompanying language training. More broadly, hearing-impaired retarded persons have needs in the areas of self-care, mobility, social behavior, and vocational development which are interlocked with communication needs. Manuals directed toward primary care personnel are available and suggest specific training areas and sequences appropriate for the hearing-impaired retarded (e.g., Griffing and Huffman, 1969; Marion County Association for Retarded Children, 1973; Watson and Nicholas, 1973).

TRAINING AND SUPERVISING SUPPORTIVE PERSONNEL

For the potential of supportive staff to be realized, the professional must devote considerable effort to training them and maintaining their performance over long periods of time. In schools and residential facilities, it is important for supportive personnel to be oriented to the communication problems of students and to communication program objectives; as previously suggested, direct-care staff require orientation to hearing-impaired, mentally retarded residents. A second type of training provides staff and/or volunteers with special skill training as they perform their jobs. Finally, in the context of the new careers movement, supportive personnel are trained through more formal academic programs for credit and certification.

As long ago as the early 1960's, the vast majority of institutions for the retarded offered at least inservice training for direct-care staff, but training time generally had to be squeezed into overloaded schedules (Parnicky and Ziegler, 1964). More recently, the need for training that has an enduring impact on knowledge, attitudes, and skills has been appreciated (Bensberg and Barnett, 1966). Moreover, it has become apparent that effective training that produces usable skills in trainees is not enough. In order for programs to be executed on a continuing basis, trained staff must be supervised and motivated to apply their skills.

Training Priorities and Practices

The starting point in any attempt to train staff should be a basic orientation to communication difficulties. With little investment in time and money, supportive personnel working with the deaf or hearing-impaired retarded can learn simple guidelines to effective habilitation. For example, Lloyd (1966) has offered 21 suggestions for nurses and aides working with the hearing-impaired retarded. Rules of thumb such as facing the patient when talking; gaining the patient's attention; keeping the light on one's face; remaining stationary; speaking in a natural tone of voice; and using complete, simple sentences represent easily learned behaviors that must underlie more formal training. (Appendix E presents a similar set of suggestions for speech and language development.) Broberg (1968) discussed aspects of audiology that should be part of a nurse's knowledge and that also might be presented to attendants in orientation sessions. Nober (1974) has produced a more ambitious manual to orient school personnel who may find themselves working with hearing impaired students as more of them are integrated into the public schools. Finally, Naiman (1972) and Naiman and Mashikian (1973) offer a variety of materials that can serve as a basis for staff orientation based on the efforts of the Deafness Research and Training Center at New York University to coordinate class and afterclass activities in residential schools for the deaf. A variety of such materials can provide supportive personnel, as well as professionals whose competencies are not in the area of communication programming, with basic understandings of hearing impairment, developmental disabilities, and diagnostic and treatment procedures used with these groups. Lloyd (personal communication; also see Cox and Lloyd, this volume) recommends that orientation include the playing of tapes that demonstrate how sounds are perceived by persons with various degrees and types of hearing impairment (and how speech and various environmental noises sound through hearing aids). This is a concrete way to convey the needs of the hearing impaired and dispel the mistaken impression that they often "play deaf."

A second type of training attempts to provide supportive personnel with new skills that they can apply in training and teaching activities. For example, Griffing and Huffman (1969) have developed a handbook for direct-care staff working with the deaf mentally retarded at Sonoma State Hospital; the handbook suggests how different personnel fit into a coordinated effort and outlines specific tasks to be accomplished by aides. In an intriguing use of a critical incident technique, Jacobs, Nichols, and Larsen (1969) developed a catalog of over 8000 behaviors of attendants caring for the mentally retarded in institutions, with each behavior skill exemplified by positive and negative examples collected from several institutions. Such a catalog of specific task behaviors is readily adaptable to training courses that stress "real-world" demands on the attendant. The READ Project Series (Baker et al., 1973), reported in the chapter by Baker (this volume), exemplifies a more specific training technique that can be used by parents or attendant staff. It is a clear and simple guide to the use of behavior modification in teaching basic life skills.

Another medium of training, the Associate of Arts or junior college degree, has only recently emerged in conjunction with the new careers concept. For example, Rieger and De Vries (1974) described formal training for the "child mental health specialist" as consisting of courses in child care, education, and clinical management. Junior college graduates who hold AA degrees are prepared to be assistant teachers, therapists, aides, cottage parents, and day-care center workers in settings that serve emotionally disturbed and delinquent children. Another 2-year program has been established at Miami-Dade Junior College to train mental retardation technicians

(Cortazzo and Orkin, 1970). In this program, students receive approximately 30 hours of background in liberal arts and behavioral science and approximately 35 hours of coursework and practicum in mental retardation, ranging from supervised observations of programs in the first semester to full internships in the summers. Finally, Eastfield College, in Dallas, now offers a program to train paraprofessionals for the deaf so that they can work as teacher aides, interpreters, and assistants to the multiply handicapped (Palmer, 1974). This program also has a heavy emphasis on practicum experiences interwoven with classroom instruction.

Rister (1974) reported a practical method of training teacher aides in a speech and hearing center. Teachers, at first dubious of the aide program, changed their attitudes when, asked to list their specific job duties, they recognized that many of the tasks they routinely performed could be delegated to an assistant. These same task descriptions were then arranged in order of difficulty and degree of expertise required and were taught to aides in an increasing order of difficulty. A "career ladder" concept allowed for the advancement of aide recruits from a clerical trainee level to the status of an instructional aide with a full range of teaching and auxiliary duties. At the end of the 2-year training program, which combined basic educational training with the on-the-job training sequenced from simple to complex, the instructional aide became a regular employee.

With these suggestions on the range of available training programs, one must now ask what makes for effective training. Two general themes have emerged with respect to training supportive personnel: 1) training must be concrete and structured, and 2) training must emphasize actual rehearsal of the skills being acquired. As one moves down the scale in professional training and experience, task specificity becomes more crucial, for one cannot depend on the supportive staff member's ability to generalize abstract learning and apply it in new situations. It is not uncommon for the cottage life supervisor in a state school to walk through a ward and say, "We have to toilet train these kids," expecting that general orientations to mental retardation and child development have prepared attendants to work on toilet training. For such a prescription to be implemented, it is probably necessary to meet with attendants, lay out a specific training sequence and schedule that includes methods of reinforcing behavior, and then monitor and reinforce the efforts of aides. Training is apt to be even more effective if supportive personnel have opportunities to rehearse specific skills in nonthreatening situations before they are responsible for full implementation of a program.

The need for practical, concrete training is supported by a study of training approaches for use with mental health technicians in an institution (Paul, McInnis, and Mariotto, 1973). In one training program to teach social-learning and milieu therapy approaches, aides received academic instruction from the professional staff followed by an on-the-ward practicum supervised by professionals. In a second program, they received an abbreviated academic program that was integrated with clinical observation and followed by a practicum supervised by experienced technicians rather than by professionals. The aides' performance was evaluated through observations in two 6-week periods, one while they were still under supervision and one while they were operating independently. Although the professional training model previously had been found to produce better performance on academic tests (Paul and McInnis, 1974), the program that deemphasized theoretical training and stressed observation and practicum under an experienced aide was more effective than the more traditional approach in improving on-the-floor performance.

Much the same conclusion was drawn from a study in which attendants in an institution for the mentally retarded were taught behavior modification (Gardner, 1972). The usual training format consisted of lecture and discussion on the principles of behavior modification, and a practicum in which pairs of attendants played roles, one serving as trainer, the other serving as the resident being trained. When the lecture portion of the program was compared with the role-playing portion, the lecture was found to be more effective in teaching principles of behavior modification, as evidenced by scores on a paper-and-pencil test, but role playing was more effective in teaching behavior modification skills, as evidenced by ratings of attendants as they demonstrated skills.

The role-playing approach used by Gardner (1972) actually consisted of demonstration of the skill by a master trainer, role playing of the skill by attendants, and feedback regarding performance. A similar model has been effective in training houseparents in small community homes for delinquent and disturbed youth (Maloney, 1974). A combined approach consisting of instructions regarding appropriate behavior, modeling of the behavior, and feedback was found to be more effective than instructions and feedback alone.

Whether the specific approach is demonstration followed by role playing, or instruction followed by modeling by a master trainer and then imitation by the trainee, the critical element seems to be direct involvement of the trainee in using the skills to be acquired. Lecture formats, common in inservice training, can increase knowledge, but research suggests that they are minimally effective in changing the behavior of supportive personnel.

Supervising and Motivating Supportive Staff

As already noted, the salaries of most supportive personnel are low, and in some cases, their perceptions of their own roles and professionals' perceptions of them do not foster dedication to the goals of a program. Once supportive personnel are trained to aid in diagnosis or intervention, the job of the professional is just beginning, for high levels of performance must be maintained over a long period of time, often under less than ideal working conditions. The master trainer must be a student of organizations, for organizational characteristics often constrain the extent to which trained personnel actually translate their skills into effective, ongoing programs (Brightman, 1975).

The first step is adequate supervision, which consists of teaching, administration, and evaluation (Nash and Mittlefehldt, 1975). Reinherz (1967) reported that the motivation, goals, and length of stay in service of student volunteers in mental health were affected by the quality of supervision that they received. Boone (1964) voiced the opinion that approximately 30 minutes each morning devoted to preparation of volunteers in a speech pathology-audiology clinic would yield 5 hours of service from each volunteer. Meetings between teachers and dormitory counselors have been used to promote consistency between class and afterclass programs (Lennan, 1973).

Supervision of supportive personnel is essential, although not always sufficient. The more difficult problem is to motivate supportive personnel by providing them with incentives for performance. Watson (1970) argued that, if behavior modification principles are to be applied in a residential setting, staff members up and down the organizational hierarchy must be reinforced for their efforts. Unfortunately, meaningful rewards are not always available to supportive personnel, as illustrated dramatically by the failure of many new careers programs to offer real opportunities for advancement toward professional status (Gartner, 1971).

One reward that is inexpensive and easily overlooked is knowledge of results. Prierton, Garms, and Metzger (1969) reported that attendants in a token economy cottage were highly rewarded by evidence of progress among the residents they trained. Beginning teachers have been reinforced by knowledge of their effectiveness in rewarding their students according to behavior management principles (Hall et al., 1968). In a variation on this theme, attendants can be motivated to compete with attendants in other cottages to conduct the most training sessions (Panyan, Boozer, and Morris, 1970).

Feedback regarding performance may be even more effective when it is coupled with other types of rewards. For example, Bricker, Morgan, and Grabowski (1972) offered attendants in a facility for for the mentally retarded commercial trading stamps as a reward for interacting with low functioning children. This inexpensive reward in itself was effective, but the researchers combined it with watching videotapes of attendant-resident interactions and feedback as to the behaviors that earned stamps. The combined program effectively increased the amount and quality of interaction and led to increases in behavioral teaching skills among a group of attendants selected for more intensive training.

Similar findings were reported in a residential unit for maladjusted children (Pommer and Streedbeck, 1974). Posting public notices listing tasks expected of child care aides was effective, but its impact wore off with time. Monetary rewards for performance of tasks raised staff performance to high levels again. The use of either token rewards or public notices, each used singly, improved performance above baseline, but the combination of the two was the most powerful strategy.

The combinations of feedback about performance and reward for performance even may explain the well known "Hawthorne effect," whereby workers (or students or subjects in experiments) seem to thrive in any innovative program or environment simply because it represents a change. According to a reinterpretation by Parsons (1974), workers in the original Hawthorne electrical plant experiments set goals for themselves and increased their production rates because they knew what their past performance was and they knew what monetary rewards they could expect for good performance.

The most logical way to design a reward system is to make rewards contingent on improvements in clients or residents. In a mental hospital, cash awards to psychiatric aides contingent on appropriate behavior by residents had a positive effect on resident behavior (Pomerleau, Bobrove, and Smith, 1973). This was not the case when the awards were independent of patient improvement. In this study, feedback to aides about patient improvement also produced gains among patients, as did direct supervision of patient-aide interactions. However, consultations with supervisors about patient progress were not effective. Thus, three strategies for maintaining high performance levels—reward, feedback, and direct supervision—were effective, but the more traditional tactic of holding periodic meetings was not.

A variety of rewards can have similar impacts on the performance of supportive personnel, including reinforcers that can be readily built in to any job. Parnicky and Ziegler (1964) found that most institutions for the retarded tie completion of training by attendants to salary increases or promotion. Time off from work—coupled with recognition and greater decision-making latitude—has been used to maintain attendant involvement in modifying the behavior of retarded children (Watson, Gardner, and Sanders, 1971). Direct-care staff even can be reinforced by being shown how teaching residents self-care skills and other behaviors makes their own jobs easier and less menial. The career ladder concept, if faithfully used, should reward paraprofessionals for increasing mastery of job functions. By far the most persuasive argument for the use of feedback and reinforcements in motivating supportive personnel is the simple fact that performance drops off sharply when such procedures are terminated (Pomerleau, Bobrove, and Smith, 1973; Pommer and Streedbeck, 1974). The great potential of supportive personnel in communication programming will be realized only to the extent that professionals use sound strategies of training, supervision, and motivation.

CONCLUSIONS AND FUTURE PROSPECTS

Supportive personnel—nonprofessionals who work under the direction of professionals— are a major resource in residential, school, and clinical settings if their energies are correctly channeled by professionals. Attendants and other residential care personnel, teacher aides and other paraprofessional workers, and volunteers constitute the major classes of supportive personnel, although the professional communication programmer also must work with professionals in related fields. Supportive personnel must be integrated in a coherent program in which the handicapped person's daily activities are coordinated and in which progress through a developmental sequence of programs is orderly. The "team" organizational model is more conducive than a hierarchical model to effective working relationships between professionals and supportive personnel.

Many supportive personnel, particularly direct-care staff in residential settings, have not fulfilled their potential for contributing to programming—because they lack educational background and competencies, because there is often a discrepancy between their understandings of their roles and professionals' concepts of their proper functions, and because their actual daily tasks consist more of menial maintenance and clerical work than of teaching or involvement with residents or students.

Research suggests, however, that supportive personnel can significantly improve program effectiveness. Supportive personnel are generally accepted by professionals after a period of initial skepticism; they benefit the professional by freeing his or her time for planning and work with clients; they themselves reap benefits in terms of new career goals and attainments; and most importantly, they produce positive changes in handicapped children and adults in a variety of programs and settings. In fact, supportive personnel with minimal training have, in some settings, proved to be at least as effective as professionals in working with clients and achieving positive outcomes. For the multiply handicapped, (e.g., hearing-impaired/mentally retarded persons), supportive personnel are essential in achieving proper use of hearing aids, applying communication approaches in daily activities, and providing well rounded training in self-care, mobility, communication, social behavior, and vocational development.

Training of supportive personnel has taken many forms, and several manuals and curricula for training personnel working with the multiply handicapped recently have been produced. Research suggests that the traditional lecture approach to training, while it may increase levels of knowledge, is not as effective as more practical training in changing the behavior of supportive personnel. In view of the background characteristics of supportive personnel, training that is carefully structured and that provides opportunities for skill rehearsal and feedback regarding performance is likely to be most effective. However, even the most sophisticated training techniques will have only a fleeting impact unless supportive personnel are supervised and offered incentives for their activities after training. Research indicates that high levels of performance are effectively maintained by the use of feedback regarding performance and progress and by the use of more tangible rewards, and are even more effectively maintained by the use of the two conjointly.

Three trends suggest that the role of supportive personnel will be strengthened in the future. The first is the increasingly critical element of fiscal and program accountability. Budgetary reviewers are likely to insist on the use of supportive personnel where it is demonstrated that nonprofessionals can perform as effectively as higher salaried professionals. Human services agencies increasingly will be required to use sound management principles in allocating staff resources, and cost-effective programming will require the use of supportive personnel.

A second trend is the movement toward performance-based criteria of certification, hiring, and advancement (Popham, 1971). Many observers have questioned strict reliance on the degree as the only criterion of competency and are searching for alternatives that place more emphasis on job performance. The career ladder design, if it is effectively implemented, should permit staff members who meet professional standards of performance to be certified and salaried as professionals without having to "put in time" at a college or university. Competency-based tests are difficult to design, and professional organizations may oppose such innovations where they see their self-interests jeopardized, but the concept of career ladders, still in the process of evolution, is unlikely to disappear.

Finally, the trend toward community-based services for the multiply handicapped also should be noted. Deinstitutionalization and the development of community alternatives are only parts of the process; agencies and organizations that serve discrete disability groups will be required to cooperate with one another to avoid duplication of services. The concept of developmental disabilities itself represents a trend toward interagency coordination of services in the community. The implication of this shift in service patterns is that a greater number and variety of supportive personnel will be needed to meet needs, and supportive personnel will have a greater role to play in bridging the gap between service agencies and target populations. One can expect to see more supportive personnel serving as houseparents and foster parents, home care aides, aftercare workers, and indigenous community relations personnel. As multiply handicapped persons leave institutions for the community, the task of coordinating the efforts of various supportive personnel and professionals will be more logistically complex than it was when all services were housed in a single residential setting. But institutions will not be without their own special challenges, particularly as they shift toward more "homelike" care and training. In either case, not only will efforts to recruit, train, and place supportive personnel need to be stepped up, but professional preparation programs eventually will have to face their responsibility to equip professionals with skills in mobilizing and supervising supportive personnel.

REFERENCES

Accreditation Council for Facilities for the Mentally Retarded. 1975. Standards for Residential Facilities for the Mentally Retarded. Joint Commission on Accreditation of Hospitals, Chicago.

Allen, B. J., and J. G. Foshee. 1966. Student Work Programs in Mental Retardation Facilities, 1966. Department of Special Education and Rehabilitation, Florida State University, Tallahassee.

Alpiner, J. G., J. A. Ogden, and J. E. Wiggins. 1970. The utilization of supportive personnel in speech correction in the public schools: A pilot project. Asha 12:599–604.

Baker, B. L., A. J. Brightman, L. J. Heifetz, and D. M. Murphy. 1973. The READ Project Series. Behavioral Education Projects, Cambridge, Mass.

Barrett, B. H., and J. E. McCormack. 1973. Varied teacher tutorials: A tactic for generating credible skills in severely retarded people. Ment. Retard. 11:14–19.

Bath, K. E., and S. A. Smith. 1974. An effective token economy program for mentally retarded adults. Ment. Retard. 12:41–44.

Beck, J., D. Kantor, and V. A. Gelineau. 1963. Follow-up study of chronic psychotic patients "treated" by college case-aide volunteers. Amer. J. Psychiatr. 120:269–271.

Beck, J., D. Kantor, and V. Gelineau. 1965. Impact of undergraduate volunteers on the social behavior of chronic psychotic patients. Int. J. Soc. Psychiatr. 11:96–104.

Bennett, W. S., Jr., and R. F. Falk. 1970. New Careers and Urban Schools. Holt, Rinehart and Winston, New York.

Bensberg, G. J. 1966. Job families in mental retardation. In The Community College in Mental Health Training: Report of a Conference to Explore the Role of the Community College in Training Mental Health Workers, April, 1966. Southern Regional Education Board, Atlanta.

Bensberg, G. J., and C. D. Barnett. 1966. Attendant Training in Southern Residential Facilities for the Mentally Retarded: Report of the SREB

Attendant Training Project. Southern Regional Education Board, Atlanta.

Bogdan, R., S. Taylor, B. deGrandpre, and S. Haynes. 1974. Let them eat programs: Attendants' perspectives and programming on wards in state schools. The Center on Human Policy, Syracuse University, Syracuse.

Boone, D. R. 1964. The use of volunteers in the speech pathology-audiology clinic in the medical setting. Asha 6(8):284–286.

Bowman, G. W., and G. J. Klopf. 1968. New Careers and Roles in the American School: A Study of Auxiliary Personnel in Education. Bank Street College of Education, New York.

Brannan, A. C., C. K. Sigelman, and G. J. Bensberg. 1975. The hearing impaired/mentally retarded: A survey of state institutions for the retarded. Monogr. 4, Research and Training Center in Mental Retardation, Texas Tech University, Lubbock.

Bricker, W. A., D. G. Morgan, and J. G. Grabowski. 1972. Development and maintenance of a behavior modification repertoire of cottage attendants through T.V. feedback. Amer. J. Ment. Defic. 77:128–136.

Brightman, A. J. 1975. Behavior modification in organization development. Toward planned change in five settings for retarded children. Unpublished doctoral dissertation, Harvard University, Cambridge, Mass.

Brighton, H. 1972. Utilizing Teacher Aides in Differentiated Staffing. Pendell, Midland, Mich.

Broberg, R. F. 1968. Guidelines for nurses working with hearing impaired children. Volta Rev. 70:552–558.

Butler, J. W., and R. T. Hanks. (undated). The utilization, training, and financial support of instructional para-professionals in the education of the deaf: A survey report. Southwest Regional Media Center for the Deaf, Las Cruces, N. Mex.

Butterfield, E. C. 1967a. The characteristics, selection, and training of institution personnel. In A. A. Baumeister (ed.), Mental Retardation: Appraisal, Education, and Rehabilitation. Aldine, Chicago.

Butterfield, E. C. 1967b. The role of environmental factors in the treatment of institutionalized mental retardates. In A. A. Baumeister (ed.), Mental Retardation: Appraisal, Education, and Rehabilitation. Aldine, Chicago.

Butterfield, E. C., C. D. Barnett, and G. J. Bensberg. 1966. Some objective characteristics of institutions for the mentally retarded: Implications for attendant turnover rate. Amer. J. Ment. Defic. 70:786–794.

Carkhuff, R. R. 1968. Differential functioning of lay and professional helpers. J. Coun. Psychol. 15:117–126.

Carkhuff, R. R., D. Kratochvil, and T. Friel. 1968. Effects of professional training on communication and discrimination of facilitative conditions. J. Coun. Psychol. 15:68–74.

Cortazzo, A. D., and K. H. Orkin. 1970. The mental retardation technician program at Miami-Dade Junior College. Ment. Retard. 8:7–11.

Craig, H. B. 1970. Reinforcing appropriate visual attending behavior in classes of deaf children. Amer. Ann. Deaf 115:481–491.

Cytryn, L., and A. Uihlein. 1965. Training of volunteers in the field of mental retardation: An experiment. Amer. J. Orthopsychiatr. 35: 493–499.

Dailey, W. F., G. J. Allen, J. M. Chinsky, and S. W. Veit. 1973. Attendant behavior and attitudes toward institutionalized retarded children. Amer. J. Ment. Defic. 78:586–591.

Dunn, L., J. Smith, and K. Horton. 1968. Peabody Language Development Kit. American Guidance Service, Circle Pines, Minn.

Eveslage, R. A., and A. V. Buchmann. 1973. The effect of consequences delivered contingent upon intelligible speech by deaf children. Amer. Ann. Deaf 118:446–453.

Fleming, J. W. 1962. The critical incident technique as an aid to in-service training. Amer. J. Ment. Defic. 67:41–52.

Freeman, S. W., and C. L. Thompson. 1973. Parent-child training for the mentally retarded. Ment. Retard. 11:8–10.

Gardner, J. M. 1972. Teaching behavior modification to nonprofessionals. J. Appl. Behav. Anal. 5:517–521.

Gartner, A. 1971. Paraprofessionals and Their Performance: A Survey of Education, Health, and Social Service Programs. Praeger, New York.

Glovsky, L., and C. Rigrodsky. 1963. A classroom program for auditorially handicapped, mentally deficient children. Train. School Bull. 60:56–69.

Griffing, B. L., and J. M. Huffman. 1969. Handbook for nursing personnel working with mentally retarded deaf minors. Sonoma State Hospital, Eldridge, Cal.

Guerney, L. 1974. Training parents in fostering skills: Program description and evaluation. Paper presented at the 82nd annual meeting of the American Psychological Association, August, New Orleans.

Hall, R. V., M. Panyan, D. Raborn, and M. Broden. 1968. Instructing beginning teachers in reinforcement procedures which improve classroom control. J. Appl. Behav. Anal. 1:312–322.

Hall, S. M., and L. W. Talkington. 1970. The use of resident aides in a speech and hearing program for the mentally retarded. Ment. Retard. 8:37–38.

Harris, J. M., S. W. Veit, B. J. Allen, and J. M. Chinsky. 1974. Aide-resident ratio and ward population density as mediators of social interaction. Amer. J. Ment. Defic. 79:320–326.

Haviland, R. T. 1972. A stimulus to language development: The institutional environment. Ment. Retard. 10(2):19–21.

Horton, K. B. 1974. Infant intervention and language learning. In R. L. Schiefelbusch and L. L. Lloyd (eds.), Language Perspectives—Acquisition, Retardation, and Intervention. University Park Press, Baltimore.

Jacobs, A. M., D. G. Nichols, and J. K. Larsen. 1969. Critical Behaviors in the Care of the Mentally Retarded. Vol. 2: Behavior of Attendants. American Institutes for Research, Pittsburgh.

Katkin, S., V. Zimmerman, J. Rosenthal, and M. Ginsburg. 1974. Development of a volunteer therapist after-care program: A progress report. Paper presented at the 82nd annual meeting of the American Psychological Association, August, New Orleans.

Klaber, M. M. 1969. The retarded and institutions for the retarded: A preliminary research report. In S. B. Sarason and J. Doris (eds.), Psychological Problems in Mental Deficiency. 4th Ed. Harper & Row, New York.

Kopchick, G., D. W. Rombach, and R. Smilowitz. 1975. A total communication environment in an institution. Ment. Retard. 13:22–23.

Lennan, R. K. 1973. The deaf multi-handicapped unit at the California School for the Deaf at Riverside. Amer. Ann. Deaf 118:439–445.

Lloyd, L. L., 1966. Helping your retarded patients with hearing impairments. J. Psychiat. Nurs. 4(3):255–259.

Lloyd, L. L., and B. P. Cox. 1972. Programming for the audiologic aspects of mental retardation. Ment. Retard. 10(2):22–26.

Ludtke, R. H., and A. Elliott. 1969. The changing role of volunteers in a residential facility for the mentally retarded. Ment. Retard. 7:13–16.

McCoy, D. F., and L. L. Lloyd. 1967. A hearing aid orientation program for mentally retarded children. Train. School Bull. 64:21–30.

Maloney, D. M. 1974. The use of instructions, feedback, and modeling to train the direct-care staff (teaching-parents) of group homes for disturbed youths. Western Carolina Center Papers and Reports 4(21), Morganton, N. Ca.

Mamula, R. A., and N. Newman. 1973. Community Placement of the Mentally Retarded: A Handbook for Community Agencies and Social Work Practitioners. Charles C Thomas, Springfield, Ill.

Marion County Association for Retarded Children. 1973. Curriculum Activities Guide for Severely Retarded Deaf Students. Marion County Association for Retarded Children, Indianapolis.

Mitra, S. 1971. Guidelines for hospitalized retarded-deaf children. Amer. Ann. Deaf 116:385–388.

Mitra, S. B. 1974. Language training for retarded-deaf children in a state institution. Train. School Bull. 71:41–48.

Moore, E. J., G. E. Miltenberger, and P. S. Barber. 1969. Hearing aid orientation in a state school for the mentally retarded. J. Speech Hear. Disord. 34:142–145.

Moores, D. F. 1974. Nonvocal systems of verbal behavior. In R. L. Schiefelbusch and L. L. Lloyd (eds.), Language Perspectives—Acquisition, Retardation, and Intervention. University Park Press, Baltimore.

Naiman, D. W. (ed.). 1972. Inservice training of afterclass staff in residential schools for deaf children. Deafness Research and Training Center, New York University, School of Education, New York.

Naiman, D. W., and H. S. Mashikian. 1973. Handbook for Staff Development in Residential Schools for Deaf Children. Deafness Research and Training Center, New York University, School of Education, New York.

Nash, K. B., and V. A. Mittlefehldt. 1975. Supervision and the emerging professional. Amer. J. Orthopsychiat. 45:93–101.

Nober, L. W. 1974. Hearing Impaired Formal In-service Program. University of Massachusetts, Northeast Regional Media Center for the Deaf (Grant OEG-O-73-0534-B, Bureau of Education for the Handicapped HEW), Amherst, Mass.

Osborne, J. G. 1970. Behavior modification with a deaf student: A case study. Psychol. Aspects Disabil. 17: 71–78.

Overbeck, D. 1971. Attitude sampling of institutional charge attendant personnel: Cues for intervention. Ment. Retard. 9(4):8–10.

Owens, M., and B. Harper. 1970. Sign Language: A Teaching Manual for Cottage Parents of Non-verbal Retardates. Pinecrest State School, Pineville, La.

Palmer, U. 1974. The value and training of the paraprofessional with the deaf. Paper presented at the meeting of the Texas Speech and Hearing Association, September, Forth Worth, Tex.

Panyan, M., H. Boozer, and N. Morris. 1970. Feedback to attendants as a reinforcer for applying operant techniques. J. Appl. Behav. Anal. 3:1–4.

Parnicky, J. J., and R. C. Ziegler. 1964. Attendant training: International survey. Ment. Retard. 2:76–82.

Parsons, H. M. 1974. What happened at Hawthorne? Science 183:922–932.

Paul, G. L. and T. L. McInnis. 1974. Attitudinal changes associated with two approaches to training mental health technicians in milieu and social-learning programs. J. Consult. Clin. Psychol. 42:21–23.

Paul, G. L., T. L. McInnis, and M. J. Mariotto. 1973. Objective performance outcomes associated with two approaches to training mental health technicians in milieu and social-learning programs. J. Abnorm. Psychol. 82:523–532.

Pomerleau, O. P., P. H. Bobrove, and R. H. Smith. 1973. Rewarding psychiatric aides for the behavioral improvement of assigned patients. J. Appl. Behav. Anal. 6:383–390.

Pommer, D. A., and D. Streedbeck. 1974. Motivating staff performance in an operant learning program for children. J. Appl. Behav. Anal. 7:217–221.

Pope, B., S. Nudler, M. R. Vonkorff, and J. P. McGhee. 1974. The experienced professional interviewer versus the complete novice. J. Consult. Clin. Psychol. 42:680–690.

Popham, J. W. 1971. Performance tests of teaching proficiency: Rationale, development, and validation. Amer. Educ. Res. J. 8:105–117.

Prierton, G., R. Garms, and R. Metzger. 1969. Practical problems encountered in an aide administered token reward cottage program. Ment. Retard. 7:40–43.

Reinherz, H. 1967. Professional supervision as a means of achieving volunteer program goals. In P. Ewalt (ed.), Volunteers in Mental Health. Charles C Thomas, Springfield, Ill.

Rettig, S. 1956. An investigation of behavior potentials of psychologists and supervisors toward the institutionalized patient. Amer. J. Ment. Defic. 60:714–720.

Rich, T. A., A. S. Gilmore, and C. F. Williams. 1964. Volunteer work with the mentally retarded. Rehab. Rec. 5(5):4–7.

Rieger, N. I., and A. G. De Vries. 1974. The child mental health specialist: A new profession. Amer. J. Orthopsychiatr. 44:150–158.

Rister, A. 1974. Training of Nonprofessionals in Early Childhood Education Centers. University of Texas at Austin Distinguished Staff Training Monograph Series, Vol. 1, no. 11 Austin, Tex. (Printed by Council for Exceptional Children, Handicapped Children in Head Start Series).

Scheerenberger, R. 1971. Management systems and styles in a residential facility for the mentally retarded. Ment. Retard. 9(5):22–24.

Schmidmayr, B., and W. Weld. 1971. Attitudes of institution employees toward resident oriented activities of aides. Amer. J. Ment. Defic. 76:1–4.

Shotwell, A. M., H. F. Dingman, and G. Tarjan. 1960. Need for improved criteria in evaluating job performance of state hospital employees. Amer. J. Ment. Defic. 65:208–213.

Simmons, A. A. 1964. Home demonstration teaching for parents and infants at Central Institute for the Deaf. In G. W. Fellendorf (ed.), Proceedings of International Conference on Oral Education of the Deaf. Vol. 2. Alexander Graham Bell Association for the Deaf, Washington, D.C.

Sutherland, G. F., and J. W. Beckett. 1969. Teaching the mentally retarded sign language. J. Rehab. Deaf 2:56–60.

Tarjan, G., A. M. Shotwell, and H. F. Dingman. 1955. A screening test for psychiatric technicians: A preliminary report on five years experience with the work assignment aid. Amer. J. Ment. Defic. 59:388–394.

Tharp, R. G., and R. J. Wetzel. 1969. Behavior Modification in the Natural Environment. Academic Press, New York.

Thormahlen, P. W. 1965. A study of on the ward training of trainable mentally retarded children in a state institution. California Mental Health Research Monogr. 5.

Thornhill, H. L., D. A. Ho Sang, D. Holmes, and A. D. Anderson. 1974. Rehabilitation in the ghetto. Department of Rehabilitation Medicine, Harlem Hospital Center, New York.

Truax, C. B., and J. L. Lister. 1970. Effectiveness of counselors and counselor aides. J. Coun. Psychol. 17:331–334.

Vernon, M. 1970. Potential, achievement and rehabilitation in the deaf population. Rehab. Lit. 31:258–267.

Viaille, H. D., and W. G. Hills. 1973. Management Practices in Vocational Rehabilitation District Offices. Regional Rehabilitation Research Institute, University of Oklahoma, Norman.

Vockell, K., E. L. Vockell, and P. Mattick. 1973. Language for mentally retarded deaf children: Project LIFE. Volta Rev. 75:431–439.

Warren, S. A., and L. W. Mondy. 1971. To what do attending adults respond? Amer. J. Ment. Defic. 75:449–455.

Watson, L. S., Jr. 1970. Behavior modification of residents and personnel in institutions for the mentally retarded. *In* A. A. Baumeister and E. Butterfield (eds.), Residential Facilities for the Mentally Retarded. Aldine, Chicago.

Watson, L. S., J. M. Gardner, and C. Sanders. 1971. Shaping and maintaining behavior modification skills in staff members in an MR institution: Columbus State Institute Behavior Modification Program. Ment. Retard. 9(3):39–42.

Watson, M. J., and J. L. Nicholas. 1973. A practical guide to the training of low-functioning deaf-blind children. Connecticut Institute for the Blind, Hartford.

Wills, R. H. 1973. The Institutionalized Severely Retarded: A Study of Activity and Interaction. Charles C Thomas, Springfield, Ill.

Wilson, P. S. 1974. Sign language as a means of communication for the mentally retarded. Paper presented at the meeting of the Eastern Psychological Association, April, Philadelphia.

Wolfensberger, W. 1972. Toward citizen advocacy for the handicapped, impaired, and disadvantaged: An overview. U.S. Department of Health, Education, and Welfare Publication no. (OS) 72-42.

Zeaman, D., and B. J. House. 1963. The role of attention in retardate discrimination learning. *In* N. Ellis (ed.), Handbook of Mental Deficiency. McGraw-Hill, New York.

17

PARENT INVOLVEMENT IN PROGRAMMING FOR DEVELOPMENTALLY DISABLED CHILDREN

Bruce L. Baker

CONTENTS

Roles and Responsibilities _____ 694

Parents as Teachers _____ 696

Models of Parent Training _____ 699
    Center-based individual training/699
    School-home individual training/701
    Home-based individual training/703
    Group training/706
    Training through media: the READ Project/708

Outcome: Empirical Basis _____ 710
    Does child change occur?/710
    Does change relate to intervention?/712
    Which aspects of training relate to change?/714

Parent Participation _____ 717
    Parent characteristics/717
    Siblings/719
    Child characteristics/720
    Trainer characteristics//21
    Program incentives/721

Conclusion _____ 724

Acknowledgments _____ 724

References _____ 725

Although parents of developmentally disabled children will appreciate the advances in knowledge described in this volume, their enthusiasm certainly must be tempered by the realization that professional knowledge is usually slow to translate into benefits attainable for their own children. The reality for parents is that, even when new learnings lead to new programs, these are often out of reach: *This toy-lending library is for another school district. . . . That infant screening program serves only a county upstate. . . . The local "demonstration" language program will not be refunded next year. . . . Other programs are filled up, for low income families only, too expensive, for older— or younger—children or for those with a slightly different label.* The dearth of effective, available, and continuing services is a desperately familiar reality to parents (see Greenfeld, 1970); access still depends on where one lives, whom one knows, how much money one has— and just plain luck.

Yet, however fragmented, the service delivery pattern is changing. After more than 100 years of separating the developmentally disabled from the mainstream of society, a reversal of trends is gaining force; the last two decades have seen increasing efforts to maintain and integrate these individuals in the community (Kugel and Wolfensberger, 1969; Wolfensberger, 1969). A guiding philosophy has been the principle of *normalization,* first voiced and implemented in the Scandinavian countries and then eagerly embraced in the United States. *Normalization* was delineated by Nirje (1969, p. 181) as: *"making available to the mentally retarded, patterns and conditions of everyday life which are as close as possible to the norms and patterns of mainstream society."*

The key notion is one of accepting developmentally disabled persons as an integral part of society, rather than seeking ways and means, however apparently well intentioned, to separate them from that society. When translated into practice, this philosophy calls for some accommodation on the part of individuals and social institutions to the needs of the developmentally disabled, as well as for teaching persons with developmental disabilities to adapt better to social institutions. The individual with greater adaptive skills quite likely will be more easily accepted into a community, and so the spirit of normalization calls for more broad-based learning opportunities. Yet even as a continuum of services begins to develop, providing resource rooms, sheltered workshops, teaching group homes, and the like, it becomes increasingly apparent that education, to be truly effective, must begin as early as possible. Parents cannot simply wait for this service continuum to emerge for their child because they themselves are in fact an integral part of that continuum, especially in the early years. The skills that children bring to their first school and their attitudes toward further learning are very much a product of parent teaching.

Too, meaningful progress toward an increase in available services, as well as their more equitable distribution, in large part depends on the development of more cost-effective approaches. As agencies search for ways to better use limited professional resources, parents have been "discovered" as a large, often motivated, and certainly inexpensive pool of potential teachers who, with proper training, can assume a more active role in their children's education. Indeed, it is the thesis of this chapter that the considered involvement of parents as partners in teaching their developmentally disabled children has a demonstrated promise that agencies concerned with early intervention and with cost effectiveness cannot afford to ignore.

ROLES AND RESPONSIBILITIES

The initial step in developing a program for parent involvement is to clarify objectives, to ask what changes are being sought. Would the program be judged successful if children learned additional skills? if institutionalization were prevented? if family interaction patterns changed? if parents provided useful information? if the attitudes or self-image of parents changed? if parents better understood the child's school program? if parents demanded changes in that school program? These aims are variously related to the particular role(s) implicitly ascribed to parents in the different involvements offered by agencies which serve their children.

For years a primary role for parents vis-à-vis service agencies was as *objects of study,* providers of information not only to clinicians about their developmentally disabled child but also to researchers about themselves—their own attitudes, feelings, and behavior. Emphasizing the demonstrated stresses of giving birth to and raising a handicapped child, most mental health agencies tended to view such parents as *patients,* in need of a therapeutic experience themselves. Parents' limited involvement in most special school programs has been only as informed, or more often uninformed, *spectators,* receiving just enough information about the methods being employed to be accepting of them.

Recently, though, parents have begun assuming more active roles. Many have become involved as *advocates* urging better services for their own and other children. Some school programs have welcomed parents as *volunteers,* thereby affording them both a concrete way to be helpful and the opportunity to enhance their own teaching skills. And, in the last 10 years or so, parents have been increasingly enlisted as *teachers,* with responsibilities ranging from carrying out a single program at home to learning comprehensive teaching principles and implementing a full, home-based program.

This chapter is written from the position that programs which seek only to study parents, counsel them, or generally educate them to no specific end, lack both proved effectiveness in what they aim to do and the vision to aim further. Hence, its selective focus is on programs that train parents to have an active involvement in teaching their own child. These programs tend to have a behavioral orientation and certainly have the most solid empirical basis. It is noteworthy that the role of *parents as teachers* may realize some of the aims inherent in the above roles as well. In research with families of young developmentally disabled children (Baker, Heifetz, and Brightman, 1973; Baker et al., 1975) there is some evidence, for instance, that parents trained in teaching methods feel more able to evaluate the quality of educational services that their children are receiving and are thereby prepared to be more influential advocates. Too, those parents who are able to intervene effectively on their children's behalf report enhanced self-confidence, decreased frustration, and other changes in attitudes usually sought in programs that view the parent as patient.

Conversely, though, Baker and his co-workers found that parents who had been previously involved in parent groups (in which they were most often viewed as observers, patients, or advocates) tended to develop *less well* as teachers of their own children than did parents who had had no previous group experience. Having accepted a definition of their involvement on behalf of their child in passive, self-centered, or political terms, parents seem less likely to manifest involvement in active teaching. In fact, the extent to which parents accept some responsibility for actively teaching their handicapped child emerges as a critical predictor of training program success.

The prevalent belief that any real responsibility for the child's education rests almost exclusively with agencies is not surprising. The medical or impairment model thrives around developmentally disabled children; many families soon come to accept their child's problem as too complex for them to understand and thus view the responsibility for helping to reside elsewhere. Letting go of some of the pervasive professional mystique and seeing parents as genuine co-workers is difficult for many professionals and parents alike; when both have dared such involvement, however, the results have been heartening.

PARENTS AS TEACHERS

The parents who accept responsibility for teaching their developmentally disabled child are still faced with some very real barriers. In addition to the conflicts with other home roles and responsibilities are the same difficulties that face the child's teachers: There is not one isolated and obvious target problem, but a plethora of deficiencies and often no clear starting place. Skills must be simplified and then simplified yet further, while motivating the child to perform the task usually requires imagination and persistence. With multiply handicapped children this problem of finding effective incentives is compounded. For example, Mira and Hoffman (1974), working with deaf-blind children, noted the frequent failure of social, and even food, consequences to motivate performance. Indeed, the most effective reinforcement proved to be allowing the child to engage in stereotyped behavior—the very interfering behavior which teachers were seeking to eliminate! Similarly, the use of firm contingencies and punishment, difficult with any child, is often especially problematic for handicapped children's parents and teachers, who are apt to indulge these children in ways they would not treat a nonhandicapped child, with predictable consequences in unmanageable behavior. With hearing-impaired children, the limited effectiveness of verbal control is additionally disconcerting for parents, often necessitating a reorientation toward modeling and physical guidance that requires a more conscious, patient, and well planned effort. And finally, of course, learning for the developmentally disabled child comes slowly.

Yet parents do have the advantage of usually being very reinforcing to their child and therefore ideal teachers (Tharp and Wetzel, 1969). In fact, Schopler and Reichler (1971) reported that trained parents obtained better responsiveness from their autistic children in teaching sessions than did professionals. Hence, despite the above concerns, the research literature already describes an impressive array of behaviors that have been successfully modified at home by parents of developmentally disabled children (Berkowitz and Graziano, 1972; Johnson and Katz, 1973). Behavior problems are often foremost in parent priorities, as these are usually disruptive, sometimes dangerous, and almost always obstructive of other skill learning. Examples of the many behavior problems successfully diminished by parents of severely disturbed or retarded children include a child's refusal to wear eye-glasses despite gradual loss of vision (Wolf, Risley, and Mees, 1964); an autistic girl's repeated dangerous climbing (Risley, 1968); and a 3-year-old's constant crying, screaming, aggression, and biting him-self (Peine, 1969). Among the few reports of behavior problem man-agement by parents of hearing-impaired children are a mother's co-teaching with two therapists to decrease her toddler's screaming and increase attention to an auditory task (Gerrard and Saxon, 1973) and programs to reduce the common problems of running away from an adult (Mira, 1970), refusal to wear a hearing aid, and looking away from a speaker's lips (Hoover, 1970). These programs have usually involved systematically altering the consequences of problem behavior (by removing reinforcement—e.g., ignoring—or by punishment) and have simultaneously involved the teaching of more acceptable be-havior patterns. Even seizure disorders have been reduced by parent programming (Gardner, 1967; Zlutnick, Mayville, and Moffat, 1975), dramatically demonstrating the considerable power of parent attention in maintaing and modifying troublesome child behavior.

Similarly, parents have carried out planned programs to build skills in areas of cognition, communication, motor performance, social interaction, and self-help. This teaching has usually involved parents' setting aside a fixed teaching time, presenting tasks to the child in a carefully graduated manner, and providing reinforcements for appro-priate performance. Communication programming is a good example and has an especially strong rationale. Because language development takes place in the years of infancy and early childhood, and because language skills are so central to the development of other abilities, communication programming for the developmentally disabled child must begin as early as possible. Although early programming need not mean exclusively home programming, it certainly should include the child's home. There is ample evidence that the development of child language relates to both the amount and quality of parent stimu-lation, and, while simple enrichment of a child's environment will likely have benefits, contingent stimulation seems yet more effective (Horowitz, 1968; Hursh and Sherman, 1973; Simeonsson and Wiegerink, 1974).

Much parent training has been based on recent work aimed at applying learning theory in the development of speech and language skills, especially with nonverbal or minimally verbal children (see reviews by Hartung, 1970, and Garcia and DeHaven, 1974). Usually there are two major phases to training: 1) developing imitative verbal, and perhaps motor, behavior (Peterson, 1968; Schroeder and Baer, 1972), and 2) teaching functional and spontaneous speech, generalized to a number of persons and places (Sloane, Johnston, and Harris, 1968). Examples of specific programs for parent teaching of speech and language include: increasing the intelligibility of speech in a brain-injured child (Pascal, 1973), increasing naming vocabulary and decreasing stereotyped chanting in a 6-year-old echolalic child (Risley and Wolf, 1966), and increasing receptive vocabulary in a 6-year-old blind, nonambulatory child (Watson and Bassinger, 1974). Preschool retarded children have been systematically taught to increase their imitation of movements, sounds, and words (Allen and Harris, 1964; Freeman and Thompson, 1973) while programs developed by Lovaas (1966), Risley and Wolf (1966), and MacDonald et al. (1974) build from these basic skills to longer utterances and a wider range of language forms (labels, mands, verbs, prepositions, pronouns, etc.)

The next section considers five models for training parents as teachers, models that vary both in format (individual, groups, media) and training site (center, school, home). Rather detailed examples are given for each model, to help the reader who might be interested in instituting a parent training program consider which of these models is best suited to the requirements of his or her own setting. Although the choice of a particular model often depends mainly on factors such as the service provider's preferred way of working, the orientation of the service agency, and the realities of funding, the evidence for whether a model is effective should have some bearing. Hence, the next section describing models is followed by a section on training outcome. It should be noted at the outset that some parent training programs (Bricker and Bricker, 1976) hold that no one model, regardless of its general effectiveness, can best serve every family and that to be truly helpful to parents an agency must provide several options of training format and be flexible as regards content.

MODELS OF PARENT TRAINING

Center-based Individual Training

Infant Programs   Programs for handicapped infants customarily are center based. A fairly consistent assumption in infant programs is that parents need guidance in dealing with their feelings toward themselves and their child and need education for more realistic acceptance of the infant's disability (Northcott, 1967, 1971). Beyond this, however, some programs aim to train parents to increase certain infant skills. Parents are scheduled for periodic visits with the infant, to raise questions about the infant's development and, through discussion with and modeling by staff, to learn ways to interact more effectively with the infant. An example of such a program is the Model Preschool Center for Handicapped Children in the Experimental Education Unit at the University of Washington (Hayden, 1974; Hayden and Haring, 1976). In this special program for parents of Down's syndrome infants, weekly clinic visits may begin as early as 5 weeks of age, continuing to 18 months. These 30-minute sessions focus on early motor and cognitive development, with heavy emphasis on visual and sound stimulation. As the infant grows older, self-help training is begun. Weekly goals and in-home teaching procedures are established with the mother, and progress is reviewed at the next visit. Parents often stay after their own appointment to observe a similar session being held with another parent (through a one-way mirror, with the other parent's permission) or to observe the clinic preschool classrooms. Hayden and Haring (1976) reported that, after participation in the program, infants with Down's syndrome perform very close to age norms on the Gesell Preliminary Behavior Inventory, although the authors did not include the necessary controls in their evaluation to ensure that the observed gains are attributable to the program.

Hayden (1974) argued that the individualized aspect of the center-based program best meets the parents' needs during the child's infancy, pointing out that a parent training group could not anticipate and respond adequately to individual needs. The prevalent feelings of loss and guilt, coupled with some hesitancy and inadequacy in handling and stimulating the child, are thought to be best dealt with on an individual basis. However, the opportunities within this program for parents to interact with and observe other parents seem likely to be important as well, in reducing the desperate feeling of isolation usually experienced by parents of handicapped infants.

Programs for Older Children   Reports of center-based training for families of older children tend to concentrate, at least initially, on the management of specific behavior problems. Much of the early experimental study of parents training utilized this model because data could be more readily gathered in the clinic setting. In practice, this model best suits agencies where one or several staff members wish to train parents, but where the agency as a whole has not committed itself to broader training responsibilities. After observing mother-child interactions, the clinic staff member typically instructs the mother in more effective ways to interact, often rehearsing these with her, modeling them for her and/or providing her with critical feedback that sometimes may include the review of videotaped sessions (Bernal, 1969).

An example of a brief center-based training program mainly relying on didactic instruction is reported by Allen and Harris (1966). Five-year-old Fay's excessive scratching for over a year had resulted in large sores and scabs on her forehead, nose, cheeks, chin, and one arm and leg. "The mother declared that she had come to dislike the child so intensely and to be so repelled by her appearance that she felt it might be better if Fay were placed outside the home to live" (p. 80). Indeed, clinic observations revealed that Fay's mother "spoke to the child only to criticize, direct or explain why the child should behave in a different fashion" (p. 80). During seven clinic sessions with Fay's mother a home program was developed and monitored. The primary elements were the ignoring of scratching and the reinforcing of scratch-free periods with gold stars exchangeable for inexpensive trinkets and shopping trips.

Scratching diminished sharply, the extrinsic reinforcers were gradually phased out, and, at a 4-month follow-up, the scars were barely discernible. This case, like many, analyzed and redirected parent attention while also employing extrinsic reinforcers. However, the clinic training was brief and focused on a single problem; it did not really educate the parent in the principles of effective teaching.

A somewhat more complete center-based program was reported by Forehand, Cheney, and Yoder (1974) for 7-year-old John, who demonstrated a 70-dB hearing loss (1969 ANSI) (30 dB aided) in both ears. John's targeted problem was noncompliance. He often would respond by running away from his mother, throwing a tantrum, or turning aside and acting as if he did not hear her request. Thirteen brief training sessions helped John's mother to reinforce desired behavior selectively and to establish compliance. She was taught by direct instructions, modeling, role playing, and ongoing feedback from a trainer located behind a one-way mirror (through a "bug in the ear" auditory receiver, Welsh, 1966). Improvement was maintained at a 3-month follow-up, and as in Fay's case, a questionnaire indicated that mother's attitudes toward John were much improved.

As problem behavior is brought under control in the structured clinic setting, skill teaching can be initiated, with parents observing, practicing, and then carrying the program back into the home (Gardner et al., 1968; Schopler and Reichler, 1971). For example, Gerrard and Saxon (1973) reported a clinic-based program to increase sitting and attending in a severely hearing-impaired child, in preparation for auditory training. A speech pathologist, psychologist, and the child's mother worked together, interchanging roles of teacher, observer-recorder, and signaler (cuing when to give reinforcement). In this type of approach the initial difficulties in teaching are minimized by help in the center, and the teaching situation can be arranged so that parents quickly experience success.

Center-based training is the easiest model to implement, and there is evidence for its effectiveness. However, it is a costly model, especially if it is expanded into a broader program with home visits or group sessions, as is often deemed necessary (Terdal and Buell, 1969; Freeman and Thompson, 1973). This model also can be quite inappropriate if it is implemented in isolation from the child's school program—as is too often the case.

School-Home Individual Training

An increasing number of school programs for developmentally disabled children are realizing the importance of supplementary family programming. For some learning, home and school cooperation is essential (e.g., toilet training) and for most learning it is certainly desirable (e.g., language). There are certain skills that might be best taught at home (e.g., self-help), thereby freeing school time for other teaching. It is a source of considerable frustration for the competent teacher to see skills painstakingly taught at school not encouraged at home (and, as more parents learn to be effective teachers, they too despair about school programs that fail to follow through on their efforts).

School-based parent training differs in several respects from other models. Parent training must be added into an already busy teacher schedule, and, as the school maintains its involvement with the children and their families for at least 1 year, training must be arranged as more than a brief series of meetings. But the school has the enormous advantage of working with the child daily and hence being in a good position to train parents: to offer suggestions, to choose among various teaching objectives, to model techniques, to videotape the child's behavior for viewing by parents, and to bring the parent into the classroom as an aide.

An interesting example of the school-home model is the "Lunch Box Data System" operated by Teaching Research in Monmouth, Oregon (Fredericks, Baldwin, and Grove, 1974; Fredericks et al., in press), in a school for children with all handicapping conditions. Parents in this system are asked to carry out a teaching program at home for 10 to 30 minutes daily, and data suggest that this will almost double the rate of acquisition of a skill also being taught at school. In an individual conference, parents select a skill and the teacher models the program; the parent is then asked to try, and the session is videotaped for subsequent review and discussion. The key to continuing communication is a data sheet, carried between school and home by the child. Each day the teacher indicates the step worked on at school and the number of lessons, while the parent similarly records the program at home. Every 3 to 4 weeks a parent conference reviews the program. Hence, with very little staff supervision, those parents who so choose become meaningfully involved in their child's program (about 60% of parents).

Another type of school-based training program is that offered by the time-limited, intensive residential program such as a therapeutic summer camp, 30-day respite care or a live-in school for parents and child (Jelinek and Schaub, 1973). Although still rare, these programs can offer unique training opportunities because staff are able to get to know a child throughout all aspects of daily routine. For instance, Camp Freedom, a 7-week residential program in Center Ossipee, New Hampshire, serves school-age developmentally disabled children with behavior problems (Baker, 1973a, b; Brightman, 1972, 1973). Participating families seek not only performance gains in their children but also some respite for themselves, together with strategies for post-camp programming at home. During camp, parents live in for a weekend of observation and supervised teaching. They have already learned general behavior modification principles through group meetings and readings before camp, and they continue to meet every 3 weeks or so after camp, to discuss home programming and receive further instruction. But while at camp, parents are active participants as teachers in skill-building programs that are already underway.

This involvement is particularly important because at camp parents often see dramatically what can be done for and by their child. When they are only involved as observers they tend to exalt the capabilities of the camp staff and feel even more demoralized about their own. Self-confidence can be enhanced, though, by having parents participate in classes, with successes assured by the back-up supervision of the camp staff and the controls effected by contingencies already operating in the camp program. An in-home program begun after: 1) a summer respite, 2) some programming practice, and 3) the initial modification of target behaviors, is much easier to execute and more likely to succeed.

Home-based Individual Training

Although regular home visiting is the most costly parent training model in general practice, many feel that such individual contact in the child's natural environment has sufficient advantage to justify it (McCroskey, 1967; Fraiberg, 1971). Some programs begin with weekly or less frequent visits up until about 18 months, when the child enters a clinic-based program and the parents join a clinic-sponsored group (Jew, 1974). Other programs use home visits in addition to ongoing preschool programs for the child, or even in lieu of such programs (Shearer, 1974). In justifying home visit programs, it is noted that: 1) parents learn best through direct modeling and supervision in the setting where they are going to teach; 2) trainers can instruct better because they are more aware of in-home practices, obstacles, and the like; and finally 3) participation by the teaching parent and other family members is increased by eliminating long travel and providing a personal relationship with the trainer. Unfortunately, though, most home visits are scheduled at times when only the mother can be home, thereby not fulfilling the opportunities for fuller family involvement promised by this model.

Home Visiting Programs   Perhaps the most systematic and long-term home visiting program is the Portage Project, serving 150 handicapped children between birth and 6 years, in a 3600 square mile area in south-central rural Wisconsin (Shearer, 1974; Shearer and Shearer, 1972, 1976). A unique aspect of the project is its sole reliance on parents as teachers—there is no classroom program—

both for the reasons cited above and because it costs less than one-half of what a classroom program would cost.

A home teacher visits each of 15 families for 1.5 hours each week to: 1) assess the child's performance on behaviors targeted for in-home teaching during the previous week; 2) select two to four steps to be taught the next week, and 3) model the appropriate teaching techniques. The parent then tries out the teaching program under supervision and continues to implement it (usually 30 minutes a day or less) throughout the week, recording the child's behavior on an activity sheet prepared by the home teacher. Each activity sheet contains a prescription for the specific behavioral objective to be taught (e.g., *Billy will name pictures using three word phrases*), directions for presenting the task, and a procedure for recording progress. Such individualized planning is facilitated by an Early Childhood Curriculum Guide (Shearer et al., 1972) consisting of: 1) Developmental Sequence Checklist, listing 450 behaviors in five areas: language, self-help, cognition, motor, and social development; and 2) Curriculum Cards, using behavioral objectives to describe each of the 450 skills and suggesting teaching methods. With these aids, the home teacher still must break down each skill into finer components so that the parents are able to teach a substep to mastery in 1 week. In 1 year, the average family successfully taught 91% of 128 such prescriptions.

The Portage Project seems especially exportable; it has clear procedures, limited goals, packaged curriculum guides, and lower cost than classroom programs. In fact, compared with a group of children in a classroom program, the Portage children showed significantly greater gains in measured intelligence, language, academic, and socialization skills (Shearer and Shearer, 1972). The model already has been replicated in at least nine agencies, annually serving a total of over 500 children.

The combined research-intervention program for blind infants reported by Fraiberg (Fraiberg, Smith, and Adelson, 1969; Fraiberg, 1971) is another impressive demonstration of the value of home visits. The bimonthly visits over a period of years sought developmental data specific to this handicap and, in turn, used these observations to increase parents' understanding, expectations, and skills, through specific developmental information and modeling. Clinical evidence suggested that blindness was an impediment to development in three central areas, and therefore stress was placed on helping parents understand the expression of human object relations in the absence of vision, the use of hands to receive information, and locomotor functioning. Some home-visiting programs are less extensive and are aimed more at supplementing other approaches: helping to motivate the parent, assessing the contingencies operative at home, or monitoring the parent's application of methods learned elsewhere. Most trainers feel that their own effectiveness is enhanced when they have even a cursory observation of the home situation to inform their consultation.

Simulated Home Programs   A simulated home program, while not widely utilized, is an interesting combination of the strengths of center-based and home-based models. The parent(s) and child may live together in the simulated setting for a period of training or visit there on a regular basis. The center-based advantages of having programming equipment and ancillary services available and of eliminating staff travel are preserved, while the home-based advantages of more natural interactions, a greater range of potential activities, and smoother generalization are realized as well. Wiltz and Gordon (1974) reported a brief live-in training program for a family with an extremely disruptive 9-year-old boy, diagnosed "childhood schizophrenia." For 5 days the family lived in a three-bedroom laboratory-apartment that was equipped with microphones and one-way mirrors. After several days of baseline observations, a behavior management program was instituted with ongoing feedback to parents from the staff. The parents were reported to have carried over the program very well from this brave-new-worldish environment to their own home, with a significant reduction of problem behavior.

The few reported simulated home programs, however, are almost exclusively for infants and preschool children with severe hearing loss (e.g., John Tracy Clinic, Los Angeles; Central Institute for the Deaf, St. Louis (Simmons, 1967); University of Kansas Medical Center). One such program, the Mama Lere Parent Teaching Home, has been in operation since 1966 at the Bill Wilkerson Hearing and Speech Center in Nashville, Tennessee (Knox and McConnell, 1968; Horton and McConnell, 1970; Horton and Sitton, 1970; McConnell, 1970, 1974; Horton, 1974). This is a comfortably furnished house on a residential street. Mother and child customarily visit the home weekly to engage with a teacher-counselor in many routine tasks of daily living (e.g., preparing lunch, making beds, bathing, and dressing the child) and to discover ways to stimulate the child's interest in speech and environmental sounds during these activities. Concentrating on the development of the child's residual hearing, the program sets teaching objectives that include the following (Horton and McConnell, 1970):

1.   To orient the parents to a more insightful analysis of their own auditory environment and, through parents, to orient the child to the world of sounds; for example, parents are helped to make lists of sounds in the home environment and then are shown how to (over-) react visibly to them, consistently associating all sounds with their sources (e.g., running with the child to the window to see a car that has just screeched its brakes)

2.   To assist the parents in helping their child make a successful adjustment to daily, full-time use of individual hearing aids, preferably binaural; the program loans a range of hearing aids until the audiologist determines the one most appropriate for the child[1]

3.   To teach the parents how best to talk with their child (see *39 Rules of Talking;* Lillie, 1972; *Rules of Talking* (Bill Wilkerson Hearing and Speech Center), 1974; and Appendix E). The teacher models consistent and appropriate use of short, simple sentences and phrases that relate to subjects, that have demonstrable referents in the present environment, and that have high interest value and meaning to the child (*That car stopped. It made a big noise. Now it's ready to go. See the car go.*)

The parent is encouraged to incorporate teaching into the whole daily routine rather than to set aside a given time for formal language teaching each day. The success of this program is demonstrated in heightened level of awareness for speech and improved language competency, relative both to expected gains in a given time period and to equally handicapped children who did not receive early programming (Horton, 1974; McConnell, 1974).

Group Training

The models presented thus far involve individual training. Many clinicians, however, have always preferred to work with parents in groups,

---

[1]For parents of hearing-impaired children, the hearing aid itself is a good focus for early individual or group consultation. The program can give parents concrete information about maintenance of the device and about progressively shaping the child to longer periods of use. By following through on the specific instructions regarding the hearing aid, the parent has already begun to be meaningfully involved in the child's program and has set the stage for further teaching. For a further discussion of this critical area of parental involvement for hearing-impaired children, the reader is referred to the chapters by Cox and Lloyd (this volume) and Ross (this volume).

although the approaches of parent group counseling and parent group education (Auerbach, 1968; Beck, 1973) are focused almost entirely on changing parent *attitudes* and, despite their popularity in the mental health culture, have done so with little demonstrated effectiveness (see Brim, 1965). Increased interest in parent groups has been sparked by the recent successes of these individual models that trained parents to change their *behavior* vis-à-vis their handicapped children. If parents could learn teaching methods just as well in groups, there should be considerable cost savings and hence more families served with the same limited resources. Group parent training offers other advantages: Parents can derive peer support and encouragement for their own teaching efforts as well as information from others in the group about their child-rearing practices and about available services. A group format also makes more feasible a structured curriculum utilizing films, tapes, modeling, role playing, group problem solving, and mini-lectures; some of these would be impossible in one-to-one training, others possible but cumbersome.

Group training may take place independent of the child's school program or may be conducted by school personnel and integrated with the classroom program, perhaps involving the parent in regular observation of or teaching in the classroom. Some school-related groups place few demands on parents, perhaps meeting only monthly and mainly encouraging carryover of a specific school program. Other groups, though, aim to instruct parents in broader teaching principles and to prepare them to develop and carry out their own programs (Walder et al., 1969; Baker, Heifetz, and Brightman, 1973; Bricker and Bricker, 1976). Although there is considerable variability, groups are apt to include two leaders and from three to 10 participating families, and they typically meet biweekly for six to 20 sessions. Meetings usually last 1.5 to 3 hours, with time alloted for introduction of new content as well as for feedback to parents about their teaching efforts.

An example of a very comprehensive (and operationally very expensive) group training procedure is Kozloff's (1974) program in Boston for families of autistic children. Groups of four families met for 16 weekly 3-hour sessions, supplemented by weekly 2-hour, in-home supervisory visits. During the group meetings, each family described its home teaching for the week, critiqued it, asked for suggestions, and discussed possible changes for the ensuing week. Videotape made during the weekly visit was shown to elicit feedback from, and to serve as modeling for, the other families. Each week a unit of written material was assigned and discussed at the next meeting; teaching methods involved in the unit were first demonstrated by staff and then role played by parents. Finally, each family was consulted individually by a staff member.

The Infant, Toddler, and Preschool Research and Intervention Project at George Peabody College in Nashville (Bricker and Bricker, 1973, 1976) combined the group model with components of both the clinic and school-related models. Each of the groups focuses on *one* of four skill areas (language, cognition, motor, and social development), and mothers are often involved in two groups (areas) simultaneously. The unique behavior management group reflects the composition of the classroom program, which involves equal numbers of handicapped and nonhandicapped children. The language group meets weekly and uses the first half-hour for discussing general classroom procedures, with media aids. Mothers are then subdivided, according to the developmental level of their child, into three smaller groups: function/receptive, imitation/expressive, and syntax—the target training areas of the child's classroom language programs. Mothers learn to conduct home training sessions by working with their own children and are supervised with the aid of videotape feedback.

Group training is discussed further in the *Outcome* section below, since most controlled research on training utilizes this model. Group training particularly lends itself to research because a relatively large sample of families can be studied, the involvement is time limited, and the curriculum is defined and thus amenable to controlled modification.

Training through Media: The READ Project

Almost all parent training programs make some use of media: commercially available films and center-produced videotapes (see Brightman, Baker, and Delphin, 1975: "Filmography"), audio or video feedback of teaching sessions, published "how to" books, center-prepared handouts. Recently, films and tapes have been developed specifically for use in parent training (see Benchmark Films: "Child Behavior Equals You;" Prentice-Hall: "Help for Mark;" Baker, Brightman, and Blatt, 1973: "Parents as Teachers Series"). The starred references at the end of this chapter indicate some useful media supports.[2] Yet there have been virtually no studies of the

---

[2]For additional information on audiovisual media, the reader is also referred to the chapter by Striefel, Baer, and Douglass (this volume) and to Appendices D and E.

marginal advantage of media inputs and few attempts to train parents exclusively through media (Latham, 1972; Morreau, 1972).

This is unfortunate, because the development of media packages, either as supplement to, or substitute for, other parent training models seems a worthwhile undertaking for professionals. In the author's own service programs, many of the parent training variations already discussed have been employed, but there was always the nagging concern that so few families could be included under these formats. Hence, in initiating the READ project, the author and his co-workers set out to package into self-instructional manuals those principles and guidelines that had proved useful to parents of retarded children in previous training. The aim was to produce manuals that would be informative, enjoyable to read, respectful of parental concerns, and, at the same time, directive and flexible.

The resultant *Series* (Baker et al., 1972, 1973, 1976; Baker and Heifetz, 1976) contains an Assessment Manual and 10 skill-teaching manuals in the areas of self-help, speech and language, play skills, and behavior problem management. Each manual is aimed at a particular skill area and functioning level, with general teaching strategies and specific program guidelines. Programs were carefully developed through repeated pilot testing, but are still meant to be simply guidelines.

The manuals are self-contained, so that parents with the appropriate manual (e.g., *Beginning Speech*) can pinpoint behaviors to be changed, develop a daily "lesson plan," and teach, using the skills they already have for relating to and helping the child, combined with simple teaching practices. Initial evaluation with the self-help manuals indicates that many families appreciate having useful information given them in this way and can use the manuals very well, especially if there is some eventual accountability to research or service personnel. In fact, child skill gains may be as great when parents have just manuals as teaching guides as when they have more extensive professional supervision (Baker, Heifetz, and Brightman, 1973; Baker and Heifetz, 1976), an unexpected finding discussed further below. Packaging training inputs in this way provides a more standardized means of evaluating the relative contributions of various inputs to program outcome.

The assessment of outcome—of what immediate and lasting effects training by any of these models provides—is a surprisingly complex and problematic area. As discussed next, even programs that rest on the best experimental evidence available must still rest as much on faith.

OUTCOME: EMPIRICAL BASIS

Most reports of parent training have been marked by a lack of scientific rigor. Perhaps there has been some advantage in observing parents as teachers with an eye unrestricted by methodologic blinders. And to be sure, the more recent behaviorally oriented programs such as those emphasized in this chapter are an enormous improvement in methodologic sophistication over earlier approaches. Yet the number of shortcomings in available studies compel one to temper the highly successful reports of outcome. For example, research reports of parent training programs have usually concerned but one or a small number of selected families with generally good motivation for training and limited treatment objectives. Although there are many ongoing service projects that involve larger numbers of families for a longer period and with broader training objectives, these typically have not contributed to the empirical literature. Reports that do exist often lack appropriate control procedures, leaving one unsure about how to interpret reported changes. Hence, one must be cautious about generalizing from available studies to the population of families as a whole. The success and shortcomings of research are considered here as they relate to several questions about the effects of parent training.

Does Child Change Occur?

Almost all published reports indicate positive change, but there are measurement problems that leave some doubts. Often, reports present little evidence of effectiveness other than the parents' global statements of child improvement, and these should be considered somewhat suspect. Walter (1971) for example, found that parents consistently answered "yes" to: "Has your child improved?," regardless of whether behavioral observation had indicated a decrease or an increase in targeted child problem behavior. Parent recording of the frequency or duration of discrete events seems to be more accurate, but any such measures in the privacy of the home call for some independent corroboration. Some investigators have placed observers in the home for periods of time, but one wonders whether the dubious gains in objectivity (from observers who often know what changes are demanded by the design) are offset by the unnaturalness of the situation and the questionable utility of in-home observers on a broad scale. Parent-recorded measures have obvious advantages if they can be shown to be accurate.

The assessment of change in excess behavior problems is more difficult than in deficient skills. Problem behaviors are generally not present all of the time, and require well specified and sometimes continuous measures. Too, they are more apt to vary situationally and, therefore, be influenced by the demands read by parents and child alike into the observer's presence. For example, Johnson and Lobitz (1974) have demonstrated how parents can produce greater problem behaviors in their child at will (mainly by increasing the intensity of their demands) and hence perhaps distort comparisons from pretraining (where parents claim high problem behavior) to posttraining (where parents wish to demonstrate improvements). One creative attempt to reduce the potential bias in reaction to an observer was by Bernal et al. (1971), who placed in the home a timer-operated tape recorder, which quietly turned on and registered interactions at random periods throughout the day. It remains to be seen, though, how many families would tolerate such an obvious intrusion into their privacy.

Skill deficiencies, on the other hand, are more stable, and skill level can be accurately assessed in a more limited and structured measurement period. If a checklist is sufficiently detailed, parents can report highly accurate information about their child's skill level. For example, in the READ Project (described above) parents were given a scale of 43 self-help skills, each divided into five to eight steps; a comparison of professional in-home observers' scores with parents' scores yielded very high agreement. Too, when targeting skill deficiencies, periodic progress measures can be taken by the trainer during weekly home visits or during visits to the center.

A different problem with much evaluation of group training is that the measure chosen for assessment of the whole group is not really a valid measure of the particular behaviors being programmed, and hence the intervention appears misleadingly *in*effective. For example, a standardized intelligence test might be used to assess progress, when parents are, in fact, targeting self-help or communication skills (e.g., Doernberg, 1971).

Two remaining issues related to change that are critically important but minimally studied are the *generalization of changes across settings* and the *maintenance of change over time.* The need to intentionally program for generalization is considered in many of the above models because parents are helped to carryover the program into their own home. There is usually good carryover of child change from center or school training into the home when parents make an effort to maintain the program (Schwenn, 1971; Wiltz and Gordon, 1974).

Naturally occurring generalization (and maintenance) may be greater for skills acquired than for behavior problems reduced, and some evidence supports this contention (Schwenn, 1971; Ferber, Kelley, and Shemberg, 1974). Specific skills bring a modicum of external reinforcement in most settings and afford some degree of intrinsic reinforcement; hence, a child who learns to dress or tell time or speak more clearly is likely to continue these skills unless the contingencies at home are very contrary. Behavior problems are apt to be much more situation specific because different settings encourage different coping behaviors, and children develop a repertoire from which to draw as they assess the opportunities and anticipated effects in a given situation.

Controlled follow-up studies are rare because authors do not want to keep families in a no-training condition for a long period. The few case reports of follow-up generally find child progress in specific targeted behaviors maintained, although reports of larger samples are more likely to find a proportion of relapse (Lovibond, 1964; Patterson, 1974). Also, without continuing staff intervention, parents do not typically continue to program new behaviors as one might wish. In a 1-year follow-up of the READ Project (see below) most formal teaching and data recording dropped out rather soon, although in many cases parents did continue to teach better than before in informal ways (Baker et al., 1975). Some trainers have found more successful formal parent followthrough when expectations were well structured and periodic individual or group consultation was available (Kozloff, 1974; MacDonald et al., 1974). It is likely that studies soon will begin to examine the critical question of follow-up and the conditions that facilitate or impede it.

Does Change Relate to Intervention?

Assuming that real changes have occurred in child functioning, one must ask next whether these relate to the interventions by parents, and whether these in turn relate to the training received. One can usually entertain a number of "rival hypotheses" (Campbell and Stanley,

1966) to account for observed change, such as the child's maturation, other learning experiences at home or in school, or unrelated changes in the home environment. Often such rival hypotheses hardly seem tenable if the problem behavior has been present for a long period and improvement is rapid (e.g., the 8-year-old with an uninterrupted history of bedwetting who becomes dry after 3 weeks of a program). Yet generally it is desirable to design a program so that extratraining effects are controlled for, especially if the effectiveness of the approach is not already well established. Some authors have formally taken measures on the child for a period of time before training in order to demonstrate greater change in the same time period during training. Many authors concerned about extratraining effects introduce other "child-as-his-own control" designs within the training to demonstrate that behavior is under the control of intervention manipulations.[3]

---

[3]The most commonly employed own-control design is a *reversal*. In this procedure, baseline data are first taken (A); next a program is introduced (B); then, after marked behavior change is evidenced, contingencies are reversed to resemble those originally operating during baseline (A'); and finally, if and when the behavior has also reversed toward baseline level, the program is reintroduced (B'). If behavior can be shown to vary with the experimental changes (ABA'B'), it is concluded that the intervention, rather than something else, is responsible for effects. This is the same design referred to by Spradlin, Karlan, and Wetherby (this volume) as ABAB.

It should be obvious that this reversal plan makes far more sense to the researcher than to the parent who, at last, is seeing a troublesome problem decrease. In fact, as Hartmann and Atkinson (1973) pointed out, the philosophy underlying the ABA'B' design is conceptually at odds with good treatment practice. While the researcher wants to demonstrate that the behavior change is under specific stimulus control, the therapist wants to bring the behavior under more generalized stimulus control, to promote change across many situations. The child whose behavior does not deteriorate at reversal may be an experimental failure but a clinical success! Actually, there is good reason to question the research meaning of a reversal as well. Baseline conditions cannot ever be re-created in A'. Rather, the parent-teacher strains to do something now unnatural, and the child reacts to an unexplained and seemingly irrational change. Surely some of the "deterioration" is the child's reaction to an arbitrary and ambivalently presented change.

An alternative design, less commonly used, is the *multiple baseline* (see Hall et al., 1970) where measures are taken simultaneously on: 1) several behaviors, and/or 2) the same behavior in several situations. If the targeted behavior changes and others do not, or changes are in evidence only in the treatment setting, stimulus control is demonstrated. Although more ethical and practical than the withdrawal of program in the ABA'B' design, the multiple baseline is equally open to Hartmann and Atkinson's criticism regarding generalization. For a further discussion of ABA'B' and multiple baselines the reader is referred to the chapter by Spradlin, Karlan, and Wetherby (this volume).

Some of the problems in own-control designs are avoided in larger studies, where "no-treatment" control groups are employed. It is often possible and even necessary, given limited resources, to deny or delay training for some families; and, if assignments are at random, changes in these untrained families can serve as a comparison base for trained families. Wiltz (1969) for example, randomly assigned 12 families with conduct-disordered boys to a training or waiting list; by the end of 4 weeks, problem behaviors of boys in trained families had already decreased by 48% while waiting list boys remained unchanged. With self-help skills in retarded children, Baker, Heifetz, and Brightman (1973) reported a 4-month gain of 3.1 skills for children in trained families versus 1.3 for children in a randomly assigned waiting list control group. This latter study shows the importance of a control comparison, to indicate the extent to which skills develop from maturation, schooling, or other factors—a base rate that must be bettered if specific parent intervention is to be worthwhile.

Which Aspects of Training Relate to Change?

Training programs vary considerably in curriculum inputs (e.g., group training, use of media, professional supervision), and it is important to determine how much each of these inputs relates to change. Also, training programs inherently have a number of nonspecific factors (e.g., status of attending a prestigious clinic or university, attention from professionals, expectancy of success, support from other parents, opportunity to vent feelings), and it is likewise important to ascertain how much these account for obtained outcomes. To date there have been few of the more complex and controlled studies necessary to partial out these relative effects, but those that are available for review are useful. They generally run counter to the skeptical view that nonspecific aspects of training account for success, but they also tend to question the generally held assumption that "more is better" in selecting training inputs.

Nonspecific Aspects of Training   Walter (1971, p. 2) noted that, "the placebo elements of status attention and expectancy common to all therapies have been demonstrated to be powerful psychological components of therapy processes." Posing this, she compared a 10-week behavior modification training program for parents of conduct-disordered boys (after Patterson, Cobb, and Ray, 1972) with a very believable placebo treatment, the same in most respects but omitting the essential behavior modification content. Parents in both conditions had equally high expectancies for success throughout and reported equally good improvement. However, *specific* in-home observations and parent-completed symptom checklists revealed notable improvement among children in the trained condition and actually increased deviance in the placebo condition children.

Similarly, Tavormina (1975) compared training programs for parents of mentally retarded children. Reflective group counseling (emphasizing "parent awareness, understanding and acceptance of the child's feelings: Auerbach, 1968; Ginott, 1957") was compared with behavioral group counseling (emphasizing "actual observable behavior and the environmental variables that maintain certain behavior patterns"). Because both groups met for eight sessions under very similar conditions, many of the nonspecific aspects of being in a program were controlled, and differences therefore would reflect differential effectiveness of training. Although both counseling models were generally effective relative to a (nonrandom) waiting list control group, the behavioral method produced greater change than the reflective, in parent attitudes, parents views of the child's behavior, and parent behavior vis-à-vis the child.

These studies suggest that measured changes in behaviorally oriented parent training are at least in part attributable to the specific inputs of the training program. The nonspecific factors, of course, may result in effects not measured. Also, some of these factors may be essential in motivating parent involvement and, in this sense, may be necessary while still not sufficient conditions for change.

Curriculum Inputs   Several studies have examined the relative effectiveness of different training models or formats, within a general behavioral orientation. Most of these studies bear on the question of cost effectiveness; they seek ways to maintain effects while decreasing the amount of staff time per family. Comparisons with parents of brain-injured children using individual versus group training (Salzinger, Feldman, and Portnoy, 1970) or groups of five versus groups of 10 parents (Hirsh and Walder, 1969) have found the less costly alternative equally effective.

Still other programs have explored increasing cost effectiveness by using written or visual media for training (Nay, 1971; Saslow, 1972; Watson and Bassinger, 1974). The relative effects of the READ Project manuals were assessed over 4 months of training (Baker, Heifetz, and Brightman, 1973). Families of 128 retarded and severely disturbed children (ages 3 to 13) were randomly assigned to one of the following training conditions: 1) manuals only, 2) manuals plus eight biweekly telephone consultations, 3) manuals plus nine biweekly group meetings, and 4) manuals plus nine biweekly group meetings and six home visits. On measures of parent information acquired and child *skill* development, the families in each of the training approaches were superior to those in a randomly assigned untrained control condition. Yet significant differences were not found among training conditions; the least costly condition—manuals only—was at least as effective as the others. In the area of *behavior problem* management, however, it seemed that greater professional contact (conditions 3 and 4) did have a facilitative value.

This possibility that training inputs will differentially effect various outcome measures has been addressed in other studies. Several comparisons have been made of lecture or manual presentation versus modeling and role playing. On *information acquired,* the more didactic approach has been found at least as effective (Nay, 1971) or more so (Watson and Bassinger, 1974; Gardner, 1972–with ward attendents). With *ability to apply* teaching methods Nay (1971) found modeling and role playing superior in an analog measure (response to videotaped situations) while Watson and Bassinger (1974) and Gardner (1972) found these more active methods superior on the Training Proficiency Scale (Gardner, Brust, and Watson, 1970), which rates proficiency in role play teaching of behavior modification.

Hence, the common clinical assumption that training should involve considerable staff input and individual consultation to be effective must be questioned from the available empirical evidence. Too, it seems that the choice of a given model or input should depend in part on the types of child behavior to be taught (e.g., skills versus behavior problem management) and in part on the parent skills to be acquired (e.g., information versus action). Curriculum decisions also relate to characteristics of the families being trained, and these are considered in the next section. In conclusion here, though, it is appropriate simply to repeat the caution that, although parent training has been generally demonstrated to be effective, the empirical basis for specific procedural decisions remains fragmented at best. Any parent training program should make a methodologically sound effort to assess its effects. To do so is not a luxury but a basic component of service if that service is to be responsible and ethical.

PARENT PARTICIPATION

Most of the teaching approaches presented in parent programs are relatively easy to learn and to carry out; few families make a consistent and serious effort to carry out programs and still fail. Hence, encouraging participation becomes the paramount issue. From reading case reports, one might imagine mistakenly that parents are immediately receptive to and continually involved in training programs. Yet trainers of larger and less selected samples soon find that training is not for everyone—that perhaps even a majority of parents choose not to enter training, or maintain poor attendance, fail to complete assignments, or drop out altogether. Morris' (1973) experience is not atypical. Of 80 families invited to participate in a free group training program, 41 agreed to do so, only 14 attended the initial meeting, and 11 completed the program. Fredericks et al. (1974) noted that the school-home "Lunch Box" program described earlier will do well in the average setting to involve one-half of the families.

The relatively high involvement in the READ Project (described above) may highlight some correlates of participation. Only 5% of parents who attended an introductory explanatory meeting failed to begin training, and an additional 8% dropped out during training; 87% of families completed the 4-month program. This *volunteer* sample of predominantly *middle-class* and reasonably *well educated* parents of *retarded* children participated in a *structured, research* training program which was lead by *experienced trainers;* there is some evidence that each of these characteristics may have contributed to participation.

Parent Characteristics

Parents who voluntarily join a program in response to media publicity are likely to be better motivated on the average than parents who are offered training as part of a school or clinic program. Too, lower socioeconomic status (SES) families are less apt to join and more apt to drop out of training, for many reasons, including: the other more pressing priorities of these families, some possible clash in values with (customarily) middle-class trainers, a lack of time to get to meetings, a lack of funds for babysitters and/or transportation, and a tendency to be less comfortable with the usual classroom-type format.

As noted above, information may be acquired as well or even better with didactic training, while actual skills in teaching are perhaps best taught through an action-oriented approach. It seems that the choice of the latter approach may be especially appropriate for increasing participation and benefits for lower SES and/or less well educated families. Schwenn (1971) found better attendance at (and benefit from) lecture-discussion sessions for families where the father's occupation required a higher level of verbal ability, and others found success in didactic training to be positively related to level of education and/or reading level (Salzinger, Feldman, and Portnoy, 1970; Baker, Heifetz, and Brightman, 1973). Schneiman (1972) developed alternative training approaches based on hypothesized SES differences in cognitive and communicative set. Lower SES teacher aides learned to carry out behavior modification techniques better from a "structured learning program" (employing modeling, role playing, and social reinforcement) than from a "didactic learning program" (highly verbal lecture-discussion method). For middle SES trainees, the two methods were equally effective. Hence, one could reasonably apply an action-oriented approach for all families and need not group families by SES. This is fortunate, because Rose (1974) has found that welfare mothers attended and programmed more when in mixed groups with middle-class mothers than when in separate groups.

Sustained program participation, regardless of SES, also relates to the support available within the family. Typically, one parent, usually the mother, becomes principally involved in training and carrying out teaching programs. Not unexpectedly, there are reports of fathers sabotaging mother-initiated programs either intentionally or inadvertantly, because of lack of understanding of, or disagreement with, treatment procedures (Sajwaj, 1973). However, many fathers who do not regularly teach do play an important supportive and reinforcing role, at training sessions as well as at home.

Training programs could make considerable progress toward increasing father involvement—for instance, by scheduling meetings at more accessible times and accommodating somewhat to the prevalent sex-role stereotypes that run more deeply than one brief parent program can hope to eliminate. For example, fathers sometimes can be gradually phased into teaching through assessment and record keeping roles and may be more apt to teach in areas as play and social skills (where fathers are often quite involved with their handicapped children, though not systematically so) than in self-help training or formal speech teaching sessions. In some instances, specific contracts that delineate shared responsibilities are possible to negotiate between parents (Stuart, 1971).

Not surprisingly, Bernal et al. (1972) observed that training is most beneficial for parents who participate together, cooperate with training demands, and "who have a basically stable and satisfying marriage." Certainly most other trainers would concur. In some programs (Baker, 1972) the least consistent participation in training has been with single-parent families, especially those in a state of confusion and flux (e.g., repeated separation, divorce imminent), where there is virtually no interpersonal support at home. It is likely that a single parent would participate best in a home-based program, although attendance in agency-based individual or group programs might be enhanced by encouraging the parent to attend the sessions with a friend, relative, or older child. Indeed, involvement of brothers and sisters in training efforts directed toward the developmentally disabled child is rarely considered but potentially quite advantageous, for the siblings, parents, and target child alike.

Siblings

Having a developmentally disabled child in the family certainly has a profound effect on siblings, and although research is somewhat equivocal as to the precise nature and extent of the effect, it is most often found to be an adverse one (Farber, 1959; Farber, Jenne, and Togio, 1960; Fotheringham, Skelton, and Hodinott, 1971). In one of the first reported efforts to deal therapeutically with brothers and sisters of retarded children, Grossman (1972) conducted group counseling sessions for adolescent siblings. Treatment focused on exploration and sharing of feelings, attitudes, and experiences related to the retarded child, and participants were reported to have developed a capacity to better discuss these and to be more comfortable with their retarded sibling. Consistent with recent trends away from viewing families as patients, though, sibling programs are now beginning to focus less exclusively on the siblings' feelings and to include skill training as well, so that they might interact more constructively with the disabled child (Bennett, 1973; Laviquer, 1973; Laviquer et al., 1973).

Camp Freedom has for several years conducted a sibling training program, involving adolescent siblings of younger retarded campers in a 3- to 5-day residential institute during the summer (Weinrott, 1974; Pasick, 1975). Objectives include: acquiring information about retardation and its related content areas; acquiring abilities to teach according to behavioral principles; and talking about feelings and experiences involving the retarded child and what these imply for home programming. This program is received enthusiastically and comfortably by most siblings, the exceptions generally being the youngest children (ages 10 to 12) who might be better included in a program together with their parents.

Siblings tend to model their parents' approach to the handicapped child (see Brown and Guilani, 1972), and many sibling-child interaction problems in some way reflect parental attitudes (often unexpressed) and/or management procedures. It may be that parents trained to be effective teachers provide a sufficient model for sibling interactions, hence eliminating the need for separate sibling training. A recent exploration of the marginal advantages of sibling training (over training parents only) suggests that trained siblings can indeed carry out more effective teaching procedures when asked to do so, but that their spontaneous, day-to-day experiences with the retarded child differ little from those of untrained siblings (Pasick, 1975). The overall effect on siblings may be greater when they are helped to work together with their parents to modify the handicapped child's behavior. Patterson, Cobb, and Ray (1972) noted that siblings of aggressive children were often as deviant in their behavior as the target child, and that involvement with their parents in implementing a program for the target child resulted in improved behavior for them as well. In any event, it is clear that siblings are an important, although hitherto neglected, part of the handicapped child's environment.

Child Characteristics

Although comparisons have not been made directly, it seems that parents of developmentally disabled children, especially those classified as "organic" rather than "cultural-familial," are more apt to become productively involved in training than parents of children with more normal intelligence but who display oppositional behavior. Cohen et al. (1970) reported that group attendance by mothers of deliquent boys dropped as low as 19% when programming requests were made. Too, Reid and Hendricks (1973) reported that, of 27 families who sought help for their sons' stealing, only five decided to enter the well established and highly regarded program at Oregon Research Institute, and that the course of treatment even for these was characterized by missed appointments and incomplete assignments. In many cases, the child's oppositional behavior is a reflection of family disorganization, and it in turn leads more to unproductive conflict, fixing blame, or denial than to a concerted effort to help. Changing oppositional child behavior clearly involves changing family behavior.

For the family of the developmentally disabled child, the changes required to increase skills are less of a challenge to established patterns. There is, of course, much variability among developmentally disabled children, and some are naturally easier for parents to teach than others. It is especially difficult to present material to the multiply handicapped child, to find reinforcers for the "autistic-like" child, or even to address some learning needs of the retarded adolescent, such as sex education. Yet with young retarded children, for example, skill teaching objectives and approaches are reasonably clear and parents are more apt to be gratified by their involvement in a training program.

Trainer Characteristics

In some programs, poor participation in part must be attributed to inappropriate content or less-than-adequate trainers. Many nonbehavioral groups are too lacking in substance and structure to generate real changes in parent behavior; it is also the case that some behavioral curricula are presented in too dogmatic, or conversely, too ambivalent a manner to inspire credibility. Although the quality of programs cannot be readily judged from the literature, some authors do mention their trainers' lack of previous experience with parent training and/or with the programming methods being taught. The issue is not professionalism, but rather adequate training, structure, and interpersonal skills. There is some evidence that nonprofessionals, in fact, can train parents as well as or even better than professionals, provided they are given specific training in the requisite skills for conducting parent training and are provided ongoing supervision (Tharp and Wetzel, 1969; Schortinghuis and Frohman, 1974).

Program Incentives

Even with the most carefully and creatively designed program, child progress is apt to be uneven and sometimes painfully slow. Indeed, "seeing progress" is not an entirely sufficient sustainer of parent performance. Fortunately, the introduction of additional incentive for parents seems, predictably, to increase participation.

One class of incentive are those that utilize *social pressure and social support:* the writing and signing of specific performance contracts with the trainers, the praise for success inherent in the group, and the expectations engendered by agreeing to participate in a research program. A second class of incentives involves *money*. In some programs a "contract deposit" is required; the deposit is refunded according to certain prior agreed-upon performance. Hirsch and Walder (1969), for example, refunded a $50 deposit in its entirety if eight of nine sessions were attended, with no refund at all if fewer sessions were attended (all 30 mothers maintained perfect attendance). Benassi and Benassi (1973) modified this strategy, refunding according to a schedule of points earned for attendance, completed assignments, and participation in the group meetings. In other programs the fee is reduced or parents are paid according to the number of sessions attended and/or data recorded (Patterson et al., 1967; White, 1972; Gilbert, 1973).

A third type of incentive arranges for *family members to reinforce each other,* contingent on some specific gain in child performance. The trainer can help to arrange an agreement whereby certain successful programming will mean, for example, the whole family going out to a movie or mother getting breakfast in bed—the possibilities are limitless and need not cost anything.

A final class of incentive involves *contingent professional resources.* For example, Donahue (1973) gave as reinforcement to parents a card allowing them to check out toys from a lending library (for attendance), a reference book (for completed assignments), and a certificate of completion (for handing in evaluations). In a controlled study, Eyberg and Johnson (in press) compared the typical Oregon Research Institute individual consultation program to one utilizing several of the above incentives: a refundable contract deposit, contingent telephone time, and contingent training time (parents could not attend a consultation session without data!). Parents in the incentive condition were found to complete more assigned data recording, treat a greater number of child problems, and receive a higher cooperation rating from the staff.

It seems well established that incentives for parents promote greater participation. Quite apart from the inherent desirability of the incentives themselves, their provision may impress upon parents the expectations held for them and concretize an agreement with the trainers that then becomes more difficult to break. However, there is virtually no follow-up data reported in studies that have increased participation through incentives, and it remains to be examined whether increased involvement ends with the end of training and its accompanying incentives. Yet, well managed incentives may maintain participation long enough for parents to realize the value of their involvement and consequently may become less necessary. For example, a group of second-year parents at Camp Freedom recently advised continuation of the $25 tuition rebate plan for first-year parents, but preferred to forgo it for themselves; they were now teaching their children well, and perhaps did not want the merit of their efforts diminished by being partly attributable to incentives they would gain.

Programmatic implications drawn from the programs and studies reviewed above are summarized below. These guidelines for structuring parent training are oriented primarily toward group training. They presuppose that the trainer is competent and clinically sensitive, able to inform parents and encourage them, while also understanding the many real restraints that at times may interfere with their teaching ambitions. The guidelines are:

1.   Seek some homogeneity in child functioning and types of problems
2.   Seek some diversity in parents' background
3.   Have two trainers in the group—one male, one female, if possible; make certain one is thoroughly experienced in parent training and child programming as well as familiar with the type of disabilities represented in the group
4.   Schedule some groups to meet in evenings, so that fathers can attend
5.   Schedule groups to meet in easily accessible locations
6.   Provide supervision for children during daytime meetings; if possible, include children in the training
7.   Encourage single parents to bring a friend
8.   Have an organized plan for training sessions but be prepared to depart from it as seems necessary
9.   Present objectives of training clearly at the outset: what you will do, what you will expect of parents, what you will not do
10.   State parameters of training clearly at the beginning (e.g., how many sessions, schedule of inputs)
11.   Have parents assist in assessing their child and selecting target goals (thereby shaping them into record keeping)
12.   Begin with skills that parents want to teach and that the child is ready to learn

13.   Minimize lectures; use action-oriented inputs such as modeling, role playing, and group planning sessions

14.   Practice in training everything you expect parents to do at home

15.   Provide some information through written books and manuals; use trainer time less to provide information and more to model and give feedback

16.   Require record keeping only as much as it is really needed

17.   Model your interest in record keeping by reviewing records carefully with parents

18.   Structure occasions for parents to consult with one another

19.   Provide incentives for parents' attendance and programming

20.   Provide ways for parents to give feedback about the training program, and be responsive to it

CONCLUSION

To be the parent of a handicapped child not only means to struggle with the feelings and against the odds generated by the child's limitations, but also to confront the painful limitations in the service delivery system. However, the programs and effects reviewed herein should give some substance to the claim that parents, themselves, can do much to increase their child's learning opportunities.

Although dealing at some length with ways to increase parent participation in training, this author would be remiss not to point out the obvious: that parents already "participate" with their handicapped child in a multitude of meaningful if less formal ways. The parents of a retarded, hearing-impaired, or other developmentally disabled child did not choose this role, nor can they leave it behind as they exit the agency at 5:00 p.m. or close the cover of this book. Each day calls for considerable strength and imagination if a parent is to see what might be possible and to go beyond just coping to actually teaching. It is a small wonder that parents ask for concrete guidance, and one must applaud the growing movement to provide this.

ACKNOWLEDGMENTS

The author is grateful to Drs. Alan J. Brightman and Louis J. Heifetz for critical readings of earlier drafts of this chapter.

REFERENCES

*Allen, K. E., and F. R. Harris. 1964. Speech Development in a Retarded Child Using Reinforcement Techniques. University of Washington Developmental Psychology Lab Pre-School, Seattle. (16mm film).

Allen, K. E., and F. R. Harris. 1966. Elimination of a child's excessive scratching by training the mother in reinforcement procedures. Behav. Res. Ther. 4:79–84.

Auerbach, A. B. 1968. Parents Learn through Group Discussion: Principles and Practices of Parent Group Education. John Wiley & Sons, New York.

Baker, B. L. 1972. Training in behavior modification for retarded children. Progress Report, SRS Training Grant.

Baker, B. L. 1973a. Parents as teachers: Promise and pitfalls. Paper presented at the American Psychological Association Convention, September, Montreal.

Baker, B. L. 1973b. Camp Freedom: Behavior modification for retarded children in a therapeutic camp setting. Amer. J. Orthopsychiatr. 43:418–427.

*Baker, B. L., A. J. Brightman, and J. Blatt. 1975. Parents as Teachers Video Series: Self-Help Skills for Children with Special Needs. New Hope–New Horizons, Keene, N. Hamp.

*Baker, B. L., A. J. Brightman, L. J. Heifetz, and D. Murphy. 1972, 1973. READ Project Series: Ten Instructional Manuals for Parents. Behavioral Education Projects, Cambridge, Mass.

*Baker, B. L., A. J. Brightman, L. J. Heifetz, and D. Murphy. 1976. Steps to Independence Series: Behavior Problems; Early Self-Help; Intermediate Self-Help; Advanced Self-Help. Research Press, Champaign, Ill.

Baker, B. L., and L. J. Heifetz. 1976. The READ Project: Teaching manuals for parents of retarded children. In T. D. Tjossem (ed.), Intervention Strategies for High Risk Infants and Young Children. University Park Press, Baltimore.

Baker, B. L., L. J. Heifetz, and A. J. Brightman. 1973. Parents as Teachers. Manuals for Behavior Modification of the Retarded Child: Studies in Family Training. Cambridge, Mass: Behavioral Education Projects, Inc.

Baker, B. L., D. Murphy, L. J. Heifetz, and A. J. Brightman. 1975. Parents as Teachers: Follow-up after 18 Months. Behavioral Education Projects, Cambridge, Mass.

Beck, H. L. 1973. Group Treatment for Parents of Handicapped Children. U.S. Government Printing Office, Washington, D.C.

*Becker, W. 1971. Parents are Teachers. Research Press, Champaign, Ill.

Benassi, V. A., and B. Benassi. 1973. An approach to teaching behavior modification principles to parents. Rehab. Lit. 34:134–137.

*Benchmark Films Inc. 1975. Child Behavior Equals You. Benchmark Films Inc., Briar Cliff Manor, N.Y. (16mm Film).

---

*Media references, useful in parent training programs.

Bennett, C. W. 1973. A four-and-a-half year old as a teacher of her hearing impaired sister: A case study. J. Commun. Disord. 6:67–75.

Berkowitz, B. P., and A. M. Graziano. 1972. Training parents as behavior therapists: A review. Behav. Res. Ther. 10:297–317.

Bernal, M. E. 1969. Behavioral feedback in the modification of brat behaviors. J. Nerv. Ment. Disord. 148:375–385.

Bernal, M. E., D. M. Gibson, D. E. Williams, and D. I. Pesses. 1971. A device for automatic audio tape recording. J. Appl. Behav. Anal. 4:151–156.

Bernal, M. E., D. E. Williams, W. H. Miller, and P. A. Reogor. 1972. The use of videotape feedback and operant learning principles in training parents in management of deviant children. In R. Rubin, H. Fensterheim, J. Henderson, and L. Ullman (eds.), Advances in Behavior Therapy. Academic Press, New York.

Bricker, D. D., and W. A. Bricker. 1973. Infant, Toddler and Preschool Research and Intervention Project Report: Year III. IMRID Behavioral Monogr. 23, Institute on Mental Retardation and Intellectual Development, George Peabody College, Nashville.

Bricker, W. A., and D. D. Bricker. 1976. The Infant, Toddler, and Preschool Research and Intervention Project. In T. D. Tjossem (ed.), Intervention Strategies for High Risk Infants and Young Children. University Park Press, Baltimore.

Brightman, A. 1972. Toward the non-issues of retardation. Syracuse Law Rev. 23(4):1091–1108.

Brightman, A. 1973. Behavior modification training: From word to deed. Paper presented at the American Psychological Association Convention, September, Montreal.

Brightman, A. 1975. Behavior modification in organization development: Toward the implementation of planned change in settings for retarded children. Unpublished doctoral dissertation, Harvard University, Cambridge, Mass.

*Brightman, A., B. L. Baker, and J. Blatt. 1975. Parents as Teachers Video Series: Play Skills for Children with Special Needs. New Hope–New Horizons, Keene, N. Hamp.

*Brightman, A., B. L. Baker, and J. Delphin. 1975. Filmography: Audio-Visual Materials for Use in Training Parents as Teachers of their Developmentally Disabled Children. New Hope–New Horizons, Keene, N. Hamp.

Brim, O. G., Jr. 1965. Education for Child Rearing. (Russell Sage Foundation, New York, 1959). Free Press (paper with new introduction), New York.

Brown, N., and B. Guilani. 1972. Siblings as behavior modifiers. Paper presented at the meeting of the Association for the Advancement of Behavior Therapy, New York.

*Caldwell, B. Home Teaching Activities. Center for Early Development and Education, University of Arkansas, Little Rock.

Campbell, D. T., and J. C. Stanley. 1966. Experimental and Quasi-experimental Designs for Research. Rand McNally, Skokie, Ill.

Cohen, H. L., J. Filipezak, J. Slavin, and D. Green. 1970. The PICA Project, Year 2. Project Interim Report. Programming interpersonal curricula for adolescents.

Doernberg, N. L. 1971. The differential effect of parent-directed and child-directed part-time educational intervention on the level of social functioning of young mentally ill children on waiting lists. Unpublished doctoral dissertation, New York University, New York.

*Donahue, M. J. 1973. Home Stimulation of Handicapped Children: Parent Guide. (ERIC ED 079 921). Marshall-Poweshiek Joint County School System, Marshalltown, Iowa.

*Esche, J., and C. Griffen. 1973. A handbook for parents of deaf-blind children. (ERIC ED 067 803). Michigan School for the Blind, Lansing.

Eyberg, S., and S. M. Johnson. Multiple assessment of behavior modification with families: The effects of contingency contracting and order of treated problems. J. Consult. Clin. Psychol. In press.

Farber, B. 1959. Effects of a severely mentally retarded child on family integration. Monogr. Soc. Res. Child Dev. 24 (2, whole no. 71).

Farber, B., W. Jenne, and R. Togio. 1960. Family crises and the decision to institutionalize the retarded child. Council for Exceptional Children Research Monogr. Ser. no. A1.

Ferber, H., S. M. Kelley, and K. M. Shemberg. 1974. Training parents in behavior modification: Outcome of and problems encountered in a program after Patterson's work. Behav. Ther. 5:415–419.

Forehand, R., T. Cheney, and P. Yoder. 1974. Parent behavior training: Effects on the non-compliance of a deaf child. J. Behav. Ther. Exp. Psychiatr. 5:281–283.

Fotheringham, J. B., M. Skelton, and B. A. Hodinott. 1971. The Retarded Child and His Family. Monogr. Ser. 2, Ontario Institute for Studies in Education, Toronto.

Fraiberg, S. 1971. Intervention in infancy: A program for blind infants. J. Amer. Acad. Child Psychiatr. 10:381–405.

Fraiberg, S., M. Smith, and E. Adelson. 1969. An educational program for blind infants. J. Spec. Educ. 3:121–139.

Fredericks, H. D., V. L. Baldwin, and D. Grove. 1974. A home-center based parent training model. In J. Grim (ed.), Training Parents to Teach: Four Models. First Chance for Children 3:11–24.

Fredericks, H. D., V. L. Baldwin, D. Grove, and W. Moore. A Data Based Preschool for the Multiple Handicapped. Charles C Thomas, Springfield, Ill. In press.

Freeman, S. W., and C. L. Thompson. 1973. Parent-child training for the mentally retarded. Ment. Retard. 11(4):8–10.

Garcia, E. E., and E. D. DeHaven. 1974. Use of operant techniques in the establishment and generalization of language: A review and analysis. Amer. J. Ment. Defic. 79:169–178.

Gardner, J. E. 1967. Behavior therapy treatment approach to a psychogenic seizure case. J. Consult. Psychol. 31:209–212.

Gardner, J. E., D. T. Perason, A. N. Bercovici, and D. E. Bricker. 1968. Measurement, evaluation and modification of selected social interactions between a schizophrenic child, his parents and his therapist. J. Consult. Clin. Psychol. 32:537–542.

Gardner, J. M. 1972. Teaching behavior modification to nonprofessionals. J. Appl. Behav. Anal. 5:517–521.

Gardner, J. M., D. J. Brust, and L. S. Watson. 1970. A scale to measure proficiency in applying behavior modification skills to the mentally retarded. Amer. J. Ment. Defic. 74:633–636.

Gerrard, K. R., and S. A. Saxon. 1973. Preparation of a disturbed deaf child for therapy: A case description in behavior shaping. J. Speech Hear. Disord. 38(4):502–509.

Gilbert, E. M. 1973. Effectiveness of incentives for kindergarten children and parents in a reading readiness program. Unpublished doctoral dissertation, Arizona State University, Tempe.

Ginott, H. G. 1957. Parent education groups in a child guidance clinic. Ment. Hygiene 41:82–86.

Greenfeld, J. 1970. A Child Called Noah. Holt, Rinehart and Winston, New York.

Grossman, F. K. 1972. Brothers and Sisters of Retarded Children. Syracuse University Press, Syracuse.

Hall, R. V., C. Cristler, S. S. Cranston, and B. Tucker. 1970. Teachers and parents as researchers using multiple baseline designs. J. Appl. Behav. Anal. 3:247–255.

Hartmann, D. P., and L. Atkinson. 1973. Having your cake and eating it too: A note on some apparent contradictions between therapeutic achievements and design requirements in N=1 studies. Behav. Ther. 4:589–591.

Hartung, J. R. 1970. A review of procedures to increase verbal imitation skills and functional speech in autistic children. J. Speech Hear. Disord. 35:203–217.

Hayden, A. H. 1974. A center-based parent training model. In J. Grim, (ed.), Training Parents to Teach: Four Models. First Chance for Children 3:11–24.

Hayden, A. H., and N. G. Haring. 1976. Early intervention for high risk infants and young children: Programs for Down's syndrome children at the University of Washington. In T. D. Tjossem (ed.), Intervention Strategies for High Risk Infants and Young Children. University Park Press, Baltimore.

Hirsch, I., and L. Walder. 1969. Training mothers in groups as reinforcement therapists for their own children. In Proceedings of the 77th Annual Convention of the American Psychological Association 4(2)561–562.

Hoover, L. 1970. Teaching behavior modification techniques to parents of hearing handicapped children. In J. B. Miller (ed.), A Demonstration Home Training Program for Parents of Preschool Deaf Children. (ERIC ED 058 697). University of Kansas Medical Center.

Horowitz, F. D. 1968. Infant learning and development: Retrospect and prospect. Merrill-Palmer Q. Behav. Dev. 14:101–120.

Horton, K. B. 1974. Infant intervention and language learning. *In* R. L. Schiefelbusch and L. L. Lloyd (eds.), Language Perspectives—Acquisition, Retardation, and Intervention, pp. 469–491. University Park Press, Baltimore.

Horton, K. B., and F. McConnell. 1970. Early intervention for the young deaf child through parent training. *In* Proceedings of the International Congress on Education of the Deaf (Stockholm) 1:291–296.

Horton, K. B., and A. B. Sitton. 1970. Early intervention for the young deaf child. South. Med. Bull. 58:50–57.

Hursh, D. E., and J. A. Sherman. 1973. The effects of parent-presented models and praise on the vocal behavior of their children. J. Exp. Child Psychol. 15:328–339.

Jelinek, J. A., and M. T. Schaub. 1973. A model of parent involvement in programming for communicatively handicapped children. Rehab. Lit. 34:231–234.

Jew, W. 1974. Helping handicapped infants and their families. Child. Today 3(3):7–10.

Johnson, C. A., and R. C. Katz. 1973. Using parents as change agents for their children: A review. J. Child Psychol. Psychiatr. Allied Disc. 14(3): 181–200.

Johnson, S. M., and G. K. Lobitz. 1974. Parental manipulations of child behavior in home observations. J. Appl. Behav. Anal. 7:23–31.

*Joseph, R., H. Klebanoff, et al. 1974. Exploring Materials. Massachusetts Department of Mental Health, Division of Mental Retardation: Media Resource Center, Waltham, Mass.

Knox, L. L., and F. McConnell. 1968. Helping parents to help deaf infants. Children 15(5):183–187.

Kozloff, M. 1974. Parents as teachers (2). Forum 15:8–12.

Kugel, R., and W. Wolfensberger (eds.). 1969. Changing Patterns in Residential Services for the Mentally Retarded. U.S. Government Printing Office, Washington, D.C.

Latham, G. I. 1972. A systematic media approach to teaching parents to train their pre-school mentally retarded children. Unpublished doctoral dissertation, Utah State University, Logan.

Laviquer, H. 1973. The use of siblings as an adjunct to the behavioral treatment of children in the home with parents as therapists. Diss. Abst. Int. 35(12):6214-B.

Laviquer, H., R. Peterson, J. Sheese, and L. Peterson. 1973. Behavioral treatment in the home: Effects on an untreated sibling and long-term follow-up. Behav. Ther. 4:431–441.

Lillie, D. (ed.). 1972. Parent programs in child development centers. Technical Assistance Development System (TADS), Chapel Hill, N.C.

Lovaas, O. I. 1966. A program for the establishment of speech in psychotic children. *In* J. K. Wing (ed.), Childhood Autism, pp. 115–144. Pergamon Press, Oxford, England.

*Lovaas, O. I. 1968. Behavior Modification: Teaching Language to Psychotic Children. Prentice-Hall, Englewood Cliffs, N.J. (16mm film).

Lovibond, S. H. 1964. Conditioning and Enuesis. Pergamon Press, Elmsford, N.Y.

MacDonald, J, D., J. P. Blatt, K. Gordon, B. Spiegel, and M. Hartmann. 1974. An experimental parent-assisted treatment program for preschool language delayed children. J. Speech Hear. Disord. 39(4):395–415.

McConnell, F. 1970. A new approach to the management of childhood deafness. Ped. Clin. N. Amer. 17:347–362.

McConnell, F. 1974. The parent teaching home: An early intervention program for hearing impaired children. Peabody J. Educ. April:162–170.

McCroskey, R. L. 1967. Early education of infants with severe auditory impairments. In G. F. Fellendorf (ed.), Proceedings of International Conference on Oral Education of the Deaf, pp. 1891–1905. Vol. 2. Alexander Graham Bell Association for the Deaf, Washington, D.C.

Mira, M. 1970. Results of a behavior modification training program for parents and teachers. Behav. Res. Ther. 8:309–311.

Mira, M., and S. Hoffman. 1974. Educational programming for multi-handicapped deaf-blind children. Except. Child 40:513–514.

Morreau, L. E. 1972. Televised parent training program: Reinforcement strategies for mothers of disadvantaged children. (ERIC ED 73 670).

Morris, R. J. 1973. Issues in teaching behavior modification to parents of retarded children. Paper presented at the American Psychological Association Convention, September, Montreal.

Nay, W. R. 1971. Written, lecture, lecture modelling and modelling-role-playing as instructional techniques for parents. Unpublished doctoral dissertation, University of Georgia, Athens.

Nirje, B. 1969. The normalization principle and its human management implications. In R. B. Kugel and W. Wolfensberger (eds.), Changing Patterns in Residential Services for the Mentally Retarded. President's Committee on Mental Retardation, Washington, D.C.

Northcott, W. N. 1967. Counseling parents of preschool hearing-impaired children. In Proceedings of the International Conference on Oral Education of the Deaf, pp. 424–442. Alexander Graham Association for the Deaf, Washington, D.C.

Northcott, W. N. 1971. Infant education and home training. In L. E. Conner (ed.), Speech for the Deaf Child: Knowledge and Use, pp. 311–334. Alexander Graham Bell Association for the Deaf, Washington, D.C.

Pascal, C. E. 1973. Application of behavior modification by parents for treatment of a brain damaged child. In B. A. Ashem, and E. G. Poser (eds.), Adaptive Learning: Behavior Modification with Children, pp. 299–309. Pergamon Press, Elmsford, N.Y.

Pasick, R. S. 1975. Inclusion of siblings of the retarded in a family training program in behavior modification. Unpublished doctoral dissertation, Harvard University, Cambridge, Mass.

Patterson, G. R. 1974. Retraining of aggressive boys by their parents: Review of recent literature and follow-up evaluation. Can. Psychiatr. Assoc. J. 19:142–157.

Patterson, G. R., J. A. Cobb, and R. S. Ray. 1972. A social engineering technology for retraining the families of aggressive boys. In H. Adams, and L. Unikel (eds.), Georgia Symposium in Experimental Clinical Psychology. Vol. 2 Charles C Thomas, Springfield, Ill.

*Patterson, G. R., and M. E. Gullion. 1968. Living with Children: New Methods for Parents and Teachers. Research Press, Champaign, Ill.

Patterson, G. R., S. McNeal, N. Hawkings, and R. Phelps. 1967. Reprogramming the social environment. J. Child Psychol. Psychiatr. Allied Disc. 8:181–195.

Peine, H. 1969. Programming the home. Paper presented at the meetings of the Rocky Mountain Psychological Association, Albuquerque, N.Mex.

Peterson, R. F. 1968. Imitation: A basic behavioral mechanism. In H. N. Sloane and B. D. MacAulay (eds.), Operant Procedures in Remedial Speech and Language Training. Houghton Mifflin, Boston.

*Prentice-Hall. Help for Mark. Prentice-Hall, Englewood Cliffs, N.J. (16mm film).

Reid, J. B., and A. F. Hendricks. 1973. Preliminary analysis of the effectiveness of direct home intervention for the treatment of predelinquent boys who steal. In L. A. Hamerlynck, L. C. Handy, and E. J. Mash (eds.), Behavioral Change: Methodology, Concepts and Practice, pp. 209–219. Research Press, Champaign, Ill.

Risley, T. 1968. The effects and side effects of punishing the autistic behaviors of a deviant child. J. Appl. Behav. Anal. 1:24–34.

Risley, T., and M. M. Wolf. 1966. Experimental manipulation of autistic behaviors and generalization into the home. In R. Ulrich, T. Stachnik, and J. Mabry (eds.), Control of Human Behavior, pp. 193–198. Scott, Foresman, Glenview, Ill. (First read at American Psychological Association meeting, Los Angeles, 1964.)

Risley, T., and M. Wolf. 1967. Establishing functional speech in echolalic children. Behav. Res. Ther. 5:73–88.

Rose, S. D. 1974. Group training of parents as behavior modifiers. Social Work 19:156–162.

*Rules of Talking. 1974. Bill Wilkerson Speech and Hearing Center, Nashville.

Sajwaj, T. 1973. Difficulties in the use of behavioral techniques in changing child behavior: Guides to success. J. Nerv. Ment. Disord. 156(6): 395–403.

Salzinger, K., R. S. Feldman, and S. Portnoy. 1970. Training parents of brain-injured children in the use of operant conditioning procedures. Behav. Ther. 1:4–32.

Saslow, J. A. I. 1972. Four therapeutic programs compared through training mothers to increase children's verbal behavior. Diss. Abst. Int. 32:9-B, 5458–5459.

Schneiman, R. S. 1972. An evaluation of structured learning and didactic learning as methods of training behavior modification skills to low and middle socio-economic level teacher-aides. Unpublished doctoral dissertation, Syracuse University, Syracuse.

Schopler, E., and R. J. Reichler. 1971. Parents as co-therapists in the treatment of psychotic children. J. Autism Child. Schizo. 1:87–102.

Schortinghuis, N., and A. Frohman. 1974. A comparison of professional and paraprofessional success with preschool children. J. Learn. Disabil. 7:245–247.

Schroeder, G. L., and D. M. Baer. 1972. Effects of concurrent and serial training on generalized vocal imitation in retarded children. Dev. Psychol. 6:293–301.

Schwenn, M. R. 1971. The effects of parent training on generalization of therapeutic behavior change in retarded children from an educational camp to home. Unpublished senior honors thesis, Harvard University, Cambridge, Mass.

Shearer, D., J. Billingsky, A. Frohman, J. Hilliard, F. Johnson, and M. Shearer. 1972. Portage Checklist and Curriculum Guide to Early Education, Cooperative Educational Service Agency No. 12, Portage, Wisc.

Shearer, D. E., and M. S. Shearer. 1976. The Portage Project: A model for early childhood education. In T. D. Tjossem (ed.), Intervention Strategies for High Risk Infants and Young Children. University Park Press, Baltimore.

Shearer, M. S. 1974. A home based parent training model. In J. Grim (ed.), Training Parents to Teach: Four Models. First Chance for Children 3:49–62.

Shearer, M. S., and D. E. Shearer. 1972. The Portage Project: A model for early childhood education. Except. Child. 39:210–217.

Simeonsson, R. J., and R. Wiegerink. 1974. Early language intervention: A contingent stimulation model. Ment. Retard. 12(2):7–11.

Simmons, A. A. 1967. Home demonstration teaching for parents and infants at Central Institute for the Deaf. In Proceedings of International Conference on Oral Education of the Deaf, pp. 1863–1873. Vol. 2. Alexander Graham Bell Association for the Deaf, Washington, D.C.

Sloane, H. N., M. K. Johnston, and F. R. Harris. 1968. Remedial procedures for teaching verbal behavior to speech deficient or defective young children. In H. N. Sloane and B. D. MacAulay (eds.), Operant Procedures in Remedial Speech and Language Training. Houghton Mifflin, Boston.

Stuart, R. 1971. Behavioral contracting with the families of delinquents. Behav. Ther. Exp. Psychiatr. 2:1–11.

Tavormina, J. B. 1975. Relative effectiveness of behavioral and reflective group counseling with parents of mentally retarded children. J. Consult. Clin. Psychol. 43:22–31.

Terdal, L., and J. Buell. 1969. Parent education in managing retarded children with behavior deficits and inappropriate behaviors. Ment. Retard. 7(3):10–13.

Tharp, R. G., and R. J. Wetzel. 1969. Behavior Modification in the Natural Environment. Academic Press, New York.

Walder, L. O., S. I. Cohen, D. E. Breiter, P. G. Daston, I. S. Hirsch, and J. N. Leibowitz. 1969. Teaching behavioral principles to parents of disturbed children. In B. G. Guerney, (ed.), Psychotherapeutic Agents:

New Roles for Nonprofessionals, Parents and Teachers, pp. 443–449. Holt, Rinehart and Winston, New York.

Walter, H. 1971. Placebo versus social learning effects in parent training. Unpublished doctoral dissertation, University of Oregon, Eugene.

Watson, L. S., and J. F. Bassinger. 1974. Parent training technology: A potential service delivery system. Ment. Retard. 12(5):3–10.

Weinrott, M. R. 1974. A training program in behavior modification for siblings of the retarded. Amer. J. Orthopsychiatr. 44(3):362–375.

Welsh, R. S. 1966. A highly efficient method of parental counseling. Paper presented at the meetings of the Rocky Mountain Psychological Association, Albuquerque, N.Mex.

White, T. D. 1972. Training parents in a group situation to use behavior modification techniques to reduce frequency of maladaptive behavior in their learning disabled child. Diss. Abst. Int. 33(4):1776-B.

Wiltz, N. A. 1969. Modification of behaviors in deviant boys through parent participation in a group technique. Unpublished doctoral dissertation, University of Oregon, Eugene.

Wiltz, N. A., and S. B. Gordon. 1974. Parental modification of a child's behavior in an experimental residence. J. Behav. Ther. Exp. Psychiatr. 5:107–109.

Wolf, M. M., T. Risley, and H. Mees, 1964. Application of operant conditioning procedures to the behavior problems of an autistic child. Behav. Res. Ther. 1:305–312.

Wolfensberger, W. 1969. The origin and nature of our institutional models. In R. Kugel and W. Wolfensberger (eds.), Changing Patterns of Residential Services for the Mentally Retarded. U.S. Government Printing Office, Washington, D.C. (Also: Human Policy Press, Syracuse, 1975, as a separate monograph.)

Zlutnick, S., W. J. Mayville, and S. Moffat. 1975. Modification of seizures: The interruption of behavior chains. J. Appl. Behav. Anal. 8:1–12.

18

AUDIOVISUAL MEDIA AND MATERIALS

Sebastian Striefel, Richard Baer, and Vonda Douglass

CONTENTS

Audiovisual Approaches _____ **737**
    Definition/737
    Advantages/737
    Limitations/738
    Selection/739

Television and Videotapes _____ **739**
    Assessment/740
    Intervention/742
    Training/748

Films _____ **751**
    Assessment/751
    Intervention/753
    Training/754

Teaching Machines _____ **754**
    Assessment/755
    Intervention/756
    Training/763

Materials _____ **764**

Summary _____ **769**

References _____ **769**

This chapter presents information on the uses of audiovisual media and materials for the assessment, intervention, and training of the communicatively handicapped. Audiovisual media (television, videotape, film, and teaching machines) are only beginning to be exploited as communication aids for the hearing-impaired, mentally retarded, and other developmentally disabled persons. Obviously, not everything can be covered in one chapter. The chapter is designed to introduce teachers and clinicians of the communicatively handicapped to the broad range of teaching alternatives made possible through audiovisual technology.

AUDIOVISUAL APPROACHES

Definition

Audiovisual (AV) devices are pieces or combinations of equipment that have components for providing both visual and auditory stimuli. For education or training, the stimuli, or information, presented via the audiovisual device consist of a program that is produced on a medium. A program is a sequential organization of the content to be presented. The medium is the tape, slide, or film used to present the information. The production of the program requires three steps. First, a decision is made regarding who is going to use the material and what information is to be presented. Next, a choice is made on the medium for presentation. Third, with the most skilled persons and techniques available, the information is put onto the medium. The combination of AV devices, the materials, and the media used is what is known as AV technology, and instruction or training conducted using AV technology is called AV instruction. It is realized that other definitions for the above terms exist, as well as other terms with similar meanings; however, the above definitions serve the purposes of this chapter.

Advantages

Shelhass (1968) reported three primary advantages of audiovisual presentations. First, an AV presentation is precise. This precision is accounted for by material that is permanent and invariant, presents the same stimuli each time, and provides behavior that is "realistic" inasmuch as it is in the context of other behavior rather than in isolation. Second, the presentation can be administered to persons of different educational backgrounds. Third, an AV presentation seems to involve the respondent actively.

In addition, specific stimuli can be selected for AV presentation, thus limiting the stimuli to those considered important. For example, Burkland (1967) reported the use of TV close-up shots of the mouth during articulation training, thus exposing the child to the correct mouth-tongue movements.

The use of AV media very clearly has the advantage of making available appropriate models in a variety of environments. It is well known that new patterns of behavior can be acquired on the basis of film-mediated model observation (Bandura, 1965; Hicks, 1965; Bandura and Menlove, 1968; O'Conner, 1969; Striefel, 1972a) and that mentally retarded persons, particularly those living in institutions, often live in environments that are devoid of appropriate models to imitate (Spradlin, 1966). Withrow (1975) reported the use of closed-circuit TV in classrooms and in living areas to stimulate activity. In some cases, activities were planned to stimulate imitation and provide models; in other cases, questions were asked of the learner via TV. This system has been combined with a two-way TV system similar to the one discussed later in this chapter.

Stepp (1970) reported some additional advantages of AV media, specifically multimedia approaches. These advantages included: 1) increasing the use and effectiveness of coordinated visual stimuli in the classroom; 2) providing more appropriate vocabulary and language in the same amount of time; 3) using various new media to provide ample, interesting repetitions of information (because repetitions enhance learning); and 4) providing the child with the opportunity to practice and then use language.

Also, the availability of good AV materials allows the individual to develop a degree of independence. The individual becomes responsible for much of his own learning, with the "teacher" serving only as a guide or counselor (Stepp, 1970). To encourage independence, each individual should have his own cubicle for training. Each cubicle should be equipped with the appropriate AV equipment, and the training materials should be readily available.

Limitations

Except when fully automated AV devices are used, AV stimulus materials for assessment, training, or intervention have one severe limitation: They continue regardless of the behavior of the audience.

This limitation could be alleviated through the availability of a monitor who deals with any difficulties that arise. In some cases, it might be necessary only for the person monitoring the client to reinforce successes; in other cases the monitor may need to provide physical prompts or to give verbal feedback for correction of errors. For many of these activities, the monitor could be a person with limited technical training, thus freeing the professional staff for other activities. Another alternative is the use of the two-way TV system discussed later in this chapter.

Selection

There are numerous AV approaches; however, they should be related to existing needs of students and teachers. A diversity of approaches may increase the motivation of the students involved. Much of the focus in using AV media has been on the teacher; yet the person who is to learn from the materials should be the prime consideration and should be involved in the selection process.

In accounting for the needs of students, the needs of teachers also must be considered. Lange, Mattson, and Thomann (1974), summarizing the findings of over 250 studies on media and materials for handicapped learners, reported a need for media and materials. Teachers working with the trainable mentally retarded consistently expressed greater needs than did regular classroom teachers. Armstrong and Senzig (1970) reported that the filmstrip projector and chalkboard are seen as the equipment most appropriate for regular classroom use. Most teachers did not use, have access to, or express a desire for items such as a still camera or TV equipment. Besides cost, the lack of an expressed need for AV materials may be attributable to a lack of familiarity with the uses and potential uses of AV media.

TELEVISION AND VIDEOTAPES

Commercial TV is one of the foremost influencers and entertainers of our time. Available in almost every home in America, it daily bombards its viewers with news, weather, sports, and entertainment, but its educational potential is just beginning to be realized. To date, attempts to use it successfully for educational purposes have been scarce. An exception is the well known *Sesame Street* (Bogatz and Ball, 1971), which has succeeded in teaching 3- to 5-year-olds a variety of simple and complex skills.

Individuals dealing with the communication problems of the handicapped are likely to find closed-circuit television (CCTV) useful. A simple CCTV system consists of a videocamera, a monitor (TV screen), and a videocorder. This equipment can be operated by people with little or no technical skill if they follow the instructions contained in the operations manual. Dawson's (1973) booklet, *Instrumentation in the Speech Clinic,* includes much information on the components, uses, and operating instructions for AV equipment such as CCTV, tape recorders, and delayed feedback instruments.

Assessment

Several uses of TV as an assessment device exist. Hopkins, Lefever, and Hopkins (1967) conducted a study comparing the results of a standardized achievement test when administered by a teacher versus when presented via TV. The test scores for the two groups were very similar and attested to the validity of the test being presented via TV. TV administration of tests is appealing because it frees the teacher for proctoring and provides control over several variables of test administration, thus contributing to increased reliability. Certain factors are constant no matter how many times the test is administered, to whom it is administered, or where it is administered. Audiovisual media are used only for presentation of the stimulus materials. The individuals tested can record their responses in test booklets, on answer sheets, or by pushing a button if a video teaching machine is used. With some subjects or with some tests, a second person may have to record the subject's responses.

Videotape has been used to investigate observer reliability in behavior observation audiometry (see Cox and Lloyd, this volume). For example, Moncur (1968) compared ratings—made by audiologists, pediatric audiologists, and laymen—of infants' responses to auditory stimuli. Each group of judges viewed 96 videotape sequences. The two groups of audiologists were only slightly more consistent in their ratings from test to retest than were laymen. All judges reversed themselves on at least 18% of the items. These findings suggest that trained laymen can be used effectively as monitors to conduct assessments in areas previously considered to be the domain of the professional.

Another process being developed to administer assessment instruments is called a two-way telecommunication TV system

(Baldwin, Greenberg, and Muth, 1975). In this system, the individual being assessed can communicate directly with the source presenting the test stimuli via a console of five to 12 buttons. A computer then monitors the responses made on the buttons. Wheelden (1972) reported the use of a two-way TV system for diagnostic testing of patients at the Veterans Administration Hospital in Bedford, Massachusetts, with the computer located at the Massachusetts General Hospital in Boston. Some of the tests successfully administered via this system included the Schuell Minnesota Test for Differential Diagnosis of Aphasia, subtests of Eisenson's Examination for Aphasia, Peabody Picture Vocabulary Test, Goldman-Fristoe Articulation Test, Templin-Darley, Iowa Pressure Subtest, an auditory discrimination test, voice evaluations, stuttering evaluations, and collections of case histories.[1] This same system was used to provide therapy for aphasic, dysarthric, apraxic, dysphonic, dyslalic, dysfluent, and alaryngeal patients.

Assessment via two-way cable TV has the advantages of: 1) facilitating early detection because large numbers of clients can be screened easily; 2) providing screening of a large number of people using only a minimal number of professionals; 3) encouraging the involvement of parents, who are valuable training resources; 4) allowing contact with parents to relieve their anxiety and to clarify instructions previously given by clinicians; 5) allowing for mutual and specific feedback; 6) allowing for pacing of parents as they test or work with their child; and 7) allowing easy test scoring because the computer gives scores automatically and provides immediate feedback.

Videotapes of a client's behavior also can be useful. The client's behavior can be analyzed to find examples of appropriate or inappropriate behavior. An intervention program can be designed, based on the data accumulated from the tapes and geared to the specific needs of that client. Periodic videotaping during therapy can provide a means of gauging progress and can be used to modify the initial program as necessary. In addition, tapes can be shown to concerned parents, particularly when the child's new behavior patterns occur only in the presence of the clinician and are not yet being used in

---

[1]The clinician must be aware that, when one deviates from the standardized administration of a test, the published norms for the test no longer may be valid and new norms may need to be established.

the home. Clients also can keep track of their success by observing the tapes.

Videotape is preferrable to film because it does not have to be processed, costs less, and is more readily available. It is particularly useful in teaching communication skills that require visual stimuli, such as manual communication, receptive language, or symbol systems (see Wilbur; Kopchick and Lloyd; Carrier; Vanderheiden and Harris-Vanderheiden, this volume). However, to improve sound fidelity, an audiotape should be used in cases where only the production of speech sounds is important.

Intervention

Intervention with the communicatively handicapped can be conducted by trained teachers and clinicians or by supportive personnel or parents (or other family members). Intervention also can occur with minimal supervision, with heavy reliance on media and developed materials, or with some combination of the two. New methods for using TV for intervention programs with handicapped children are continuously being developed and seem to be limited only by the imagination of the developers and the availability of adequate financial resources.

TV Uses with the Deaf A captioned tape is one in which the material presented by the auditory channel is either supplemented or replaced by printed words. The application of captioned films and videotapes for the hearing impaired was initially for entertainment purposes but now is being used for educational purposes. Boston's educational station (WGBH) presents the day's news in caption form at 11:00 p.m. The news program is available to other local stations along the east coast.

Efforts are underway to develop a system for providing regular TV programs with captions. A special decoder was demonstrated at a National Conference on TV for the deaf and hearing impaired at the University of Tennessee in 1971. The device, attached to a TV set, makes captions visible on the screen. Before such a system can be used extensively, several things must occur: 1) the compatibility of different systems needs to be developed or else a single captioning system needs to be established; 2) an effective decoder needs to be developed; 3) field tests need to be conducted; 4) cost factors and economic feasibility must be determined; and 5) an efficient way for captioning films needs to be developed. The Public Broadcasting

System is refining such a system now. An alternative would be to provide open captions, visible to everyone, on all TV shows. For example, a sequence of 26 programs of *The French Chef* has open captions, and the Public Broadcasting System plans additional captioned programs in the future. The availability of captioned materials should greatly enhance the learning of hearing-impaired individuals. It also could be used as an aid to reading.

News programs have been developed in which a person (shown in one corner of the screen) signs what is being presented orally. Such a system also should have utility for teaching other skills to those with communication handicaps. In another endeavor, O'Neill and Oyer (1961) described a series of TV programs that they and others have developed to teach lipreading skills. The programs described have had varying degrees of effectiveness in teaching new sounds, words, and sentences.

Instant Replay   The use of the instant replay feature is probably the most common use of TV for intervention purposes. The clinician videotapes live intervention sessions and stops the tape and replays all or portions of it for the client (Greelis, 1974). During replay, the client observes and hears his behavior in the context in which it occurred. Such vivid confrontations provide a rare opportunity for gaining information about one's own communication behaviors —information that can be used to change undesirable behaviors. The exact point of occurrence of errors can be recaptured so that the individual can be taught how to correct them. Later replays can provide feedback on whether or not progress is being made.

The instant replay feature also can be used by the client to practice specific communication skills. For example, after a clinician has pointed out a particular error pattern, has instructed the client on how to correct it, and is assured that the client understands and can carry out the instruction with practice, the clinician might leave the client to practice alone. Such use requires the clinician to show the client how to use the video equipment. However, the clinician is then free to spend time with other clients.

Live Self-Observation   Live self-observation via TV has several advantages over the use of a mirror: 1) the TV can focus on the desired part(s) of the body; 2) the body parts can be magnified; 3) sound can be included; and 4) the tape can be replayed. A modified TV camera has been developed by Apollo Lasers in Los Angeles. It has a zoom lens with magnification from 4× to 40×

and can be applied to a number of communication needs, such as teaching signs.

Animated Puppets   Greelis (1974) reported the use of animated puppets for therapeutic purposes. The child watches the puppet on a TV monitor. The puppet operator, who is able to observe the child without being observed, has the puppet instruct the child on what to do (i.e., request imitation of sounds, words, or actions) and reinforce the child for appropriate behavior. If a clinician is in the room with the child, the clinician's influence over the child can be increased by having the puppet model behaviors requested by the clinician. The puppet thus serves the functions of teacher, model, and dispenser of reinforcers. The puppet, because of its strong appeal to most children (Baer and Sherman, 1967), also can serve as a motivational device for obtaining and maintaining the child's attention so that intervention can occur with a minimal loss of time.

Prerecorded Videotapes   Prerecorded videotapes can be used as language intervention aids (Greelis, 1974). The tapes could be selected from those that are commercially available or could be made by a clinician for use in therapy sessions. For example, a tape might include a sequence of appropriately modeled behaviors that the child is to imitate. The sequence could be followed by potential reinforcers such as a cartoon strip, by a sequence of inappropriate behaviors, or by a blank period during which the child can engage in other behaviors. In such use, the videotape is in a programmed format similar to that used with teaching machines.

Lombardi and Poole (1968) developed a series of videotapes for use in a state institution for the mentally retarded. The tapes were a part of a speech and language development program. Lombardi and Poole reported paying particular attention to developing tapes that would be visually and auditorily stimulating because many videotapes do not seem to be so.

Cypreansen and McBride (1956) described a series of 16 speechreading lessons given over a Nebraska Educational TV station. Individuals could register for credit with the university and could obtain a manual to accompany the programs. The last lesson included a test. Returned tests indicated that persons both with hearing impairment and with normal hearing learned from the programs.

Larkey and Brownstein (1974) are compiling a library of existing TV tapes, films, filmstrips, and slide presentations concerned with parent education on child development, facilitating developmental skills, community adaptation, self-care, and job readiness skills. They plan to review these existing materials to help in the development of new materials.

Two-Way Telecommunication System In the two-way telecommunication system, an individual at home can tune in to a special TV channel and can respond to information presented via the TV by pressing buttons on a console connected to the TV. The viewer responses are monitored by a computer at the TV station. Larkey and Brownstein (1974) are developing such a system to deliver services to mentally and/or physically handicapped children and adults and for their caregivers (parents, etc.) in urban areas. They plan to collect data on various potential use areas. Such a system might be even more useful in rural areas where few, if any, services exist. In addition, such a TV system could provide additional services for individuals who: 1) are already involved in existing service programs, 2) cannot get to service agencies, 3) are on waiting lists for existing services, 4) are living in areas where few, if any, services exist, 5) will not seek services for fear that a stigma will be attached to their child, or 6) have been discharged from programs where no follow-up services are provided. Larky and Brownstein (1974) plan to include comparisons of live versus one- and two-way TV systems in their research effort, as well as keeping data on the effectiveness of such a system for various purposes. Baldwin, Greenberg, and Muth (1975) plan to collect similar data on a two-way system concerned with both assessment and intervention processes. If such systems prove to be effective and economically feasible, their impact will be limited only by imagination.

Dual Audio Television Borton (1971) has proposed a system called Dual Audio Television. The system consists of a commercial TV program with a second announcer weaving comments in between the verbal script and music of the regular program. The comments of the second announcer could be received by the child from a transistor radio through an "ear bug." From the radio, the child would receive a broadcast aimed at helping him understand the particular TV program being broadcast. The narrator could define words, ask questions, repeat words shown visually on the screen (but not presented auditorily, such as show titles and actor's names), and explain plots. Borton (1971) tested such a system with 200 children and reported that the experimental group learned more than the control group and was more actively involved in what happened.

The drawback of such a system is that what needs to be explained varies from age to age and from child to child. However, if such a system is effective, it also would be feasible for a parent or teacher to serve the role of the second announcer by being present and explaining to the child the things with which the child specifically needs help. This person also could increase the child's communication skills by having the child repeat words and sentences out loud, by repeating definitions of words, and by using new words in sentences constructed by the child himself. Another way of dealing with the problem would be to have different levels of explanations; e.g., one radio station would present the material at a first-grade level, another at a second-grade level, and so on. While such an approach would be useful with many children, the clinician must be careful to avoid perceptual overload with many developmentally disabled children.

Reading by Television   Torr (1974) reported using television to increase the reading rate of a young deaf student who was losing his vision. The TV camera was mounted on a stand so that the lens pointed straight down. Lights were placed on each side. The reading material was placed under the camera, and the child read the material by looking at it under magnification on the TV monitor. The student also could write under the camera and see the results on the screen. It would be feasible to expand such a system for teaching reading and language skills to children with communicative problems by adding an audio portion to materials presented via TV. Thus, the child could see a word and its referent object while simultaneously hearing the word itself. Such materials could be available on prerecorded tapes.

Delayed Video Feedback   Delay auditory feedback devices often have been used to deal with communication problems such as stuttering. In using such a device, individuals monitor their own voice as they speak. However, a delay is inserted between the speaking and hearing of what was said. The length of the delay can be varied by changing the distance between the record and playback heads of the tape recorder. Sometimes this is done with commercially available machines and other times by running a tape from the record head on one tape recorder to the playback head on another recorder.

To date, no one has tried to add a visual component to such a delayed feedback system; however, it seems both feasible and useful. Theoretically, a videocorder could be used in the same manner as a delayed audio feedback device. In dealing with problems like articulation therapy, clients not only would hear their performance shortly after speaking, but also would be able to see the visible aspects of the mouth and tongue movements they used. It seems easier to analyze one's own speech after a brief delay than to analyze it while also producing it. A clinician even might present the stimuli to clients on videotape. Thus, clients could hear and see a correct model and compare that with their own performance. The same result could be accomplished by a delayed feedback audio device if the individual were seated in front of a mirror. One also might use a delayed video feedback system with individuals learning sign language.

Stimulation and TV Preference   Friedlander (1970) has developed an apparatus called the Playtest. It consists of a pair of large response switches, a loudspeaker, an electronic control and response recording unit, and a stereo tape player with a preprogrammed selection of two audio channels. The apparatus is placed by a baby's crib. When the baby pushes either switch, he automatically records the frequency and duration of his responses and simultaneously turns on one channel of the audio tape. Different stimulus materials are programmed on the two audio channels; thus, one can determine the type of stimulation preferred by the baby. His response rate for preferred types of stimulation (e.g., his mother's voice) should increase. Babies in the 11- to 15-month age range show clear preferences for certain types of stimulation although such preferences differ from baby to baby. Such a device could be readily used to provide stimulation for children with communication handicaps. In fact, one could expand the stimulation provided by replacing the audio tape player with a TV set. The baby then could receive both audio and visual stimulation.

Striefel and Smeets (1974) and Striefel (1974a) reported the use of a procedure similar to Friedlander's for determining the TV preference of older retarded children. The technique used three videocorders all in continuous motion, each with a different program attached to one of four response keys. Depression of any one of three keys resulted in the presentation, on the TV monitor, of the auditory and visual stimuli associated with a specific program. The fourth key had no programmed consequence. The simultaneous depression of more than one key, a failure to respond, and the depression of the blank key (the key with no programmed consequences) resulted in no audio or video being presented. To eliminate the possibility of position responding, the consequence associated with each of the four keys was switched periodically during the session. The duration, in seconds, that the child depressed the key associated with each consequence was recorded. From these data, the child's program preference was determined. The technique was used by Striefel (1974a) to isolate the preferred variables within a program, e.g., a program in color versus black and white. The technique could be used to determine an individual's TV program preference and then deliver that program contingent on other behaviors, e.g., sounds emitted correctly. It also could be used to determine what type of programs and program variables are most reinforcing for a particular individual or type of audience. Such information could be used to develop videotapes (or films) for use for educational or therapeutic use.

In summary, TV has been used in a variety of ways for intervention purposes, yet many other possible uses probably will be developed in the future. The potential use of TV for intervention in communication problems has only begun to be realized.

Training

TV has great potential for changing the attitudes of professional and paraprofessional personnel, and the public in general, toward handicapped people. TV also can be used to teach such groups specific intervention skills and provide them with feedback on their own performance (Boone and Prescott, 1972).

Attitude Changes   Austin (1969) reported using videotapes to modify the attitudes of persons working with the mentally retarded. Accepting the mentally retarded and other persons with handicaps as human beings with feelings, emotions, problems, and potential probably fosters progress in providing them with the skills they need. Well developed videotape presentations have the potential for educating those working with the handicapped as well as the public in general.

A series of films, tapes, and slide shows concerned with modifying the attitudes of the public concerning the mentally retarded, hearing impaired, and other handicapped groups is currently available (see Appendix G). Efforts should be made to broadcast some of this information on a regular basis on national television, possibly in the form of 30-second "spot" announcements. Such an endeavor might begin eroding the old stereotypes and stigmas that have for so long plagued the handicapped. Moore (1955) presented a series of 12 TV programs concerned with changing attitudes. Unfortunately, the effectiveness of the programs in changing attitudes is unknown. It often has been stated that a person who is told something often enough will soon begin to believe it. The area of attitude changes might well be the ideal testing ground for such an idea.

Continuous loop films, videotapes, and slide sound presentations concerned with changing attitudes could be made available in supermarkets, laundromats, and lobbies of public buildings and thus could serve as a vehicle for changing public attitudes.

Videotapes could be made about the feelings and adjustments of a family who discovers that their child has a handicap such as retardation. These tapes then could be shown to other families in similar situations. After seeing the tapes, the content could be discussed with a family as a preliminary means of coping with the family's emotions.

Training Tapes   Videotapes that teach people from various backgrounds to work with handicapped children are limited in number and content. Videotapes could be designed and sequenced to teach, particularly through demonstration, some of the specific skills used in remediation of communication problems. Well developed tapes can be reused and can provide a teaching method that is probably easier to learn from than a verbal or written format. Such training tapes are now being developed by Murry Sidman at the Shriver Center in Boston. The tapes are designed to teach many of the applied behavior analysis skills such as the application of consequences of behavior, conditioned reinforcement, fading, shaping, and stimulus control procedures. The videotapes allow the trainee to see the small changes in behavior that are followed by the delivery of a reinforcer. The format used in Sidman's tapes is also of interest. It is an interactive system between the viewer and the tape. At critical points, the tape presents questions to the viewer about what has been presented. The tape is then stopped while the viewer answers the question on an interaction sheet. Such a system has several advantages including: 1) active involvement of the viewer,

2) self-pacing for the viewer, and 3) use of a programmed format.

Videotape Feedback   Many of the comments and issues discussed in the previous section on instant replay apply to the use of videotapes for training intervention personnel. Thus, they are not reiterated here. Holvoet (1974) stated that the majority of studies involving videotape feedback used the trainees themselves as models and then gave oral feedback on their performance (Gibbs, 1970; Marshall and Hegrenes, 1970; Eisenberg, 1971; Fauguet, 1971; Greenberg, 1973). Feedback on one's behavior clearly can result in behavioral changes, but using the trainees as their own model also results in variance that may preclude the possibilities of predicting later success or failure. A more useful initial step would be to have trainees watch a videotape of another person, possibly with the other person also getting feedback. Koran, Snow, and McDonald (1971) reported that observing a videotape of another model resulted in higher performance levels than did the use of written models or the use of no models at all. After the individual observes various models performing a task, asks questions, and discusses the different levels of performance, then the individual should perform the various tasks while being videotaped. This procedure should save time and money in training personnel and should be a morally defensible way of screening applicants for jobs that require that specific procedures be followed.

Nardine (1974) observed that parents are a valuable teaching resource. They are motivated to help their own child acquire communication skills. However, they must master specific skills if they are to be effective. As parents learn to work with their child, they must be able to analyze their own teaching behavior in terms of what is and what is not effective. Watching videotapes of other teachers often helps them learn to discriminate effective from ineffective techniques. It may be advisable for clinicians or teachers to review the tape with the parents, pointing out factors that the parents are not yet able to discriminate on their own.

Videotapes (and audiotapes) also can be used by clinicians to improve their own skills. Clinicians can analyze the content and sequence of events in therapy by replaying the tapes (Boone and Goldberg, 1969; Boone and Stech, 1970). Boone and Prescott (1972) reported that audiotapes may be more practical than videotapes for such purposes in many clinical settings. However, the use of audiotapes results in an average loss of about 15% of the information in a speech and hearing session. This loss does not occur with videotapes. The basic content and sequence analysis used by Boone and Prescott consist of:

1. Recording the middle 20 minutes of a therapy session
2. Selecting for playback and analysis a 5-minute segment of the recording
3. Having the clinician view and hear the 5-minute segment with no attempt to score the content on sequence of events
4. Replaying the segment and having the clinician score it using Boone and Prescott's Ten Category System Analysis
5. Summarizing the content and sequence of events on a therapy and scoring form

Boone and Prescott (1972) reported a maximum of 2 hours to teach clinicians to use the system and a maximum of 20 minutes to replay, score, and summarize the data from a 5-minute therapy segment. This system enables clinicians in training to study the therapy techniques of a master clinician, to examine the various parameters of the clinical process, and to confront themselves and analyze their own therapy skills. The use of a therapy content and sequence analysis procedure also provides a supervisor with a systematic technique for evaluating the progress of clinicians in training.

Because of the limited time needed to train clinicians in the use of such a system and the limited time needed to apply the system, it seems highly probable that such a system also could be utilized to improve the skills of parents and other paraprofessionals involved in training individuals with communication difficulties.

FILMS

Many of the advantages and uses described in the previous section on TV are also pertinent to the use of films. Although the uses are not reiterated here, it is suggested that the reader remember that videotapes and films often can be used interchangeably to accomplish the same goals. The following material is selected to represent current applications of films to the communications problems of the handicapped. Proposals for future applications are also presented.

Assessment

O'Neill and Oyer (1961) described a standardized testing format that employs 16mm film. The test is the Mason Multiple Choice

Test for Children, developed by Marie K. Mason of the Hearing and Speech Clinic at Ohio State University. It assesses whether or not a preschool deaf child can recognize a spoken word visually by choosing from a set of four the picture that corresponds to the word spoken by a person on the screen. The testing format is separated into three phases, each of which is presented on 16mm film. The first film shows a teacher seated at a table flanked by two children: there is a set of five objects in front of her. She picks up each object sequentially, turns to one child and pronounces the name of the object, turns to the second child and pronounces the name again, and finally pronounces the name directly into the camera. In a second film, the teacher pronounces the name of an object but does not identify it. The children who flank her identify the object by marking an X through a picture of their choice on a large chart containing several sets of four pictures. Before observing the third film, the child being tested is given a test form containing several sets of four pictures. As the child watches, the teacher in the third film pronounces words corresponding to the pictures on the form. The child's task is to mark an X through the correct picture.

As O'Neill and Oyer pointed out, a film testing format offers advantages over more traditional formats because: 1) each child views and responds to the same films so that standardization is assured; 2) the simplicity of the testing format allows the most unsophisticated of examiners to administer the test: the films only need to be started and stopped with the child being given test materials at appropriate times; 3) the testing of groups of children is allowed for, thus economizing examiner time; and 4) the modeling of peers may be an advantage when attempting to assess difficult-to-treat children. From the work of Bandura (1965) and others, it is well documented that children have a high probability of modeling the film-mediated behavior of peers. Having difficult-to-test children imitate the test-taking behavior of peers may save the examiner lengthy time periods for establishing rapport. An alternative to presenting peers as models might be to use puppets, cartoon characters, or clowns. Testing films also might be developed in which such characters assume the role of the examiner. Baer and Sherman (1964) have commented that children seem to relate quite naturally to puppets.

Intervention

Many films have been developed as intervention aids for improving the communication problems of the handicapped. The following paragraphs describe a sample of films available. (Sources of other films are listed in Appendix G.)

Withrow (1975), working at the Illinois School for the Deaf in Jacksonville, Illinois, in the 1960's developed a series of more than 100 sound films designed to teach a vocabulary of 300 nouns to deaf children. Each of the objects represented in the films is paired with appropriate speech, speechreading, and cursive stimuli. The films are designed so that they can be used by children individually or in a group.

Driscoll (1968) described three films produced at the University of California and designed to teach retarded adolescents. One film deals with the experiences of an apparently retarded young man attempting to find a job, another with economic issues such as consumer demand, and the third with the structure of American government. The films are specifically designed in terms of their pacing and narration to impart factual information, change attitudes, and develop concepts. From an analysis of a variety of pre- and postviewing measures, Driscoll made the following conclusions:

1.   The films were effective in teaching factual information and changing attitudes
2.   The films seemed to be effective in developing concepts in all but the most retarded of the population studied
3.   Humor and audiovisual cuing were not as important as story line
4.   Animation and color were not superior to live production and black and white

Mason (1961) described a series of thiry 16mm silent color films designed to teach speechreading. The films are sequenced to proceed from simple to more complex aspects of speechreading, and each is a complete instructional unit dealing with a different phonetic element or principle. The lack of a synchronized sound track, however, seriously limits the use of these films. However, such films with a synchronized audiovisual presentation could be used in conjunction with a fading procedure to facilitate discrimination of speechreading cues. For example, a film first might be viewed with the volume on the sound track set at the optimal level to take advantage of residual hearing. Once speechreading was established under these conditions, the volume gradually could be decreased to improve visual speech discrimination using an approach similar to that described by Sidman and Stoddard (1967) to teach other types of visual discriminations.

Training

Films also have been developed for training people to deal with the communication problems of the handicapped. For example, the John Tracy Speech Clinic, in Los Angeles, produced a series of 42 films, entitled "Teaching Speech to the Profoundly Deaf" (Rowe, 1974). The first three films describe the clinic's speech model, which is designed to give teachers a systematic framework for planning appropriate learning experiences. This model represents speech training in three dimensions: the stages of learning the process, incorporation into appropriate words, and generalization. The other 39 films deal with various aspects of teaching speech to the deaf.

The Tracy Clinic also has produced a series of 19 parent education films. This series includes an introductory film, nine films dealing with the psychologic problems of parents, and nine dealing with techniques for building communication skills.

TEACHING MACHINES

The hardware of most teaching machines consists of three basic components: 1) a mechanism for presenting stimuli to a subject, 2) a mechanism that the subject can use to respond to the stimuli, and 3) a mechanism for giving the subject feedback concerning the accuracy of the response. The software consists of a program of carefully designed stimulus materials. Several steps are involved in developing a program for use with a teaching machine. First, the subject to be mastered or the skill to be taught is carefully defined in reference to a specific audience. Next, the subject or skill is broken down into bits of information that must be mastered. Subsequently, stimulus presentations designed to impart these bits of information to the subject are developed. Finally, the stimulus presentations are arranged sequentially beginning with the most basic and proceeding gradually through the most complex materials. Ideally, the information imparted by a correct response to one stimulus presentation allows the subject to respond correctly to the next stimulus presentation and without error to proceed through the program to master the subject or skill.

As Skinner (1967) pointed out, the advantages of teaching machine systems are that the user is immediately and frequently reinforced for correct responses, usually by responding correctly, and that progress occurs through a coherent sequence of active participation at the subject's own pace.

A number of teaching machine systems that incorporate audiovisual stimulus presentations have been developed. A discussion of some of these systems and their uses follows.

Assessment

To date, administering standardized tests via teaching machines has not been tried, although the idea is plausible. For example, administration of a test like the Peabody Picture Vocabulary Test easily could be adapted to a teaching machine format.[2] This test requires a child to choose from four pictures the one that best corresponds to a word spoken by the examiner. The four pictures could be presented on the visual display of the teaching machine via a paper tape or slide projector while an audiotape presented instructions and the stimulus words to the child. Clear plastic response panels could be arranged over the visual display in such a manner that, when the child touches a picture, the child's response automatically is recorded and the program advances to the next stimulus presentation. The system also could be given the capacity to move to the appropriate starting point for a particular child when certain demographic data were punched in and to automatically score the test. Such a system of test administration assures standardization and reliability of scoring and places minimal demands on the examiner.

Teaching machine programs use criterion-referenced tests for determining a "starting point" for each subject. The tests determine the skills and deficiencies of each subject. After analysis of the test results, subjects are exposed to program materials appropriate for developing the skills they do not have. Tests are readministered to provide an objective measure of the program's effects.

Audiovisual teaching machine systems developed for dealing with communication problems of the handicapped typically have not incorporated standardized criterion-referenced tests into the system. Rather, this assessment seems to occur informally as the stimulus materials are presented or other testing formats are used. One excep-

---

[2] See footnote 1.

tion to this seems to be programs developed for Project LIFE (Pfau, 1975). This project includes a set of programmed materials designed to teach basic language and reading skills to language-impaired children. Built into the program are diagnostic tests for determining a child's needs and posttests for evaluation of the program's effects.

Intervention

A variety of audiovisual teaching machine systems has been developed to improve the quality of speech of the handicapped by training various parameters of speech. Basically, these systems involve having a clinician vocalize a unit of speech into a microphone. The sound is transmitted to the client via headphones or a hearing aid and is also displayed on an oscilloscope or television screen. Clients must match the pattern created on the screen by the clinician with their own vocalization. For example, Pickett (1968a) described the Visible Speech Translator, a device developed by Bell Telephone Laboratories and used in articulation training. It represents a unit of speech on a storage oscilloscope in three dimensions: frequency, time, and energy. Frequency corresponds to the height of columns of lights on the oscilloscope screen, time is represented horizontally, and energy is represented by the brightness of the lights.

Berg and Fletcher (1970) described a similar piece of apparatus called the Video Articulator, which represents phonemes as distinct patterns on a television screen as an individual speaks. For example, the /s/ sound appears as a dark swirl and the /n/ sound as a circular pattern with two loops in it. This device also has the capacity for training pitch. Controls on the front of the apparatus can be set to represent any pitch frequency between 50 and 500 Hz as a circle of a particular diameter on the television screen. When the client sustains a vowel, its frequency also appears on the screen as a circular pattern. When the two frequencies represented are the same, they superimpose and a beating configuration is produced. Similar systems have been developed for training voiced or nonvoiced discrimination, the /s/ sound, intonation, and nasality, among other parameters. Many of these devices are described by Pickett (1968b).

Boothroyd et al. (1975) described a computer system that can be programmed to aid individuals in improving articulation skills. They pointed out that such a system offers several advantages: 1) computers, by their very nature, can make complicated speech transformations; 2) computers, once programmed, are simple for clinicians to use—most programs can be initiated by the press of a button; 3) computer programs can be modified relatively easily in comparison to modifying an existing machine or building a new one to serve a particular function. The components of the system are a microphone into which the clinician or client speaks; a computer that stores speech patterns and represents them visually on an oscilloscope; and an accelerometer (vibration detector) that can be attached to the nose, for detecting nasal vibrations, or to the throat, for detecting vocal cord vibrations. The system has the capacity for storing and freezing speech patterns and for representing those of the clinician and client simultaneously.

Currently, four programs are available for use with the system. One program is designed to train the following speech parameters: loudness, pitch, voicing, nasality, tongue position in vowels, aspirations, and certain combinations of these parameters. The parameter to be trained is selected from a "menu" displayed on the oscilloscope screen. Once a program is selected, it is used by having children match their own speech pattern display to a sample of the clinician's speech displayed on the screen. A second program allows for the matching of a speech spectrum. Vocalizations are displayed in two dimensions. Frequency is represented along the vertical axis of the display with low frequencies at the bottom and high frequencies at the top. The width of the image corresponds to the energy at each frequency. Two game programs that have been found to be highly motivating when used with children are also available. One involves a cartoon face. The size of the mouth is controlled by loudness, and the height of its adam's apple is controlled by pitch. The other game involves having the subject move basketballs across the screen past obstacles and into a basket. Control of the ball's movement is determined by the pitch of the child's voice.

Dawson (1973) described a device called the Language Master, which can be used in a number of ways including training in articulation, language, and reading. For example, the Central Arkansas Education Center has used this device to improve reading skills in retarded persons. The apparatus employs cards with a word and/or picture printed on them and two strips of magnetic tape fixed along the bottom. The child views the word and/or picture as the card is fed through the Language Master and, at the same time, hears the word or words pronounced. After hearing the word, the child repeats it and the device auditorily feeds back that response for comparison with the standard. Standard or blank cards can be purchased for use with the device. The blank cards are quite versatile in that pictures or photographs may be fixed to them or words printed on them while appropriate auditory stimuli are recorded on the magnetic tape.

Project LIFE (Pfau, 1975) developed an extensive set of programmed materials for establishing basic language and reading skills in the repertoires of language-impaired children. The materials are designed to train skills in three core areas: 1) perceptual training, including visual properties, additions and omissions, spatial relations, positions in space, and figure-ground relationships; 2) perceptual thinking, including object memory, color memory, sequencing according to size, simple pattern analysis, picture analysis, picture absurdities, and figural transformations; and 3) language/reading, where language principles and concepts and basic sentence patterns are introduced. In addition to these core materials, many other support materials are currently available and still others are continually being developed. All materials are carefully sequenced and their content is selected to be particularly motivating to children.

Project LIFE materials are designed to be used with two sets of teaching machine hardware developed by General Electric. Both systems allow for viewing of stimulus presentations via a filmstrip projector. One of these, the PAL System (Programmed Assistance to Learners), is a self-contained unit that the child works on independently. The other system, the Student Response Program Master, is designed for use with a remote control filmstrip projector. This system allows the teacher to present the same stimuli on individual monitors to a group of children. With both systems, the child responds to the presentation by pressing one of four buttons on a console. A correct response causes the illumination of a green "go" light and the advancing of the filmstrip. Errors are automatically recorded, and the filmstrip does not advance until the correct response is made. With the PAL system, children can move at their own pace through the program but must reach a criterion of 80% correct responses to the stimuli presented by any one filmstrip before being allowed to move to the next filmstrip. Both systems can be used in conjunction with other visual devices, such as slide projectors, and both have audio capacity.

Withrow (1975) designed a series of pilot materials to teach the passive and active voices. The materials have a style similar to that used on *The Electric Company,* a childrens' TV show, but include response items about every 90 seconds. Responses are multiple choice and can be made, via interactive cable TV techniques, in conjunction with a PAL program master or in response booklets. Withrow also produced some pilot materials using computer graphics to emphasize verbs and prepositions. The words change into the action or object as the audio narration is made. For example, in the sentence, *The butterfly is flying,* the word *butterfly* animates into a butterfly as it is said and flies away as the words *is flying* are said. Withrow reported that young children are fascinated with such sequences and that their attention is almost 100%. The use of such sequences is a good example of intrinsic motivation, which Pfau (1972) suggested must be included in language materials for the deaf and which probably applies equally to other groups with communication handicaps.

Spradlin, Cotter, and Baxley (1973), researching the development of language concepts in retarded children, used a match-to-sample apparatus in which a sample is delivered either visually or auditorily and is followed by the presentation of several choices in the form of pictures, words, etc., displayed on illuminated panels. The child responds by pushing on the panel displaying one of the choices. Using this procedure, Spradlin, Cotter, and Baxley have been able to establish response classes by sequentially training members of the classes until the children generalize the concept and respond correctly to items not yet trained. This match-to-sample strategy for training communication skills has just begun to prove its utility.

Sidman and his colleagues (Sidman and Cresson, 1973; Sidman, Cresson, and Willson-Morris, 1974) have developed a teaching machine system that employs a variety of matching tasks to teach basic reading and reading related skills to retarded children. In this system, the child is seated before a display of nine panels, eight of which are response panels arranged in a circle around a central panel. Each trial is begun by presenting the child with a sample stimulus either visually via the central panel or auditorially via a speaker. For example, the child might be presented with the printed word *car* on the central panel or the sound of the word *car* over the speaker. After presentation of the sample stimulus, the child is required to make a response by touching the central panel. Completion of that response causes other response choices to be presented on the response panels. For example, pictures of a car, an axe, a saw, a cap, a man, a cow, an ear, and a hat might be presented. Using the printed word *car* as the sample stimulus, the child could make a correct response by touching the response panel on which a picture of a car was displayed. Correct responses cause a chime to sound and are reinforced by delivery of a toy, candy, or token. The reading and reading-related skills this system has been employed to teach are:

1.   Identity matching—the child is presented with a printed word as a sample stimulus and must respond by touching the same printed word on the response panel
2.   Picture naming—the child is presented with a picture as a sample stimulus and must respond by saying the word that corresponds to the picture
3.   Oral reading—the child is presented with a printed word as a sample stimulus and must respond by saying the word
4.   Auditory receptive reading—the child is presented with the sound of a word as a sample stimulus and must respond by touching the same printed word on the response panel
5.   Auditory comprehension—the child is presented with the sound of a word as a sample stimulus and must respond by touching the picture corresponding to it on the response panel
6.   Reading comprehension I—the child is presented with a picture of a sample stimulus and must respond by touching the corresponding printed word on the response panel
7.   Reading comprehension II—the child is presented with a printed word as a sample stimulus and must respond by touching the corresponding picture on the response panel

Interestingly, the developers of this system found that each skill does not have to be taught independently. Instead, generalization of skills occurs: Once one skill is learned, performance on the others is improved. For example, Sidman, Cresson, and Willson-Morris (1974) found that one child's performance on reading comprehension II, auditory receptive reading, and oral reading tasks improved after training on identity matching, auditory comprehension, and reading comprehension I tasks.

Wyman (1969) described an overhead projector system that is designed to improve small group interaction between teacher and students and that incorporates a number of teaching machine features. The system is referred to as MIRV, Mediated Interaction Visual Response system. According to Wyman, in a small group interaction the teacher presents a question and calls on one child in the group to respond orally while the rest of the children observe. With the MIRV system, the teacher faces the students and presents a question via an overhead projector on to a screen in front of the students. All members of the group then respond on individual transparencies, and their answers appear on a screen behind them via overhead projectors. For example, the teacher presents a picture of a ball on the screen and asks the children to spell the word *ball* on their transparencies. The teacher then checks the children's responses, projected on the screen behind them, and gives each child feedback on the correctness of the response.

The system is quite flexible in that it allows the teacher to present questions and the children to respond in a wide variety of ways. The question could be presented orally, via records, slides, or transparencies. Children could respond on their transparencies by underlining the correct word in a sentence or by pointing to the appropriate object among choices (recognition responses) or filling in the blanks (recall responses). This system, like all good teaching machine systems, ensures that each child responds actively to each stimulus presentation and receives immediate feedback regarding responses. Materials used with the MIRV system typically have been designed to suit the needs of both teacher and student. Sequentially programmed materials have not been developed although they are certainly possible.

Kant, Ramos, and Shanks (1970) reported on the use of a "talking" typewriter to teach reading skills to emotionally disturbed children. This system, produced by Thomas A. Edison Laboratories, incorporates a computerized electric typewriter, tape recorder, speaker, viewing screen, and slide projector that is housed within a small booth. The system is capable of operating on three levels:

1. As a typewriter with large print
2. As a system for feeding back information to the child about the key just pressed; the system can be programmed to feed back to the child auditorily the name of the letter, the phonetic sound, or the color associated with any key pressed
3. As a programmed system: programs are fed into the system on cards with a strip of magnetic tape fastened onto the back. The tape gives instructions to the computer regarding what stimuli to present to the child. For example, a program might be fed in whereby the computer instructs the child to type the name of the picture projected on the screen. The cards also may be used to present stimulus materials, e.g., typed messages, drawings, photographs

In addition, the teacher can observe the child through a small window in the booth and, from a control panel, control variables such as the type, delay, and repetition of cues. Kant, Ramos, and Shanks (1970) have developed individualized prescriptive programs for remediation of the reading difficulties of emotionally disturbed children. These authors have emphasized the importance of this type of programming for emotionally disturbed children. They also have suggested that the impersonal, infinitely patient manner of presentation offered by this talking typewriter in an advantage in working with this population.

Upton (1968) adapted some of the elements of teaching machine technology to a unique pair of eyeglasses that are used in conjunction with a hearing aid and speechreading to enable a hearing-impaired individual to understand spoken language. Five incandescent lamps are bonded into the lenses of a pair of eyeglasses. The lamps form a V around the pupil, and each lamp lights in correspondence with different parameters of phonemes. The parameters that the device is sensitive to are frication, stop, voicing, voiced frication, and voiced stop. Upton pointed out, however, that the device is not 100% reliable. It does not respond at all to some of the more difficult phonemes and makes errors on others. It takes time for an individual to learn to use the device and become accustomed to the lamps, but once the device is mastered, its use becomes automatic. Upton cited two advantages. First, the device allows deaf or hearing-impaired persons to view their own speech in the same channel that they view other people's, therefore serving as a training device; and second, it can indicate sounds such as a telephone ringing or a vehicle approaching and thus help to create some of the "sense of awareness" present in individuals with normal hearing.

Another related system, not designed as a teaching machine, is the TV phone developed by Phonics Corporation to enable the deaf and hearing impaired to communicate over long distances. The system employs a special crystal to interpret sounds by means of a telephone typewriter that displays the typewritten message on a TV screen. If provided with a feedback mechanism, it could be developed as a teaching machine for the hearing impaired. Additional related systems are described in the annotated bibliography of communication aids by Luster and Vanderheiden (1974).

Training

With proper training and supervision, supportive personnel, aides, and parents can be taught to conduct intervention procedures. One approach is to rely on media and materials that have been developed for this purpose.

The CAMS (Computer Assisted Monitoring System) Project at Utah State University's Exceptional Child Center consists of a curriculum and monitoring system to assist professionals, paraprofessionals, and parents in teaching handicapped children (Casto et al., 1975). To date, this system consists of three basic programs, one each in receptive and expressive language and one in motor development. The Receptive Language Program is a sequential set of instructions and criteria for guiding parents, paraprofessionals, and teachers in teaching skills ranging from responding to auditory symbols through relatively complex concepts such as identifying plurals. The Expressive Language Program is designed to teach skills ranging from increasing verbalizations to use of relatively complex sentences. The motor program is designed for use with children who are primarily "slow developers" or mentally retarded. It begins with behaviors such as raising the head and terminates with behaviors such as running and skipping.

The use of these materials is taught through slide-sound presentations in a format similar to that used with teaching machines. Each presentation describes the procedures, requires the individual to make a paper-and-pencil response to questions, and provides feedback as to the correctness of the response. This has proved to be a very effective means of training professionals and nonprofessionals to follow the program's procedures. Additionally, these presentations have the advantage of being relatively inexpensive to produce and highly transportable. The materials have been designed to be relatively self-contained and to provide services to children in rural areas where other services are scarce or unavailable.

Many sequenced programs have been written to train individuals to deal with the communication and communication related problems of the handicapped, and the majority employ a programmed text format. However, it would be quite possible to adapt them to various audiovisual formats. For example, Striefel (1974b) developed a step-by-step method for teaching retarded children to imitate motor behaviors; the method is outlined in a programmed booklet designed to train others to use it. Within the training program itself, behaviors are broken down into a sequence of small steps and each step is described for the trainer. A sequence of pictures accompanies the description for the purpose of illustration. Because written training procedures are often tedious to read and comprehend, Striefel (1972b) also made a 16mm sound film of the procedures. The training procedures also could have been made available in the form of a slide sound show or videotape. The availability of training programs in a variety of formats increases their versatility by allowing organizations that may have only certain equipment (e.g., only a slide projector or only a videotape player) access to the programs. A listing of sources of information is available in Appendix G.

MATERIALS

Lance (1973) has pointed out that each individual child cannot have his own special teacher, but that media can help individualize each child's instruction. Individualization of programs could be accomplished by matching learner variables with the instructional techniques used. The critical variables include:

1.   How the child reacts to media that utilize various input and output modes
2.   What curriculum areas require materials that differ from those being used by the majority of the individual's peers
3.   What interactive aspects of the learning environment must be modified to enhance learning

Individualization of instruction requires active involvement in the learning process by including the learner *in* media, not just having the learner *use* the media.

The main reasons why individualized instruction systems are not yet available are that most teachers:

1.   Lack the time needed to individualize instruction
2.   Are not prepared to diagnose, prescribe, or implement on an individual basis
3.   Lack access to an effective system
4.   Find that instructional materials are not available
5.   Lack access to a specially designed classroom

6. Lack access to equipment that is permanently located in their classroom (checking equipment in and out each time it is needed is time consuming and limits flexibility)

Aserlind (1966) postulated that the shortage of materials exists because:

1. Teachers are accustomed to developing their own materials
2. The market for such specialized materials is small, so that few publishers and producers of audiovisual media have invested in it
3. No agency has been given the task of evaluating materials
4. Researchers are more interested in basic than in applied research

The situation is changing, however. Over the past years, the availability of instructional materials has changed dramatically. The large variety of resources currently available for developing instructional materials and their accessibility to teachers will continue to make drastic changes in the teaching-learning process with handicapped children (Stepp, 1970). The development of instructional materials has placed the teacher in a different, more demanding role. The very term *instructional* materials indicates that the purpose of the materials is to provide a basis for learning (Belland and Rothenberg, 1973).

Teachers no longer regard media and their associated materials as being only for use by the teachers as aids in their presentations; they also see a need for student involvement. Students are becoming much more involved, not only in operating and using the equipment but also in choosing the curriculum materials they would like to learn. In this type of classroom setting, the teacher's role becomes one not only of instructing but also of advising, monitoring, and guiding the learning experience (Stepp, 1970).

Teachers must know how and when to use individualized programs and how and when to use interactive and group instruction methods. Teachers also must be aware of what materials are appropriate and available for their students as a group or as individuals. This includes the ability to know when not to use AV materials and media, such as when their use actually may be handicapping to certain children. For example, certain children with hearing impairments or language deficits may be unable to understand the auditory instructions and/or information accompanying the curriculum materials. In addition, the signal-to-noise ratio resulting from use of the equipment may cause reception problems for children with hearing aids.

Children who are mentally retarded or who have attention span or figure-ground problems also may have difficulty learning from standard AV materials. The teacher's strategy then becomes one of providing a prescriptive program for the students. This type of teaching strategy generates new needs in educational media and materials.

A review of current needs assessment studies for media and materials in special education programs (Lange, Mattson, and Thomann, 1974) indicated that most of the reviewed studies were limited to small geographic areas and that much of the information included was part of existing records or was reported within broader studies. The reviewers categorized the needs identified by the studies into the following four categories: 1) need for instructional materials, 2) need for training in the use of instructional media and materials, 3) need for information about existing media and materials, and 4) need for methods and strategies of distributing media and materials. Within the reviewed studies, most needs were identified by teachers of the handicapped. Lange, Mattson, and Thomann mentioned that teachers' perceived needs may not be the same as that of other groups such as administrators and that teachers who have not used or had access to such materials did not express a need for them. Needs were identified only when the teacher was aware of a service or material and had used it or had seen its use demonstrated.

Across studies, needs in only a few academic content areas appeared. These were language arts, social studies, science, and mathematics. The only content area that was identified as a high priority need was for new or revised materials in language arts. A high need for mathematics was not reported, and the social studies were in the low to moderate need level. Teachers of the trainable mentally retarded reported a greater need for media and materials than did teachers of children with other handicapping conditions. Responses to format needs were very consistent and indicated that the greatest needs were in instructional games and manipulative materials. A need for supplementary and individualized materials was also indicated.

This type of needs assessment summary is very informative. However, there still exists a great need for a more comprehensive assessment of needs that could provide valid descriptions of currently available resources and identify the discrepancies between those resources and the existing need (White, 1974). White summarized the needs perceived by special educators. These are:

1.   Development of a communication system between teacher, local school district, state-regional resource and materials center, state department of special education, and the National Center for Educational Media and Materials for the Handicapped (NCEMMH)

2.   Field testing of instructional materials developed by teachers, special education organizations, or commercial organizations

3.   Development of instructional materials for teachers in all areas of education for the handicapped

4.   Development of a training system for improving organizational and management skills of Instructional Resource Center coordinators

5.   Development of a system for identifying and reporting needs in the field of special education

An endeavor to bring together media, materials, and techniques has resulted in the establishment of national and regional media centers. Future planning includes the development of a Learning Resources System composed of: the Special Education Instructional Materials Centers already in existence, Regional Media Centers for the Deaf, Regional Resource Centers, and the NCEMMH. The intent of this system is to help the state provide identification, diagnosis, program prescription, development of instructional materials, and delivery of support services to handicapped learners (Norwood, 1974).

The programmatic areas in the new network consist of the Regional Resource Centers (RRC) and the Area Learning Resource Centers (ALRC). Each will work with State Education Agencies. The RRC's assure effective appraisal and educational programs for all handicapped children, and the ALRC's assure effective instructional materials and service to the same population (Norwood, 1974). For the addresses of these centers, see Appendix G.

The development and use of materials is of vital concern to those involved in assessment and intervention procedures for the handicapped. Begun first in the area of deaf education, the application of technology to instructional media and materials has expanded to encompass the education of children with other handicapping conditions. As McDonald, Blum, and Barker (1971) pointed out, most materials developed for the handicapped are not unique to one condition and have broader application.

Materials that are being used to instruct handicapped learners are usually either commercially developed materials, which may or may not fit the needs of specific learners, or materials developed by teachers that are specific to the learning problem but are not designed for replication by others.

In order to assist professionals in special education in developing and distributing materials to others, the NCEMMH developed a manual that contains information about planning, producing, and assessing materials. It also includes information on copyrights, patents, and other legal considerations. (See Appendix G for the address.)

To assist professionals in developing learning systems in the area of programmed instruction, Hofmeister (1971) listed the following eight steps for the development of this type of programming:

1. Select and define the task to be learned
2. Prepare the instructional sequence
3. Develop the instructional materials
4. Develop a feedback loop
5. Conduct formal field testing
6. Place learners in the instructional sequence
7. Monitor the progress of the learners
8. Conduct a final evaluation using the criterion measures developed earlier

Hofmeister has used this technique in developing child training packages for use by parents. Several of the packages use a combination of audio cassettes and paper-pencil materials to teach skills such as the blending of sounds.

Dailey (1971) described a unique program that uses AV media. It is located in a Special Experience Room at the Everett A. McDonald Comprehensive Elementary School in Warminster, Pennsylvania. The Special Experience Room is circular with a 40-foot diameter and a hemispheric dome. The floor is carpeted and free of fixed furniture. In the center is audiovisual equipment capable of projecting slides or films on all 360 degrees of the walls. Dr. Henry Ray (1971), director of Teaching and Learning Resources for the Centennial School District, is largely responsible for the project. The program grew out of his concern over the relationship between the environment and learning and the development of children's perceptual abilities. The Special Experience Room provides a technique for simulating environments and allowing children to experience them as they might be experienced in the real world. For example, the Eiffel Tower might be projected on the wall so that it towers above the children watching it just as it would if they were standing at its base in Paris. It also can include sounds and smells to simulate reality.

The concept of the Special Experience Room offers some interesting possibilities for training individuals with many kinds of problems. It provides a technique for representing the world the way it is along a number of dimensions and offers tremendous potential as an aid for remediating the perceptual and conceptual problems often encountered by individuals with communication difficulties.

SUMMARY

This chapter presents an overview of AV media and materials in dealing with the communication problems of hearing-impaired, mentally retarded, and other developmentally disabled individuals. It focuses specifically on the uses of media in client assessment and intervention and in staff training activities. In summary:

1.   A variety of AV media and materials is available
2.   AV media and materials have been used for a variety of assessment, intervention, and training purposes
3.   The use of AV media and materials is limited only by imagination and availability of resources (including money and time)
4.   Many professionals currently lack the information and skills needed to use AV media and materials effectively
5.   The skills needed for using most AV media and materials require a minimum of training
6.   The use of AV media and materials is increasing rapidly
7.   The current use of AV media and materials is just a glimpse of their future use
8.   Many sources of information and help are available for those interested in using AV media and materials
9.   AV media and materials add several advantage to face-to-face involvement
10.   Although more teachers and clinicians are using AV media and materials, there is a paucity of research on their effectiveness

REFERENCES

Armstrong, J. R., and K. Senzig. 1970. Educational Materials: Instructional materials used and preferred by Wisconsin teachers of the mentally retarded. Educ. Train. Ment. Retard. 5:73–86.

Aserlind, L. 1966. Audiovisual instruction for the mentally retarded. Audiovis. Instruct. 11:727–730.

Austin, J. T. 1969. Videotape as a teaching tool. Excep. Child. 35:557–558.

Baer, D. M., and J. A. Sherman. 1967. Reinforcement control of generalized imitation. *In* S. W. Bijou and D. M. Baer (eds.), Child Development: Readings in Experimental Analysis, pp. 66–78. Appleton-Century-Crofts, New York.

Baldwin, T. F., B. T. Greenberg, and T. A. Muth. 1975. Experimental applications of two-way cable communications in urban administration and social service delivery. NSF Grant, Michigan State University, East Lansing.

Bandura, A. 1965. Influence of model's reinforcement contingencies on the acquisition of imitative responses. J. Personal. Soc. Psychol. 1:589–595.

Bandura, T., and F. L. Menlove. 1968. Factors determining vicarious extinction of avoidance behavior through symbolic modeling. J. Personal. Soc. Psychol. 8:99–108.

Belland, J., and S. Rothenberg. 1973. Developing Instructional Materials for the Handicapped: Guidelines for Preparing Materials Suitable for Wide Distribution. Developers Guide, NCEMMH, Ohio State University, Columbus.

Berg, F. S., and S. G. Fletcher. 1970. The Hard of Hearing Child. Grune & Stratton, New York.

Bogatz, G. A., and S. Ball. 1971. Some things you've wanted to know about "Sesame Street." Amer. Educ. 7:12–25.

Boone, D. R., and A. Goldberg. 1969. An experimental study of the clinical acquisition of behavior principals by videotape self-confrontation. Final Report, Project 4071, Grant OEG 8-071319-2814, U.S. Department of Health, Education, and Welfare, Division of Research, Bureau of Education for the Handicapped, Office of Education, Washington, D.C.

Boone, D. R., and T. E. Prescott. 1972. Content and sequence analysis of speech and hearing therapy. Asha 14:58–72.

Boone, D. R., and E. L. Stech. 1970. The development of clinical skills in speech pathology by audiotape and videotape self-confrontation. Final Report, Project 1381, Grant OEG 9-071318-2814, U.S. Department of Health, Education, and Welfare, Division of Research, Bureau of Education for the Handicapped, Office of Education, Washington, D.C.

Boothroyd, A., P. Archambault, R. E. Adams, and R. D. Storm. 1975. Use of a computer based system of speech training aids for the deaf. Volta Rev. 77:178–193.

Borton, T. 1971. Dual audio television. Harvard Educ. Rev. 41:64–78.

Burkland, M. 1967. Use of television to study articulatory problems. J. Speech Hear. Disord. 32:80–81.

Casto, G., V. Douglass, J. Jones, and A. Peterson. 1975. A curriculum monitoring system for young handicapped children. Paper presented at the Council for Exceptional Children, April, Los Angeles.

Cypreansen, L., and J. McBride. 1956. Lipreading lessons on television. Volta Rev. 58:346–348.

Dailey, R. F. 1971. Media in the round: Learning in the special experience room. Teach. Except. Child. 4:4–9.

Dawson, W. L. 1973. Instrumentation in the Speech Clinic: A Handbook for Clinicians. Interstate Printers & Publishers, Danville, Ill.

Driscoll, J. 1968. Educational films and the slow learner. Ment. Retard. 6:32–34.

Eisenberg, S. 1971. Implications of video simulation of counseling. Educ. Tech. 11:50–52.

Fauguet, M. 1971. Orientation of research on the use of closed circuit television for teacher training. Educ. Media Int. 1:11–17.

Friedlander, B. F. 1970. Receptive language development in infancy: Issues and problems. Merrill-Palmer Q. Behav. Dev. 16:7–51.

Gibbs, O. 1970. Investigation into presentation of videotapes to college of education students. Educ. TV Int. 4:94–102.

Greelis, M. 1974. Media stimulation and exceptional children. Ment. Retard. 12:30–31.

Greenberg, J. S. 1973. How videotaping improves teaching behavior. J. Health Phys. Educ. Rec. 44:36–37.

Hicks, D. J. 1965. Imitation and retention of film-mediated aggressive peer and adult models. J. Personal. Soc. Psychol. 2:97–100.

Hofmeister, A. 1971. Programmed instruction revisited: Implications for educating the retarded. Educ. Train. Ment. Retard. 6:172–176.

Holvoet, J. F. 1974. Monitoring trainer effectiveness using videotape model sequences. Working paper, Parsons Research Center, Parsons, Kan.

Hopkins, K. D., D. W. Lefever, and B. R. Hopkins. 1967. TV vs. teacher administration of standardized tests: Comparability of scores. J. Educ. Meas. 4:35–40.

John Tracy Clinic Educational Materials. Parent Education Film and Record Services, Los Angeles.

Kant, T., G. Ramos, and R. Shanks. 1970. The talking typewriter. In The Role of Media in the Education of Emotionally Handicapped Children. New York Education Department, Albany.

Koran, M. J., R. E. Snow, and F. J. McDonald. 1971. Teacher aptitudes and observational learning of a teaching skill. J. Educ. Psychol. 62:219–228.

Lance, W. D. 1973. Instructional Media and the handicapped. Stanford Center for Research and Development in Teaching, School of Education, Stanford University, Stanford, Cal. (ED084853, 7DRS price microfiche 65¢)

Lange, R. R., C. T. Mattson, and J. B. Thomann. 1974. Needs for instructional media and materials services for handicapped learners: A summary of extant information. National Center on Educational Media and Materials for the Handicapped, Ohio State University, Columbus.

Larkey, A. I., and C. N. Brownstein. 1974. Implementation of urban telecommunication experiments. Proposal submitted to the National Science Foundation, December.

Lombardi, T. P., and R. G. Poole. 1968. Utilization of videosonic equipment with mentally retarded. Ment. Retard. 6:7–9.

Luster, M. J., and G. C. Vanderheiden. 1974. 1974 Preliminary Annotated Bibliography of Communication Aids. Cerebral Palsy Communication Group, University of Wiscon, Madison.

McDonald, P. L., E. R. Blum, and P. E. Barker. 1971. Kaleidoscope: Emerging Patterns in Media. Council for Exceptional Children, Arlington, Va.

Marshall, N. R., and J. R. Hegrenes. 1970. The application of video tape replay in academic and clinic settings. Ment. Retard. 8:17–19.

Mason, M. K. 1961. Visual Hearing Films. In J. J. O'Neill and H. J. Oyer (eds.), Visual Communication for the Hard of Hearing, pp. 147–153. Prentice-Hall, Englewood Cliffs, N.J.

Moncur, J. P. 1968. Judge reliability in infant testing. J. Speech Hear. Res. 11:348–357.

Moore, L. 1955. Television as a medium for teaching speech reading and speech. Volta Rev. 57:346–348.

Nardine, F. E. 1974. Parents as a teaching resource. Volta Rev. March, 76:172–177.

Norwood, M. . 1974. "Future trends" update '74: A decade of progress. Amer. Ann. Deaf. 119(5).

O'Conner, R. D. 1969. Modification of social withdrawal through symbolic modeling. J. Appl. Behav. Anal. 2:15–22.

O'Neill, J. J., and H. J. Oyer. 1961. Visual Communication for the Hard of Hearing. Prentice-Hall, Englewood Cliffs, N.J.

Pfau, G. S. 1972. Built-in motivation. Hear. Speech News 40:16–17, 24, 26, 28.

Pfau, G. S. 1975. Kids and teachers love LIFE. Hear. Speech Action 13:20–23.

Pickett, J. M. 1968a. Recent research on speech-analyzing aids for the deaf. IEEE Trans. Audio Electroacoust. AV-16:227–234.

Pickett, J. M. (ed.). 1968b. Proceedings of the conference on speech-analyzing aid for the deaf. Amer. Ann. Deaf 113:116–326.

Ray, H. W. 1971. Designing tomorrow's school today: The multi-sensory experience center. Child. Educ. 47:254–258.

Rowe, L. 1974. The speech model. Volta Rev. 76:107–112.

Shelhass, M. 1968. Motion pictures for stimulus presentation: Development and uses for opinion-attitude research interviews. Psychol. Rept. 22:689–692.

Sidman, M., and O. Cresson, Jr. 1973. Reading and crossmodel transfer of stimulus equivalencies in severe retardation. Amer. J. Ment. Defic. 77:515–523.

Sidman, M., O. Cresson, Jr., and M. Willson-Morris. 1974. Acquisition of matching to sample via mediated transfer. J. Exp. Anal. Behav. 22:261–273.

Sidman, M., and L. T. Stoddard. 1967. The effectiveness of fading in programming a simultaneous form discrimination for retarded children. J. Exp. Anal. Behav. 11:3–15.

Skinner, B. F. 1967. Why we need teaching machines. *In* S. W. Bijou and D. M. Baer (eds.), Child development: Readings in Experimental Analysis, pp. 274–294. Appleton-Century-Crofts, New York.

Spradlin, J. E. 1966. Environmental factors and the language development of retarded children. *In* S. Rosenberg (ed.), Developments in Applied Psycholinguistic Research, Macmillan, New York.

Spradlin, J. E., V. W. Cotter, and N. Baxley. 1973. Establishing a conditioned discrimination without direct training: A study of transfer with retarded adolescents. Amer. J. Ment. Defic. 77:556–566.

Stepp, R. E. 1970. Utilization of educational media in the education of the acoustically handicapped student. *In* F. S. Berg and S. G. Fletcher (eds.), The Hard of Hearing Child, pp. 245–274. Grune & Stratton, New York.

Striefel, S. 1972a. Television as a language training medium with retarded children. Ment. Retard. 10:27–29.

Striefel, S. 1972b. Graduation Day. Film produced by Media Support Services, Parsons State Hospital and Training Center, Parsons, Kan.

Striefel, S. 1974a. Isolating variables which affect the TV preference of retarded children. Psychol. Rept. 35:115–122.

Striefel, S. 1947b. Managing Behavior, Part 7: Teaching a Child to Imitate. H & H Enterprises, Lawrence, Kan.

Striefel, S., and P. M. Smeets. 1974. TV preference as a technique for selection of reinforcers. Psychol. Rept. 35:107–113.

Torr, D. V. 1974. Comment: Reading by television. Amer. Ann. Deaf 119:6–7.

Tweedie, D. 1975. Videoaudiometry: A possible procedure for difficult to test populations. Volta Rev. 77:129–134.

Upton, H. H. 1968. Wearable eyeglass speech reading aid. Amer. Ann. Deaf 113:222–229.

Wheelden, J. A. 1972. Speech therapy via interactive television. Paper presented at the Annual Convention of American Speech and Hearing Association, November, San Francisco.

White, A. H. 1974. NCEMMH Report on Needs in Special Education, NCEMMH, Ohio State University, Columbus.

Withrow, F. B. 1975. Personal communication. (Special assistant to the deputy Commissioner, Bureau of Education for the Handicapped, U.S. Department of Health, Education, and Welfare, Washington, D.C.)

Wyman, R. 1969. A visual response system for teacher group interaction in the education of deaf children. Volta Rev. 71:155–160.

APPENDICES

CONTENTS

APPENDIX A/Language Assessment Procedures ———————— 777
  Anthony Cicciarelli, Patricia A. Broen, and Gerald M. Siegel

**APPENDIX B/International Phonetic Association
(IPA) Alphabet Pronunciation Key** ———————————— 801

**APPENDIX C/Standards for Speech Pathology
and Audiology Services** ———————————————— 803

**APPENDIX D/Language Intervention Systems:
Programs Published in Kit Form** ——————————— 813
  Macalyne Fristoe

APPENDIX E/Rules of Talking ———————————————— 861

APPENDIX F/A Functional or Basic Vocabulary ——————— 863

APPENDIX G/Audiovisual Information Sources ——————— 867

APPENDIX A / Language Assessment Procedures

Anthony Cicciarelli,
Patricia A. Broen,
and Gerald M. Siegel

Included in this appendix are brief descriptions of a number of tests that are either commercially available or have been described in the literature. The list is in no way exhaustive but is intended to be suggestive of the range of tests that attempt to sample language behaviors. The tests differ in the extent of their standardization. For a fuller characterization, the tests themselves must be consulted. The literature also should be consulted to see the ways in which the tests have been used and to find additional data concerning the tests.

ASSESSMENT OF CHILDREN'S LANGUAGE COMPREHENSION (ACLC; 1969, 1973)

Rochana Foster, Jane Giddan, and Joel Stark

Publisher

Consulting Psychologists Press, Inc.
577 College Avenue
Palo Alto, California 94306

Price: $42.25 for the complete ACLC kit (includes series of plates, manual, and response sheets)

Purpose

To assess the child's ability to identify lexical items in syntactic sequences.

Description

Age Level 3,0 to 6,11 years.

Response Items The ACLC is composed of four parts. Part A is a 50-item vocabulary test consisting of common count nouns, adjectives, present progressive form of verbs, and prepositions. These single elements serve as the core vocabulary for the other parts (B, C, and D). The test is discontinued if the child responds incorrectly to more than five items on Part A. Parts B, C, and D consist of 10 multielement combinations each. Examples of response items from each part are presented below:

Part B (two critical elements)—"horse standing"

Part C (three critical elements)—"ball under the table"

Part D (four critical elements)—"broken boat on the table"

Administration   This untimed test requires approximately 10 to 15 minutes to administer. No specialized preparation is required of the examiner.

Scoring   The number of correct items in each part is converted into a percentage score.

Standardization   The normative group consisted of 365 nursery school and kindergarten children living in California or Florida. The greatest proportion of subjects were white. However, blacks, Asian-American, and Mexican-American children were represented. Mean percentage scores are presented by age at 6-month intervals from 3,0 to 6,11 years. The test authors recommend that these mean scores should be treated as suggestive only since they are based on the experimental edition (1969). Preliminary mean scores were also presented for children diagnosed as neurologically or educationally handicapped in these age groups.

Reliability   Internal consistency was assessed by comparing the scores for odd and even numbered items. The correlation coefficients were 0.86 and 0.80 for Parts A, and B through D, respectively.

Validity   No discussion of validity is presented.

THE BASIC CONCEPT INVENTORY (BCI; 1967)

Siegfried E. Engelmann

Publisher

Follett Educational Corporation
Department DM
P.O. Box 5705
1010 West Washington Boulevard
Chicago, Illinois 60607

Price: $19.32 (includes manual, test materials, and scoring booklets)

Purpose

To assess the child's knowledge of "certain beginning, academically related concepts." The BCI is designed as a "criterion-reference" measure as contrasted with "norm-reference" tests. That is, the test items were "selected according to an absolute criterion of performance" without reference to average performance.

Description

Age Level   Preschool to 10 years.

Task   The BCI consists of three parts: 1) basic concepts, 2) statement repetition and ocmprehension, and 3) pattern awareness.

Basic Concepts (10 items)   Items 1 through 9 use picture stimuli and require either a pointing or a yes-no response. The child is required to identify the object or aspect of the picture stimulus that best illustrates the statement spoken by the examiner. The response items include: identifying object names and their properties ("Find the balls that are black"); compound selection criteria ("Find the ball that is big *and* black"); full statements as criteria ("Find the right picture: The man is chopping down the tree"); and problem solving (The child is shown an illustration of three boxes of varying proportions and is told, "There is a ball in one of these boxes. The ball is not in this box. Do you know where the ball is?"). Item 10 assesses the child's ability to follow directions involving body parts ("Touch your ear").

Statement Repetition and Comprehension (8 items)   This part assesses the child's ability to repeat sentences modeled by the examiner and to answer questions implied by the statement. For example, the child is asked to repeat the statement, "Puppies are baby dogs," and then is asked the following question, "Are puppies baby dogs?" The child's response may be verbal or gestural.

Pattern Awareness (3 items)   The first item requires the child to identify a particular movement pattern as being the same or different from the initial stimulus pattern. The stimulus pattern consists of the examiner first slapping the table then clapping his hands. The second item consists of digit repetition, and the third item evaluates sound blending ability; e.g., the examiner says "M–ilk" and asks the child to repeat what he said.

Administration   The BCI is untimed; the average administration time is 20 minutes; no special preparation is required of the examiner.

Scoring   Binary, correct or incorrect. The total number of *incorrect* responses is tallied for each part separately and for the composite test. No age norms are provided. The test author provides guidelines for interpreting errors.

Reliability   Not provided.

Validity   Only content validity is discussed.

BERRY-TALBOTT EXPLORATORY TEST OF GRAMMAR (1966)

Mildred Berry and Ruth Talbott

Publisher

Berry Language Test
4332 Pine Crest Road
Rockford, Illinois 61107

Price: $12.00 (includes a series of plates and test records)

Purpose

To assess the child's knowledge of English inflectional morphology in the context of nonsense syllables.

Description

Age Level   5 to 8 years.

Task   The child is required to supply the proper word and its inflection in response to a sentence frame provided by the examiner. The 30 response items represent the following morphophonemic forms: the plural and two possessives of the noun, the third person singular of the verb, the progressive and the past tense, and the comparative and superlative of the adjective.

Administration   The test is untimed, and administration time is approximately 15 minutes. No special preparation is required of the examiner; the book of plates and record sheets are provided.

Scoring and Standardization   The test author provides some tentative guidelines for interpreting scores.

Reliability and Validity   This information is not provided.

BOEHM TEST OF BASIC CONCEPTS (BTBC; 1969, 1971) FORMS A AND B; SPANISH EDITION AVAILABLE

Ann Boehm

Publisher

Psychological Corporation
304 East 45th Street
New York, New York 10017

Price: $5.90 for 30 tests; $0.50 for the manual; and $1.00 per specimen set

Purpose

To assess the child's knowledge of concepts considered necessary in the first years of school; to identify individual children with deficiencies in concept mastery; and to identify individual concepts which may be unfamiliar to a number of children in a given class.

Description

Age Level   5 to 8 years.

Task   A child (or group of children) is instructed to mark an "X" on the number of a set of three pictures which best illustrates the statement read by the examiner.

Fifty pictoral items are arranged in ascending order of difficulty. Fifty-six percent of the items deal with spatial concepts; 36% pertain to quantity; 26% to time; and 10% miscellaneous. Some of the items test more than one concept. The item tested is embedded in a short sentence and is emphasized by the examiner. The total number correct provides a raw score which may be compared to normative data.

Administration   This is an untimed test; the total administration time is approximately 30 to 40 minutes. The test may be given in two sessions. No specialized preparation is required of the examiner.

Scoring and Standardization   The normative sample consisted of a total of 9737 children enrolled in kindergarten, first, and second grade in 16 cities across the United States. An attempt was made to represent children in high, middle, and low socioeconomic classes. The norm tables include the percentage of children passing each item by grade and socioeconomic level at the beginning level and at the middle of the school year. The percentile equivalent of the raw score by grade and socioeconomic level is also provided. No cut-off scores are presented. The percentage of children passing each item at the second-grade level is very high, indicating that the test may be too easy for this group. Form B appears to be more difficult than Form A.

Reliability   Alternate form reliability coefficients ranged from 0.55 to 0.92. Split-half reliability for Form A ranged from 0.68 to 0.94, and from 0.12 to 0.94 for Form B. Test-retest reliability is not provided.

Validity   The relevance of the test items to school curriculum is the only validity discussed.

CARROW ELICITED LANGUARE INVENTORY (CELI; 1974)

Elizabeth Carrow

Publisher

Learning Concepts
2501 North Lamar
Austin, Texas 78705

Price: $39.50 (includes manual, training tape with a guide, and scoring forms)

Purpose

To provide a means for measuring the child's productive control of grammar.

Description

Age Level   3,0 to 7,11 years.

Task   The test contains 51 sentences and one phrase that range in length from two to 10 words. The sentences are read to the child, who is asked to repeat each sentence. The child's responses are recorded on audiotape and scored on a special form from the tape. Of the 51 sentences, 47 are in the active voice and four are passive. The sentence modalities include declarative statements, negatives, imperatives, yes-no interrogatives, and wh- questions.

The following grammatical categories and features are evaluated: articles; adjectives; nouns, singular and plural; pronouns; verbs; negatives; prepositions; adverbs; contractions; demonstratives; and conjunctions.

Administration and Scoring   The administration and scoring of this untimed test requires approximately 45 minutes. Errors are scored as substitutions, omissions, additions, transpositions, or reversals. A separate, more detailed analysis of verbs is also available. Both the total error score and the grammatical subscores may be converted into percentile ranks or compared with the means and standard deviations for various age levels. A *stanine* scale is provided for the total test score.

Standardization The normative sample consists of 475 white children between the ages of 3,0 and 7,11 years. These children were drawn from middle socioeconomic level homes in Houston, Texas, and standard American English was the sole language spoken. Children with apparent speech or language disorders were excluded.

Reliability and Validity Interexaminer reliability for transcribing and scoring 10 randomly selected tapes was 0.98. A test-retest reliability coefficient of 0.98 was reported. This reliability coefficient was obtained by retesting 25 children from the normative group after a 2-week interval. Construct and criterion-related validity data were presented while differences in total error scores between age groups in the normative sample were significant. The performance of the 5- through 7-year-olds was relatively homogeneous, indicating that the CELI is most stable for 3- to 4-year-old children. Significant positive correlations were found between the total score and each grammar subscore. An unpublished study by Cornelius (1974) indicated that the CELI distinguishes between a group of children with normal language development and a group diagnosed as language deviant. In this same study, the correlation between the CELI and the DSS was found to be −0.79, "indicating a high relationship between these two methods in obtaining grammatical data."

COMPREHENSION TESTS FOR SYNTACTIC CONSTRUCTIONS (1971)

Ursula Bellugi-Klima

Reference

Bellugi-Klima, U. 1971. Some language comprehension tests. *In* C. Lovateli, (ed.), Language Training in Early Childhood Education. University of Illinois Press, Urbana-Champaign.

Purpose

To assess the child's comprehension of syntactic structures.

Description

The child is given familiar objects and toys and asked to act out a sentence spoken by the examiner. The syntactic structures tested are active sentences, singular/plural nouns, possessives, negative/affirmative statements and questions, singular/plural with noun and verb inflections, and adjectival questions, negative affix, reletivization, comparatives, passives, and self-embedded sentences. The test items themselves are only suggested examples and may be supplemented by the examiner.

Administration This test is untimed; administration time varies with the number of test items presented. The basic test materials are not provided but are common to most school situations.

Standardization This is not a standardized test, and normative data are not presently available.

Reliability and Validity No information is provided.

DEVELOPMENTAL SENTENCE ANALYSIS (DSA; 1974)

Laura Lee

Reference

Lee, L. L. 1974. Developmental Sentence Analysis. Northwestern University Press, Evanston, Ill.

Purpose

To assess and quantify syntactic development on the basis of spontaneous speech. The author proposes that this analysis provides the basis for the selection and planning of appropriate remedial instruction.

Description

Task The DSA consists of two separate procedures: Developmental Sentence Types chart (DST) and Developmental Sentence Scoring (DSS). The DSS method evaluates the grammatical structure of complete sentences; i.e., the subject (noun) and verb are both spoken. The DST chart evaluates presentences; i.e., utterances which do not contain both a subject and a verb. Both methods evaluate the child's use of the grammatical rules of standard adult English. Developmental sentence analysis is not appropriate for use with children from bilingual homes or speech communities with significant dialect variation.

Developmental Sentence Types The DST procedure classifies presentences. It is based on a speech sample of 100 different, intelligible utterances. The DST chart classifies presentences according to length (horizontal level) and grammatical type or form (vertical level). The horizontal level distinguishes between utterances consisting of single words, two-word combinations, and multiword constructions. The vertical classification describes five "types" of utterances that are posited to follow different lines of grammatical development: 1) noun phrase; 2) designative sentence, which names, points out, or identifies a subject of conversation (e.g., "There a truck"); 3) predictive sentence, which "names the topic and proceeds to predicate something about it" (e.g., "The car broken"); 4) verb phrase, which represents the development of the subject-verb sentence (e.g., "Eat the cookies"), and 5) fragments or vocabulary items that contain neither subject nor a verb.

Various methods are proposed for evaluating the child's language development from the DSA, including: 1) counting the number of utterances at each DST level; 2) looking at the variety of sentence types; and 3) examining the grammatical development within levels, such as the presence of negatives, questions, pronouns, etc. The basic assumption of the DST chart is that increasing length signifies increasing grammatical complexity.

Standardization DST classifications of speech samples of 40 normally developing children are presented to serve as a basis of comparison with clinical children. Five boys and five girls were evaluated at each 3-month interval between 2,0 and 2,11 years. The children were from middle-income homes. No other normative data are available for the DST.

Developmental Sentence Scoring This is the second revision of the DSS procedure originally introduced by Lee and Canter in 1971. The DSS is used to evaluate the grammatical structure of complete sentences. Complete sentences are defined by the presence of the subject and verb. For the DSS analysis, a corpus of 50 complete, consecutive, different, and intelligible sentences is required. The sentences are scored according to eight grammatical categories: 1) indefinite pronoun or noun modifier, 2) personal pronoun, 3) main verb, 4) secondary verb, 5) negative, 6) conjunction, 7) interrogative reversal, and 8) wh- question. Certain grammatical forms, such as articles, adverbs, and prepositions, are excluded from the analysis. The child's sentences are entered on the DSS record form, and weighted scores (from one to eight) are assigned to the structures within each grammatical category. The weighting of grammatical structures provides higher scores for later-occurring structures. For example, in the pronoun category, a first or second person pronoun is weighted at one, while a reflexive pronoun is weighted at five.

The 50 sentences are scored. The total mean score on the DSS is obtained. An individual child's DSS score can be compared with the DSS scores of the group. Selected percentiles for the DSS scores of the normative sample are presented graphically.

Standardization The normative data are based on the DSS language samples of 200 white children, five girls and five boys at each 3-month age interval between 2,0 and 6,11. (Note that these are cross-sectional, not longitudinal, data). All the children were from monolingual homes where standard English was spoken, and resided in Illinois, Maryland, Michigan, or Kansas. All except three were from middle-income homes. The subject group excluded children with "unusual development or social histories." Children older than 3,0 years were screened with the PPVT, and only children within one standard deviation from the mean score for their age level were included. Children younger than age 3 were also screened with the PPVT; however, an extrapolated set of criteria was constructed to determine average performance.

Reliability and Validity Over a 2-week interval, the mean DSS score for 10 subjects increased progressively from 6.90 to 8.22 for the fourth sampling. This increase in DSS scores is equivalent to a 9-month increase according to the normative data. For longer time intervals (4 months) the increase in overall scores was consistent with the performance of the normative sample. The split-half reliability was 0.73. Studies of the DSS indicate that two interviewers obtain similar language samples from children of the same age, and stimulus material differences do not significantly affect the overall DSS score (for children ages 4,0 to 5,6 years). However, four of the grammatical categories do show significant score changes with different stimulus materials. Interjudge reliability was not discussed; however, a study by Johnson and Tomblin (1975) reported an interscorer reliability coefficient of 0.94.

Construct validity was discussed in terms of an overall increase in DSS scores throughout the 2,0 to 6,11 age levels. The overall DSS revealed significant differences in syntax between all successive 1-year age levels. The developmental scores within specific DSS component categories do not necessarily evidence increases between successive age levels. The most discriminating grammatical category was main verbs, whereas interrogative reversal was the least discriminating. Each of the grammatical categories correlate significantly with the overall DSS score. In addition, computer analysis of the speech samples of the normative group generally confirmed the rank order of grammatical structures within the categories.

FULL RANGE PICTURE VOCABULARY TEST (FRPVT; 1948) FORMS A AND B

Robert A. Ammons and Helen S. Ammons

Publisher

Psychological Test Specialists
Box 1441
Missoula, Montana 59801
Price: $15.00

Purpose

To provide an index of vocabulary comprehension.

Description

Age Level   2,0 years to adult.

Task   To indicate by word or gesture which of four pictures best illustrates the meaning of a given word.

Response Items   Eighty-five vocabulary items are distributed among 16 plates with each plate containing four black-and-white pictures. The vocabulary items for each plate are arranged in ascending order of difficulty. The items are also given approximate chronologic age placement. The test words include nouns, adjectives, and verbs, with the greatest emphasis on nouns.

Administration   This is a nontimed test, requiring approximately 10 to 15 minutes to administer. No specialized preparation is required of the examiner.

Scoring   Total number correct gives the raw score, which may be converted into a mental age for subjects under 16.5 years or a percentile rating for adult subjects.

Standardization   Normative groups consisted of 589 whites, ranging from 2 years to adulthood, living around the Denver area. Separate norms were provided for a white farm population from a rural area of Nebraska, and for Spanish-American children and black children and adults.

Reliability   Reliability and validity data appear in a series of articles presented by the authors. Forms A and B correlate 0.93. The median odd-even reliability coefficient for the various age levels was 0.81.

Validity   The FRPVT was correlated with the Stanford-Binet vocabulary subtest to assess its validity as a measure of verbal intelligence. For Form A of the FRPVT, the correlation with the Stanford-Binet was 0.91 and for Form B, it was 0.93.

THE HOUSTON TEST OF LANGUAGE DEVELOPMENT (HTLD; 1958, 1963)

Margaret Crabtree

Publisher

Houston Test Company
P.O. Box 35152
Houston, Texas 77035

Price: $27.00 (for Parts I and II; includes manual, test materials, and score sheets); Parts I and II may be purchased separately at $9.50 and $20.00, respectively

Purpose

To evaluate the "language functioning" of children.

Description

Age Level   6 to 36 months (Part I); 3,0 to 6,0 years (Part II).

Task   The test consists of two parts, which may be used separately or conjointly. Part I is an observational device for assessing the presence of various behaviors that are considered to be representative of normal child development. Response items for Part I are arranged according to age levels. The language behaviors evaluated include: the vocalization of back vowels; sound imitations; use of two to three words; identifying parts of a doll; and use of pronoun "I" among others. Many behaviors are obviously prelinguistic, such as "use of vocal grunts," while others are sensorimotor, such as "will pat-a-cake." Scoring for Part I is generally binary. The behavior in question is present or absent, and the examiner must determine subjectively the response accuracy. The scoring procedures for many items allow credit for only one response during the testing period. For example, the child who produces only one back vowel during the session is given the same credit as the child who produces 10 such sounds. The number of items passed at each 6-month age level is multiplied by the particular value for that age level. These age level subscores are added to give a total "language age" in months. The norms for Part I are based on a sample of 113 white children living in Houston, Texas. Children with observable mental or physical handicaps were excluded. An interexaminer reliability coefficient of 0.84 was reported. Validity data were restricted to the observation that age scores increased for each successive age group.

Part II of the HTLD consists of 18 subtests that are designed to evaluate the language status of normal and language deviant children. The various aspects of behavior sampled include, among others: self-identity; expressive vocabulary; geometric drawing; counting, and syntactic complexity and sentence length in spontaneous speech (sample is limited to 10 utterances). Scoring for Part II is binary, correct or incorrect. The total score is converted into a language age. Adequate performance is defined as a score within 1 year of the norm score for that age.

Administration Both parts of the HTLD are untimed; the average administration time for each part is 30 minutes; no special preparation is required.

Standardization Norms for Part II are based on a sample of 102 white children between the ages of 3 and 6 years living in Houston, Texas. Handicapped children were excluded.

Reliability Not provided.

Validity Validity data are restricted to the observation of increasing language age scores for successive age groups.

ILLINOIS TEST OF PSYCHOLINGUISTIC ABILITIES (ITPA; 1961, 1968)

Samuel A. Kirk, James J. McCarthy, and Winifred D. Kirk

Publisher

University of Illinois Press
Urbana, Illinois 61801

Price: $43.50 (includes manual, test materials, 25 record forms, and carrying case)

Purpose

To assess the psycholinguistic abilities and disabilities of children who are encountering learning difficulties. The diagnostic profile obtained from the ITPA may serve as a model for selecting and programming remedial instruction.

Description

Age Level 2,0 to 10,0 years.

Task The ITPA consists of 10 basic subtests and two optional tests which measure communication at two levels of organization, the representational and the automatic levels.

Tests at the Representational Level Six tests assess the child's ability to deal with the reception, expression, and the internal manipulation (organization) of auditory and visual symbols.

Auditory Reception (50 items)   This test assesses the child's ability to comprehend the spoken word. The child is requested to respond yes or no, verbally or by gesture, to a series of questions of the form, "Do dogs eat?"

Visual Reception (40 items)   This test measures the child's ability to comprehend pictures. The child is required to select from a set of four pictures the one that is perceptually similar or associated categorically with a previously exposed stimulus picture.

Auditory Association (42 items)   This test assesses the child's ability to relate spoken lexical items by requiring the child to supply the appropriate word to an analogous sentence, e.g., "Soup is hot; ice cream is ———."

Visual Association (42 items)   This picture-associated test assesses the child's ability to relate concepts presented visually. The child is required to select from a set of four pictures the one that is conceptually similar to the stimulus picture, such as a sock belonging to a shoe. The upper-level test items consist of visual analogies.

Verbal Expression   This test assesses the ability to express concepts verbally. The child is asked to describe four familiar objects.

Manual Expression (15 items)   The child is shown pictures of objects (e.g., a hammer) and is asked, "Show me what you do with this."

Tests at the Automatic Level   Six tests measure the child's ability to perform "nonsymbolic" tasks. This level, in contrast to the representational level, presumably mediates less complex, more highly organized (in the sense of overlearned) processes. The automatic level involves two types of abilities: 1) ability to effect linguistic and perceptual closure, and 2) ability to repeat a sequence of auditory and visual symbols from memory.

Grammatic Closure (33 items)   The child is required to supply the appropriate grammatical form to an incomplete statement spoken by the examiner. Pictures representing the content of the verbal expression accompany the test item. An example of a test items is, "Here is a dog; here are two ———."

Visual Closure   The test consists of four scenes each containing 14 or 15 objects in varying degrees of concealment. The child is required to point to particular objects within a specified time limit.

Auditory Closure (30 items)   This supplementary test is optional. The examiner presents an incomplete word, such as *tele–one,* and asks the child to produce the complete word.

Sound Blending (32 items)   This supplementary test is optional. In this test the sounds of words are spoken singly at half-second intervals, and the child is required to tell what the word is.

Auditory Sequential Memory (28 items)   The child is required to reproduce from memory digit sequences ranging in length from two to eight digits. The digits are presented at half-second intervals.

Visual Sequential Memory (25 items)   The child is shown a sequence of geometric forms varying in length from two to eight figures for 5 seconds and is asked to duplicate the design with a set of chips.

Administration   The ITPA tests are untimed tests with the exception of the Visual Closure Subtest. Administration time is about 45 to 50 minutes. The examiner is required to administer and score a minimum of 10 practice tests before being considered a valid examiner. Each subtest has its own administration and scoring procedures, and the tests are presented in a prescribed order.

Scoring   Scoring procedures including basal levels and ceilings vary from one subtest to another. Scores for individual subtests can be converted into a scaled score or an age score. An overall language age can be obtained from the total raw score.

Standardization   The normative sample consisted of 962 children, approximately 120 children in eight age groups, who were of average intelligence (IQ 84 to 116), average school achievement, no emotional disturbances or sensorimotor problems. The children were drawn from predominately English-speaking families in five midwestern communities. Four percent of the sample was black.

Reliability and Validity   Reliability and validity data for the ITPA are presented by Paraskevopoulos and Kirk (1969). The available information is extensive and should be evaluated for both the individual subtest and the test as a whole. Reliability is generally very satisfactory, but validity is more problematic and less completely analyzed.

THE MILLER-YODER TEST OF GRAMMATICAL COMPREHENSION, EXPERIMENTAL EDITION (M-Y TEST, 1972)

Jon Miller and David Yoder

Reference

University of Wisconsin, Madison (Bookstore)

Purpose

To assess children's grammatical comprehension.

Description

Age Level   3,0 to 6,0 years.

Task   The childs' task is to point to the picture from a set of four that represents the sentence spoken by the examiner.

Response Items   Forty-two sentence pairs test the following grammatical forms: 1) active; 2) prepositions; 3) possessive; 4) negative/affirmative statements; 5) pronouns; 6) singular/plural, noun and verb; 7) verbal inflections; 8) adjective modifiers; 9) passive reversible; and 10) reflexivizations. Stimulus sentences are controlled for length (four or five words) and stated in the present tense unless tense itself is being assessed. The lexical items used in the test are considered common to the expressive vocabulary of a 5-year-old child, but are not tested separately.

Administration   This is an untimed test; plates are provided.

Standardization   This test is currently available only in an experimental edition and its distribution is limited. Standardization and normative information are not provided with the test. However, an unpublished study (Owings, 1972) established tentative age norms for 120 normal subjects ranging in age from 3 to 6 years of age.

Reliability and Validity   Owings (1972) obtained data supporting the internal consistency of the M-Y test (0.93 Hoyt reliability index).

NORTHWESTERN SYNTAX SCREENING TEST (NSST; 1969, 1971)

Laura Lee

Publisher

Northwestern University Press
1735 Benson Avenue
Evanston, Illinois 60201

Price: $10.00 (includes set of plates and record forms)

Purpose

To screen for comprehension and expression of morphologic and syntactic forms.

Description

Age Level   3 to 8 years.

Task   In the receptive section, the child is requested to match a sentence spoken by the examiner with the proper reference picture from a set of four line drawings.

Stimulus Mode   Auditory and visual.

Response Mode   Pointing, in the comprehension portion, and speech in the expressive.

Response Items   The task consists of 20 sentence pairs arranged in increasing order of difficulty. The grammatical items tested include: prepositions, personal pronouns, plurals, negatives, verb tenses, reflexive pronouns, possessives, wh- questions, yes-no questions, passives, and indirect objects.

Administration   This is an untimed test, requiring approximately 15 minutes to administer. Test plates and response sheets are provided. No special preparation is required of the examiner.

Scoring   Binary, correct or incorrect. Each sentence is scored as a single item. In the expressive portion, any response containing a grammatical error is considered incorrect. Scores are discussed in terms of means, standard deviations, and percentiles for chronologic ages. Guidelines for interpreting scores are presented.

Standardization   The normative sample consisted of 344 normal children (3,0 through 7,11 years) from middle and upper-middle income communities. The children were drawn from nursery public schools, and presumably children with atypical language were excluded from the sample.

Reliability and Validity   No reliability and validity data are presented with the test, but Ratusnik and Koenigsknecht (1975) obtained data supporting the internal consistency and validity of the NSST. The reliability coefficients were 0.78 and 0.81 for the expressive section, and 0.67 and 0.55 for the receptive section. These data are based on scores obtained from 20 mentally retarded children and 20 children with severe expressive language delay. The validity of the test was substantiated somewhat in terms of its ability to distinguish between children with normal and deviant language.

PEABODY PICTURE VOCABULARY TEST (PPVT; 1959, 1965)

Lloyd M. Dunn

Publisher

American Guidance Service, Inc.
Publishers' Building
Circle Pines, Minnesota 55014

Price: $13.25 for the complete PPVT kit (includes a series of plates that are used with Form A and Form B, a manual, and 50 score sheets)

Purpose

To measure receptive vocabulary development.

Description

Age Level   Between 2,6 and 18,0 years.

Task   The subject is instructed to indicate which of a set of four pictures best depicts a word spoken by the examiner. The subject either may point to the appropriate picture or indicate the number of the picture.

Administration   An untimed test that can usually be administered in about 15 minutes. No special preparation or materials are required.

Scoring   Within the test 150 words—nouns, verbs, and adjectives— are arranged in order of increasing difficulty. The raw score may be converted into a percentile score, a mental age, or an intelligence quotient.

Standardization   The normative group consisted of 4012 white children between 2,6 and 18 years living in or around Nashville, Tennessee. Age norms were extrapolated to 1,9, and the 18 year norms can be used for adults.

Reliability and Validity   Eleven reliability studies are reported in the manual including studies with retarded and handicapped groups. Alternate form reliability coefficients range from 0.61 to 0.97, and test-retest reliability coefficients range from 0.54 (over 2 years) to 0.88.

THE PARSONS LANGUAGE SAMPLE (PLS; 1963)

Joseph E. Spradlin

Reference

Spradlin, J. E. 1963. Assessment of Speech and Language of Retarded Children: The Parsons Language Scales. J. Speech Hear. Disord. monogr. suppl. 10.

Purpose

To assess the verbal and nonverbal language behavior of mentally retarded children according to concepts derived from Skinner's work, *Verbal Behavior* (1957); thus, emphasis is placed on the environmental conditions which evoke or control the occurrence of language behavior.

Description

The PLS consists of seven subtests. Three sample the child's speech behavior: tact, echoic, and intraverbal. The Echoic Gesture, Comprehension, and Intraverbal Gesture Subtests sample nonvocal communication, and the Mand samples vocal and nonvocal behavior.

Vocal Subtests

TACT (28 items) The child is required to name objects or pictures. The controlling stimuli are visual, a picture or an object.

Echoic Gesture (22 items) The echoic response is the repetition of a stimulus. The child is asked to repeat 10 words and sentences of varying length, and 12 series of digits from one to six digits in length.

Intraverbal Gesture (29 items) Intraverbal responses are responses elicited by verbal stimuli. Seven items require the child to respond to open-ended questions of the form, "What do we do when we are hungry?" Sixteen items require the child to supply the appropriate lexical item to an incomplete statement, such as, "The flag is red, white, and ———." The remaining items require responses to verbal analogies, such as, "In what way are dog and cat alike?"

Nonvocal Subtests

Echoic Gesture (13 items) This measures the child's ability to mimic motor behavior. The child is asked to repeat a series of motor acts or gestures modeled by the examiner.

Comprehension (18 items) This taps the child's ability to execute motor acts in response to verbal, gestural, or a combination of vocal and gestural commands. Thus, the controlling stimulus may be vocal or nonvocal.

Intraverbal Gesture (24 items) The child is required to respond with gestures to a series of questions, such as, "Where is your ear?" "What do you do with a handkerchief?" Only gestural behavior is judged.

Vocal and Nonvocal Subtest

Mand (5 items) Mand behavior includes gestural or verbal behaviors which demand or request. For items one through four, either vocal or gestural responses are acceptable. However, only a vocal response is acceptable on the fifth item. Mand items are interspersed among the other subtests.

Administration This is an untimed test. The subtests are presented in a prescribed order. No special preparation is required of the examiner. Test materials are not provided.

Scoring Binary, correct or incorrect. The number of accurate responses on each subtest gives the composite PLS score. Percentile ranks may be derived. Means and standard deviations for each of the subtests except the Mand are presented. Subsection scores are also provided. Scores are converted to standard scores.

Standardization The PLS was standardized on a group of 275 ambulatory mentally retarded children between the ages of 7,11 and 15,8 years.

Reliability Reliability of the PLS subtests was evaluated by split-half (odd-even) and test-retest reliability procedures. The odd-even reliability coefficients for the vocal subtests and the nonvocal subtests were all above 0.90. The Mand subtest reliability coefficients were low, 0.25 for vocal scoring and 0.17 for nonvocal scoring. The temporal stability of the PLS was assessed by retesting 40 children within 2 to 5 months after the initial testing. (The Mand subtest was not included in the analysis because of its very low split-half reliability coefficients.) For the vocal subtests, the correlation coefficients ranged from 0.86 to 0.99 with a median correlation of 0.92, and for the nonvocal tests, the correlations ranged from 0.64 to 0.92 (median = 0.80).

Validity The lack of independency between the subtests, with the exception of the Intraverbal Gesture Subtest, fails to support the theoretical construct on which the PLS is based. However, internal consistency is somewhat supported since the subtests correlate substantially with their respective subsections and with the total PLS (with the exception of the Intraverbal Gesture Test). A median correlation of 0.64 (range, 0.33 to 0.86) was found between the ranking of the children's communication skills by psychiatric aides and their PLS vocal performance. The correlation between aid ranking and PLS nonvocal performance was positive but only fair (medial correlation of 0.40).

PORCH INDEX OF COMMUNICATIVE ABILITY IN CHILDREN (PICAC; 1974)

Bruce E. Porch

Publisher

Consulting Psychologist Press, Inc.
577 College Avenue
Palo Alto, California 94306
Price: $43.00

Purpose

To assess general communication ability in terms of certain verbal, gestural, and graphic skills.

Description

Age Level   Preschool to 5 years (Basic Battery); first-grade level to 12 years (Advanced Battery).

Types   The PICAC is divided into two batteries: Basic and Advanced. There are 15 subtests in the Basic and 20 in the Advanced. All subtests (except the geometric form tests) use 10 common objects as stimuli (toothbrush, key, comb, brush, fork, spoon, crayon, pencil, ring, and scissors) and require the child to respond verbally, graphically, and by gesture.

Basic Battery Subtests

Verbal Function   The child is required to describe with a complete sentence the function of the objects.

Gestural Function   The child is asked to demonstrate gesturally the function of the objects.

Verbal Naming   This requires the child to name the objects.

Verbal Completion   The child supplies the name of the object to an incomplete sentence frame that describes the function of the object (e.g., "You lock a door with a ————.")

Reading Names   This requires the child to match the written name of the object with the object.

Auditory Commands   The child is directed to perform certain gestural responses to verbal commands (e.g., "Point to the key," "Touch the toothbrush").

Visual Pictures   The child is directed to match a picture of the object with the object.

Auditory Naming   The child points to the object named by the examiner.

Verbal Imitation   The child repeats the name of the object as modeled by the examiner.

Visual Matching   The child is directed to match identical objects.

Graphic Tests   These include four subtests: 1) writing the name of the object after spoken by the examiner, 2) writing the name after it is spelled, 3) copying the name, and 4) copying geometric forms.

Advanced Battery   The majority of the subtests for the Advanced Battery are similar to those presented in the Basic Battery; however, additional tests are included which assess more complex skills. For example:

Verbal Description   This requires the child to describe the object in terms of three categories—color, shape, and composition.

Reading (Function)   The child is required to read a card that describes the function of an object and then match the card to the appropriate object.

Reading Backwards   This requires the child to read words printed in reverse letter order.

Verbal Imitation   This requires the child to repeat short sentences (four to five words in length) spoken by the examiner. The sentence modalities include interrogatives, imperatives, negatives, and declaratives.

Graphic Function   The child is directed to write a sentence describing the function of the objects.

Administration   The Battery is untimed; the average administration time is 1 hour. Forty hours of study and supervised practice in admintration and scoring are required.

Scoring   The responses are described using a multidimensional scoring system rather than the plus-minus dichotomy that is generally employed by other tests. The child's response to a given item is recorded in terms of a 16 category rating scale. Mean scores for each subtest, each modality (gestural, verbal, and graphic), and the entire test (Overall Score) are converted into percentiles.

Standardization, Reliability, and Validity   This information is unavailable at present.

PRESCHOOL LANGUAGE SCALE (PLS; 1969)

Irla L. Zimmerman, Violette G. Steiner, and Roberta L. Evatt

Publisher

Charles E. Merrill Publishing Co.
1300 Alum Creek Drive
Columbus, Ohio 43216

Price: $4.95 (includes manual, picture book, and record booklet; $3.95 per 10 record booklets)

Purpose

To evaluate auditory comprehension and verbal ability with respect to normal stages of development. The authors emphasize that this is a scale and not a test.

Description

Age Level   1,6 to 6,11 years.   The Scale consists of a series of age-graded auditory comprehension and verbal language tasks. The task items are given age placement on the basis of age levels suggested by Gesell, Binet, Templin, McCarthy, and others.

Auditory Comprehension Scale   There are a total of 40 response items, with four tasks at each age level. The task items include pointing to parts of a doll and pictures when named, color recognition, distinguishing between prepositions, number concepts, and texture differentiation. Only nonverbal responses are required.

Verbal Ability Scale   Forty response items are distributed equally across the 10 age levels (from 18 months to 7 years). The test items include: use of 10 words (this may be based on either observation or caretaker report), digit and sentence repetition, naming members of a category (e.g., animals), articulation, and sentence building (i.e., the ability to construct a sentence from three words provided by examiner). Scoring instructions and citations of relevant research accompany each item.

Administration   The scale is untimed, with the exception of particular test items; the average administration time is reportedly under 30 minutes; no special preparation is required of the examiner.

Scoring and Standardization   The child receives credit, in terms of months, for each item passed; an auditory comprehension age, a verbal ability age, and a total language age may be derived. The scale is not standardized.

Reliability and Validity   Data are not provided.

TEST FOR AUDITORY COMPREHENSION OF LANGUAGE (1968, 1973) ENGLISH/SPANISH VERSIONS

Elizabeth Carrow

Publisher

Urban Research Group
306 West 16
Austin, Texas 78701

Price: $37.50 (includes test manual, book of plates, and response sheets)

Purpose

To: 1) measure auditory comprehension of vocabulary and linguistic structures, and 2) diagnose specific areas of linguistic difficulty to provide basis for therapeutic intervention.

Description

Age Level   3,0 to 6,11 years.

Task   The child is requested to point to the picture from a set of three that best depicts the word or statement spoken by the examiner.

Stimulus mode   Auditory and visual.

Response mode   Pointing.

Test items   The test consists of 101 plates, each with three pictures representing referential categories and contrasts that can be signaled by form classes and function words (nouns, verbs, adjectives, adverbs, and prepositions), morphologic constructions (comparative and superlative morphemes), grammatical categories (case, number, tense, voice, and mood), and syntactic structures. The plates represent the linguistic form being tested (e.g., "The lion *has eaten*") and two alternate pictures representing the referents for the contrasting linguistic forms (e.g., "The lion *is eating*," and "The lion *will eat*"). The test items are sequenced by grammatical category and not by level of difficulty.

Administration   This test is untimed; administration time is approximately 20 minutes. The tester should have a B.A. in education, psychology, or sociology and significant testing experience.

Scoring   Binary, correct or incorrect. The total raw score may be converted into an age-score equivalent and percentile rank. An analysis section for studying an individual child's performance on specific classes of items (vocabulary, morphology, grammar and syntax) is provided.

Standardization   The standardization sample consisted of 200 middle-class black, Anglo-American, and Mexican-American children between the ages of 3 and 6 years. Geographic information is not provided. Normative data are presented for the English version only.

Reliability   Test-retest reliability coefficients (0.93 and 0.94) are presented for both the Spanish and English versions of the test.

Validity   Construct and criterion-related validity are discussed. Test scores significantly increase with age, and the test reportedly distinguishes between normal and linguistically handicapped children.

UTAH TEST OF LANGUAGE DEVELOPMENT
(UTLD; REVISED EDITION, 1967)

Merlin J. Mecham, J. Lorin Jex, and J. Dean Jones

Publisher

Communication Research Associated, Inc.
P.O. Box 11012
Salt Lake City, Utah 84111

Price: $16.50 (includes manual, set of testing materials, and record sheets)

Purpose

To measure the expressive and receptive verbal language skills in both normal and handicapped children.

Description

Age Level   1,6 to 14,5 years.

The Utah test was constructed by assembling behavioral items from original standardized developmental tests such as the Stanford-Binet and the Gesell Developmental Scales. These items were arrangd in accordance with the age norms from the original sources.

Response Items   The test contains 51 items arranged in increasing order of difficulty. Items include: recognizing body parts when named, responding to simple commands (e.g., "Give me the ball!"), naming common pictures and colors, repeating digits, copying geometric forms, and decoding written words.

Administration   This test is untimed, but the average administration time is 30 to 45 minutes; no special preparation is required of the examiner.

Scoring The total number of correct responses may be converted into a language age equivalent in 1-year intervals. Standard scores and percentile ranks are not provided for the original standardization sample. However, percentile norms from a sample of 989 kindergarten children are provided by Mecham, Jones, and Jex (1973).

Standardization The original normative sample consisted of 273 normal, white children drawn from four sections of Salt Lake County, representing high, middle, and low socioeconomic levels. Approximately 20 children are represented at each age level from 1,6 to 12,5 years; 30 children represent the age range from 12,6 to 14,5 years.

Reliability Split-half reliability correlation is high (0.94).

Validity The test authors consider that the test has good face validity since all the items were selected from previously standardized sources. Also, the correlation between the item-age levels for the Utah sample and the original test sources was 0.98. In their 1973 article, the test authors reviewed three studies which compared the performance of subjects on the UTLD and the ITPA. The correlation coefficients were relatively high, 0.86, 0.87 and 0.91.

References

Ammons, R., and A. Aguero. 1950. The Full-Range Picture Vocabulary Test: VII. Results for a Spanish-American school age population. J. Soc. Psychol. 32:3 10.

Ammons, R., P. Arnold, and R. Herrmann. 1950. The Full-Range Picture Vocabulary Test: IV. Results for a white school population. J. Clin. Psychol. 6:164–169.

Ammons, R., and J. Holmes. 1949. The Full-Range Picture Vocabulary Test: III. Results from a preschool-age population. Child Dev. 20:5–14.

Ammons, R., and R. Huth. 1949. The Full-Range Picture Vocabulary Test: I. Preliminary scale. J. Psychol. 28:51–64.

Ammons, R., W. Larson, and C. Shearn. 1950. The Full-Range Picture Vocabulary Test: Results with an adult population. J. Consult. Psychol. 14:150–155.

Ammons, R., and N. Manahan. 1950. The Full-Range Picture Vocabulary Test: VI. Results for a rural population. J. Educ. Res. 44:14–21.

Ammons, R., and L. Rachiele. 1950. The Full-Range Picture Vocabulary Test: Selection of items for final scales. Educ. Psychol. Meas. 10:307–319.

Coppinger, N., and R. Ammons. 1952. The Full-Range Picture Vocabulary Test: VIII. A normative study of Negro children. J. Clin. Psychol. 8:136–140.

Cornelius, S. 1974. A comparison of the elicited language inventory with the developmental sentence scoring procedures in assessing language disorders in children. Unpublished masters thesis, University of Texas, Austin.

Johnson, M., and B. Tomblin. 1975. The reliability of developmental sentence scoring as a function of sample size. J. Speech Hear. Res. 18:372–380.

Lee, L., and S. Canter. 1971. Developmental sentence scoring: A clinical procedure for estimating syntactic development in children's spontaneous speech. J. Speech Hear. Disord. 36:315–340.

Mecham, M., J. Jones, and J. Jex. 1973. Use of Utah Test of Language Development for screening language disabilities. J. Learn. Dis. 6:65–68.

Owings, N. 1972. Internal reliability and item analysis of the Miller-Yoder Test of Grammatical Comprehension. Unpublished masters thesis, University of Wisconsin, Madison.

Paraskevopulos, J., and S. Kirk. 1969. The Development and Psychometric Characteristics of the Revised Illinois Test of Psycholinguistic Abilities. University of Illinois Press, Urbana.

Ratusnik, D., and R. Koenigsknecht. 1975. Internal consistency of the Northwestern Syntax Screening Test. J. Speech Hear. Disord. 40: 59–68.

Skinner, B. 1957. Verbal Behavior. Appleton-Century-Crofts, New York.

APPENDIX B / International Phonetic Association (IPA) Alphabet Pronunciation Key

Each symbol stands for only one speech sound, and each speech sound has only one symbol to represent it. In accord with the practice of many British and American users of this alphabet the accented sounds ʌ, ɜ, ɝ are considered to be separate speech sounds from the unaccented sounds ə and ɚ. Diphthongs are regarded as single sounds and their symbols (aɪ, aʊ, ɔɪ, etc.) as single symbols. The same is true of tʃ, dʒ.

In using the phonetic alphabet the reader must be careful to give only the one designated sound to those letters which in ordinary spelling represent more than one sound. Thus the symbol g has only the sound in *get* gɛt, never that in *gem* dʒɛm; s has only the sound in *gas* gæs, never that in *wise* waɪz or that in *vision* 'vɪʒən. The dotted i has only the sound in *machine* mə'ʃin, never that in *shin* ʃɪn; ordinary e always has the sound in *gate* get, never that in *met* mɛt. Below is the list of symbols with key words. The notes after the table give fuller information and additional symbols. The accent mark (') always precedes the syllable accented.

Vowels

Sym-bol	Spelling	Spoken Form	Sym-bol	Spelling	Spoken Form
i	bee	bi	ʊ	full	fʊl
ɪ	pity	ˈpɪtɪ	u	tooth	tuθ
e	rate	ret	ɝ	further	ˈfɝðɚ *accented syllable only, r's sounded*
ɛ	yet	jɛt			
æ	sang	sæŋ	ɜ	further	ˈfɜðə *accented syllable only, r's silent*
a	bath	baθ *as heard in the East, between æ (sang) and ɑ (ah)*	ɚ	further	ˈfɝðɚ *unaccented syllable only, r's sounded*
ɑ	ah far	ɑ fɑr	ə	further	ˈfɜðə *unaccented syllable only, r's silent*
ɒ	watch	wɒtʃ *between ɑ (ah) and ɔ (jaw)*		custom above	ˈkʌstəm *unaccented syllable* əˈbʌv *lable*
ɔ	jaw gorge	dʒɔ gɔrdʒ	ʌ	custom above	ˈkʌstəm *accented syllable* əˈbʌv *ble*
o	go	go			

Diphthongs

aɪ	while	hwaɪl	ju	using	ˈjuzɪŋ
aʊ	how	haʊ		fuse	fjuz
ɔɪ	toy	tɔɪ	ɪu	fuse	fɪuz

Consonants

Sym-bol	Spelling	Spoken Form	Sym-bol	Spelling	Spoken Form
p	pity	ˈpɪtɪ	dʒ	jaw	dʒɔ
b	bee	bi		edge	ɛdʒ
t	tooth	tuθ	m	custom	ˈkʌstəm
d	dish	dɪʃ	m̩	keep 'em	ˈkipm̩
k	custom	ˈkʌstəm	n	vision	ˈvɪʒən
g	go	go	n̩	Eden	ˈidn̩
f	full	fʊl	ŋ	sang	sæŋ
v	vision	ˈvɪʒən		angry	ˈæŋ·grɪ
θ	tooth	tuθ	l	full	fʊl
ð	further	ˈfɝðɚ	l̩	cradle	ˈkredl̩
s	sang	sæŋ	w	watch	wɒtʃ
z	using	ˈjuzɪŋ	hw	while	hwaɪl
ʃ	dish	dɪʃ	j	yet	jɛt
ʒ	vision	ˈvɪʒən	r	rate	ret
h	how	haʊ		very	ˈvɛrɪ
tʃ	watch	wɒtʃ		far	fɑr
	chest	tʃɛst		gorge	gɔrdʒ

APPENDIX C / Standards for Speech Pathology and Audiology Services

It is strongly recommended that speech pathology and audiology services be accredited by the American Board of Examiners of Speech Pathology and Audiology (ABESPA). Complete information about their guidelines and the accreditation process may be obtained by writing ABESPA, 9030 Old Georgetown Road, Washington, D.C. 20014. The same address may be used for obtaining information about the certification of clinical competence of speech pathologists and audiologists. Those concerned with standards and guidelines for the delivery of services in speech pathology and audiology also should be aware of the speech pathology and audiology section of the Standards of the Accreditation Council for Facilities for the Mentally Retarded (AC/FMR). These standards were originally very specific guidelines for services for the retarded; however, they provide a number of specific recommendations applicable to speech pathology and audiology service in any type of facility. Those concerned specifically with the facilities of the retarded may wish to obtain a copy of the completed standards from AC/FMR (Joint Commission on Accreditation of Hospitals, 875 North Michigan Avenue, Chicago, Illinois 60611). However, for the convenience of those primarily concerned with communication disorders, below is reprinted the "Special Report" that appeared in the October 1971 *Asha* (pp. 607–610), which describes the development of the standards as well as the specific standards for speech pathology and audiology services:

The Establishment of Standards for Speech Pathology and Audiology Services in Facilities for the Retarded

The purpose of this report is to provide the ASHA membership with information about the standards for accrediting facilities for the mentally retarded adopted by the Accreditation Council for Facilities for the Mentally Retarded (AC/FMR) of the Joint Commission on Accreditating Hospitals (JCAH) in May, 1971. In addition to the immediate relevance to all speech pathologists and audiologists working in (or serving as consultants to) facilities for the mentally retarded, these standards provide operational guidelines that have implications for speech pathology and audiology services in other types of facilities.

Although the ABESPA Professional Services Board's 1970 guidelines were generally incorporated and ASHA was officially represented in the final drafting of the guidelines, publication in *Asha* at this time does not represent official endorsement of the Association.

The AC/FMR standards relate to all professional and special services needed by the retarded. This report presents the standards of direct relevance to speech pathology and audiology services quoted directly from the total standards document titled *Standards for Residential Facilities for the Mentally Retarded.* This has been published in two editions: (1) a soft-cover bound edition including all standards adopted by the AC/FMR in May 1971 may be obtained from AAMD, 5201 Connecticut Avenue, N.W., Washington, D.C. 20015 for $1.00; and (2) a looseleaf binder edition including all standards and a two-year updating service of revisions as issued may be obtained from AC/FMR, 645 North Michigan Avenue, Chicago, Illinois for $6.00. (Both editions are sent postpaid, but prepayment is requested. The price covers only partial cost, since the publication is partially supported by the Federal grants.) The AAMD edition is for general information, but the AC/FMR edition is needed for accreditation and self-survey use.

A brief history of the establishment of these standards seems indicated. In 1952 the American Association on Mental Deficiency (AAMD) first published the report of its special committee on standards for institutions. Seven years later AAMD, supported by a grant from the National Institute of Mental Health, undertook a major standards development project which culminated in the 1964 publication of *Standards for State Residential Institutions for the Mentally Retarded.*

The 1964 AAMD Standards were presented as minimal, as generally attainable within five to ten years, and as a basis for evaluation and accreditation activities. Concurrent with their publication, the AAMD established a committee to continue review and revision of the standards and to encourage their implementation by developing an evaluation instrument based upon them, by providing an evaluation service to institutions requesting it, and by planning for the eventual establishment of a formal accreditation program. In 1965 a grant from the Mental Retardation Branch of the U.S. Public Health Service (subsequently the Division of Mental Retardation and recently the Division of Development Disabilities in the Social and Rehabilitation Service) enabled development of the evaluation instruments. A second grant, in 1965, provided for the evaluation, over the ensuing three years, of 134 state institutions for the mentally retarded, which represented three-quarters of such institutions and housed 90% of the residents of public facilities in the United States. Along with this project the AAMD instigated the formation of the National Planning Committee on Accreditation of Residential Centers for the Retarded, composed of representatives of AAMD, the American Psychiatric Association, the Council for

---

Lyle L. Lloyd, Ph.D., Chairman of the ASHA Mental Retardation Committee, prepared this Special Report.

Exceptional Children, the United Cerebral Palsy Associations (the five national organizations that now constitute the AC/FMR), plus the American Medical Association (which is a member organization of the JCAH). The National Planning Committee continued the review and revision of the 1964 standards and developed the structure of an accrediting agency, which in 1969 culminated in the establishment of the AC/FMR within the JCAH.

The AC/FMR enlisted participation of over 200 individuals representing 42 organizations (in addition to the five member organizations of the AC/FMR) working in 20 committees. These committees, representing all the disciplines and interests that must be involved in providing fully adequate programs for the retarded, were selected and functioned according to the five fundamental principles as stated in the standards document as follows:

1.   Since all of the problems associated with mental retardation do not fall within the purview of any one discipline, but require for their alleviation the knowledge and skills of many professions, the philosophy of the entire project, and of all its associated committees, must be thoroughly interdisciplinary in concept.

2.   Consequent to this philosophy, while each committee should be charged with primary responsibility for that section of the Standards pertaining to the activities of its particular discipline, no area of the Standards is the exclusive property of any discipline and, therefore, the Standards as a whole must be subject to review and criticism by every committee.

3.   Since standards for services to the mentally retarded must, at this point in time, be derived from the consensus of experienced leaders in the field as to what constitutes an adequate program, rather than from empirical data relating program provisions to desired outcomes, representation on committees must be as broad as possible in terms of variety of current viewpoints and program approaches, as well as in terms of levels of administrative responsibility.

4.   Inasmuch as identical standards must apply to the level of professional services rendered, whether within or without a residential setting, and since the Standards are intended to be applicable to both public and private facilities, representatives of nonresidential as well as public facilities must be included on committees.

5.   In order to broaden participation in standards development, to obtain the latest information and thought, and to secure the widest possible consensus while, at the same time, maintaining continuity with earlier endeavors, committees should include representatives of college and university programs and of research activity, as well as representatives of operating programs, and no more than one member of a committee should have served on previous standards committees.

The AC/FMR extended committee membership invitations to individuals on the basis of their known expertise, experience, and viewpoints in addition to asking national professional organization to name official representatives to the committees pertinent to their areas of interest. Twenty committees were selected with concern for administration, architecture, business management, dentistry, dietetics and nutrition, education, library services, medicine, nursing, pharmacy, physical and occupational therapies, psychology, records, recreation, religious services, resident living, social work, speech pathology and audiology, vocational rehabilitation, and volunteer services. In keeping with the interdisciplinary philosophy, most of the committees were multidisciplinary in composition.

The committee for speech pathology and audiology consisted of: Gerald G. Freeman, Alfred Hirschoren, Edwin A. Leach, John R. Olson, Paul A. Rittmanic, Boyd V. Sheets, Joseph E. Spradlin, and Lyle L. Lloyd, Chairman. The committee's audiologists, educators of the deaf, educators of the retarded, psychologists, and speech pathologists represented administrative, classroom, clinic, and research experience in community clinics, day schools, hospitals, residential facilities, and university settings. This committee's drafting of standards represents several years of activity of the AAMD's Speech Pathology and Audiology Subdivision and the ASHA Mental Retardation Committee. In addition to AAMD and ASHA representation, the CEASD and CEC were officially represented on the committee.

Audiologists and speech pathologists responsible for programs in facilities for the retarded should become familiar with the total standards document, but those standards of most direct relevance to speech and hearing services for the retarded and with general implications for all service-oriented ASHA Members are presented below:

**SECTION 3. PROFESSIONAL AND SPECIAL PROGRAMS
AND SERVICES**

3.1 Introduction

3.1.1 In addition to the resident-living services detailed in Section 2, residents *shall* be provided with the professional and special programs and services detailed in this Section, in accordance with their needs for such programs and services.

3.1.1.1 The professional and special programs and services detailed herein may be provided by programs maintained or personnel employed by the residential facility, or by formal arrangements between the facility and other agencies or persons, whereby the latter will provide such programs and services to the facility's residents as needed.

3.1.1.2. In accordance with the normalization principle, all professional services to the retarded should be rendered in the community, whenever possible, rather than in a residential facility, and where rendered in a residential facility, such services *must* be at least comparable to those provided the nonretarded in the community.

3.1.1.3 Programs and services provided by the facility, or to the facility by agencies outside it, or by persons not employed by it, *shall* meet the Standards for quality of service as stated in this Section.

3.1.1.3.1 The facility *shall* require that services provided its residents meet the Standards for quality of services as stated in this Section, and all contracts for the provision of such services *shall* stipulate that these Standards will be met.

3.1.2 Individuals providing professional and special programs and services to residents may be identified with the following professions, disciplines, or areas of service:

    a. Audiology [see 3.14];

    b. Dentistry (including services rendered by licensed dentists, licensed dental hygienists, and dental assistants) [see 3.2];

    c. Education [see 3.3];

    d. Food and Nutrition (including services rendered by dietitians and nutritionists) [see 3.4];

    e. Library Services [see 3.5];

    f. Medicine (including services rendered by licensed physicians, whether doctors of medicine or doctors of osteopathy, licensed pediatrists, and licensed optometrists) [see 3.6];

    g. Music, art, dance, and other activity therapies [see 3.11];

    h. Nursing [see 3.7];

    i. Occupational Therapy [see 3.9];

    j. Pharmacy [see 3.8];

    k. Physical Therapy [see 3.9];

    l. Psychology [see 3.10];

    m. Recreation [see 3.11];

    n. Religion (including services rendered by clergy and religious educators) [see 3.12];

    o. Social Work [see 3.13];

    p. Speech Pathology [see 3.14];

    q. Vocational Rehabilitation Counseling [see 3.15];

    r. Volunteer Services [see 3.10].

3.1.2.1 Interdisciplinary teams for evaluating the resident's needs, planning an individualized habilitation program to meet identified needs, and periodically reviewing the resident's response to his program and revising the program accordingly, *shall* be constituted of persons drawn from, or representing, such of the aforementioned professions, disciplines, or service areas as are relevant in each particular case.

3.1.2.2 Since many identical or similar services or functions may competently be rendered by individuals of different professions, the Standards in the following subsections *shall* be interpreted to mean that necessary services are to be provided in efficient and competent fashion, without regard to the professional identifications of the persons providing them, unless only members of a single profession are qualified or legally authorized to perform the stated service. Services listed under the duties of one profession may, therefore, be rendered by members of other professions who are equipped by training and experience to do so.

3.1.2.3 Regardless of the means by which the facility makes professional services available to its residents, there *shall* be evidence that members of professional disciplines work together in cooperative, coordinated, interdisciplinary fashion to achieve the objectives of the facility.

3.1.3 Programs and services and the pattern of staff organization and function within the facility *shall* be focused upon serving the individual needs of residents and should provide for:

3.1.3.1 Comprehensive diagnosis and evaluation of each resident as a basis for planning programming and management;
3.1.3.2 Design and implementation of an individualized habilitation program to effectively meet the needs of each resident;
3.1.3.3 Regular review, evaluation, and revision, as necessary, of each individual's habilitation program;
3.1.3.4 Freedom of movement of individual residents from one level of achievement to another, within the facility and also out of the facility, through training, habilitation, and placement;
3.1.3.5 An array of these services that will enable each resident to develop to his maximum potential.

3.14 Speech Pathology and Audiology Services
3.14.1 Speech pathology and audiology services *shall* be available, in order to:
3.14.1.1 Maximize the communication skills of all residents;
3.14.1.2 Provide for the evaluation, counseling, treatment, and rehabilitation of those residents with speech, hearing and/or language handicaps.

3.14.2 The specific goals of speech pathology and audiology services *shall* be:
3.14.2.1 Appropriate to the needs of the residents served;
3.14.2.2 Consistent with the philosophy and goals of the facility;
3.14.2.3 Consistent with the services and resources offered by the facility;
3.14.2.4 Known to, and coordinated with, other services provided by the facility.

3.14.3 Speech pathology and audiology services *shall* be rendered through:
3.14.3.1 Direct contact between speech pathologists and audiologists and residents;
3.14.3.2 Participation with administrative personnel in designing and maintaining social and physical environments that maximize the communication development of the residents;
3.14.3.3 Working with other personnel, such as teachers and direct-care staff, in implementing communication improvement programs in environmental settings.

3.14.4 Speech pathology and audiology services available to the facility *shall* include, as appropriate:
3.14.4.1 Audiometric screening of:
3.14.4.1.1 All new residents;
3.14.4.1.2 Children under the age of ten, at annual intervals;
3.14.4.1.3 Other residents at regular intervals;
3.14.4.1.4 Any resident referred;
3.14.4.2 Speech and language screening of:
3.14.4.2.1 All new residents;
3.14.4.2.2 Children under the age of ten at annual intervals;
3.14.4.2.3 All residents, as needed;
3.14.4.3 Comprehensive audiological assessment of residents, as indicated by screening results, to include tests of pure-tone air and bone conduction, speech audiometry, and other procedures, as necessary, and to include assessment of the use of visual cues;
3.14.4.4 Assessment of the use of amplification;
3.14.4.5 Provision for procurement, maintenance, and replacement of hearing aids, as specified by a qualified audiologist;
3.14.4.6 Comprehensive speech and language evaluation of residents, as indicated by screening results, including appraisal of articulation, voice, rhythm, and language;

3.14.4.7 Participation in the continuing interdisciplinary evaluation of individual residents for purposes of initiation, monitoring, and follow-up of individualized habilitation programs;

3.14.4.8 Treatment services, interpreted as an extension of the evaluation process, that include:

3.14.4.8.1 Direct counseling with residents;

3.14.4.8.2. Speech and language development and stimulation through daily living activities;

3.14.4.8.3 Consultation with classroom teachers for speech improvement and speech education activities;

3.14.4.8.4 Direct contact with residents to carry on programs designed to meet individual needs in comprehension (e.g., speech reading, auditory training, and hearing aid utilization) as well as expression (e.g., improvement in articulation, voice, rhythm, and language);

3.14.4.8.5 Collaboration with appropriate educators and librarians to develop specialized programs for developing the communication skills of multiply handicapped residents, such as the deaf retarded and the cerebral palsied;

3.14.4.9 Consultation with administrative staff regarding the planning of environments that facilitate communication development among residents in:

3.14.4.9.1 Living areas;

3.14.4.9.2 Dining areas;

3.14.4.9.3 Educational areas;

3.14.4.9.4 Other areas, where relevant;

3.14.4.10 Participation in inservice training programs for direct-care and other staff;

3.14.4.11 Training of speech pathology and audiology staff;

3.14.4.12 Training of speech pathology and audiology graduate and/or undergraduate students, interns, supportive staff, and volunteer workers;

3.14.4.13 Consultation with, or relating to:

3.14.4.13.1 Residents (e.g., self-referral);

3.14.4.13.2 Parents of residents;

3.14.4.13.3 Medical (otological, pediatric, etc.), dental, psychological, educational and other services;

3.14.4.13.4 The administration and operation of the facility;

3.14.4.13.5 The community served by the facility;

3.14.4.14 Program evaluation and research.

3.14.5 Comprehensive evaluations in speech pathology and audiology *shall* consider the total person and his environment. Such evaluations should:

3.14.5.1 Present a complete appraisal of the resident's communication skills;

3.14.5.2 Evidence concern for, and evaluation of, conditions extending beyond observed speech, language, and hearing defects;

3.14.5.3 Consider factors in the history and environment relevant to the origins and maintenance of the disability;

3.14.5.4 Consider the effect of the disability upon the individual and the adjustments he makes to the problem as he perceives it;

3.14.5.5 Consider the reaction of the resident's family, associates, and peers to the speech and/or hearing problem.

3.14.6 Evaluation and assessment results *shall* be reported accurately and systematically, and in such manner as to:

3.14.6.1 Define the problem to provide a basis for formulating treatment objectives and procedures;

3.14.6.2 Render the report meaningful and useful to its intended recipient and user;

3.14.6.3 Where appropriate, provide information useful to other staff working directly with the resident;

3.14.6.4 Conform to acceptable professional standards, provide for intra-individual and interindividual comparisons, and facilitate the use of data for research and professional education;

3.14.6.5 Provide evaluative and summary reports for inclusion in the resident's unit record.

3.14.7 Treatment objectives, plans, and procedures *shall*:

3.14.7.1 Be based upon adequate evaluation and assessment;

3.14.7.2 Be based upon a clear rationale;

3.14.7.3 Reflect consideration of the objectives of the resident's total habilitation program;

3.14.7.4 Be stated in terms that permit the progress of the individual to be assessed;

3.14.7.5 Provide for periodic evaluation of the resident's response to treatment and of treatment effectiveness;

3.14.7.6 Provide for revision of objectives and procedures as indicated;

3.14.7.7 Provide for assistance or consultation when necessary.

3.14.8 Continuing observations of treatment progress *shall* be:

3.14.8.1 Recorded accurately, summarized meaningfully, and communicated effectively;

3.14.8.2 Effectively utilized in evaluating progress.

3.14.9 There *shall* be established procedures for evaluating and researching the effectiveness of speech pathology and audiology services, including:

3.14.9.1 Utilization of adequate records concerning resident's response and progress;

3.14.9.2 Time schedules for evaluation that are appropriate to the service being evaluated;

3.14.9.3 Provision for using evaluation results in program planning and development;

3.14.9.4 Encouragement of speech pathology and audiology staff to participate in research activities;

3.14.9.5 Provision for dissemination of research results in professional journals.

3.14.10 There *shall* be available sufficient, appropriately qualified staff, and necessary supporting personnel, to carry out the various speech pathology and audiology services, in accordance with stated goals and objectives.

3.14.10.1 A speech pathologist or audiologist, who is qualified as specified in Item 3.14.10.2, and who, in addition, has had at least three years of professional experience, *shall* be designated as being responsible for maintaining standards of professional and ethical practice in the rendering of speech pathology and audiology services in the facility.

3.14.10.2 Staff who assume independent responsibilities for clinical services *shall* possess the educational and experiential qualifications required for a Certificate of Clinical Competence issued by the American Speech and Hearing Association (ASHA) in the area (speech pathology or audiology) in which they provide services.

3.14.10.3 Staff not qualified for ASHA certification *shall* be provided adequate, direct, active, and continuing supervision by staff qualified for certification in the area in which supervision is rendered.

3.14.10.3.1 Supervising staff *shall* be responsible for the services rendered by uncertified staff under their supervision.

3.14.10.3.2 Adequate, direct, and continuing supervision *shall* be provided nonprofessionals, volunteers, or other supportive personnel utilized in providing clinical services.

3.14.10.4 Students in training and staff fulfilling experience requirements for ASHA certification *shall* receive direct supervision, in accordance with the requirements of the American Board of Examiners in Speech Pathology and Audiology.

3.14.10.5 All speech pathology and audiology staff *shall* be familiar with, and adhere to, the Code of Ethics published by the American Speech and Hearing Association.

3.14.11 Appropriate to the nature and size of the facility and to the speech pathology and audiology service, there *shall* be a staff development program that is designed to maintain and improve the skills of speech pathology and audiology staff, through methods such as:

3.14.11.1 Regular staff meetings;

3.14.11.2 An organized inservice training program in speech pathology and audiology;

3.14.11.3 Visits to and from the staff of other facilities and programs;

3.14.11.4 Participation in interdisciplinary meetings;

3.14.11.5 Provision for financial assistance and time for attendance at professional conferences;

3.14.11.6 Provisions for encouraging continuing education, including educational leave, financial assistance, and accommodation of work schedules;

3.14.11.7 Workshops and seminars;

3.14.11.8 Consultations with specialists;

3.14.11.9 Access to adequate library resources, which include current and relevant books and journals in speech pathology and audiology, mental retardation, and related professions and fields.

3.14.12 Space, facilities, equipment, and supplies *shall* be adequate for providing efficient and effective speech pathology and audiology services, in accordance with stated objectives, including:

3.14.12.1 Adequate and convenient evaluation, treatment, counseling, and waiting rooms;

3.14.12.2 Specially constructed and sound-treated suites for audiological services, meeting U.S.A.S.I. standards;

3.14.12.3 Design and location such as to be easily accessible to all residents, regardless of disability;

3.14.12.4 Specialized equipment needed by the speech pathologist;

3.14.12.5 Specialized equipment needed by the audiologist, including an audiometer, with provisions for sound field audiometry, and equipment capable of performing at least the following procedures; hearing screening, pure-tone air and bone conduction with contralateral masking, speech audiometry, site-of-lesion battery, nonorganic hearing loss battery and hearing aid evaluation;

3.14.12.6 Provisions for adequate maintenance of all areas, facilities, and equipment, including;

3.14.12.6.1 Electroacoustic calibration of audiometers at regular, at least quarterly, intervals;

3.14.12.6.2 Calibration logs on all audiometers.

3.14.12.7 Appropriate speech pathology and audiology consultation *shall* be employed in the design, modification, and equipage of all speech pathology and audiology areas and facilities.

APPENDIX D / Language Intervention Systems: Programs Published in Kit Form

Macalyne Fristoe

What programs of language training are presently in use with the retarded in the United States? This was one of the first questions that arose when the Lurleen B. Wallace Developmental Center at Decatur, Alabama, and the Center for Developmental and Learning Disorders at the University of Alabama in Birmingham, joined forces to design a language training program for the L. B. Wallace Center. It seemed desirable to select several programs that would provide maximal benefit for the residents with the limited personnel and funds available. Relatively few programs were known, and attempts to find an extensive review of such programs, both published and unpublished, were fruitless. It was decided, therefore, that it would be desirable to start the project by determining what had been published and what is currently being developed in the way of language programs for the retarded, especially the lower level retarded. In recognition of the realities of economic restrictions in even the best funded programs, special attention would be given to programs that can be carried out by aides or supportive personnel working under professional supervision, an economical way of providing services. Since programs that have been published would probably represent only a small fraction of what is being used, a special effort would be made to locate unpublished programs that are in use in one or more locations. Supported by an ESEA Title III grant from the State of Alabama Department of Education (Elementary and Secondary Education Act of 1965, Public Law 89-10), a national survey of language programs in use with the retarded was undertaken.

The first step in the survey was the creation of a detailed plan of operation. According to this plan, all the state directors of mental health, mental retardation, and special education would be written to request a

Published simultaneously by the Council for Exceptional Children's Division for Children with Communication Disorders in their *Journal of Childhood Communication Disorders*.

list of individuals and facilities providing speech, hearing, and language services for the retarded in their respective states. To decrease the likelihood that anyone would be overlooked, the director of the speech and hearing division at each University Affiliated Facility (UAF) in the country and the president of each state speech and hearing association also would receive a similar request. The organizations identified on the lists would be asked for information about the services that they provide; this information would be made into a directory of speech, hearing, and language services for the retarded throughout the country. In addition, they would be asked what programs they use. Those that appeared to be using original or novel programs would be written again for detailed information. A description of each novel or original program thus identified would be included in a small catalog. There was one basic flaw in this plan, however; few state officials had the information about speech, hearing, and language services for the retarded that was expected, and so they could not provide the desired lists.

The plan had to be modified. It was necessary to take the much more difficult approach of writing to all of the day and residential facilities for the retarded that could be located to ask whether or not they provided speech/hearing/language services. Help in locating the most up-to-date lists was sought from national organizations such as the American Association on Mental Deficiency, the Council for Exceptional Children, the National Institute of Mental Health, and the American Speech and Hearing Association. The information available from these sources was far from being complete and in many cases was outdated; however, it did provide a beginning. The appropriate agencies that could be identified were sent a questionnaire that asked, among other things; 1) Do you provide speech/hearing/language services for the retarded at your facility? 2) Can you give the names of persons or organizations in your state that you think may be providing such services? 3) What programs, published or unpublished, do you use for language training? On the basis of the names obtained in response to these questionnaires, additional questionnaires were sent out; these secured more names, and another round of questionnaires was sent out, etc. By this rather cumbersome method, information about most of the major programs in each state was obtained. The directory was prepared from information in the returned questionnaires.

The task had become much bigger and more difficult than originally anticipated. At this point almost 700 completed questionnaires had been returned and approximately 200 programs that appeared to be original had been identified. It seemed desirable to obtain expanded information about these original approaches for presentation in the catalog, and it would enhance the value of the catalog to obtain information from the authors themselves whenever possible. In most cases this was accomplished—the desired information was secured from the authors or their designated representatives. In the remainder, information was obtained from materials that had been sent by the authors or by their publishers.

Detailed information on 187 programs out of the 229 identified has been published in *Language Intervention Systems for the Retarded* (Fristoe, 1975). (For the remaining programs this information could not be obtained before the publication deadline.) Of the 187 programs, 39 are in the form of kits, 31 have been reported in books or journals, 66 have been published privately, either in experimental or "in-house" limited editions, and 51 are in preparation or else are not currently available. This appendix, which focuses on the first category—programs that are available in kit form—summarizes some of the information in the catalog (Fristoe, 1975) and adds other details. Additional articles examining other aspects of this survey are scheduled for publication in the next several months.

Information about each program is arranged under the headings that are explained below. Except in the case of Auditory Perceptual Training and Language Lotto, for which the descriptive information was derived directly from the programs, the information in the program descriptions between the double lines was abstracted from that provided by the authors or their designated representatives. An asterisk (*) indicates that no information was provided. Items in brackets were not provided by the program author but were supplied by the present writer.

Above the first double line is the identifying information—the formal title of the program, followed in parentheses by other names by which it is known. The alternative names are included because a program may be referred to by more than one name or be commonly called by a name other than its formal name. The names of the authors are next, followed by the publisher's name and address. Most kits are available from commercial publishers, a few from nonprofit organizations.

TARGET—What was the original target group, the population that the program was designed to serve? In some cases a program might not have been developed for use with the retarded in particular but, for example, may have been designed as a treatment program for children with learning disabilities or as a developmental program for normal children. Since some survey respondents indicated that they used it with retarded persons and found it beneficial, it is therefore included. The abbreviations used are: MR, mentally retarded; LD, learning disabled; DIS, disadvantaged; CP, cerebral palsied; and All, all persons needing this type of language therapy.

LEVEL—This refers to the level of retardation for which the program is most applicable. (Since the survey was concerned with language intervention systems used with the retarded, a category of normal was not included.) In most cases, a borderline, mild, moderate, severe, or profound level of retardation was designated; in other instances, programs were described as most applicable for a grade or age range (MA, mental age; CA, chronologic age; LA, language age) or for an educational classification (EMR, educable mentally retarded; TMR, trainable mentally retarded; SMR, severely mentally retarded).

TYPE—Programs are classified as operant or nonoperant in type. They also are classified as being designed either for use as a stimulation program or for remedial purposes. Some programs are classified as both; this may reflect a theoretical point of view, i.e., that the best remedial approach is to provide an increased amount of stimulation.

MODEL—The models to which a program is most closely related are presented here. The choices given on the questionnaire were behavioral, cognitive, developmental, functional language, information processing, medical, and other. Some approaches are based on more than one model; for example, a Piagetian approach could be classified as both cognitive and developmental. The use of some combinations that do not seem intuitively compatible may be due to a difference of opinion regarding what these commonly used terms mean.

EMPHASIS—This section deals with the relative emphasis of the program in terms of expressive language development (listed as "expressive"), receptive language development ("receptive"), motor imitation development ("motor imitation"), and nonverbal communication by manual language, communication board, or other means. (Use of the term *nonvocal* might be better than *nonverbal* because it is more specific, more descriptive of communication by some means other than the spoken word.) Major emphasis is represented by (1), moderate emphasis by (2), and minor emphasis by (3).

STRUCTURE—The amount of structure in the program is given. High, moderate, slight, and unstructured were the choices available on the questionnaire; all kit programs were classified as either high or moderate. After this is the number of lessons or steps that are available and the format (script, activity cards, cassettes, etc.).

BASELINES—If the program includes a way of obtaining baseline data before beginning the first instructional step or lesson, then this is indicated.

USERS—The users for which the program is appropriate are given. They could be professionals—persons with graduate training in the area of language development and intervention, such as speech pathologists, special educators, or psychologists—or they could be classroom teachers, parents, volunteers, aides working under professional supervision, etc. Presumably, when a program is designated as one that can be used by aides (and the requirement for professional supervision is implied with the use of the term *aides* unless otherwise indicated), then it is also suitable for parents to use under similar conditions in most cases. A percentage figure in parentheses after *aides* refers to the amount of the total program that can be administered by aides.

SETTING—The setting in which a program can be used effectively is indicated. The choices included were individual therapy (a one-to-one relationship in a separate room), group therapy, (a one-to-several relationship), a classroom, the home, or a residential setting (cottage, ward, group home, etc.).

COST—The approximate 1975–1976 price of the program kit is given. In some cases it is itemized to show the cost of units, extra workbooks, etc.

COMMENTS—The miscellaneous comments below the second double line were added by the present writer. They include information about the theoretical basis for the program, kit contents, equipment requirements, and special applications of the program not given elsewhere. Some of the information in this section is derived from that provided by the program author; the remainder is abstracted from the program itself.

For more extensive information about these kit programs, as well as about the remainder of the programs identified in the survey, the reader is referred to the catalog (Fristoe, 1975).

No prepared program, packaged or otherwise, can be expected to provide all of the intervention assistance necessary to aid a specific person or even to fill all the needs of that person at a given time. Ideally, an alert, well trained clinician should be able to generate for each language-handicapped person an individualized program that would provide the greatest opportunity for that person's improvement. In instances where the facilities and personnel are not readily available for designing and executing an individualized program for each person and for preparing all the necessary materials, a prepared program can offer varying amounts of assistance in closing the gap between the ideal and the possible.

REFERENCE

Fristoe, M. 1975. Language Intervention Systems for the Retarded: A catalog of original structured language programs in use in the U.S. State of Alabama Department of Education, Montgomery, Ala. (Copies of this book can be obtained by writing to: Language Intervention Systems for the Retarded, L. B. Wallace Developmental Center, P.O. Box 2224, Decatur, Alabama 35601.)

NAME	Auditory Perception Training; Figure Ground; Memory; Motor; Discrimination; Imagery (A.P.T.)
AUTHOR	Rosemarie Willette Brenda Jackson Irwin Peckings
PUBLISHER	Developmental Learning Materials 7440 Natchez Avenue Niles, Illinois 60648

TARGET	LD, All
LEVEL	Borderline–moderate
TYPE	*; stimulation, remedial
MODEL	Cognitive, functional language, information processing
EMPHASIS	Receptive (1), motor imitation (1)
STRUCTURE	High; 140 lessons in script format
BASELINES	Informal
USERS	Professionals, classroom teachers, parents, aides (100%)
SETTING	Individual, group, classroom, home
APPROXIMATE COST	$275.00

COMMENTS

This program is based on the belief that auditory perception is fundamental to success in learning. For each area named in the title, 18 to 36 lessons are provided. The kit contains spirit masters, cassettes, teacher's manuals. Cassette recorder is required.

NAME	Auditory Perceptual Training Program (APT)
AUTHOR	Belle Ruth Witkin Katharine G. Butler Donna Lea Hedrick Charlie C. Manning
PUBLISHER	Alameda County School Department 224 West Winton Avenue Hayward, California 94544

TARGET	Grades 1–3 for auditory perceptual problems; grades 2–6 for learning or language problems
LEVEL	*
TYPE	Not operant; stimulation, remedial
MODEL	*
EMPHASIS	*
STRUCTURE	High; 39 lessons on cassettes
USERS	Classroom teachers, aides (100%), qualified students
SETTING	Individual, group, classroom
APPROXIMATE COST	$49.75+

COMMENTS

This program is designed for children who experience difficulty in learning or reading due to inadequate or faulty processing of auditory information. It is not applicable in the presence of gross language delay.

The program is divided into four units. Unit I: Listen for Sounds includes selective attention, speech sound discrimination and analysis and temporal sequencing. Unit II: Listen for Words and Speakers includes auditory closure and synthesis, temporal sequencing, voice identification and attention to intonation patterns. Unit III: Listen to Remember covers recognition of the number of sounds and syllables in words and phrases and selective attention or "figure-ground discrimination" activities in the presence of competing messages. Unit IV: Listen to Learn includes recognition of subject-verb agreement, active and passive voice, complex syntactic structure, and more difficult competing message tasks. A review lesson for each unit samples the most difficult items from lessons in that unit. The lessons in each unit are designed so that the auditory tasks grow in complexity while visual/motor responses remain at the same simple level throughout the unit.

The basic APT program includes 39 audio cassette lessons, 43 consumable student listening booklets per student, four review lessons, and a teacher's manual. Also available are the composite auditory perceptual test (CAPT) for diagnostic and pre- and posttesting and a film strip and cassette introduction to the program. A cassette recorder and red and blue markers are required.

NAME	BKR Educational Projects, Inc.
AUTHOR	Louise M. Bradtke William J. Kirkpatrick, Jr. Katherine P. Rosenblatt
PUBLISHER	BKR Educational Projects, Inc. 1970 S.W. 43rd Way Fort Lauderdale, Florida 33317

TARGET	All persons with severe language problems [especially the multiply handicapped severely or profoundly retarded child]
LEVEL	Moderate–profound
TYPE	Operant; stimulation
MODEL	Developmental
EMPHASIS	Receptive (1), expressive (1), nonverbal communication by sign (3)
STRUCTURE	High; 75% of program in detailed lessons in activity card format
BASELINES	Development and Trainability Assessment (DATA)
USERS	Professionals, classroom teachers, parents, aides (75%)
SETTING	Individual, classroom, home
APPROXIMATE COST	$25.00 per kit, plus postage and handling $15.00 for 25 additional copies of assessment (DATA)

COMMENTS

Fifteen "basic language" lessons are included in the program, which also contains sections labeled cognition, visual skills, auditory (nonverbal) fine motor gross motor, social self, personal skills acquired, and direction. The authors state that they wish to have each user take the lesson plans and adapt them to create individualized programs to suit the needs of each child rather than following a set program.

The materials to be used with this program are listed but are not included in the kit; they must be supplied by the user.

NAME	Concepts for Communication (CFC; Concept 7-9)
AUTHOR	J. Wright R. A. Norris F. J. Worsley
PUBLISHER	Developmental Learning Materials 7440 Natchez Avenue Niles, Illinois 60648

TARGET	All
LEVEL	Borderline–moderate
TYPE	Operant; stimulation, remedial
MODEL	Cognitive, functional language, information processing
EMPHASIS	Receptive (1), expressive (1), motor imitation (1)
STRUCTURE	Moderate; about 50% written out (Units II and III are open ended); script format
BASELINES	*
USERS	Classroom teachers, parents, aides, LD teachers, speech clinicians
SETTING	Partly for whole class, partly for large and small group, partly for individuals
APPROXIMATE COST	$125.00—Total program $ 40.00—Unit I $ 50.00—Unit II $ 55.00—Unit III

COMMENTS

CFC is divided into three units; Unit I, Listening with Understanding; Unit II, Concept Building; Unit III, Communication. The course from England, "Concept Seven-Nine," has been modified for use in America. It stresses concept building, language, and reasoning. Some of the material is designed for use with a whole class throughout the school year, some for large or small groups with varying amounts of teacher involvement. Unit I is for individual children working by themselves.

NAME	Developmental Syntax (Coughran-Liles Syntax Program)
AUTHOR	Lila Coughran Betty V. Liles
PUBLISHER	Learning Concepts 2501 North Lamar Austin, Texas 78705

TARGET	All, primarily LD, DIS, and those with syntactic disorders
LEVEL	Borderline–moderate; EMR; Prekindergarten to 5th grade
TYPE	Operant; remedial
MODEL	Behavioral, developmental, functional language
EMPHASIS	Expressive (1), receptive (2), motor imitation (3)
STRUCTURE	High; 8 programs written out in detailed lessons in script format
BASELINES	50 utterance sample using pictures
USERS	Professionals, parents (for homework carryover), aides (100%)
SETTING	Individual, group (2–4)
APPROXIMATE COST	$30.00—Kit $ 3.75—Score Record Sheets (25)

COMMENTS

Emphasis is on the remediation of problems of syntax that the authors have found to be most common in children they have seen. It is designed for children with normal conceptual development and normal receptive language but with expressive problems of a syntactic nature. It is based on structured therapy techniques de-scribed by Siegfried Engelmann, Edgar Garrett, and Margaret H. Powers. There are three phases of training: ear training, production, and carryover. The kit contains a manual in looseleaf notebook form and a box of eight sets of cards with black and white drawings. A mental age of at least 3 years is required.

NAME	Distar Language I
AUTHOR	Siegfried Engelmann Jean Osborn
PUBLISHER	Science Research Associates, Inc. 259 East Erie Chicago, Illinois 60611

TARGET	All
LEVEL	Bright to [below normal]
TYPE	Operant; stimulation, remedial
MODEL	Behavioral, information processing
EMPHASIS	Receptive (1), expressive (1), motor imitation (1)
STRUCTURE	High; entire program written out in script format
BASELINES	No
USERS	Professionals, classroom teachers, parents, aides (100%)
SETTING	Individual, group, classroom
APPROXIMATE COST	$175.00

COMMENTS

Most users report that this program is of value with the higher level retarded but must be modified for use with the moderately retarded. Distar Language I is currently being revised and should be out at the beginning of 1976.

NAME	Distar Language II
AUTHOR	Siegfried Engelmann Jean Osborn
PUBLISHER	Science Research Associates, Inc. 259 East Erie Chicago, Illinois 60611

TARGET	All
LEVEL	Bright to [below normal]
TYPE	Operant; stimulation, remedial
MODEL	Behavioral, information processing
EMPHASIS	Receptive (1), expressive (1), motor imitation (1)
STRUCTURE	High; entire program written out in script format
BASELINES	No
USERS	Professionals, classroom teachers, parents, aides (100%)
SETTING	Individual, group, classroom
APPROXIMATE COST	$175.00

COMMENTS

Most users report that this program is of value with the higher level retarded but must be modified for use with the moderately retarded.

NAME	Fokes Sentence Builder Kit
AUTHOR	Joann Fokes
PUBLISHER	Teaching Resources 100 Boylston Boston, Massachusetts 02100

TARGET	All, especially deaf, LD, hearing impaired, foreign language
LEVEL	Borderline, mild; EMR
TYPE	Not operant; stimulation, remedial
MODEL	Cognitive, psycholinguistic
EMPHASIS	Receptive (1), expressive (2), nonverbal communication—sign (3)
STRUCTURE	High; entire program written out, 50 lessons in script format
BASELINES	Response sheet used as guide
USERS	Professionals, classroom teachers, parents (supervised), aides (25%)
SETTING	Individual, group, classroom, home, any structured setting
APPROXIMATE COST	$40.00–$50.00

COMMENTS

This program, designed to teach syntactic structures, requires language development beyond the two-word stage and the ability to attend to pictures. It is designed to teach syntactic structures but not rote responses. The kit contains the manual and all necessary materials.

NAME	General Electric/Project LIFE Program (Project LIFE)
AUTHOR	Glenn S. Pfau
PUBLISHER	Instructional Industries, Inc. Executive Park Ballston Lake, New York 12019

TARGET	All, especially deaf, emotionally disturbed, DIS, MR
LEVEL	Borderline–moderate; EMR; IQ range 60–100; grades K–6
TYPE	Operant; stimulation, remedial
MODEL	Behavioral, cognitive, developmental, functional language
EMPHASIS	Receptive (1), expressive (3)
STRUCTURE	Moderate; about 75% of program written out; 500 lessons [filmstrips, cassettes, teaching machines]
BASELINES	*
USERS	Classroom teachers, parents, aides, (100%)
SETTING	Individual, classroom, home, dormitory, library, media resource room
APPROXIMATE COST	$8.00 per filmstrip. Write company for equipment (PAL) information

COMMENTS

Presently available filmstrips include approximately 30 in perceptual training (prereading level), 100 in perceptual thinking (prereading level through grade three), 350 in language reading (grades one to five). Optional cassettes to go with some filmstrips and several equipment options are also available.

NAME	GOAL: Language Development—Games Oriented Activities for Learning
AUTHOR	Merle B. Karnes
PUBLISHER	Milton Bradley and Co. Springfield, Massachusetts 01101

TARGET	All, including normal
LEVEL	Borderline–moderate; EMR-TMR; normals age 3–5, older for language handicapped
TYPE	Not operant; stimulation, remedial
MODEL	Developmental, information processing
EMPHASIS	Receptive (1), expressive (1), motor imitation (1)
STRUCTURE	High; 337 lessons on cards
BASELINES	Yes
USERS	Professionals, classroom teachers, aides (100%), volunteers, older students
SETTING	Individual, group, classroom, home
APPROXIMATE COST	$125.00

COMMENTS

GOAL is built on the clinical model of the Illinois Test of Psychological Abilities (ITPA). The kit contains 337 model lesson plans on 8″ × 9″ cards (35 in auditory reception, 35 in visual reception, 47 in verbal expression, 35 in manual expression, 47 in auditory association, 35 in visual association, 23 in auditory sequential memory, 35 in visual sequential memory, 11 in auditory closure, 23 in grammatic closure, and 11 in visual closure). Each lesson plan has five parts: 1) language processing category, 2) lesson objectives, 3) materials, 4) procedure, 5) criterion activities, and, in some plans, 6) reinforcement activities.

Lessons are in a game format. Other materials in the kit are those to be used with the lesson plans.

There are eight sets of Picture Cards with 42 cards in each. These include categories such as family, home, things that go together, food, opposites, alikes, everyday objects, and picture dominos. Thirty-six Situation Pictures illustrate impossible situations, actions, emotion as expressed by facial expression, and nursery rhyme scenes. In the category, What is Missing?, there are 12 posters and 12 templates that can be used for identification of missing parts or for visual closure activities. There are six simple animal puzzles, three hand puppets, and patterns for making "paper dolls" with clothing for use in lessons. Eight picture overlays that use the same plastic spinner are provided with the Spin and Find Games. Materials are included for lotto games that permit object to object and word to object matching. Twelve large posters ("murals") are also included. The kit contains all the materials needed for the program, but suggestions are given for using other materials that are not included in the kit for supplementary lessons.

The objectives do not designate an exact level of attainment, which must be selected by the user. Criterion activities are described, but decisions regarding when to move to another activity and when to repeat an activity in a similar form are left up to the user to a great degree. The GOAL program is designed to be "flexible rather than totally complete."

NAME	Goldman-Lynch Sounds & Symbols Development Kit (G-L Program)
AUTHOR	Ronald Goldman Martha Lynch
PUBLISHER	American Guidance Service Circle Pines, Minnesota 55014

TARGET	All, especially LD, DIS, normal
LEVEL	Borderline–mild; preschool through 4th grade
TYPE	Not operant; stimulation, remedial
MODEL	Cognitive, developmental
EMPHASIS	Expressive (1), receptive (2), motor imitation (1)
STRUCTURE	High; 64 lessons in script format
BASELINES	No
USERS	Professionals for articulation problems, classroom teachers, aides (100%)
SETTING	Group, classroom, home
APPROXIMATE COST	$120.00

COMMENTS

This program is designed to make children familiar with the relationships between American English phonemes and their most common graphemic representations. It also serves to accelerate articulatory development. The kit contains word cards, picture cards, sentence strips, a pocket chart, 27 colored posters, two illustrated books with 39 High Hat stories, 38 character cards and flash cards, two hand puppets, 40 magnetic symbols, two sound and song cassettes, 805 colored picture cards and other program accessories in a metal case. The set of workbooks, which is ordered separately, contains an orientation record that gives instructions and examples for untrained users such as parents.

NAME	Karnes Early Language Activities
AUTHOR	Merle B. Karnes
PUBLISHER	GEM
	P.O. Box 2339, Station A
	Champaign, Illinois 61820

TARGET	MR, LD, DIS, language lag
LEVEL	Borderline–profound; EMR-SMR; 18–36 months functional level
TYPE	*; stimulation
MODEL	Developmental, information processing, functional language
EMPHASIS	Receptive (1), expressive (1), motor imitation (1)
STRUCTURE	Moderate, 75% written out; 200 model lessons, 1000 activities on cards
BASELINES	Yes
USERS	Professionals, classroom teachers, aides, parents, volunteers
SETTING	Individual, group, classroom, home
APPROXIMATE COST	$40.00

COMMENTS

Built on the ITPA clinical model, this program is a downward extension of the GOAL Program but is not sequential. Materials are to be provided by the user.

NAME	Language Lotto
AUTHOR	Lassar G. Gotkin
PUBLISHER	New Century Education Corp. 440 Park Avenue South New York, New York 10016

TARGET	Normal preschool and 1st grade children
LEVEL	Mild; EMR
TYPE	Not operant; remedial
MODEL	*
EMPHASIS	Receptive (1), expressive (1)
STRUCTURE	Slight; not written out
BASELINES	No
USERS	Classroom teachers, aides (100%)
SETTING	Group
APPROXIMATE COST	(No longer available)

COMMENTS

Six programmed games—Objects, Prepositions, Actions, More Actions, Compound Sentences, Relationships— are designed to develop visual and aural discrimination and stimulate language growth. Each game is designed for use on different levels, moving from concrete to abstract, from single word names to complex sentences. Supplemental games can be introduced if the child has particular difficulty moving to a sequence. The kit contains the six games and a teacher's manual.

NAME	Learning to Develop Language
AUTHOR	Merle B. Karnes
PUBLISHER	Milton Bradley and Co. Springfield, Massachusetts 01101

TARGET	[MR, LD]
LEVEL	Moderate; EMR; age range: 3–7
TYPE	*
MODEL	*
EMPHASIS	Receptive (1), expressive (1), motor imitation (1), nonverbal communication (1)
STRUCTURE	Moderate; 150 lessons
BASELINES	No
USERS	Professionals, classroom teachers, parents, aides (100%), volunteers [Written for nonprofessionals]
SETTING	Individual, group, classroom, home
APPROXIMATE COST	Under $50.00

COMMENTS

This program follows the same general format as the lessons in GOAL. It was designed to train teachers to interact appropriately with children. Lessons are written so that they can be easily understood by persons without professional training. The kit contains lessons in booklet and materials.

NAME	Merkley Developmental Approach to Speech and Language (Merkley Adaptation of the Barry Slate System)
AUTHOR	Frances A. Merkley
PUBLISHER	Project A.D.A.P.T. Tri-Counties Regional Center 22 W. Michetorena Santa Barbara, California 93101

TARGET	Deaf, LD, CP, MR, all developmentally disabled
LEVEL	Mild, moderate; EMR, TMR; age range: 2–8
TYPE	Not operant; stimulation
MODEL	Developmental, cognitive
EMPHASIS	Receptive (1), expressive (1), motor imitation (2), nonverbal communication (3)
BASELINES	Yes
STRUCTURE	High; script format
USERS	Professionals, classroom teachers, aides (100% with the child)
SETTING	Individual, group, classroom
APPROXIMATE COST	(Program still in press)

COMMENTS

Programming is planned according to cognitive and motor development status. Formal programming begins at the sixth stage of the sensorimotor period (Piaget). The kit contains materials or sample materials.

NAME	Michigan Language Program (Michigan Successive Discrimination Reading Program)
AUTHOR	Donald E. P. Smith Judith M. Smith
PUBLISHER	Random House, Inc. 201 East 50th Street New York, New York 10022

TARGET	Anyone who wishes to read and write
LEVEL	Severe [?]; IQ range: 50+; grade range: kindergarten +
TYPE	Operant; stimulation
MODEL	Information processing
EMPHASIS	Receptive (2), expressive (2)
STRUCTURE	No
BASELINES	High; 440 lessons in script format
USERS	Classroom teachers, parents, aides (100%), high school students
SETTING	Classroom
APPROXIMATE COST	$ 25.00 per child $650.00 per class

COMMENTS

This program stresses the written (or printed) form of language rather than the spoken. The kit contains the book and all necessary materials. A tape player is required.

NAME	Missouri State Department of Education Speech and Language Kit
AUTHOR	John B. Heskett Jess A. LaPuma
PUBLISHER	Speech and Hearing Services State Schools for Severely Handicapped P.O. Box 480 Jefferson City, Missouri 65101

TARGET	MR
LEVEL	TMR
TYPE	Not operant; stimulation
MODEL	Developmental, functional language
EMPHASIS	Receptive (1), expressive (1), motor imitation (3), nonverbal communication—communication board (3)
BASELINES	Yes
STRUCTURE	Slight; sample lessons provided, individualized
USERS	Professionals, classroom teachers, aides
SETTING	Individual, group, classroom
APPROXIMATE COST	(No longer available)

COMMENTS

This kit is designed to assist the teacher of TMR pupils in planning lessons involving speech and/or language development activities. It contains a speech workbook with suggested lesson plans to serve as a beginning point for the teacher, an auditory training series workbook with sample lesson plans, general information regarding auditory training and worksheets, four recorded tapes for use in auditory discrimination training, and 509 large colored photographs (stimulation pictures). The parts are enclosed within a plastic carrying case. A tape recorder is required for the auditory training portion. Unfortunately, this kit, which was produced as part of a project, is no longer available.

NAME	Monterey Language Program (Programmed Conditioning for Language)
AUTHOR	Burl B. Gray Bruce P. Ryan
PUBLISHER	Monterey Learning Systems 900 Welch Road Palo Alto, California 94304

TARGET	All
LEVEL	Borderline–profound
TYPE	Operant; remedial
MODEL	Behavioral
EMPHASIS	Receptive (1), expressive (1)
BASELINES	Yes
STRUCTURE	High; 40 lessons with approximately 25 steps each in coded script format
USERS	Professionals, classroom teachers, aides (100%); all users must take training, pass performance and written tests, and be certified by the distributor
SETTING	Individual, group, classroom
APPROXIMATE COST	$150.00; may not be purchased "off the shelf" unless user is certified

COMMENTS

The program consists of 40 individualized language training units. Each unit has a screening test, a pretest, a posttest, a criterion test and an automatic branching feature which gives alternatives for each step to be used if the student experiences difficulties. To qualify for using this program, one must be trained by a certified trainer, pass both performance and written tests, and be certified by the distributor. Monterey Learning Systems maintains a directory of all certified users and trainers. Currently there are approximately 1500 certified users.

No other program provides more data concerning program effectiveness than the Monterey program. This is particularly true in areas of transfer to nontherapy settings and maintenance of changes over time. The goals, steps, criteria, etc., are unambiguously stated. A program that is this highly structured does not give the user much opportunity to wax creative but it does result in known changes in language skills. Within its extremely structured format, however, it offers the maximal opportunity for individualization or prescriptive programming because of the pre- and posttests, well stated criteria, placement tests, branching provisions, etc. With the present focus on accountability and learner verification, the Monterey program is receiving increasing attention.

NAME	Motivation and Learning Centered Training Programs for Language Delayed Children (Mecham Program)
AUTHOR	Merlin J. Mecham
PUBLISHER	Word Making Productions P.O. Box 1858 Salt Lake City, Utah 84110

TARGET	All with language delay or language below their age level
LEVEL	Severe; TMR; preschool; IQ range 30–60
TYPE	Operant; remedial
MODEL	Behavioral, cognitive, developmental
EMPHASIS	Expressive (1), motor imitation (2), receptive (3), nonverbal communication—gestures (3)
BASELINES	Yes
STRUCTURE	High; 30 lessons in script format
USERS	Professionals, classroom teachers, parents, aides (100%)
SETTING	Individual, home
APPROXIMATE COST	$14.00

COMMENTS

This program was designed to develop a minilanguage, a readiness program for children without "sufficient language to benefit from such programs as Distar." It covers 15 units of language instruction: gesture language (three units; language and nonlanguage gestures); basic verbal language (six units; name and action words, two- to five-word sentences); transformations (five units; verb inflections; modification; adjectival; adverbal; negative; passive). The kit contains a manual, a picture packet of 47 black and white cartoon drawings, and books of 25 recording worksheets (tasks × trial).

NAME	MWM Program for Developing Language Abilities
AUTHOR	Esther H. Minskoff Douglas E. Wiseman J. Gerald Minskoff
PUBLISHER	Educational Performance Associates 563 Westview Avenue Ridgefield, New Jersey 07657

TARGET	LD; all with language problem
LEVEL	Borderline–moderate; EMR-TMR; grade range: primary and intermediate level MR
TYPE	Not operant; remedial
MODEL	Cognitive (ITPA)
EMPHASIS	Receptive (1), expressive (1), organizing processes (1)
BASELINES	Yes
STRUCTURE	High; script format, number of lessons depends on child and task
USERS	Professionals, classroom teachers, aides (75%)
SETTING	Individual, group, classroom
APPROXIMATE COST	$195.00—Level I, full kit with materials $150.00—All materials, but only single copies of workbooks $ 50.00—Specimen kit with all teaching manuals but no teaching materials Level II is available to selected users at cost in experimental form

COMMENTS

Based on the model of the ITPA and designed for use in a variety of settings, MWM is designed for use with or without an ITPA diagnosis. Its primary purpose is to remedy learning disabilities in each of 12 areas of language; its secondary purpose is for developmental teaching of language to children age 3 to 7 who are not learning disabled.

The kit has many parts. There is an Inventory of Language Abilities, a screening device for use by classroom teacher ("NOT a test"). There are six teaching manuals which include the developmentally arranged activities to be used with children that have learning disabilities. Each teaching manual is divided into subareas, which are not arranged in a hierarchial order. For each activity there is a list of prerequisites and related activities. Materials are identified according to whether they are included in the MWM kit or must be obtained from other sources (actual objects are not part of the MWM). A detailed description of each teaching activity is given along with specific directions for the teacher to use when a child cannot cope with a given activity. The kit includes five each of five workbooks: Reception (auditory reception and visual reception), Association (visual association), Expression (verbal and manual), Memory (visual), and Closure (grammatic and visual). A 33⅓ rpm record is provided to teach sound blending; it can be used by the children or to instruct the teacher. Other materials are 150 picture cards (nouns, verbs, descriptive words); six portraits, 20 sorting cards and 15 large stimulus scenes for use in a variety of teaching activities. A word book is included that contains a basic vocabulary of 1018 words that are appropriate for children, divided according to function (nouns, verbs, descriptive words, prepositions) and age level (3 to 4 LA or 5 to 6 LA). Instructions for teaching each word are given, along with a notation of specific kit materials that are to be used. There is a book of 37 stories to be used for auditory reception, verbal expression, and auditory association activities. Teaching scripts are in the teaching manuals. Careful study of the teacher's guide is necessary before beginning to use the program. The manual states that the program was field tested to determine "if teachers could understand and use teaching activities with their students" and cautions that careful study of the teacher's guide is necessary before beginning to use the program.

NAME	Natural Language Learning—English
AUTHOR	Harris Winitz James Reeds Paul Garcia
PUBLISHER	General Linguistics Corp. P.O. Box 7172 Kansas City, Missouri 64113

TARGET	All
LEVEL	Borderline–severe; IQ range: all; grade range: all
TYPE	Not operant but behavioral; stimulation, remedial
MODEL	Cognitive, developmental
EMPHASIS	Receptive (1)
BASELINES	Yes
STRUCTURE	High
USERS	Professionals, classroom teachers, parents, aides (100%)
SETTING	Individual, group, home
APPROXIMATE COST	$13.95—2 hours of cassette tapes and workbook $22.95—4 hours of cassette tapes and workbook

COMMENTS

The kit contains a book of picture frames and either 2 (440 programmed frames) or 4 hours (800 programmed frames) of listening tasks on cassettes. Each frame displays three pictures from which the listener selects the correct picture to correspond to what he has heard. Lessons begin with words and build up to conversation. The program is based upon "experiencing language rather than studying it." Full programs are available in English and Spanish, less extensive programs in Hebrew and German. This program is said to be useful for the language-disabled child and adult as well as for the person desiring to learn a "foreign" language.

NAME	Non-Speech Language Initiation Program (Non-SLIP)
AUTHOR	Joseph Carrier Tim Peak
PUBLISHER	H & H Enterprises, Inc. Box 3342 Lawrence, Kansas 66044

TARGET	Retarded; also deaf, emotionally disturbed, LD, DIS, CP, aphasic adults, (all with language problem)
LEVEL	Severe–profound; IQ range: 0–50
TYPE	Operant; remedial
MODEL	Behavioral, cognitive, functional language, information processing
EMPHASIS	Expressive (1), receptive (3), motor imitation (3), nonverbal communication by plastic words [abstract symbols] (3)
STRUCTURE	High; 188 lessons in script format
USERS	Professionals, teachers, parents, aides (100%)
SETTING	Individual, home
APPROXIMATE COST	$238

COMMENTS

Designed to teach the nonspeaking retarded to generate original seven-word spoken sentences with correct grammar and vocabulary in the training environment. Abstract plastic shapes are used to represent words, and position in sentence is colored coded. There are 188 highly structured lessons with pre-, post-, and probe tests. In addition to the plastic word symbols, record sheets and graphs are included in the kit. The program grew out of Premack's experiences in teaching chimpanzees to communicate through manipulation of similar abstract plastic forms.

NAME	Peabody Early Experiences Kit (PEEK, Peabody Kit)
AUTHOR	Lloyd M. Dunn L. T. Chunn D. C. Crowell Liota M. Dunn L. G. Slevy E. R. Yackel
PUBLISHER	American Guidance Service Circle Pines, Minnesota 55014

TARGET	All with a given level of language development
LEVEL	Borderline, EMR; MA, 2.5–4.5 years
TYPE	Partially operant; stimulation
MODEL	Developmental
EMPHASIS	Receptive (2), expressive (2), motor imitation (2), nonverbal communication (3)
BASELINES	No
STRUCTURE	Highly structured; 250 lessons
USERS	Professionals, classroom teachers, parents, aides
SETTING	Classroom
APPROXIMATE COST	$260.00

COMMENTS

PEEK activities are designed to focus about 50% on cognitive development, 25% on affective development, and 25% on oral language development. The kit contains enough instructional materials to accommodate a group of 12 children. It includes a teacher's guide, two lesson manuals containing 125 lessons each, four hand puppets, a pocket chart and easel, six decks of colored picture cards, flat "beads" in several shapes, sizes, and colors, "shape-pictures" to be used with the beads, eight colored posters, 335 colored photographs, four cassettes (or seven records) containing 27 songs, song cards, sound makers, and many other objects and materials to be used in the program.

NAME	Peabody Language Development Kit—Level P (Peabody Kit; PLDK)
AUTHOR	Lloyd M. Dunn J. O. Smith Katherine B. Horton
PUBLISHER	American Guidance Service Circle Pines, Minnesota 55014

TARGET	All with a given level of language development
LEVEL	Borderline, EMR; MA, 3–5 years
TYPE	Not operant; stimulation
MODEL	Developmental
EMPHASIS	Receptive (2), expressive (2), motor imitation (2), nonverbal communication (3)
BASELINES	No
STRUCTURE	High; 180 lessons in script format
USERS	Professionals, classroom teachers, parents, aides
SETTING	Classroom
APPROXIMATE COST	$186.00

COMMENTS

This program starts with "labeling language" and then includes emphasis on syntactic and grammatic structures of language and on stimulation of logical thinking. The kit contains a manual of 180 lessons, 393 colored stimulus cards, 20 family and home cards, six large colored story posters, 10 records of songs, stories and sounds, 240 colored interlocking plastic chips, three hand puppets, 21 fruit and vegetable models, three manikins, 45 magnetic geometric shapes, 22 magnetic strips, and a variety of other materials needed to carry out the program. Materials are enclosed in two metal cases.

NAME   Peabody Language Development Kit—
                  Level 1 (Peabody Kit; PLDK)

AUTHOR   Lloyd M. Dunn
                  J. O. Smith

PUBLISHER   American Guidance Service
                  Circle Pines, Minnesota 55014

TARGET	All with a given level of language development
LEVEL	Borderline; EMR; MA, 4.5 years
TYPE	Not operant or partially; emphasizes stimulation
MODEL	Developmental
EMPHASIS	Receptive (2), expressive (2), motor imitation (2), nonverbal communication (3)
BASELINES	No
STRUCTURE	Highly structured; 180 lessons in script format
USERS	Professionals, classroom teachers, parents, aides
SETTING	Classroom
APPROXIMATE COST	$70.00

COMMENTS

Level 1 is designed for oral language and intellectual stimulation. It has more auditory and visual stimuli and fewer tactual stimuli than Level P. The kit contains a manual with 100 daily lessons, 130 colored stimulus cards, 10 large colored posters, either a 5-inch magnetic tape or a cassette of stories and folk tales, songs and music, 350 colored plastic chips, and two hand puppets.

NAME	Peabody Language Development Kit—Level 2 (Peabody Kit; PLDK)
AUTHOR	Lloyd M. Dunn J. O. Smith
PUBLISHER	American Guidance Service Circle Pines, Minnesota 55014

TARGET	All with a given level of language development
LEVEL	Borderline; EMR; MA, 4.5–6.5 years
TYPE	Not operant or partially; emphasizes stimulation
MODEL	Developmental
EMPHASIS	Receptive (2), expressive (2), motor imitation (2), nonverbal communication (3)
BASELINES	No
STRUCTURE	High; 180 lessons in script format
USERS	Professionals, classroom teachers, parents, aides
SETTING	Classroom
APPROXIMATE COST	$84.00

COMMENTS

Level 2 puts more emphasis on stimulation of the intellect, with problem solving, brain storming, and other activities sequenced to stimulate divergent thinking. The kit contains a teacher's manual of 180 daily lessons, two character puppets, 404 colored stimulus cards, 560 colored plastic chips, 12 colored posters, either a 5-inch magnetic tape or a cassette, and a "Teletalk" two-way communication system.

NAME	Peabody Language Development Kit—Level 3 (Peabody Kit; PLDK)
AUTHOR	Lloyd M. Dunn J. O. Smith
PUBLISHER	American Guidance Service Circle Pines, Minnesota 55014

TARGET	All with a given level of language development
LEVEL	Borderline; EMR; MA, 7.5–9.5 years
TYPE	Not operant, or partially; emphasizes stimulation
MODEL	Developmental
EMPHASIS	Receptive (2), expressive (2), motor imitation (2), nonverbal communication (3)
BASELINES	No
STRUCTURE	High; 180 lessons in script format
USERS	Professionals, classroom teachers, parents, aides
SETTING	Classroom
APPROXIMATE COST	$63.00

COMMENTS

Level 3 emphasizes idea and concept formulation, manipulation, and creativity. The kit contains a teacher's manual with 180 daily lessons, 214 colored stimulus cards, 18 colored posters, two character puppets, four 7-inch sound recordings and 560 plastic chips in a metal carrying case.

NAME	Peabody Rebus Program (Rebus)
AUTHOR	Richard W. Woodcock Charlotte R. Clark Cornelia Oakes Davies
PUBLISHER	American Guidance Service Circle Pines, Minnesota 55014

TARGET	MR; all with a given type of language problem; deaf, LD, DIS, normal kindergarten
LEVEL	EMR, TMR
TYPE	Operant; stimulation
MODEL	Cognitive, developmental
EMPHASIS	Receptive (1), expressive (1)
BASELINES	No
STRUCTURE	High; 184 frames in script format with additional supplementary lessons
USERS	Professionals, classroom teachers, parents, aides (100%)
SETTING	Individual, group, classroom, home
APPROXIMATE COST	$42.00 for Supplementary Lessons Kit

COMMENTS

Rebus, a programmed approach to beginning reading, uses a vocabulary of pictures to represent words. As the program progresses spelled words are substituted for the rebuses. The Rebus Supplementary Lessons Kit is designed for group work. It contains a manual of 17 lessons, Books One and Two, 13 picture cards, 251 Rebus word cards, 69 large sentence cards, 31 large answer strips, and other materials, all confined in a metal case. A Teacher's Guide, transitional workbooks, Rebus Glossary, 1110 Rebus Glossary Cards, and Rub-On Rebuses are also available. Workbooks are designed to give immediate feedback.

NAME	Portage Guide to Early Education— Experimental Edition (Portage Curriculum Guide)
AUTHOR	David E. Shearer James Billingsley Alma Frohman Jean Hilliard Frances Johnson Marsha Shearer
PUBLISHER	Portage Project Cooperative Educational Service Agency #12 412 E. Slifer Portage, Wisconsin 53901

TARGET	All with MA 0–5 and a language problem; used with children with all kinds and degrees of handicapping conditions
LEVEL	Normal–profound; EMR-SMR; IQ range: full range; grade range: preschool; MA, 0–5
TYPE	Operant; stimulation, remedial
MODEL	Behavioral, developmental
EMPHASIS	Receptive (1), expressive (1), motor imitation (1), nonverbal communication by gesturing and pointing (2)
BASELINES	Yes
STRUCTURE	High (but modifiable); 88 lessons in language section; card format
USERS	Professionals, classroom teachers, parents, aides (100%)
SETTING	Individual, classroom, home
APPROXIMATE COST	$21.00, for 10 checklists and 1 deck of cards— Experimental edition $32.00—Revised edition

COMMENTS

Portage Guide to Early Education is a sequential curriculum and criterion-referenced assessment for multiply handicapped children in the following areas of development: cognitive, self-help, motor, socialization, and language. This program makes use of behavioral checklists giving behaviors in sequential order. Existing behaviors can be identified and emerging skills targeted.

Portage was not intended to be

used as a complete language program. The term *Guide* was very carefully chosen; while the materials presented are highly structured, the counselors have found it necessary to write individualized activities for specific children in a high proportion of cases. The information presented in the guide shows the type of activities and general categories of activities that can be used and provides a model for creating the individualized programs. The Guide provides a beginning structure for users to build on; the goal is to get the user to modify the program to suit the individual child. The 410 behaviors listed on the checklist are printed on individual cards. The newly revised edition of the Portage Guide carries these up through the 6-year level.

NAME	Project MEMPHIS
AUTHOR	Alton D. Quick Thomas Little Ann Campbell
PUBLISHER	Fearon Publishers 6 Davis Drive Belmont, California 94002

TARGET	MR, DIS, multiply handicapped
LEVEL	Borderline–profound
TYPE	Stimulation
MODEL	Developmental
EMPHASIS	Receptive (2), expressive (2), motor imitation (2), nonverbal communication (2) Language and communication skills is one of five areas considered.
BASELINES	Yes
STRUCTURE	Moderate; 260 lessons plans
USERS	Professionals, classroom teachers, parents, aides
SETTING	Individual, group, classroom, home
APPROXIMATE COST	Text —$4.00 ($3.00 for schools) Packets—$1.50 each, 10 for $5.00

COMMENTS

Kit includes a guide to programming and samples of the three components of the program. These components represent the three steps of the system: 1) developmental evaluation (Comprehensive Developmental Scale); 2) individual educational program planning (Developmental Skill Assignment Record); 3) educational evaluation (Continuous Record for Educational Gain). These components are designed to provide teachers with a method of planning, implementing, and evaluating this early childhood education program, which includes language development. The 152-page manual includes information about the Project MEMPHIS study that was used as the basis for developing this program and information about the individual programs for exceptional children and for their parents. Also included are lesson plans, case examples, a bibliography of selected readings, and appendices that list educational equipment, parent assessment references, and child assessment references. Materials for the program are to be selected and provided by the user.

NAME	Santa Cruz Behavioral Characteristics Progression (BCP)
AUTHOR	Laurie Duckham Shoor
PUBLISHER	Vort Corp. 385 Sherman Avenue Palo Alto, California 94306

TARGET	All with a given type of language problem; autistic, aphasic, educationally handicapped, LD, etc.
LEVEL	Borderline–profound; EMR, SMR; IQ range: all; grade range: all
TYPE	Operant; stimulation, remedial
MODEL	Behavioral, developmental
EMPHASIS	Receptive (1) and expressive (1), one strand each; motor imitation (3), nonverbal communication by sign and fingerspelling (3)
BASELINES	Yes
STRUCTURE	Moderate; 50 steps per strand
USERS	Professionals, classroom teachers, parents, aides (up to 75%)
SETTING	Individual, group, classroom, home
APPROXIMATE COST	$3.95—1 set of charts $6.95—booklet

COMMENTS

Language development is only one small part of the entire BCP. The BCP, a criterion-referenced tool, emphasizes definition of behavioral objectives for exceptional children and adults, leading to the construction of "a workable management system."

The BCP chart displays a non-standardized continuum of 2400 observable traits called behavioral characteristics. These have been grouped into categories of behavior referred to as behavioral strands. The use of a chart to display these behavioral characteristics permits perception of behavioral relationships. The BCP chart provides a "gestalt" of the child. BCP does not indicate how to get from one objective to another; it is purposely method free. Selection of methods to be used to obtain learner objectives is left up to the teacher, who may need to consult with support staff.

NAME	Sound/Order/Sense (SOS)
AUTHOR	Eleanor Semel
PUBLISHER	Follett Publishing Co. 1010 W. Washington Blvd. Chicago, Illinois 60607

TARGET	LD and normal 1st and 2nd graders
LEVEL	EMR
TYPE	Not operant; stimulation
MODEL	Developmental
EMPHASIS	Receptive (1), expressive (2)
STRUCTURE	High; entire program in 160 lessons in script format
BASELINES	No
USERS	Professionals, classroom teachers, parents, aides (100%)
SETTING	Individual, classroom, group

APPROXIMATE COST	Level 1/Developmental Program $27.00
	Level 2/Developmental Program $27.00
	Pupil Response Books 1, 2, 3, 4 $ 1.14 each
	Replacement Materials
	    Box of 36 markers $ 7.20
	    Teacher's Guide $ 3.33
	    Records: 5 for Level 1 $ 3.33 each
	    Records: 6 for Level 2 $ 3.33 each
	Sample Set $ 2.10

COMMENTS

SOS is a 2-year auditory perception program designed to develop auditory skills. Level 1 is designed for use in first grade; Level 2 follows Level 1. SOS, which can also be used for older children with perceptual difficulties, is designed to include the sounds that make up speech (SOUND), the sequence of sounds in words and words in groups (ORDER), and the attributes that give meaning to words (SENSE). The kit includes a teacher's guide for each level, two pupil response books for each level, 160 color-coded activity cards for each level, five 7-inch 33⅓ RPM records for Level 1 and six records for Level 2. The response books give immediate feedback through the use of special marking crayons.

NAME	Spacetalk
AUTHOR	Don Kurth Niel Verhoef
PUBLISHER	The Economy Company 1901 North Walnut Oklahoma City, Oklahoma 73125

TARGET	All persons with a given type of language problem
LEVEL	Borderline–mild; EMR; grade range: pre–3rd
TYPE	Operant; stimulation
MODEL	Developmental
EMPHASIS	Receptive (1), motor imitation (2), expressive (3)
BASELINES	*
STRUCTURE	High; 40 lessons on cassettes
USERS	Classroom teachers, parents, aides (75%)
SETTING	Individual, classroom, home, but always on an individual basis
APPROXIMATE COST	$65.00 per kit, without tape recorder

COMMENTS

Spacetalk takes a totally auditory approach to speech and language development. The program is designed to teach phonetic comparisons and provide needed skills for speech improvement and reading readiness. It concentrates on nine of the most frequently misarticulated consonant sounds. One goal is for a child to be able to listen to a three-element phonemic word and identify a given phoneme as being initial, medial, or final. The entire program is built around a series of space explorations and adventures. The authors stress that the program is success oriented.

The kit contains 40 lessons on 20 Spacetapes, 40 reusable response folders, a lesson index, a teacher's handbook, and crayons.

Two editions of Spacetapes are available: the Green Edition, which may be played on any cassette tape player, and the Red Edition, which is used with the Pacer, an audio cassette player with an automatic stop feature for individualized instruction.

NAME	Speech and Language Development for the Mentally Retarded
AUTHOR	Michaela Nelson Carolyn F. Saville
PUBLISHER	ESU #14 Box 414 Sidney, Nebraska 69162

TARGET	MR; all with language problems
LEVEL	TMR; IQ range: 10–70
TYPE	Operant; stimulation
MODEL	Behavioral, developmental, functional language
EMPHASIS	Receptive (2), expressive (2), motor imitation (2), nonverbal communication by gesture (3)
BASELINES	Yes
STRUCTURE	High; 15 packets, each containing 12 lessons in script format
USERS	Classroom teachers, parents, aides (100%)
SETTING	Individual, home
APPROXIMATE COST	Kit 1: Teacher's Guides, packets, recording and graph forms Kit 2: All of Kit 1 plus all materials needed Between $30 and $40, depending on which plan is used. In addition two options are available for in-service training using slide, tape, overhead presentation

COMMENTS

Designed for TMR children, this program was field-tested in five locations in Nebraska. The kit contains 16 curriculum packets (eye contact, motor imitation, visual discrimination, auditory discrimination, imitation of consonant and vowel sounds, nouns, action words, positional words, polar words, phrase chaining, plural words, pronouns, yes/no, auditory memory, visual memory), a packet placement test to be used to determine which packet is appropriate for each student and a teacher's guide which deals with concepts of reinforcement, special techniques to be mastered to use the instructional packets, a teacher's guide to graphing, and recording and self-checking exercises for the teacher. Samples of graphs and recording forms are included in each packet along with a description of the objectives and materials needed for that topic. The indicated materials must be supplied by the user.

NAME	Suggestions for Teaching Language Skills to Use with Language Making Action Cards
AUTHOR	Barbara A. Lippke
PUBLISHER	Word Making Productions 60 West 400 South Street Salt Lake City, Utah 84101

TARGET	All with language problems
LEVEL	Borderline–moderate; EMR, TMR
TYPE	Stimulation
MODEL	Developmental
EMPHASIS	Receptive (1), expressive (1), nonverbal communication by sign (2), motor imitation (3)
BASELINES	No
STRUCTURE	Moderate, program written out in general way only
USERS	Professionals, classroom teachers, parents, aides (100%, after diagnosis and prescription)
SETTING	Individual, group, classroom, home
APPROXIMATE COST	$ 5.00—Booklet only $30.00—Entire kit

COMMENTS

This is not a language program per se but is designed to serve as a resource book describing the use of language materials and presenting activities which can be adapted to use with any language program.

NAME	SYNPRO (The Syntax Programmer)
AUTHOR	Harold A. Peterson Rosemary Brener Linda Lea Williams
PUBLISHER	Mercury Co., Division of E.M.T. Labs 8564 Airport Road St. Louis, Missouri 63100

TARGET	Language-delayed children and aphasic adults; all persons with language problems, LD
LEVEL	Borderline–moderate
TYPE	Operant; remedial
MODEL	Functional language, information processing
EMPHASIS	Receptive (1), expressive (1)
BASELINES	*
STRUCTURE	High; procedure is described in detail and examples of sentences are given
USERS	Professionals, aides (speech pathologist must set lesson plans and complexity order but aides can carry out program after this has been done)
SETTING	Individual, group
APPROXIMATE COST	$100.00

COMMENTS

The basic unit of the language code used by both children and adults is the sentence or phrase. SYNPRO is designed to help retrain aphasic adults and train children who have not acquired language to use such syntactic strings, based on the assumption that practice aids performance. The kit contains a manual, a 30-inch long unit assembly tray, 19 base pieces, 33 insert pieces which fit into the base pieces, picture-symbols and the words they represent, colored cards, and colored tabs. This kit provides the components for producing an almost endless number of sentence types. Although the selection of words and pictures to be used is left to the user, the teaching sequence is outlined. Multiple cues (color, shape, pictorial symbol, printed word), designed to aid correct syntactic sequencing, are reduced one at a time to permit assessment of understanding at each level. Practical restrictive keys prevent incorrect ordering.

NAME	TRY: Experiences for Young Children
AUTHOR	George Manolakes Marie Jepson Scian Robert Weltman Louis Waldo
PUBLISHER	Noble and Noble Publishers, Inc. Dag Hammarskjold Plaza New York, New York 10017

TARGET	All with language problems
LEVEL	All children; normal, MR
TYPE	Operant; stimulation
MODEL	Developmental
EMPHASIS	Expressive (1), receptive (2), motor imitation (2); language stimulation is accompanied by appropriate manipulative experiences
BASELINES	Yes
STRUCTURE	Moderate; about 50% of the program gives in detailed lessons (manipulative tasks are structured, expressive language activities on reverse side of pages are not structured)
USERS	Professionals, classroom teachers, aides (75%)
SETTING	Individual, group, classroom
APPROXIMATE COST	$37.60 list price; $28.20 school price: Individual set/complete $27.60 list price; $20.70 school price: Plastic set/manipulative materials only

COMMENTS

TRY is a reading readiness program designed for children ages 4 to 6. It is divided into three tasks. Task 1 involves matching geometric forms to drawings on a page; Task 2 includes making designs with plastic cubes that match designs on a page; in Task 3 plastic letters are used for matching and to reproduce words, phrases, and sentences. All use matching-to-sample techniques.

Manipulative tasks are structured; expressive language activities on reverse side of each page are not structured.

The kit contains for Task 1 a tray, 24 geometric shapes, an activity book, and a teacher's guide. For Task 2 are a tray, 20 blocks, an activity book, and a teacher's guide. A tray, letter tiles, alphabet cards, activity books, and a teacher's guide are included for Task 3.

NAME	Visually Cued Language Cards (VCLC)
AUTHOR	Rochana Foster June Giddan Joel Stark
PUBLISHER	Consulting Psychologists Press 577 College Avenue Palo Alto, California 93400

TARGET	All with language problems
LEVEL	Borderline–profound; EMR, SMR
TYPE	Not operant; stimulation, remedial
MODEL	Functional language
EMPHASIS	Receptive (1), expressive (1)
BASELINES	No
STRUCTURE	Slight; program written out in a general way only
USERS	Professionals, classroom teachers, parents, aides
SETTING	Individual, home
APPROXIMATE COST	$19.75—Series I with instructions $20.00—(tentative price) Series II with instructions $21.00—(tentative price) Series III with instructions

COMMENTS

Visually Cued Language Cards are pictorial representations for use in teaching basic vocabulary and grammatical forms and constructions. This program can be used for training after testing with the Assessment of Children's Language Comprehension (ACLC), produced by the same authors. Five series of cards eventually will be available. Series 1, for the single-word level, contains 300 cards picturing objects by categories with suggestions for their use. Series 2 contains instructions and approximately 275 cards, to be used with 10 two-element constructions. Series 3 contains instructions and approximately 200 cards illustrating 15 three-element constructions. Series 4 will contain four-element constructions, and Series 5 will be a miscellaneous grouping of cards to use in teaching grammatical rules such as plurals, noun/verb agreement, is/are verbing, etc. The 5″ by 7″ pictures are printed in beige tones.

NAME	Wilson Initial Syntax Program (WISP)
AUTHOR	Mary S. Wilson
PUBLISHER	Educators Publishing Service 74 Moulton Street Cambridge, Massachusetts 02138

TARGET	All with problem primarily with syntax
LEVEL	TMR (especially cultural-familial retardation)
TYPE	Not operant; stimulation
MODEL	Rationalist
EMPHASIS	Receptive (1), expressive (1)
BASELINES	No
STRUCTURE	Moderate; 25 lessons in script format
USERS	Aides (100%)
SETTING	Anywhere, individual, group, classroom, home
APPROXIMATE COST	$42.00

COMMENTS

Theories of Chomsky have contributed to the formulation of this approach to language programming. It is based on the ideas that "certain basic grammatical concepts must be comprehended for the process of language acquisition to occur," and that when receptive language development is used to increase competence, it should result in increased expressive ability if confounding problems are absent. All emphasis is placed on improving receptive syntactic skills; no oral response is required. Improvement in both receptive and expressive syntactic skills has been reported for children who have completed the program. It can be incorporated with vocabulary and sound acquisition programs. The program has been used with children in a number of settings in Vermont.

APPENDIX E / Rules of Talking

CREATING THE CLIMATE FOR COMMUNICATION
Because children must want to communicate before they will learn language, we must provide a maximum of opportunities which encourage children to use language—to listen to and send language messages . . .

Get down on your child's level.
Tune into your child's interests.
Let your child participate. Language is best learned while doing.
Let your face and voice tell your child you're interested.

LISTENING FOR A CHILD'S MESSAGE
Because children must develop confidence in their ability to use language, we must develop our capability to fully understand their messages . . .

Show your child you want to understand.
Listen to your child's tone of voice. Voices reflect feelings.
Watch the face, the body, the hands. They help you understand your child's message.

MAKING YOUR TALK RELEVANT
Because children learn language from hearing language, and because children listen to language that is obvious, meaningful, and interesting to them . . .

Talk about the here and now.
Talk about the obvious—what your child is doing, hearing, seeing, smelling, or tasting.
At times talk for your child.
Put your child's feelings into words.

ENCOURAGING A CHILD TO USE VOICE TO MAKE SOUNDS
Because sounds are the building blocks of speech and language, children must be encouraged to vocalize—to play with, practice, and use the sounds of speech . . .

Reward your child for using his or her voice.
Chant and sing simple rhymes and songs.
Add voiced sounds to accompany the child's repeated movement.

Produced by Language Development Programs, Bill Wilkerson Hearing and Speech Center, Nashville, Tennessee. Copyright 1976 by the Bill Wilkerson Hearing and Speech Center; reprinted by permission. Special acknowldegment is accorded Sue M. Lillie and the teaching staff of the Mama Lere Home. Funded by the Bureau of Education for the Handicapped.

Vary the sounds you make to your child. Make yourself interesting to listen to.

Encourage your child to use voiced sounds to get your attention.

Imitate the sounds your child makes and add new sounds.

HELPING A CHILD UNDERSTAND WORDS

Because children learn words from hearing them hundreds and thousands of times in different ways, and because words comprise the cornerstone of language . . .

Everything has a name. Use the name.

Use short simple sentences. Avoid using single words.

Use natural gestures when you talk.

Tell, then show your child what you want him or her to do.

Use repetition. Say it again and again. Give your child a chance to show he or she understands.

TALKING WHEN A CHILD BEGINS TO USE WORDS

Because the process of children's language learning depends on their hearing adult feedback, correct and expand their words, their phrases, and their sentences . . .

Reward your child when he or she attempts to say a word.

When your child uses a single word, repeat it and put it back into a sentence.

When your child uses incomplete or incorrect language or speech, repeat the message correctly.

Expand your child's vocabulary by adding new words.

Let your child hear new and more difficult sentence forms.

When your child expresses an idea, repeat it and then expand his or her thoughts by adding new information.

APPENDIX F / A Functional or Basic Vocabulary

This appendix delineates the functional vocabulary developed by Kopchick, Rombach, and Smilowitz (1975)[1] for use in a total communication environment at Pennhurst State School and Hospital. Note that some words on the list may not be appropriate for all facilities. For example, in some environments, "pop" or "ward" are likely to be used instead of "soda" and cottage." There are other words on the list such as "New Horizons Building" which are quite meaningful for the clients at Pennhurst, but would have no meaning to clients in any other environment. It is critical that the functional or basic vocabulary lists be individualized to the needs of particular clients and particular environments.

I. Self-help objectives

A. Grooming

1. After shave lotion
2. Bed
3. Blanket
4. Clean
5. Clothes
6. Coat
7. Comb
8. Dentist
9. Deodorant
10. Dirty
11. Glasses
12. Gloves
13. Hat
14. Hearing aid
15. Mirror
16. Mouthwash
17. Pants
18. Razor/shave
19. Sheet
20. Shirt
21. Shoe
22. Shower
23. Sink
24. Soap
25. Sock
26. Sweater
27. Sweep/broom
28. Teeth
29. Toilet
30. Toothbrush
31. Toothpaste
32. Towel
33. Wash
34. Water
35. Underwear

B. Mealtime training

1. Apple
2. Banana
3. Bowl
4. Bread

---

[1]Kopchick, G. A., D. W. Rombach, and R. Smilowitz. 1975. A total communication environment in an institution. Ment. Retard. 13:22–23.

5.	Breakfast	28.	Lettuce
6.	Butter	29.	Lunch
7.	Cake	30.	Meat
8.	Candy	31.	Milk
9.	Chair	32.	Orange
10.	Chicken	33.	Pepper
11.	Coffee	34.	Pie
12.	Cookie	35.	Plate
13.	Cup	36.	Potatoes
14.	Dinner	37.	Pretzel
15.	Drink	38.	Salt
16.	Eat	39.	Sandwich
17.	Egg	40.	Soda
18.	Fish	41.	Soup
19.	Fork	42.	Spaghetti
20.	Glass	43.	Spoon
21.	Grape	44.	Stringbeans
22.	Hamburger	45.	Table
23.	Hot dog	46.	Tea
24.	Ice cream	47.	Tomato
25.	Jello	48.	Turkey
26.	Juice	49.	Vegetable
27.	Knife		

II. Educational objectives

A. Community orientation (people)

1.	Dentist	5.	Policeman
2.	Doctor	6.	Secretary
3.	Names of staff	7.	Teacher
4.	Nurse		

B. Community orientation (places)

1.	Administration Building	6.	New Horizons Building
2.	Cottage	7.	School
3.	Dining Room	8.	Store
4.	Home	9.	Town
5.	Hospital	10.	Workshop

C. Number concepts

1.	Give	3.	Number
2.	1–12	4.	Take

D. Time concepts

1.	Clock	3.	Monday–Sunday
2.	Day	4.	Night

5.	School	9.	Week
6.	Time	10.	Work
7.	Today	11.	Yesterday
8.	Tomorrow		

E. *Money concepts*

1.	Buy	5.	Nickel
2.	Dime	6.	Pay
3.	Dollar	7.	Penny
4.	Money	8.	Quarter

F. *Sex and age differences*

1.	Birthday	5.	Old
2.	Boy	6.	Woman
3.	Girl	7.	Young
4.	Man		

G. *Relationships*

1.	Aunt	6.	Grandmother
2.	Brother	7.	Mother
3.	Father	8.	Sister
4.	Friend	9.	Uncle
5.	Grandfather		

H. *Animals*

1.	Bear	9.	Horse
2.	Bird	10.	Lion
3.	Cat	11.	Monkey
4.	Cow	12.	Pig
5.	Deer	13.	Rabbit
6.	Dog	14.	Snake
7.	Duck	15.	Squirrel
8.	Elephant		

I. *Colors*

1.	Black	5.	Purple
2.	Blue	6.	Red
3.	Brown	7.	White
4.	Green	8.	Yellow

J. *Adjectives*

1.	Good	7.	Fast
2.	Bad	8.	Slow
3.	Clean	9.	Happy
4.	Dirty	10.	Sad
5.	Different	11.	Hot
6.	Same	12.	Cold

K. *Verbs*

1.	Answer	10.	Make
2.	Ask	11.	Play
3.	Come	12.	See
4.	Fight	13.	Sit
5.	Get	14.	Stand
6.	Give	15.	Stop
7.	Go	16.	Understand
8.	Help	17.	Walk
9.	Hurt	18.	Want

L. *Adverbs*

1.	Not	4.	Where
2.	What	5.	Who
3.	When	6.	Why

M. *Prepositions*

1.	Down	5.	Over
2.	In	6.	Out
3.	Off	7.	Under
4.	On	8.	Up

III. Leisure time and recreational objectives

1.	Baseball	6.	Football
2.	Basketball	7.	Movies
3.	Bowling	8.	Music
4.	Boxing	9.	TV
5.	Dance/party	10.	Zoo

APPENDIX G / Audiovisual Information Sources

INFORMATION AGENCIES

1. Bureau of Education for the Handicapped[1]
    Division of Media Services
    B.E.H.
    United States Office of Education
    400 Maryland Avenue, S.W. ROB 2020
    Washington, D.C. 20202

2. Coordinating Office for Regional Resource Centers
    Bradley Hall
    University of Kentucky
    Lexington, Kentucky 40506
    Telephone: (606) 258-4671

3. Specialized Office for the Deaf and Hard of Hearing
    University of Nebraska
    175 Nebraska Hall
    Lincoln, Nebraska 68508
    Telephone: (402) 472-2141

4. Specialized Office for Material Distribution
    Indiana University
    Audio-Visual Center
    Bloomington, Indiana 47401
    Telephone: (812) 337-2853

5. National Center on Educational Media Materials for the
    Handicapped
    Ohio State University
    220 West Twelfth Avenue
    Columbus, Ohio 43210
    Telephone: (614) 422-7596

---

[1]Information and addresses for National and Regional Learning Resource
Centers can be obtained from this address.

INSTRUCTIONAL MATERIALS CENTERS

Location and Address	Region Served
1. Instructional Materials Reference Center American Printing House for the Blind 1839 Frankfort Avenue Louisville, Kentucky 40206	National
2. New England Special Education Instructional Materials Center Boston University 704 Commonwealth Avenue Boston, Massachusetts 02215	Connecticut, Maine, Massachusetts, New Hampshire, Rhode Island, Vermont
3. Instructional Materials Center for Special Education University of Southern California 1031 South Broadway Suite 623 Los Angeles, California 90015	Arizona, California, Nevada
4. Rocky Mountain Special Education Instructional Materials Center University of Northern Colorado Greeley, Colorado 80631	Colorado, Montana, New Mexico, Utah, Wyoming
5. CEC Information Center on Exceptional Children (CECERIC) The Council for Exceptional Children 1920 Association Drive Reston, Virginia 22091	National
6. Instructional Materials Center Office of the Superintendent of Public Instruction 1020 South Spring Street Springfield, Illinois 62706	Illinois
7. Special Education Instructional Materials Center University of Kansas 1115 Louisiana Lawrence, Kansas 66044	Iowa, Kansas, Missouri, Nebraska, North Dakota, South Dakota
8. University of Kentucky Regional Special Education Instructional Materials Center 641 South Limestone Street Lexington, Kentucky 40506	Kentucky, North Carolina, Tennessee, West Virginia

Location and Address	Region Served
9. USOE/MSU Instructional Materials Center for Handicapped Children and Youth 213 Erickson Hall Michigan State University East Lansing, Michigan 48823	Indiana, Michigan, Ohio
10. Special Education Instructional Materials Center New York State Education Department 55 Elk Street Albany, New York 12224	New York State and Central New York Region
11. Northwest Regional Special Education Instructional Materials Center University of Oregon Clinical Services Building Eugene, Oregon 97403	Alaska, Hawaii, Idaho, Oregon, Washington, Guam, Trust Territory of the Pacific Islands, American Samoa
12. Special Education Instructional Materials Center University of Texas 304 West Fifteenth Street Austin, Texas 78701	Arkansas, Oklahoma, Texas
13. Mid-Atlantic Regional Special Education Instructional Materials Center George Washington University Washington, D.C. 20006	Delaware, District of Columbia, Maryland, New Jersey, Pennsylvania, Virginia
14. Special Education Instructional Materials Center University of Wisconsin Waisman Center on Mental Retardation 2605 Marsh Lane Madison, Wisconsin 53706	Minnesota, Wisconsin
15. Southern States Cooperative Learning Resources System Auburn University at Montgomery Montgomery, Alabama 36104	Alabama, Florida, Georgia, Louisiana, Mississippi, South Carolina

REGIONAL MEDIA CENTERS

Midwest Regional Media Center for the Deaf
University of Nebraska
Lincoln, Nebraska 68508

Southern Regional Media Center for the Deaf
College of Education
University of Tennessee
Knoxville, Tennessee 39716

Northeast Regional Media Center for the Deaf
University of Massachusetts
Amherst, Massachusetts 01003

Southwest Regional Media Center for the Deaf
New Mexico State University
P.O. Box 3AW
Las Cruces, New Mexico 88001

OTHER SELECTED SOURCES OF INFORMATION

1. *Learning Directory 1970–71,* 7 volumes, Westinghouse Learning Corporation, New York, New York, $90.

2. John A. Molstad, *Sources of Information on Educational Media,* U.S. Government Printing Office, Superintendent of Documents, Washington, D.C. 20402, 1963, as document OE-34024.

3. *National Audio Tape Catalog,* Association for Educational Communications and Technology, AECT Publication Sales Section, National Education Association, 1201 16th Street, N.W., Washington, D.C. 20036, 1967, $3 (Order No. 071-02836).

4. *First Chance Products.* Media information department, TADS, 625 West Cameron Avenue, Chapel Hill, North Carolina 27514.

    This 156-page catalog includes instructional and evaluative materials developed by 100 preschool demonstration projects known as the First Chance Network. All projects are funded by the Bureau of Education for the Handicapped. The materials available include films, videotapes, 35mm slide presentations, and a diversity of paper and pencil items. A wide variety of areas are covered by the materials including: parent training items, language training related activities, infant activities, lesson plans, behavioral prescription guides to communication, testing and evaluating materials, methods for dealing with specific handicapping conditions, and many more items.

5. Media Services and Captioned Films for Deaf
    Bureau of Education for the Handicapped
    U.S. Office of Education
    Department of Health, Education, and Welfare
    Washington, D.C. 20202

6. *The Audio-Visual Equipment Directory.* National Audio-Visual Association, Inc., 3150 Spring Street, Fairfax, Virginia 22030, Twentieth Edition, 1974–75 ($12.50).

7. Ann Arbor Publishers, Inc.
   P.O. Box 1446
   Ann Arbor, Michigan 48104

   This company has available sequences of books with accompanying audio tapes dealing with the blending of sounds. The sequence is entitled, "Visual Aural Discriminations."

8. Programmed Assistance to Learning (PAL)
   Instructional Industries, Inc.
   Executive Park
   Ballston Lake, New York 12019

   Under contract with General Electric, the PAL system was developed for use with filmstrips prepared by Project LIFE. The Project LIFE materials are basic language and reading programmed instruction materials.

9. John Tracy Clinic
   806 West Adams Boulevard
   Los Angeles, California 90007

   A sequence of films concerned with parent education and teaching speech to the deaf are available from the Tracy Clinic.

10. A guide to media symposium papers. *American Annals of the Deaf,* 1974, 119(5).

    A bibliography that covers publications on media uses with the deaf from 1965 through 1974.

11. Bill Wilkerson Hearing and Speech Center
    1114 19th Avenue South
    Nashville, Tennessee 37212

    The Wilkerson Center has available a variety of films, videotapes, and slide presentations developed out of their language development program. Some of the materials are concerned with the difficulties and techniques used in providing services for the deaf and hard of hearing. Other materials are concerned with the attitudes, feelings, and training of parents of language-delayed children. Still other materials are concerned with speech and language development, rules of talking, and training others in detecting and dealing with the problems of the language-delayed child.

12. Propp, G. Media Methods and Materials for Special Educators. Michigan State Department of Education, Lansing, Michigan, 1972, EDRS microfiche, price 65¢, hardcopy $3.29.

    The paper provides information on how to use multi-media and approaches to enhance learning and how to make films and videotapes.

13. Tarling, M. E. Teacher training bibliography. Los Angeles: USC, Instructional Materials Center for Special Educators, 1972.

   This bibliography contains references for 229 packaged programs. Several of the items referred to deal with communication skills.

14. Thiagarajan, S., M. Semmel, and D. S. Semmel. *Sourcebook on Instructional Development for Training of Exceptional Children.* (Field Test Version). Instructional Programming Association, Bloomington, Indiana.

Author Index

Abbs, J. H., 6, 25, 29
Accreditation Council for Facilities for the Mentally Retarded (AC/FMR), 127, 176, 183, 413, 511, 518, 660, 684
Adams, R. E., 756, 770
Adelson, E., 704, 727
Aguero, A., 798
Ahlström, K. G., 478, 491
Aikins, D. A., 238, 263
Allen, B. J., 657, 665, 666, 668, 684, 686
Allen, K. E., 698, 700, 725
Allen, N., 450, 491
Alpert, H. , 573, 605
Alpiner, J. G., 402, 413, 656, 665, 667, 684
Altshuler, K., 480, 498
American Academy of Ophthalmology and Otolaryngology (AAOO), 129, 183
American Academy of Pediatrics (AAP), 129, 183
American Association on Mental Deficiency (AAMD), 45, 66
American Organization for the Education of the Hearing Impaired, 403, 405, 413
American Speech and Hearing Association (ASHA), 151, 183
American Standards Association (ASA), 48, 66
Ammons, R., 798
Amon, C., 402, 413
Amoss, H., 209, 221
Anastasi, A., 82, 85, 118
Anderson, A. D., 670, 689
Anderson, J., 51, 66
Anderson, R. M., 58, 60, 66, 72, 406, 413

Andreas, J., 516, 518,
ANSI, 48, 66, 127, 128, 143, 165, 170, 171, 183
Anthony, D., 426, 451, 453, 492
Antilla, R., 554, 600
Aran, J. M., 174, 175, 183
Arangio, A. J., 41, 66
Archambault, P., 756, 770
Armas, J. A., 377, 392, 416
Armbruster, V. B., 297, 321
Armstrong, J. R., 739, 769
Arnold, P., 798
Aronson, A. E., 172, 187
Arthur, G., 210, 221
Ascher, R., 526, 546
Aserlind, L., 765, 770
ASHA Committee on Audiometric Evaluation, 141, 184
Atkinson, L., 713, 728
Auerbach, A. B., 707, 715, 725
Ault, M. A., 228, 260
Austin, J. T., 748, 770

Babbidge, H., 297, 320
deBaca, P. D., 272, 293
Bach, E., 96, 100, 118
Baer, A. M., 231, 232, 259
Baer, D. M., 231, 232, 233, 234, 235, 243, 244, 245, 259, 260, 261, 272, 292, 330, 367, 389, 416, 505, 520, 525, 545, 546, 698, 732, 744, 752, 770
Bailey, C-J., 450, 492
Baker, B. L., 676, 684, 695, 702, 707, 709, 709, 712, 714, 715, 718, 719, 725, 726
Baker, C., 438, 492
Baker, E., 543, 546
Baker, R. L., 337, 358, 369, 525, 546

Baldwin, T. F., 741, 745, 770
Baldwin, V. L., 702, 703, 717, 727
Ball, S., 739, 770
Ball, T. S., 267, 273, 292
Baltaxe, C., 487, 498
Balthazar, E. E., 39, 66
Baltzer, S., 378, 413
Bandura, A., 243, 260, 738, 752, 770
Bandura, T., 738, 770
Bannatyne, A. D., 562, 600
Barber, P. S., 178, 189, 409, 419, 508, 520, 671, 687
Barclay, J. R., 482, 493
Barker, P. E., 767, 772
Barnard, K. E., 395, 413
Barnett, C. D., 662, 665, 666, 675, 684, 685
Barnhart, C. L., 559, 600
Barr, B., 51, 66
Barrett, B. B., 235, 260
Barrett, B. H., 669, 684
Bartoshuk, A. D., 174, 184
Bassinger, J. F., 698, 715, 716, 733
Bateman, B., 382, 383, 389, 390, 413
Bath, K. E., 669, 684
Battison, R., 435, 441, 442, 443, 487, 492
Baubergertell, L., 51, 68
Baumeister, A. A., 290, 292
Baxley, N., 245, 247, 262, 288, 294, 759, 773
Beck, H. L., 707, 725
Beck, J., 669, 670, 684
Becker, W., 725
Beckett, J. W., 503, 521, 672, 689
Beckwith, L., 330, 367
Beedle, R. R., 172, 192
Belkin, M., 140, 184
Bell, D., 516, 518
Belland, J., 765, 770
Bellugi, U., 77, 96, 119, 120, 391, 415, 432, 435, 443, 444, 446, 448, 481, 485, 492, 495, 496, 782
Benassi, B., 722, 725
Benassi, V. A., 722, 725

Bench, R. J., 131, 184
Benchmark Films Inc., 725
Bennett, C. W., 719, 726
Bennett, W. S., Jr., 668, 684
Bensberg, G. J., 43, 63, 66, 67, 408, 409, 410, 414, 505, 519, 657, 662, 665, 666, 671, 675, 684, 685
Bensburg, G., 510, 515, 518
Benson, R. W., 156, 157, 187
Bentley, J., 516, 518
Berberich, J. P., 243, 261
Bercovici, A. N., 701, 727
Berg, F. S., 756, 770
Berger, K. W., 182, 298, 299, 321
Berger, S. L., 184, 407, 408, 413, 414, 503, 509, 513, 518, 519
Bergman, M., 140, 184
Berieter, C., 525, 545
Berko, J., 79, 96, 118, 470, 492
Berkowitz, B. P., 697, 726
Berlin, C. I., 166, 175, 184, 197, 222
Bernal, M. E., 700, 711, 719, 726
Berry, M. F., 76, 96, 118
Berry, T., 543, 546
Bialer, I., 247, 260
Biddle, R., 62, 72
Bijou, S. W., 228, 260
Billingsky, J., 704, 732
Bill Wilkerson Hearing and Speech Center, 178, 184
Bilski-Hirsch, R., 51, 68
Birch, J. W., 62, 66, 398, 422, 478, 479, 499
Blanton, R. L., 447, 484, 485, 486, 497
Blatt, J. W., 708, 712, 725, 726, 730
Bliss, C. K., 635, 640, 647
Block, J. R., 574, 600
Bloom, L., 98, 118, 361, 367, 383, 384, 387, 388, 389, 393, 414, 448, 469, 492
Bloomfield, L., 558, 559, 600
Blott, J. P., 98, 120, 383, 385, 388, 389, 395, 418, 698
Blum, E. R., 767, 772

Bobrove, P. H., 681, 688
Boehm, A. E., 112, 118
deBoer, E., 310, 311, 322
Bogatz, G. A., 739, 770
Bogdan, R., 664, 685
Bolinger, D., 526, 545
Bolton, B., 59, 67
Bond, G. L., 564, 573, 600
Bonvillian, J. D., 472, 476, 478, 492
Boone, D. R., 657, 679, 685, 748, 750, 751, 770
Boothroyd, A., 312, 321, 756, 770
Boozer, H., 263, 680, 688
Boozer, R., 256, 263
Bordley, J. E., 55, 67, 68, 174, 191
Borley, M., 182, 187
Bornstein, H. A., 426, 434, 451, 452, 453, 455, 457, 463, 464, 492, 493, 512, 519, 594, 595, 597, 600, 601
Børrild, K., 312, 321, 468, 471, 493
Borton, T., 745, 770
Boscak, N., 131, 184
Bosley, S., 537, 545
Botkin, P. T., 113, 115, 119
Bowerman, M., 361, 367, 388, 414
Bowman, G. W., 668, 685
Boyes, P., 443, 493
Boyes-Braem, P., 9, 29, 443, 448, 449, 493, 496
Bradford, L. J., 174, 184, 191
Bradley, D. P., 380, 383, 417
Bragg, B., 426, 493
Braine, M. D. S., 383, 414
Brannan, A. C., 63, 67, 408, 409, 410, 414, 505, 515, 518, 519, 671, 685
Bransford, J. D., 482, 493, 494
Brasel, K., 451, 475, 476, 493
Bray, D. W., 46, 68
Breiter, D. E., 707, 732
Brenner, L. O., 205, 212, 221
Bricker, D. D., 165, 184, 374, 375, 379, 380, 382, 385, 386, 389, 391, 392, 393, 394, 395, 396, 414, 415, 503, 519, 525, 545, 698, 701, 707, 708, 726, 727

Bricker, W. A., 165, 184, 334, 335, 367, 374, 375, 379, 380, 382, 383, 385, 386, 391, 392, 395, 396, 414, 415, 525, 545, 680, 685, 698, 707, 708, 726
Bridges, A., 173, 185
Brigham, T. A., 245, 246, 262
Brightman, A. J., 676, 679, 684, 685, 695, 702, 707, 708, 709, 712, 714, 715, 718, 725, 726
Brighton, H., 656, 685
Brill, R. G., 198, 222
Brim, O. G., Jr., 707, 726
Brink, J., 412, 416
Briskey, R. J., 297, 310, 321, 323
Brison, D. W., 43, 67
Broadbent, D. E., 5, 29
Broberg, R. F., 675, 685
Broden, M., 680, 686
Broen, P. A., 116, 119
Brookhauser, P. E., 55, 67
Brookner, S. P., 503, 519
Brooks, D., 167, 184
Brown, A., 209, 222, 484, 493
Brown, D. W., 205, 211, 215, 216, 223
Brown, L., 252, 260
Brown, M., 564, 601
Brown, N., 720, 726
Brown, R., 77, 78, 83, 98, 108, 119, 374, 384, 387, 388, 391, 415, 470, 492, 505, 519
Brown, W. P., 412, 422, 503, 521, 610, 635, 636, 639, 647
Brownstein, C. N., 744, 745, 771
Brust, D. J., 716, 727
Bryan, K. S., 238, 263
Buchanan, C. A., 330, 367
Buchanan, C. D., 590, 601
Buchmann, A. V., 669, 686
Buck, G., 516, 518
Buck, J., 215, 222
Budden, S. S., 53, 67
Buell, J., 701, 732
Burkland, M., 738, 770
Burney, P., 171, 187
Burros, O. K., 82, 119
Burrows, N., 515, 519

Bush, W. J., 88, 119
Butler, J. W., 667, 685
Butterfield, E. C., 9, 29, 184, 381, 415, 662, 666, 685
Butterfield, G. A., 174, 184
Byrne, D., 300, 321

Cairns, G. F., 9, 29
Caldwell, B., 726
Calvert, D. R., 163, 190, 312, 321
Cambon, K. G., 53, 67
Campbell, B., 526, 545
Campbell, D. T., 712, 726
Campbell, I. D., 311, 324
Canter, S., 799
Cardwell, V. E., 40, 67
Carhart, R., 145, 184, 313, 324
Carkhuff, R. R., 670, 671, 685
Carrell, J. A., 179, 180, 182, 192
Carrier, J. K., Jr., 7, 12, 13, 29, 277, 285, 286, 287, 288, 292, 293, 519, 525, 527, 528, 529, 530, 533, 536, 537, 538, 540, 543, 545, 546, 547, 597, 601
Carroll, J. B., 14, 29
Carrow, E., 76, 77, 85, 90, 97, 99, 119
Carter, A. Y., 482, 497
Carver, P. W., 312, 324
Casterline, D. C., 434, 441, 455, 499
Casto, G., 763, 770
Chafe, W. L., 98, 119
Chall, J., 486, 493
Charrow, V. R., 426, 434, 450, 472, 473, 476, 478, 490, 492, 493
Cheney, T., 700, 727
Chesser, E. S., 234, 261
Cheney, T., 700, 727
Chinchor, N., 437, 495
Chinsky, J. M., 665, 666, 686
Chomsky, N., 75, 95, 96, 119, 545
Chow, K. L., 269, 292
Christensen, N. J., 179, 184, 191
Christopher, D. A., 512, 519

Christovich, L. A., 359, 368
Church, J., 4, 29
Cinnamond, M. J., 58, 69
Clark, C. R., 584, 585, 586, 589, 591, 601, 605
Clark, M. K., 590, 602
Clifton, R. K., 174, 184
Coatsworth, J. J., 41, 67
Cobb, J. A., 714, 720, 731
Coggins, K., 503, 519
Cohen, B. D., 115, 121
Cohen, H. L., 720, 727
Cohen, S. I., 707, 732
Coleman, R. F., 318, 321
Coles, R. R. A., 310, 322
Colpoys, B. P., 63, 67
Conley, R. W., 45, 60, 67
Conlin, D., 447, 493
Conn, T. F., 515, 520
Connor, L. E., 397, 415
Conrad, R., 446, 481, 482, 494
Cooper, C., 81, 116, 119
Cooper, F. S., 25, 30
Cooper, L., 54, 67
Cooper, L. Z., 54, 67
Copeland, R. H., 379, 381, 421
Coppinger, N., 798
Cornelius, S., 798
Cornett, R. O., 468, 494
Cortazzo, A. D., 677, 685
Costello, J. M., 323, 377, 382, 392, 395, 422
Costello, M. R., 316, 323
Cotter, V. W., 245, 247, 262, 288, 294, 759, 773
Cotton, J. C., 162, 184
Covington, J .R., 574, 604
Covington, V., 438, 439, 494
Cox, B. P., 48, 126, 127, 131, 136, 139, 141, 143, 188, 381, 417, 508, 520, 660, 687
Crabtree, M., 83, 119
Craig, H. B., 669, 686
Craighead, W. E., 346, 368
Cranston, S. S., 713, 727
Creedon, M. P., 394, 415, 503, 519
Cresson, O., Jr., 246, 247, 248, 249, 253, 262, 278, 279, 280,

282, 283, 287, 288, 294, 759, 760, 772
Crickmay, M. C., 410, 415
Cristler, C., 713, 727
Critcher, C., 537, 545
Cromer, R. F., 374, 375, 380, 390, 415, 489, 494
Croneberg, C. A., 434, 441, 455, 499
Crosby, K., 375, 376, 415
Crowder, R. G., 482, 494
Cruickshank, W. M., 267, 293
Crump, B. 171, 187
Cullen, J. K., 175, 184
Curry, E. T., 162, 185
Cypreanson, L., 744, 771
Cytryn, L., 668, 686

Dahle, A. J., 131, 166, 185, 189
Dailey, R. F., 768, 771
Dailey, W. F., 665, 686
Dale, P. S., 78 , 119, 279, 292, 367
Daly, D. A., 166, 185
Damashek, M., 312, 321
Danaher, E. M., 305, 321
Daniel, Z., 179, 190
Danish, J. M., 197, 222
Darley, F. L., 76, 114, 120, 128, 185, 341, 370
Daston, P. G., 707, 732
Davies, C. O., 584, 585, 586, 591, 601, 605
Davis, H., 156, 157, 172, 179, 180, 185, 187, 300, 321, 542, 546
Davis, L. G., 576, 601
Davis, P., 172, 185
Dawson, W. L., 740, 757, 771
Decker, T. N., 137, 163, 166, 192
DeHaven, E. D., 392, 416, 698, 727
Deich, R., 542, 546
Delauney, J., 175, 183
Delk, M. T., 47, 50, 51, 53, 57, 58, 71
Delphin, J., 708, 726
DeMeyer, M., 272, 293
Dempsey, C., 404, 415
Denmark, F. G. W., 162, 185

Dennison, L., 389, 393, 414
Derbyshire, A., 173, 185
Desmedt, J. E., 6, 29
Desmond, M. M., 57, 67
Devine, J. V., 272, 293
De Vries, A. G., 676, 689
Dewey, G., 333, 367
Dickerson, D. R., 54, 72
Dickerson, M. V., 361, 367
Dill, A. C., 166, 184
Dingman, H. F., 662, 663, 689
Dingman, J. R., 44, 67
Diringer, D., 554, 556, 601
Dirks, D. D., 299, 310, 321, 323
Dix, M. R., 162, 185, 260
Dixon, L. S., 238, 239, 260
Dixon, M., 245, 246, 247, 260
Doctor, P. V., 58, 67
Dodds, E., 308, 316, 319, 321, 322
Dodds, W. G., 563, 601, 602
Doerfler, L., 51, 67
Doernberg, N. L., 711, 727
Doke, L., 391, 420
Dolan, Sister M. E., 559, 601
Doll, E. A., 42, 67, 222
Dollard, J., 247, 261
Donahue, M. J., 722, 727
Donnelly, K., 299, 321
Dorland's Illustrated Medical Dictionary, 39, 67
Douglas, V. I., 376, 415
Douglass, V., 763, 770
Downs, M. P., 129, 130, 131, 137, 138, 139, 142, 169, 175, 179, 185, 190, 299, 307, 319, 323, 399, 404, 419
Downing, J. A., 572, 573, 574, 601
Dreyfuss, H., 584, 601
Driscoll, J., 753, 771
Dunn, L. M., 77, 109, 119, 269, 292, 673, 686
Durr, W. K., 577, 601
Dvald, J., 53, 72
Dykstra, R., 564, 573, 600

Eagles, E., 51, 67
van den Eeckhaut, J., 403, 415

Eilers, R. E., 166, 185
Eimas, P. D., 9, 29
Eisenberg, S., 750, 771
Elberling, C., 175, 192
Eldert, E. G., 156, 157, 187
Eliott, L. S., 503, 519
Ellenberger, R., 434, 495
Elliott, A., 673, 687
Elliot, L. L., 297, 321
Ellis, M. S., 175, 184
Elo, O., 55, 71
Elveback, L. R., 36, 68
Emrick, L. L., 77, 119
Eng, D., 503, 519
Engelmann, S., 525, 545
Engmann, D. L., 336, 369
Erber, N. P., 316, 321
Erting, C., 449, 500
Ervin, S. M., 391, 415
Ervin-Tripp, S., 367
Esche, J., 727
Estes, W. K., 269, 270, 292
Etzel, B. C., 238, 239, 260
Evans, M. L., 185
Evans, P., 185, 318, 323
Eveslage, R. A., 669, 686
Ewing, A. W. G., 131, 137, 138,
    139, 162, 185, 186
Ewing, I. R., 131, 137, 138, 139,
    186
Eyberg, S., 722, 727

Fairbanks, G., 179, 187
Faircloth, M. A., 336, 337, 359,
    361, 367
Faircloth, S. R., 336, 337, 359, 367
Falck, V. 155, 190
Falk J. S., 551, 556, 557, 601
Falk, R. F., 668, 684
Fant, G. M., 336, 355, 367, 368
Fant, L. J., Jr., 425, 426, 431, 452,
    453, 463, 494, 512, 519
Farber, B., 719, 727
Farmer, A., 408, 416, 512, 520
Farrell, M. J., 62, 69
Fauguet, M., 750, 771
Fay, T. H., 174, 191

Fein, A., 172, 188
Feinmesser, M., 51, 68, 175, 192
Feldman, R. S., 715, 718, 731
Ferber, H., 712, 727
Ferster, C. B., 39, 68, 233, 260,
    272, 293
Fifield, D., 300, 321
Filipezak, J., 720, 727
Filler, J., 395, 420
Fillmore, C. J., 99, 119
Findlay, R. D., 318, 321
Firestone, I., 525, 546
Fisch, L., 52, 53, 68
Fischer, S., 435, 439, 440, 447,
    492, 494
Fisher, E., 318, 323, 442
Fitch, W. J., 179, 180, 182, 192
Fjellstedt, N., 229, 260
Flavell, J. H., 113, 115, 119
Fleming, J. W., 655, 662, 686
Fletcher, J. D., 426, 493
Fletcher, S., 304, 321, 756, 770
Flint, R. W., 399, 415
Fodor, J., 97, 119
Folsom, A. T., 41, 68
Ford, R. R., 56, 58, 68
Forehand, R., 700, 727
Foshee, J. G., 657, 668, 684
Fotheringham, J. B., 719, 727
Fouts, R., 488, 495
Fox, J. P., 36, 68
Fraiberg, S., 703, 704, 727
Frankenpohl, H., 110, 122
Franks, J. J., 482, 493, 494
Fraser, A., 173, 185
Fraser, C., 77, 119
Fraser, F. C., 54, 72
Fraser, G. R., 53, 68, 197, 198, 222
Fredericks, H. D., 702, 717, 727
Freeman, S. W., 668, 686, 698,
    701, 727
Friedlander, B. F., 747, 771
Friedman, I., 55, 68
Friedman, L., 436, 437, 494
Friedman, M., 247, 253, 258, 260,
    262
Friel, T., 671, 685
Fries, C. C., 560, 601

Frishberg, N., 432, 435, 438, 441, 447, 494, 495
Frisina, R., 478, 480, 497
Fristoe, M., 158, 186, 341, 363, 367, 373, 394, 408, 416, 503, 504, 512, 519
Frohman, A., 704, 721, 732
Fry, C. L., 113, 115, 119
Fry, D. B., 7, 29, 304, 324
Fry, E. B., 564, 573, 601, 602
Fuerst, J. T., 54, 72
Fulton, R. T., 143, 145, 146, 155, 160, 161, 162, 165, 166, 167, 172, 186, 236, 260, 262, 274, 293, 403, 416
Fulwiler, R., 488, 495
Furth, H., 472, 473, 474, 495

Gaeth, J. H., 318, 321
Gagné, R. M., 252, 253, 260
Gaines, J. A., 162, 186
Gallagher, J. J., 39, 68
Garber, H., 379, 380, 416
Garcia, E. E., 392, 416, 525, 546, 698, 727
Gardner, B. T., 277, 293
Gardner, H., 543, 546
Gardner, J. E., 697, 701, 716, 727
Gardner, J. M., 678, 681, 686, 690, 728
Gardner, R. A., 277, 293
Garms, R., 680, 688
Garrett, E. R., 338, 346, 358, 367
Garrett, M., 97, 119
Gartner, A., 656, 665, 666, 667, 686
Gattegno, C., 563, 602
Gazzaniga, M., 287, 293, 543, 547
Gelb, I. J., 551, 554, 555, 579, 602
Gelineau, V. A., 669, 670, 684
Gengel, R. W., 313, 321
Gentile, A., 50, 68
Gerrard, K. R., 697, 701, 727
Gerwitz, J. L., 330, 370
Gibbs, E., 172, 189
Gibbs, F., 172, 189

Gibbs, O., 750, 771
Gibson, D. M., 711, 719, 726
Gibson, E. J., 579, 602
Giddoll, A., 172, 186
Gilbert, E. M., 722, 727
Giles, M. T., 88, 119
Gill, M., 503, 519
Gill, T. V., 594, 604
Gilmore, A. S., 662, 689
Ginott, H. G., 715, 727
Ginsburg, M., 670, 687
Ginzberg, E., 46, 68
Giolas, T. G., 157, 186, 312, 324
Girardeau, F. L., 238, 239, 260
von Glaserfeld, E. C., 594, 604
Glass, A., 287, 293
Gleason, H. A., 557, 579, 581, 602
Gleitman, L. R., 579, 582, 602
Glorig, A., 49, 68, 178, 179, 186, 187
Glovsky, L., 673, 686
Glucksberg, S., 113, 115, 119, 120
Goehl, H., 380, 393, 394, 421, 503, 521
Goetzinger, C. P., 297, 322
Goldberg, A., 750, 770
Goldberg, L., 561, 602
Goldiamond, I., 242, 245, 260
Goldman, R., 158, 186, 341, 363, 367
Goldstein, R., 56, 68, 129, 131, 173, 186, 192
Goodenough, F., 222
Goodhill, V., 48, 56, 68
Goodman, K. S., 558, 562, 602
Goodman, L., 503, 504, 521
Goodwin, M. W., 399, 400, 401, 405, 419
Gordon, K., 388, 389, 395, 418, 698, 712, 730
Gordon, S. B., 705, 712, 733
Gorman, P., 426, 453, 497
Gottsleben, R. H., 62, 72
Gough, B., 438, 439, 440, 441, 494, 495
Grabowski, J. G., 680, 685
Graham, J. T., 383, 416, 490, 495
Graham, L. W., 383, 416, 490, 495

deGrandpre, B., 664, 685
Gray, B., 390, 391, 392, 395, 396,
    416, 525, 546
Gray, W., 579, 602
Graziano, A. M., 697, 726
Grazini, L., 173, 190
Grecco, R., 512, 520
Greco, J. A., 589, 601
Greelis, M., 743, 744, 771
Green, D., 720, 727
Green, D. S., 162, 186
Green, R., 311, 322
Greenbaum, S., 102, 121
Greenberg, B. T., 741, 745, 770
Greenberg, J. S., 750, 771
Greenfeld, J., 693, 727
Griffen, C., 727
Griffing, B. L., 674, 676, 686
Griffing, T. S., 140, 186
Griffith, F. A., 358, 368
Griffiths, H., 346, 368
Groht, M. A., 180, 186
Grosjean, F., 438, 495
Grossman, F. K., 719, 727
Grossman, H. J., 43, 45, 68
Grove, D., 702, 703, 717, 727
Guerney, L., 662, 686
Guess, D., 243, 244, 245, 259,
    260, 389, 416, 505, 520
Guggenheim, P., 58, 68
Guilani, B., 720, 726
Guilford, R., 162, 186
Gullion, M. E., 731
Gustason, G., 426, 452, 453, 459,
    460, 495

Hagen, C., 412, 416
Hahn, H. I., 573, 602
Hall, E. E., 36, 68
Hall, F. A., 561, 602
Hall, J., 162, 184
Hall, R. V., 228, 230, 260, 261,
    680, 686, 713, 727
Hall, S. M., 408, 416, 503, 512,
    514, 516, 520, 521, 673, 686
Hallahan, D. P., 267, 293
Halle, M., 25, 31, 333, 368

Hallpike, C. S., 162, 185
Hamilton, L. B., 426, 434, 452,
    453, 455, 464, 493, 512, 513,
    519, 595, 597, 600, 601
Hanks, R. T., 667, 685
Hanners, B. A., 178, 187, 319, 322,
    404, 416, 508, 520
Hanson, B., 115, 120
Hardy, J. B., 55, 68
Hardy, M. P., 54, 55, 68, 182, 187
Hardy, W. G., 54, 55, 68
Harford, E., 155, 178, 187, 308,
    316, 319, 321, 322
Haring, N. G., 699, 728
Harper, B., 516, 521, 672, 688
Harrington, S., 379, 380, 416
Harris, A. J., 590, 602
Harris, F. R., 261, 698, 700, 725,
    732
Harris, J. M., 666, 686
Harris, K. S., 359, 368
Harris, R. R., 272, 292
Harrison, M., 573, 602
Harris-Vanderheiden, D., 610, 635,
    636, 639, 647
Hart, B., 391, 420
Hartmann, D. P., 713, 728
Hartmann, M., 388, 389, 395, 418,
    698, 712, 730
Hartung, J. R., 382, 392, 416, 698,
    728
Harvey, E., 172, 185
Haskins, H. L. 54, 55, 68, 157, 187
Haspiel, G., 156, 157, 191
Hasse, K., 50, 68
Hatten, J. T., 77, 119
Haug, O., 162, 186
Haviland, R. T., 380, 381, 416,
    511, 520, 666, 686
Hawk, S. S., 349, 370
Hawkins, N., 722, 731
Hayden, A. H., 699, 728
Hayes, R. B., 573, 602
Haynes, S., 664, 685
Heber, R. G., 45, 68, 379, 380,
    416, 542, 546
Hedgecock, L. D., 140, 179, 180,
    182, 186, 192

Hegrenes, J. R., 377, 380, 391, 392, 416, 418, 750, 772
Heifetz, L. J., 676, 684, 695, 707, 709, 712, 714, 715, 718, 725
Hemenway, W. G., 129, 185
Hendricks, A. F., 720, 731
Henniges, M. P., 311, 324
Herrmann, R., 798
Hicks, D. J., 738, 771
Higgins, E. T., 113, 115, 119
Higgins, W. P., 37, 38, 40, 41, 45, 59, 71
High, W., 179, 187
Hill, F. G., 563, 602
Hilliard, J., 704, 732
Hillis, J. W., 162, 190
Hills, W. G., 661, 689
Hind, J. E., 172, 187
Hinds, L. R., 563, 602
Hine, W. D., 297, 322
Hirsch, I. S., 707, 722, 728, 732
Hirsh, I. J., 156, 157, 187, 312, 715
Hiskey, M. S., 206, 209, 222
Hobart, G., 172, 185
Hockett, C. F., 428, 495, 526, 546
Hodges, P., 542, 546
Hodgins, A., 401, 417
Hodgson, W. R., 55, 68
Hodinott, B. A., 719, 727
Hoemann, H. W., 433, 495
Hoffman, C., 379, 380, 416
Hoffman, H. S., 359, 368
Hoffman, S., 696, 730
Hoffmeister, R. J., 408, 416, 434, 495, 512, 520
Hofmeister, A., 768, 771
Hogan, D. D., 61, 63, 68, 172, 174, 187
Hollis, J. H., 241, 261, 269, 271, 272, 277, 285, 286, 293
Holmes, D., 670, 689
Holmes, J., 798
Holvoet, J. F., 750, 771
Hom, G. L., 236, 262
Homme, L. E., 272, 293
Hoock, W. C., 84, 85, 122
Hoover, L., 697, 728
Hopkins, B. R., 740, 771

Hopkins, K. D., 740, 771
Horner, R. D., 252, 253, 254, 261
Horowitz, F. D., 698, 728
Horowitz, S. L., 54, 72
Horton, K. B., 7, 30, 379, 380, 401, 402, 416, 673, 674, 686, 705, 706, 729
Ho Sang, D. A., 670, 689
House, B. J., 375, 422, 674, 690
Huey, E. B., 583, 602
Huffman, J. M., 674, 676, 686
Hughes, J., 594, 602
Huizing, J., 49, 68
Hunt, M. F., 311, 324
Hursh, D. E., 698, 729
Huston, K., 336, 369
Huth, R., 798
Hutton, C. L., Jr., 316, 322

Illingworth, R. S., 40, 68, 201, 222
Imaoka, N., 503, 520
Ingalls, T. H., 54, 68
Ingram, D., 17, 30
Inhelder, B., 7, 31, 375
International Phonetic Association, 602
Ipsen, J., 35, 36, 70
Irwin, J. V., 76, 77, 120, 172, 187, 338, 358, 368, 370
Ishisawa, H., 162, 187
ISO, 69
Itakura, S., 172, 193
Itard, J. M. G., 267, 273, 293

Jacobs, A. M., 676, 686
Jacobziner, H., 140, 184
Jakobovits, L. A., 390, 417
Jakobson, R. C., 333, 336, 368
Jarvis, P. E., 113, 115, 119
Jeffers, J., 182, 187
Jeffrey, D. B., 396, 417
Jeffrey, W. D., 562, 604
Jelinek, J. A., 702, 729
Jenne, W., 719, 727
Jensema, C., 406, 417
Jerger, J. F., 145, 155, 167, 169, 171, 184, 187

Jerger, S., 167, 187
Jesperson, O., 106, 120
Jew, W., 703, 729
Jex, J., 799
John Tracy Clinic, 402, 417, 771
Johnson, C. A., 697, 729
Johnson, D. J., 179, 190
Johnson, F., 704, 732
Johnson, M., 799
Johnson, P. W., 62, 69
Johnson, S. M., 711, 722, 727, 729
Johnson, W., 76, 114, 120
Johnston, M. K., 698, 732
Johnston, R., 142, 187
Jones, B., 573, 601
Jones, J., 763, 770, 799
Jones, J. K., 563, 603
Jones, M. L., 9, 31, 448, 449, 466, 499
Joseph, R., 729
Jusczyk, P., 9, 29

Kahn, J. V., 488, 489, 495
Kallmann, F., 480, 498
Kannapell, B. M., 426, 452, 453, 455, 464, 493, 513, 519, 595, 597, 600
Kant, T., 761, 762, 771
Kantor, D., 669, 670, 684
Kaplan, E., 16, 30
Kaplan, G., 16, 30
Kaplan, H. F., 188
Kaplan, J., 256, 261
Karlan, G. R., 161, 150, 251, 252, 263
Karnes, M. B., 401, 417
Kates, B., 610, 614, 635, 639, 640, 647
Kates, S., 483, 484, 495
Katkin, S., 670, 687
Katz, J., 142, 155, 188, 299, 322
Katz, R. C., 697, 729
Keane, V. E., 60, 69
Keaster, M. J., 162, 188
Kegl, J. A., 437, 495
Keith, R., 167, 188
Keller, F. S., 233, 261

Kelley, S. M., 712, 727
Kellogg, W. N., 526, 546
Kelly, V. C., 58, 69
Kendler, T. S., 245, 247, 261
Kennedy, W. A., 46, 69
Kennedy, W. P., 52, 69
Kent, L. R., 377, 382, 391, 417, 503, 504, 512, 520, 525, 546
Kerr, A. G., 58, 69
Kessler, M. E., 311, 316, 317, 322, 324
Kinde, S. W., 172, 192
Kirk, S. A., 46, 69, 76, 86, 88, 99, 110, 120, 278, 279, 293, 799
Kirk, W. D., 76, 99, 110, 120, 278, 279, 293
Klaber, M. M., 665, 687
Kladde, A. G., 412, 417
Klebanoff, H., 729
Klee, D., 516, 518
Kleffner, F. R., 297, 322
Klijn, J. A., 312, 322
Klima, E. S., 96, 120, 444, 448, 492, 495
Klingberg, M. A., 54, 69
Klopf, G. J., 668, 685
Knox, E. C., 164, 188
Knox, L. L., 705, 729
Kodman, F., 172, 188
Kodman, R., 62, 69
Koegel, R., 39, 70
Koenigsknecht, R., 799
Koh, S. D., 478, 480, 499
Kolers, P. A., 562, 603
Konigswork, B. W., 52, 69, 197, 222
Kopchick, G. A., 503, 505, 512, 516, 520, 659, 687, 863
Koran, M. J., 750, 771
Kozhevnikov, V. A., 359, 368
Kozloff, M., 707, 712, 729
Kratochvil, D., 671, 685
Krauss, R. M., 113, 115, 119, 120
Kroeber, A. L., 430, 495
Krugman, S. C., 54, 67
Krzywicki, D. F., 62, 72
Kuczaj, S. A., II, 77, 120
Kugel, R., 693, 729

Kuntz, J. B., 286, 287, 288, 293, 544, 546, 591, 603
Kurtzrock, G. H., 162, 185
Kuyper, P., 310, 311, 322

LaBerge, D., 482, 495
LaBert, G., 174, 183
Labov, W., 91, 120
Lackner, J. R., 383, 417
LaCroix, Z., 529, 537, 545, 546
Lacy, R., 435, 436, 437, 441, 449, 495, 496
Lamb, L. E., 167, 186, 188, 191
Lance, W. D., 764, 771
Landes, B., 157, 189
Lane, A., 574, 603
Lane, H., 438, 443, 495, 496
Lane, H. S., 206, 222
Langacker, R. W., 554, 603
Lange, R. R., 739, 766, 771
Langford, G. G., 298, 309, 322
LaPlace, V., 59, 71
Larkey, A. I., 744, 745, 771
Larsen, J. K., 676, 686
Larson, W., 798
Lashinger, D. R., 559, 605
Latham, G. I., 709, 729
Laviquer, H., 719, 729
Lee, L. L., 77, 79, 90, 99, 100, 101, 120, 783, 799
Leech, G., 102, 121
Leenhouts, M., 60, 70
Lefever, D. W., 740, 771
Lehtinen, L. E., 376, 421
Leibowitz, J. N., 707, 732
Lennan, R. K., 407, 410, 417, 679, 687
Lenneberg, E., 6, 7, 30, 379, 383, 417, 476, 477, 488, 496, 546
Lennox, W., 42, 70
Lenoir, J., 175, 184
Leonard, L. B., 80, 86, 120
Lerman, J. W., 158, 179, 191, 301, 316, 324
Lerner, J. W., 293
Levin, H., 561, 579, 602, 603
Levine, E. S., 206, 217

Levine, H., 51, 67
Levitan, M., 197, 222
Levitt, H., 355, 368
Lewis, D., 310, 322
Liberman, A. M., 9, 25, 30, 359, 368
Lieberman, A. T., 174, 191
Lillie, D., 706, 729
Lilly, D. J., 167, 188
Lillywhite, H. S., 380, 383, 417
Lindsay, J. R., 53, 58, 70
Lindsley, O. R., 228, 233, 261, 269, 270, 271, 272, 274, 293
Ling, D., 304, 312, 322
Lingoes, J. C., 256, 261
Lipscomb, D. M., 52, 70
Lister, J. L., 670, 689
Lloyd, L. L., 7, 30, 31, 47, 48, 60, 61, 63, 64, 70, 126, 127, 129, 131, 136, 137, 139, 141, 143, 144, 145, 146, 147, 155, 156, 157, 159, 160, 161, 162, 163, 164, 165, 166, 178, 186, 188, 189, 192, 236, 261, 262, 274, 293, 319, 322, 378, 381, 400, 403, 406, 409, 410, 416, 417, 418, 503, 504, 505, 508, 515, 519, 520, 521, 660, 671, 675, 687
Lobitz, G. K., 711, 729
Locke, B. J., 236, 262
Locke, J. L., 446, 482, 483, 496
Locke, V. L., 446, 483, 496
Lombardi, T. P., 744, 772
Long, J. S., 447, 496
Long, L., 338, 345, 347, 358, 368
Longhurst, T. M., 81, 115, 120
Loomis, A., 172, 185
Lounsbury, A., 318, 321
Lousteau, R. J., 175, 184
Lovass, O. I., 39, 70, 243, 261, 729
Lovibond, S. H., 712, 730
Lowell, E., 379, 417
Lucker, W. G., 376, 418
Ludtke, R. H., 673, 687
Luster, M. J., 614, 647, 762, 772
Luterman, D. M., 311, 322
Lybarger, S. F., 298, 299, 309, 319, 322

Lydon, W. T., 378, 418
Lynch, L., 383, 399, 418
Lynes, G., 640, 647

McAlonie, M. L., 591, 605
McBride, J., 744, 771
McCall, E., 434, 496
McCarthy, J. J., 76, 86, 88, 99,
    110, 111, 120, 278, 293
McChord, W., 318, 323
McClintick, O. F., 577, 603
McConnell, F., 7, 30, 379, 418,
    705, 706, 729, 730
McCormack, J. E., 669, 684
McCoy, D. F., 178, 189, 319, 322,
    409, 418, 508, 671, 687
McCracken, G., 561, 603
McCroskey, R. L., 403, 418, 703,
    730
McCulloch, B. F., 140, 189
McDermott, M., 173, 185
McDonald, E. T., 354, 368, 411,
    412, 418, 610, 614, 639, 647
McDonald, F. J., 750, 771
McDonald, P. L., 767, 772
McGhee, J. P., 671, 688
McGinnis, M. A., 525, 546
McGovern, F. J., 51, 72
McGraw, M. L., 378, 418
McInnis, T. L., 678, 688
McIntire, M. L., 9, 30, 448, 449,
    496
McIntyre, C. K., 447, 484, 485,
    486, 497
McLean, J. E., 338, 343, 345, 346,
    347, 356, 358, 362, 368, 369,
    505, 520, 525, 542, 546
McLean, L., 542, 546
McNaughton, S., 610, 614, 635,
    639, 640, 647
McNeal, S., 722, 731
McNeill, D., 384, 418
McNeill, N. B., 384, 385, 418
McRandle, C. C., 56, 68
McReynolds, L. V., 330, 336, 369
Mabel, S., 116, 121

MacDonald, J., 75, 98, 120, 383,
    385, 388, 389, 395, 418, 698,
    712, 730
Machover, K., 214, 222
Macht, J., 274, 293
MacKeith, N. W., 310, 322
MacKenzie, P., 412, 422, 503, 521,
    610, 635, 636, 639, 647
MacLean, C. D., 53, 67
MacLeish, A., 557, 603
MacMahon, B., 35, 36, 70
MacNeilage, P. F., 359, 368
MacPherson, J. R., 162, 179, 189,
    192
Magrab, P., 142, 187
Maison, E. P., 542, 546
Makita, K., 579, 603
Malone, J. R., 576, 577, 603
Maloney, D. M., 678, 687
Mamula, R. A., 662, 687
Manahan, N., 798
Maratsos, M. D., 77, 120
Marcus, R., 172, 189
Marion County Association for
    Retarded Children, 674, 687
Mariotto, M. J., 678, 688
Markides, A., 301, 322
Markowicz, H., 441, 442, 449, 450,
    487, 492, 496, 500
Marshall, N. R., 377, 380, 391,
    392, 416, 418, 750, 772
Martin, E. S., 179, 190
Martin, J. G., 17, 30
Martin, M. C., 300, 322
Mashikian, H. S., 659, 661, 675,
    687
Mason, M. K., 753, 772
Mast, R., 173, 190
Mathews, M. M., 570, 603
Matkin, N. D., 297, 312, 318, 324
Matthews, J., 59, 62, 66, 70
Mattick, P., 407, 422, 674, 689
Mattingly, I. G., 9, 25, 30
Mattson, C. T., 739, 766, 771
Mauldin, L., 167, 171, 187
Mayberry, R., 488, 496
Mayville, W. J., 697, 733

Mazurkiewicz, A. J., 572, 573, 603, 605
Meadow, K., 9, 31, 398, 421, 426, 478, 480, 481, 489, 496, 498
Mecham, M., 799
Medcalf, R. L., 577, 603
Medina, T., 426, 497
Mees, H., 39, 72, 697, 733
Melnick, W., 48, 51, 67, 70
Melrose, J., 156, 189
Mencher, G. T., 140, 189
Mengel, M. C., 197
Menlove, F. L., 738, 770
Menyuk, P., 336, 369, 485, 490, 498
Mercer, J. R., 47, 70
Merklein, R. A., 297, 323
Messier, L. P., 566, 603
Metz, J. R., 243, 261, 330, 369
Metz, O., 166, 189
Metzger, R., 680, 688
Meyer, V., 234, 261
Meyers, W. J., 174, 184
Meyerson, L., 164, 189
Michael, J. L., 164, 189
Milisen, R., 59, 70, 333, 337, 341, 356, 362, 369
Miller, A. L., 564, 565, 566, 603, 604
Miller, E. E., 565, 566, 603, 604
Miller, G. A., 334, 335, 369
Miller, J., 329, 380, 383, 386, 387, 391, 393, 418, 422, 505, 525, 546
Miller, M. H., 162, 189, 192
Miller, N. E., 247, 261
Miller, W. H., 726
Millichap, J. G., 42, 70
Miltenberger, G. E., 178, 189, 409, 419, 508, 520, 671, 687
Mindel, E., 197, 199, 222
Mira, M., 696, 697, 730
Miron, M. S., 390, 417
Mitra, S. B., 63, 71, 406, 419, 659, 673, 687
Mittlefehldt, V. A., 679, 688
Mixon, A., 172, 188
Moffat, S., 697, 733

Moncur, J. P., 740, 772
Mondy, L. W., 665, 689
Montanelli, D. S., 472, 473, 475, 498, 499
Montessori, M., 275, 293, 376, 419
Moore, E. G., 60, 61
Moore, E. J., 178, 189, 409, 419, 508, 520, 671, 687
Moore, J. M., 76, 77, 120, 137, 162, 163, 166, 185, 189, 192
Moore, J. P., 318, 324
Moore, L., 749, 772
Moore, W., 703, 727
Moores, D. F., 18, 30, 399, 400, 401, 405, 419, 426, 434, 441, 451, 465, 466, 468, 469, 476, 478, 479, 495, 496, 589, 591, 594, 601, 604, 672, 687
Morehead, A., 383, 419
Morehead, D. M., 383, 419
Morgan, D. E., 299, 323
Morgan, D. G., 680, 685
Morkovin, B. V., 398, 419
Morreau, L. E., 709, 730
Morris, N., 680, 688
Morris, R. J., 730
Morse, P. A., 9, 30
Mossel, M., 456, 497
Motto, J., 405, 419
Mowrer, D. E., 337, 345, 358, 369, 525, 546
Mulholland, A., 222
Muma, J. M., 76, 80, 86, 91, 121
Murphy, D. M., 676, 684, 695, 709, 712, 725
Murphy, K. P., 131, 136, 189
Murphy, N. O., 503, 519
Muth, T. A., 741, 745, 770
Myatt, B. D., 157, 190
Myklebust, H. R., 125, 190, 206, 222, 297, 323, 472, 497
Mysak, E. D., 410, 419

Nabelek, A. K., 310, 314, 323
Nagata, M., 172, 193
Naiman, D. W., 407, 419, 659, 661, 675, 687

Nakamura, F., 162, 191
Nardine, F. E., 750, 772
Nash, K. B., 679, 688
National Society for the Study of
    Education, 51, 71
Nay, W. R., 715, 716, 730
Neeley, K. K., 316, 323
Neff, W. D., 6, 30
Neisworth, J. T., 277, 293
Nelson, K. E., 329, 369, 472, 476,
    478, 492
Newby, H. A., 154, 156, 190
Newman, N., 662, 687
New York State Department of
    Mental Hygiene, 46, 71
Neyhus, A., 222
Nicely, P. E., 334, 335, 369
Nicholas, J. L., 658, 674, 690
Nichols, D. G., 676, 686
Nichols, N. J., 559, 605
Nickols, M., 75, 98, 120
Niemann, S. L., 397, 419
NINDS, 130, 189
Nirje, B., 503, 519, 693, 730
Nishikawa, H., 172, 193
Nober, L. W., 675, 688
Nodar, R., 173, 190
Nold, J. T., 577, 604
Norman, D., 436, 482, 497
Norris, T., 167, 188
Northcott, W., 379, 402, 419, 699,
    730
Northern, J. L., 131, 137, 139, 142,
    169, 175, 190, 299, 307, 318,
    319, 323, 399, 404, 419
Norwood, M., 767, 772
Nowels, M. M., 160, 190
Nudler, S., 671, 688
Nye, P. W., 355, 368

O'Connor, R. D., 738, 772
O'Connor, N., 584, 604
Odom, P. B., 447, 484, 486, 497
O'Donnell, M., 583, 604
Office of Demographic Studies, 47,
    60, 71
Ogden, J. A., 656, 665, 667, 684
Ogiba, Y., 163, 192

Ojala, P., 55, 71
Olsen, W. O., 312, 313, 318, 323,
    324
Olson, J. L., 110, 111, 121
O'Neill, J. J., 162, 180, 190, 316,
    323, 743, 751, 772
Ontario Crippled Children's Centre
    Bliss Project Team, 412, 419,
    592, 604, 640, 647
Orkin, K. H., 677, 685
O'Rourke, T. J., 426, 452, 453,
    463, 481, 497, 512, 520
Ortiz, E. R., 410, 420
Osberger, M. J., 305, 321
Osborne, J. G., 669, 688
Osgood, C. E., 76, 97, 121, 245,
    261, 278, 294
Otis, W., 179, 190
Otto, W., 561, 604
Overbeck, D., 664, 688
Owens, M., 516, 520, 672, 688
Owings, N., 799
Oyer, H. J., 162, 180, 190, 316,
    323, 743, 751, 772

Padden, C., 487, 492
Page, H. A., 59, 71
Paget, R., 426, 451, 453, 497
Palmer, U., 677, 688
Palvavi, L., 53, 72
Panyan, M., 680, 686, 688
Paradise, J. L., 54, 72
Paraskevopulos, J., 799
Paris, S. G., 482, 494
Parnicky, J. J., 661, 675, 681, 688
Parsons, H. M., 680, 688
Parsons, M. B., 402, 420
Parsons, S., 527, 547
Pascal, C. E., 698, 730
Pasick, R. S., 719, 720, 730
Patterson, G. R., 712, 714, 720,
    722, 730, 731
Paul, G. L., 678, 688
Paul, J. R., 36, 71
Pavlov, I. P., 233, 261
Peak, T., 7, 12, 29, 519, 528, 530,
    533, 537, 538, 543, 545, 547,
    597, 601

Peebles, J. D., 559, 605
Peine, H., 697, 731
Pelerin, J., 175, 184
Penrose, L. S., 44, 71
Penry, J. K., 41, 67
Perason, D. T., 701, 727
Peress, N. S., 54, 72
Perloff, B. F., 243, 261
Perrott, M. C., 233, 260
Pesses, D. I., 711, 719, 726
Peters, H. N., 279, 284, 294
Peterson, A., 763, 770
Peterson, J. L., 167, 191
Peterson, L., 719, 729
Peterson, R. F., 228, 243, 244, 259, 260, 392, 420, 525, 545, 698, 719, 729, 731
Pfau, G. S., 756, 758, 759, 772,
Pfetzing, D., 426, 452, 453, 459, 460, 495
Phelps, R., 722, 731
Philip, P. P., 62, 69
Phillips, J. W., 179, 180, 182, 192
Phillips, M. E., 316, 324
Piaget, J., 7, 8, 31, 81, 114, 121, 375, 420, 488, 497
Pickett, J. J., 305, 321
Pickett, J. L., 179, 190
Pickett, J. M., 310, 314, 323, 355, 369, 756, 772
Pitman, J., 564, 604
Polisar, I. A., 162, 192
Pollack, D., 180, 190, 397, 403, 420
Pollack, M. A., 299, 323
Pollack, M. C., 177, 190
Pomerleau, O. P., 681, 688
Pommer, D. A., 680, 681, 688
Poole, I., 333, 369
Poole, R. G., 744, 772
Pope, B., 671, 688
Popham, J. W., 683, 688
Poritsky, S., 593, 604
Porter, J., 404, 420
Porter, T. A., 318, 323
Porter, W., 412, 416
Portmann, C., 175, 183
Portnoy, S., 715, 718, 731

Powell, M. L., 395, 413
Power, D. J., 472, 473, 475, 479, 497, 498
Powers, D. J., 60, 65, 71
Powers, T. R., 62, 69
Prehm, H. J., 42, 71
Premack, A. J., 12, 13, 31, 525, 544, 547, 594, 604
Premack, D., 12, 13, 31, 271, 276, 278, 285, 287, 288, 289, 293, 294, 525, 526, 543, 544, 547, 594, 604
Prentice-Hall, 731
Prescott, T. E., 748, 750, 751, 770
Price, L. L., 155, 190
Prickett, H. T., Jr., 426, 497
Prierton, G., 680, 688
Pugh, T. F., 35, 36, 70
Purcell, G., 316, 323

Quigley, S. P., 60, 65, 71, 297, 323, 398, 420, 451, 467, 472, 473, 475, 476, 478, 480, 486, 493, 497, 498, 499
Quirk, R., 102, 121

Raborn, D., 680, 686
Rachiele, L., 798
Rafferty, J. E., 215, 223
Rainer, J., 480, 498
Rampp, D. L., 76, 77, 120, 574, 604
Ramos, G., 761, 762, 771
Randal, P., 54, 72
Randall's Island Performance Series, 210, 222
Rapin, I., 173, 190
Rasmussen, D. E., 561, 602
Ratusnik, D., 799
Ratz, M., 577, 603, 604
Raven, J., 209, 222
Ray, H. W., 768, 772
Ray, R. S., 714, 720, 731
Raymore, S., 338, 345, 346, 347, 356, 358, 362, 368, 369
Redell, R. C., 163, 190

Reese, H. W., 247, 261
Reichler, R. J., 696, 701, 732
Reid, J. B., 720, 731
Reid, M. J., 61, 63, 70, 144, 155,
    164, 165, 166, 186, 189, 236,
    261, 262
Reinen, S., 412, 422, 503, 521, 610,
    635, 636, 639, 647
Reinherz, H., 679, 688
Reneau, J., 173, 190
Reoger, P. A., 726
Resnick, L. B., 256, 261, 263
Rettig, S., 663, 689
Rheingold, H. L., 330, 370
Rich, T. A., 662, 689
Richards, J., 456, 474, 498
Richardson, S. O., 376, 378, 420
Richardson, W. L., 37, 38, 40, 41,
    45, 59, 71
Rickert, E. J., 272, 293
Rieger, N. I., 676, 689
Riekehof, L., 512, 521
Rigg, K. E., 358, 367
Rigrodsky, C., 673, 686
Risley, T. R., 39, 72, 231, 233, 238,
    260, 261, 330, 370, 391, 392,
    420, 697, 698, 731, 733
Rister, A., 405, 420, 662, 665, 677,
    689
Rittmanic, P. A., 62, 71, 408, 420
Roberts, J., 49, 68
Robertson, E. O., 167, 191
Robinett, R. F., 561, 604
Robinson, C., 395, 420
Robinson, G. C., 53, 67
Robinson, G. J., 56, 57, 71
Robinson, H. B., 42, 44, 46, 57, 71
Robinson, N. M., 42, 44, 46, 57, 71
Robinson, R. O., 40, 71
Rodman, L. B., 56, 68
Rohner, T., 574, 576, 604
Rohrer, R., 209, 222
Rombach, D. W., 503, 505, 512,
    516, 520, 659, 687
Ronnei, E. C., 404, 420
Rorschach, H., 214, 222
Rose, S. D., 718, 731
Rosen, A., 207, 222

Rosenau, H., 173, 191
Rosenbaum, R. L., 392, 421
Rosenberg, P. E., 155, 191, 297,
    323
Rosenberg, S., 113, 115, 116, 121
Rosenblatt, D., 140, 184
Rosenthal, J., 670, 687
Ross, H. W., 330, 370
Ross, M., 158, 179, 191, 297, 298,
    301, 302, 306, 309, 311, 312,
    313, 314, 315, 316, 323, 324
Rothenberg, S., 765, 770
Rotter, J. B., 215, 223
Rousey, L., 174, 191
Rowbury, T., 231, 232, 259
Rowe, L., 754, 772
Roy, H. L., 426, 452, 453, 455,
    464, 493, 512, 513, 519, 595,
    597, 600, 601
Rozin, P., 579, 582, 593, 602, 604
Rozycki, D. L., 53, 71
Ruben, R. J., 53, 71, 174, 191
Ruder, K. F., 373, 384, 391, 420
Rudolph, A., 57, 67
Rudolph, M. K., 560, 561, 601, 604
Rules of Talking, 731
Rumbaugh, D. M., 594, 604
Rupert, J., 469, 498
Rupp, R. R., 180, 191
Rush, M. L., 446, 482, 494
Rutherford, G., 244, 260
Ryan, B., 390, 391, 392, 395, 396,
    416, 525, 546

Sachs, J., 482, 498
Sailor, W., 244, 245, 260, 262,
    416, 505, 520
Sajwaj, T., 718, 731
Salzinger, K., 715, 718, 731
Samuels, S. J., 562, 563, 604
Sandel, L., 573, 605
Sanders, C., 681, 690
Sanders, D. A., 14, 20, 25, 27, 31,
    179, 180, 182, 191, 297, 316,
    324, 397, 420
Saslow, J. A. I., 715, 731

Saulnier, K. L., 426, 452, 453, 455, 464, 493, 512, 513, 519, 595, 597, 600, 601
Saunders, J. I., 512, 521
Saunders, R. R., 245, 262
Saxon, S. A., 697, 701, 727
Sayre, J. M., 412, 420
Schaeffer, B., 243, 261
Schaub, M. T., 702, 729
Scheerenberger, R., 660, 689
Scheibel, C., 412, 422, 503, 521, 610, 635, 636, 639, 647
Schein, J. D., 47, 50, 51, 53, 57, 58, 68, 71, 407, 419
Schiefelbusch, R. L., 7, 31, 379, 381, 421, 503, 505, 520, 521
Schlanger, B. B., 62, 72, 172, 179, 184, 191
Schlesinger, H. S., 9, 31, 398, 421, 426, 481, 489, 498
Schlesinger, I. M., 98, 121, 387, 388, 421
Schmidmayr, B., 663, 689
Schmidt, M. J., 527, 547
Schmitt, P., 472, 498
Schneider, J. L., 206, 222
Schneidman, E. S., 215, 223
Schneiman, R. S., 718, 731
Schneyer, J. W., 561, 604
Schoenfeld, W. N., 233, 261
Schopler, E., 696, 701, 732
Schortinghuis, N., 721, 732
Schroeder, G. L., 698, 732
Schulman, C. A., 174, 191
Schultz, A. R., 411, 412, 418, 610, 614, 639, 647
Schumaker, J., 245, 262
Schurman, J., 412, 421
Schutz, R. E., 338, 358, 369, 525, 546
Schwartz, A., 162, 191
Schwartz, D., 392, 421
Schwenn, M. R., 712, 718, 732
Scott, K. G., 245, 262
Scouten, E. L., 465, 498
Segal, P., 167, 187
Seguin, E., 267, 273, 294
Seligman, J., 411, 421

Senzig, K., 739, 769
Shaffer, T. R., 380, 393, 394, 421, 503, 521
Shanks, R., 761, 762, 771
Shankweiler, D. P., 25, 30
Shannon, C. E., 97, 121
Shearer, D. E., 395, 396, 403, 421, 703, 704, 732
Shearer, M. S., 395, 396, 403, 421, 703, 704, 732
Shearn, C., 798
Shedd, J. L., 155, 187
Sheese, J., 719, 729
Sheldon, W. D., 559, 605
Shelhass, M., 737, 772
Shemberg, K. M., 712, 727
Sherman, J. A., 243, 244, 245, 259, 262, 330, 367, 525, 545, 698, 729, 744, 752, 770
Shimiz, H., 54, 55, 68
Shimizu, H., 162, 191
Sholes, G. N., 359, 368
Shotwell, A. M., 662, 663, 689
Sidman, M., 230, 232, 237, 238, 246, 247, 248, 249, 253, 258, 262, 263, 278, 279, 280, 282, 283, 287, 288, 292, 294, 754, 759, 760, 772
Siegel, G. M., 86, 115, 116, 120, 121
Siegel, M., 54, 72
Siegenthaler, B. M., 62, 72, 156, 157, 191
Sigelman, C., 63, 67, 408, 409, 410, 414, 505, 515, 518, 519, 671, 685
Silverman, S. R., 156, 157, 179, 180, 185, 187, 300, 321, 542, 546
Simeonsson, R. J., 698, 732
Simmons, A. A., 379, 421, 674, 689, 705, 732
Simmons, J. Q., 39, 70, 487, 498
Simonton, K. M., 140, 186
Singh, S., 336, 370
Siple, P., 437, 446, 481, 485, 490, 492, 498
Siqueland, E. R., 9, 29

Sitton, A. B., 178, 187, 319, 322, 404, 416, 508, 520, 705, 729
Skalka, E. C., 318, 324
Skelton, M., 719, 727
Skinner, B. F., 81, 113, 121, 228, 233, 262, 272, 293, 391, 421, 755, 773, 799
Slavin, J., 720, 727
Sloan, W., 43, 66
Sloane, H. N., 698, 732
Slobin, D., 77, 121, 361, 370
Smeets, P. M., 747, 773
Smilowitz, R., 503, 505, 512, 516, 520, 659, 687
Smith, A. J., 205, 207, 223
Smith, C. R., 174, 191
Smith, H. L., 561, 605
Smith, J., 173, 190, 673, 686
Smith, J. O., 379, 381, 421
Smith, M., 704, 727
Smith, N. L., 472, 473, 486, 498
Smith, N. V., 104, 121
Smith, R. H., 681, 688
Smith, R. J., 561, 604
Smith, R. M., 277, 293
Smith, S. A., 669, 684
Smith, S. B., 179, 190
Smyth, G. D. L., 58, 69
Snow, R. E., 750, 771
Sohmer, H., 175, 192
Solomon, G., 175, 192
Sotsky, R., 593, 604
Southgate, V., 574, 605
Spache, E. B., 558, 572, 576, 605
Spache, G. D., 558, 572, 576, 605
Spas, D. L., 516, 521
Spicker, H. H., 401, 421
Spiegel, B., 388, 389, 395, 418, 698, 712, 730
Spitz, R., 5, 31
Spradlin, J. E., 59, 72, 76, 83, 90, 113, 116, 121, 144, 161, 164, 165, 166, 189, 236, 238, 239, 245, 247, 256, 260, 261, 262, 278, 284, 288, 294, 738, 759, 773, 792
Spriestersbach, D. C., 54, 72, 76, 114, 120

Staats, A. W., 373, 421
Stack, Sister P. M., 403, 421
Stanley, J. C., 712, 726
Statten, P., 162, 192
Stark, J., 392, 421
Stark, R., 6, 31
Stech, E. L., 750, 770
Stein, M. I., 214, 223
Stein, S., 209, 222
Steinhorst, R., 272, 293
Steinkamp, M. W., 475, 498
Stepp, R. E., 738, 765, 773
Stern, D. N., 330, 370
Stevens, C., 256, 262
Stevens, G. D., 60, 66, 406, 413
Stevens, H. A., 39, 66
Stevens, J., 39, 70
Stevens, K. N., 25, 31
Stevenson, E., 478, 479, 498
Stewart, L., 407, 419
St. John, J., 564, 604
Stinson, F., 559, 605
Stoddard, L. T., 237, 238, 263, 754, 772
Stohr, P. G., 503, 504, 516, 521
Stokes, W. T., 485, 490, 498
Stokoe, W. C., 425, 426, 434, 441, 455, 498, 499
Storm, R. D., 756, 770
Strain, B. A., 330, 370
Stratemeyer, C., 561, 605
Strauss, A. A., 376, 421
Streedbeck, D., 680, 681, 688
Stremel, K., 383, 388, 389, 421, 422, 525, 547
Streng, A., 179, 180, 182, 192
Striefel, S., 238, 250, 251, 252, 263, 738, 747, 748, 763, 764, 773
Stuart, R., 719, 732
Stuckless, E. R., 398, 422, 478, 479, 499
Studdert-Kennedy, M. G., 25, 30
Suchman, E., 140, 184
Sullivan, D., 426, 497
Sullivan, R., 162, 192
Sulzbacher, S. I., 377, 382, 392, 395, 422

Sulzer-Azaroff, B., 229, 260
Surjan, J., 53, 72
Sussman, H. M., 6, 25, 29
Sutherland, G. F., 503, 521, 672, 689
Sutsman, R., 210, 223
Suzuki, T., 163, 192
Svartvik, J., 102, 121

Tait, C., 129, 131, 186
Takei, T., 163, 192
Talkington, L. W., 408, 416, 503, 512, 514, 516, 520, 521, 673, 686
Tanyzer, H. J., 572, 573, 605
Tarjan, G., 44, 67, 662, 663, 689
Task Force on the Mentally Retared and the Deaf, 60, 65, 72
Tavormina, J. B., 715, 732
Taylor, E. M., 40, 72, 110, 122
Taylor, S., 664, 685
Templin, M., 85, 88, 101, 122, 333, 336, 341, 370
Terdal, L., 701, 732
Terrace, H. S., 237, 263
Tervoort, B., 444, 499
Teska, J. A., 401, 417
Thames, A., 426, 497
Tharp, R. G., 669, 689, 696, 720, 732
Thomann, J. B., 739, 766, 771
Thompson, C. L., 668, 686, 698, 701, 727
Thompson, G., 137, 162, 163, 189, 192
Thompson, M., 162, 189
Thompson, R. E., 205, 212, 221
Thomure, F., 297, 323
Thormahlen, P. W., 666, 689
Thornhill, H. L., 670, 689
Tillman, T. W., 313, 324
Tillson, J. K., 197, 222
Timo, V., 55, 71
Tobin, A., 399, 418
Togio, R., 719, 727
Tomblin, B., 799
Topper, S. T., 394, 422, 512, 516, 521

Torr, D. V., 746, 773
Touchette, P., 238, 263
Travis, L. E., 277, 294
Tredgold, A. F., 290, 294
Tredgold, R. F., 290, 294
Truax, C. B., 670, 689
Trybus, R. J., 406, 417
Tucker, B., 713, 728
Turton, L. J., 380, 396, 422
Turvey, M. T., 9, 25
Tweedie, D., 773

van Uden, A., 398, 422
Uihlein, A., 668, 686
Ullman, B. L., 556, 605
Upton, H. H., 762, 773
Utley, J., 162, 192

Vail, J., 516, 521
Vanderheiden, D. H., 412, 422, 503, 521
Vanderheiden, G. C., 614, 647, 762, 772
Van de Riet, V., 46, 69
VanHook, K. E., 503, 504, 516, 521
Van Riper, C., 345, 370, 516, 521
Veit, S. W., 665, 666, 686
Velletri-Glass, A., 543, 547
Vergason, G. A., 290, 294
Vernon, M., 48, 53, 55, 56, 57, 58, 72, 197, 198, 199, 200, 201, 203, 205, 211, 213, 215, 216, 222, 223, 478, 480, 481, 499, 672, 689
Viaille, H. D., 661, 689
Vicker, B., 411, 412, 422, 610, 614, 639, 648
Vigorito, J., 9, 29
Vincent-Smith, L., 389, 393, 414
Vockell, E. L., 407, 422, 674, 689
Vockell, K., 407, 422, 674, 689
Vonkorff, M. R., 671, 688

Wade, G., 174, 191
Walcutt, C. C., 561, 603
Walder, L. O., 707, 715, 728, 732
Waldrop, W. A., 162, 192

Walter, H., 710, 714, 733
Walters, R. H., 243, 260
Wampler, D., 426, 452, 453, 499
Wang, M. C., 256, 261, 263
Warburton, F. W., 574, 605
Warren, R. M., 276, 294
Warren, S. A., 665, 689
Waryas, C., 383, 388, 422
Washington State School for the
　　Deaf, 426, 452, 453, 499
Watson, C. S., 5, 6, 31
Watson, D., 452, 453, 463, 499
Watson, J., 561, 603
Watson, L., 389, 393, 414
Watson, L. S., 679, 681, 690, 698,
　　715, 716, 727, 733
Watson, M. J., 658, 674, 690
Wawrzaszek, F. J., 405, 419
Weaver, R. M., 121, 162, 192
Weaver, W., 97, 121
Webb, C., 62, 72, 172, 192
Weber, B., 62, 72
Weber, B. A., 172, 192
Weber, H. J., 51, 72
Weber, R. M., 562, 605
Webster's New Collegiate
　　Dictionary, 109, 122
Wechsler, D., 208, 223
Wedenberg, E., 51, 66
Wegner, N., 174, 193
Weiner, B. B., 46, 69
Weiner, P. S., 84, 85, 122
Weinrott, M. R., 719, 733
Weisberg, P., 330, 370
Weisinger, M., 174, 191
Weiss, K. L., 399, 400, 401, 405,
　　419
Weld, W., 663, 689
Weller, G. M., 62, 69
Welsh, C., 77, 121
Welsh, R. S., 701, 733
Wender, P. H., 269, 294
Wepman, J. M., 363, 370
Weston, A. J., 338, 358, 370
Wetherby, B., 161, 250, 251, 252,
　　263
Wetzel, R. J., 669, 689, 696, 720,
　　732

Wheelden, J. A., 741, 773
Whetnall, E., 304, 324
White, A. H., 766, 773
White, J. C., Jr., 46, 69
White, T. D., 722, 733
Wickelgren, W., 446, 481, 499
Wiegerink, R., 39, 68, 698, 732
Wiggins, J. E., 656, 665, 667, 684
Wilbur, R. B., 9, 31, 434, 446, 448,
　　449, 466, 472, 473, 475, 483,
　　486, 490, 493, 498, 499
Willard, L., 407, 422
Williams, B. J., 54, 72
Williams, C. F., 662, 689
Williams, D. E., 711, 719, 726
Willis, D., 179, 190
Wills, R. H., 666, 690
Wilson, P. S., 381, 394, 422, 503,
　　504, 512, 516, 521, 672, 690
Wilson, R. A., 299, 310, 321
Wilson, R. G., 560, 561, 601, 604
Wilson, R. H., 299, 310, 323
Wilson, W. R., 137, 163, 166, 185,
　　189, 192
Willson-Morris, M., 246, 248, 249,
　　253, 258, 278, 283, 294, 759,
　　760, 772
Wiltz, N. A., 705, 712, 714, 733
Winchester, R. A., 318, 321
Winitz, H., 17, 31
Wisan, A., 392, 421
Wishart, D. E., 162, 192
Wishik, S. M., 37, 38, 40, 41, 45,
　　51, 59, 67, 72
Withrow, F. B., 173, 192, 738,
　　753, 758, 773
Wolf, J. M., 58, 72, 591, 605
Wolf, M. M., 39, 72, 231, 233,
　　234, 238, 260, 261, 272, 292,
　　330, 370, 392, 420, 697, 698,
　　731, 733
Wolfe, W. G., 179, 192
Wolff, P. H., 330, 370
Wolfensberger, W., 658, 690, 693,
　　729, 733
Wood, M. M., 25, 31
Wood, R., 503, 504, 521

Woodcock, R. W., 158, 186, 363, 367, 574, 584, 585, 586, 589, 590, 591, 601, 605
Wooden, H. Z., 407, 422
Woodward, J. C., Jr., 426, 427, 441, 442, 443, 449, 492, 499, 500
Woodward, M., 488, 500
Wright, J. M., von, 279, 280, 294
Wright, J. W., 113, 115, 119
Wright, M. I., 55, 68
Wuest, R. C., 573, 602
Wyman, R., 760, 773

Yamamoto, K., 172, 193
Yarnall, G. D., 160, 193
Yoder, D. E., 329, 330, 369, 370, 380, 383, 386, 387, 393, 418, 422, 505, 520, 525, 546

Yoder, P., 700, 727
Yonovitz, A., 311, 324
York, R., 252, 260
Young, E. H., 349, 370

Zawolkow, E., 426, 452, 453, 459, 460, 495
Zeaman, D., 174, 193, 375, 422, 674, 690
Zenith Corporation, 137, 193
Ziegler, R. C., 661, 674, 681, 688
Zimmerman, E. H., 234, 263
Zimmerman, J., 234, 263
Zimmerman, V., 670, 687
Zink, D., 51, 72
Zink, G. D., 318, 324
Zlutnick, S., 697, 733
Zurif, E., 543, 546

Subject Index

Action, 657
Adaptive behavior
  Adaptive Behavior Scale, 45
  defined, 45
  influencing, 9
  need for, 3
Alphabets
  Fōnetic English, 574–576
  Initial Teaching, 568–574, 637
  phonemic, 567–577
  phonetic, 568
  Ten-Vowel, 576
  UNIFON, 576–577
Alphabetic systems, 556–578
American Sign Language, 425–426,
    427, 503, 512, 589, 637
  acquisition of, 448–449
  dialectal variation, 449–450
  formational constraints on,
    441–443
  historical changes in, 447–448
  history and prevalence of use,
    430
  juncture and stress in, 438–439
  linguistic rules of, 432–433
  pronouns in, 436–437
  reduplication in, 442
  syntactic structures of, 430–432
  tense formation in, 455
  time and space in, 437–438
  verbs in, 439–441
  wit and poetry in, 444–446
Ameslan, see American Sign
    Language
Aphasia, and hearing loss, 199–200
Aphasoid behavior, in hearing-
    impaired, 199–200
Applied behavior analysis, 233

Articulation, developmental errors
  of, 334–335
Articulation assessment, implications for communicatively
  delayed, 360–366
Articulation learning, components
  of, 344–347
Articulation treatment, 341–359
ASL, see American Sign
    Language
Attending behavior, 377
Audiologic assessment, see
    Hearing assessment
Audiologist, role in total communication program,
  507–508
Audiology programs, administrative factors affecting,
  126–128
Audiometry
  behavior observation, 130–131,
    161
  behaviorial vs. electro-
    physiologic, 159–161
  Békésy, 155
  conditioned orientation reflex
    (response), 163
  distraction, 131–136
  electrocardiograph, 174
  electrodermal response, 171–172
  electroencephalographic evoked
    response, 172–173
  impedance, 166–171
    in pinpointing conductive
      hearing loss, 149
  play, 162
    in screening toddlers, 137
  psychogalvanic skin response,
    171–172

pure tone, 148–155
  in screening preschoolers,
    140–141
respiration, 173–174
speech, 155–159, 166
standard, 161–162
Tangible Reinforcement Operant
  Conditioning (TROCA),
  164
tangibly reinforced, 164–166
tone decay, 155
visual reinforcement of, 162–164
Audiovisual media, in treatment of
  communicatively handi-
  capped, see Media
Auditory trainer
  hard-wire, 311–312
  radio frequency, 312
Auditory training, 180–181
Autism, 38–39
Autistic children
  in Non-SLIP, 542
  responsiveness of, and parents as
    teachers, 696
Auto-Com, 642–645

Baseline observation period, 229
Behavior
  adaptive, see Adaptive behavior
  analyses, components of, 254
    see also Design (of behavior
      analysis)
  basic principles of, 233–242
  extralinguistic, 375–377
  operant, 233
  prelinguistic, 374–375
  prerequisite, 256
  respondent, 233
Behavior measurement, 227–229
  duration measures, 228
  force measures, 229
  interval measures, 228
  latency measures, 229
  percentage measures, 228
  rate measures, 228
  "own-control" model of, 713
  parent training programs to aid
    in, 699–716

Behavior sampling, 83–84
Behavior sequence, 256–258
Behavioral equation, 270–273
Birth weight, as determinant of
  prematurity, 57
Bliss symbols, 592, 613, 635–637,
  639–640
"Brain damage," as neurologic
  myth, 269

Camp Freedom, 702, 723
CAMS Project, 763
Carryover training (phonemes),
  344–345, 356–359
Case, of pronouns, 103
Cerebral palsy, 39–40
  motor disorders associated with,
    40
  and nonvocal communication
    program, 639
Chicago Non-Verbal Examination,
  209
Children's Apperception Test, 214
Chimpanzees, 285, 288, 289
  see also Lana and Sarah
Chinese alphabetic symbols, 556
Cleft palate, and hearing
  impairment, 54
Clothing noise, 306–307
Communication
  as adaptive behavior, 3–4
  described, 11
  environmental influences on,
    8–10
  expressive or physical, 611–614
  interpersonal, 113–117
  maturational influences on, 5–6
  nonvocal (nonoral), 609–647
  requirements of, 12
  stimulus in, 10–11
  total, see Total communication
Communication aids, 625–632
Communication channels
  input, 273–275
  integrative processes, 275–276
  output, 277
Communication systems, nonoral,
  410–412

Complex performances, development of, 252–258
Components, of behavior, 254
Concept formation, 284
Concepts, description of, 107–108
Conditional discrimination, defined, 239
Conditional reinforcer, 240
Confusion matrices, for consonants, 334
Consequence, defined, 234
Consonants, acoustics of, 304
Cued Speech, description and evaluation of, 468–471

Deaf, defined, 48
Deafness
  adventitious, 48
  congenital, 48
  definition of, 48
  prevocational, 50
Deafness management quotient, 399–400
Decibels, defined, 48
Design (of behavior analysis)
  AB design, 229, 713
  multiple baseline design, 231
  reversal design, 230
Developmental adaptation, and communication, 6–8
Developmental disabilities, 36–47
  autism, 38–39
  cerebral palsy, 39–40
  defined, 227
  epilepsy, 41–42
  mental retardation, 42–47
  specific learning disabilities, 38
Developmental Sentence Scoring (DSS), 99–103
Developmentally Disabled Assistance and Bill of Rights Act, 37
DEZ, 441, 444
Diacritical Marking System, 564
Difficult-to-test, 61, 171
Direct selection communication, 621–623

Distance effects, on speech reception, 314
The Downing Readers, 572, 573
Draw-A-Person, 214
Dysarthria, and manual communication, 487
Dyslexia, 37

Early intervention, in sensory impairment, 377–380
Early-to-Read i/t/a Program, 572, 573, 590
Electroacoustic dimensions, 298–305
Electrocochleography, 174–175
Emotional disturbance, among hearing-impaired, 200–201
Encoding, 619–621
  in patterning, 15–19
  influence of, on communication, 8–10, 22–23
  and maturation, 4, 8
Epidemic, contrasted with endemic, 36
Epidemiology
  analytic, 36
  descriptive, 35
Epilepsy, 41–42
  prevalence of, 41
Equivalence, in communication, 13
Errorless discrimination, 236–237
Erythroblastosis fetalis, 56
Extralinguistic behavior, 375–377

Feedback, role of, in communication, 10
Feedback (sensory)
  capacity for, in hearing-impaired child, 21
  capacity for, in mentally retarded, 21
  channels of, 21
  external, 19–21
  influence of, 21
  internal, 19–21
Fingerspelling, 18
  description and evaluation of, 465-468

Fōnetic English, *see* Alphabets
Frequency range, 302–305
Frequency response, defined and
    described, 301–302
Functional equivalence, 245,
    250–252

Gain, defined and described,
    299–300
Gender, distinction of, 104
Generalization, in stimulus control,
    239–239
Generalized imitation, 243–244
Genetics, and hearing loss, 197–198
Gestures, as communication, 19
Goodenough Draw-A-Man Test,
    210
Grace Arthur Performance Scale,
    210
Grammar, in language assessment,
    78–80
Graphic systems
    defined, 552
    history of, 554–556
Greek alphabet, 556

Hearing aids
    BICROS, 309
    binaural, 309–311
    body-worn, 305–307
    bone conduction, 307–308
    CROS, 308–309
    ear-level, 308
    inspections of, 318–320
    malfunctions of, 317–318
    orientation, 409–410
    preventive maintenance, 508
    selection and orientation,
        177–179
    acoustic and environmental
        factors affecting, 143
    audiometric calibration checks
        in, 143
    audiometric factors affecting, 143
    developmental evaluation of
        child before, 144
    infant, 128–137

interdisciplinary input in,
    141–143
preschool, 140–141
response criteria in, 144–145
toddler, 137–140
Hearing impaired
    early amplification for, 403–404
    early detection of, 123–140, 403
    early intervention programs for,
        379
    importance of visual cues to, 23
    integration of, 404–405
    language program for, 397–410
    memory ability of, 446
    "model home" approach for,
        674
    psychologic examination of,
        202–220
Hearing-impaired retarded, and
        supportive personnel, *see*
        Supportive personnel
Hearing impairment
    classifying, 49
    and cleft palate, 54
    and congenital syphilis, 58
    definitions of, 47
    and heredity, 52–54
    and measles, 58
    and meningitis, 57–58
    and mental retardation, 60–61
    and mumps, 58
    and prematurity, 56–57
    prevalence rates of, 49, 51
    and Rh factor, 56
    and rubella, 54–55
    and scarlet fever, 58
    types
        conductive loss, 48
        sensorineural, 48
    and whooping cough, 58
Hearing loss
    bilateral, 154
    causes of, 197–198
    conductive
        causes of, 149
        defined, 149
    genetic causes, 197–198
    high risk infants for, 129–130

mixed, defined, 151
sensorineural
    causes of, 152–153
    defined, 149
unilateral, 154
Heredity, and hearing impairment,
    52–54
Hiragana, 579, 581
Hiskey-Nebraska Test of Learning
    Aptitude, 209
H. T. P. Technique, 215
Hz, defined, 48

Iconicity, of American Sign
    Language, 432–433
Illinois Test of Psycholinguistic
    Abilities (ITPA), 99–103,
    268, 278, 279
Imitation, in language intervention,
    392
Incidence, defined, 36
Information, defined, 11
Initial Teaching Alphabet, see
    Alphabets
Institutionalized retarded, language
    program for, 391
Integrative processes, 288–290
Intelligibility
    development of, in communi-
        catively delayed, 332–334
    phoneme distribution in,
        336–338
Intensity distortion, described, 22
Intermittent reinforcement, 240
Interpersonal communication,
    113–117
Interval recording, described, 228
Interval schedules, 240-241
Intervention strategies, for
    mentally retarded, 7
i.t.a., see Alphabets
ITPA, 110–112

Kanji, 579
Katakana, 579, 581

Lana, 594

Language
    basic criteria of, 427-430
    components of, 429
    comprehension and expression,
        77–78
    concepts, 80–81
    definition of, 76
displacement in, 429
    grammatical assessment of,
        78–80
    interpersonal, 81–82
    learning, 429
    morphology of, 78–79
    oral, prerequisites to, 328–329
    units of, 105
    use, 428-429
    vocabulary, 80–81
Language acquisition, 7, 105, 374
    early learning in, 476–478
    English syntax in, 472–476
    nonspecial response mode in,
        285–286
Language assessment, 76–82,
    278–279
    basis of, 76
    comprehension and expression
        in, 77–78
    formal methods, 113–115
    grammar in, 78–80
    nonstandardized, 91
    research-derived methods,
        115–117
Language-delayed child, 379
Language disorder, importance of
    defining, 93
Language intervention
    developmental approaches to,
        383–390
    manual approaches to, 393–395
    with mentally retarded, 382–397
    nondevelopmental approaches to,
        390-393
    parent involvement in, 395–397,
        401-403
    peer involvement in, 395-397
Language Master, 757–758
Language model, Osgood's,
    277–278

Language problems
  described, 76
  identification of, 92–95
  screening of, 92–95
  for hearing impaired, 397–410
  for severely retarded, 391
Language tests
  age scores, 89
  norms, 85–86
  objectivity of, 84–85
  percentage scores, 89
  reliability, 86–87
  standardization of, 84–85
  standard score, 90
  use of, 82–92
  validity, 87–89
Language training program, goals
    for, 380–382
Learning, functional analysis of,
    270-273
"Learning deficiencies," definition
    and usage of, 267–268
Learning hierarchy, defined, 253
Leiter International Performance
    Scale, 208–209
Let's Read, 559–560, 561
Linguistics of Visual English, 426
Lipreading, see Speechreading
Logographic systems, 582-599

Make-A-Picture-Story Test, 215
Manual communication
  linguistics of, 450–471
  and memory development,
    484–485
  and memory for English,
    481–484
  and memory and reading, 486
  perception in, 485–486
  and psychosocial development,
    479–481
  relationship to English, 452–456
  and speech skills, 478–479
  tense formation in, 452–456
  types of, 425–426
Manual English
  linguistics of, 462–463

tense formation in, 455
Manual English (Improved), tense
    formation in, 455–456
Masking, described, 22
Match-to-sample, 245–246
Match-to-sample task, in Non-
    SLIP, 531
Maturation
  and environment, 4
  influences on communication,
    5–6
Measles, and hearing impairment,
    58
Media
  audiovisual
    advantages of, 737–738
    definition of, 737
    limitations of, 738–739
    selection of, 739
  delayed video feedback in
    language therapy, 746–747
  films
    in communication assessment,
    752
    as intervention aids, 753–754
    in training teachers and
    parents, 754
  puppets, in therapy, 744
  teaching machines
    in communication assessment,
    755-756
    in intervention programs,
    756–762
  television
    as assessment device, 740–742
    dual audio, as intervention aid,
    745–746
    instant replay in intervention,
    743
    in live self-observation,
    743–744
    in reading programs, 746
    and stimulation, 747–748
    uses with hearing-impaired,
    742–743
  two-way telecommunication in
    home programs, 745

videotapes
  in behavior response
    audiometry, 740
  as language intervention aids,
    744–745
  in training supportive
    personnel, 748–749
Media centers, 767
Media training, through the READ
    Project, 708–712, 717
Memory, modification of, 290–291
Meningitis, and hearing impair-
    ment, 57–58
Mental retardation
  classification system, 43
  definitions of, 42
  and delayed speech, 59
  and ethnic group, 46–47
  and hearing impairment, 60–61,
    199
  prevalence of, 45–46
  and rubella, 55
  and socioeconomic status, 46
  and speech disorders, 59–60
Mentally retarded
  hearing-impaired, sign language
    system for, 512–513
  language intervention with,
    382–397
  in Non-SLIP training, 538, 542
  symbol communication for,
    639–642
Merrill Linguistic Readers, 574
Merrill Linguistic Reading
    Program, 560–561
Merrill-Palmer Scale of Mental
    Tests, 210
Miami Linguistic Readers, 561–562
Minnesota Early Language
    Development Sequence,
    589–590
MIRV system, 760–761
Morpheme training, 244
Morphology, 78–79
Motor disorders, associated with
    cerebral palsy, 40
Movement, as communication, 19
MPO, 300–301

Mr. Symbol Man, 640
Multiply handicapped, and learning
    deficiencies, 268
Multiply handicapped hearing
    impaired, programs for,
    405–410
Mumps, and hearing impairment,
    58

Negative reinforcement, 234
Noise, 313–314
  defined, 22
Nonalphabetic system, defined, 552
Nonoral physically handicapped,
    communication systems for,
    410–412
Non-SLIP, 13, 290–291, 597–598
  defined, 529
  general progress in, 539–541
  labeling training in, 531–533
  major role of, 529
  major subprograms of, summary
    of, 535
  materials necessary for, 530
  object of preposition training,
    534
  preposition training, 534–535
  recommended use of, 541–543
  sequence training in, 530–531
  subject noun training in, 533
  subjects for, 538–539
  verb training in, 533–534
Non-Speech Language Acquisition
    Program, see Non-SLIP
Normalization, defined, 693
Number, of nouns, 103–104

Ontario School Ability Examina-
    tion, 209
Operant behavior, 233
Oral apraxia, and manual
    communication, 487
ORIENTATION, 441, 444
Osgood's language model, 277–278
Output, defined and described,
    300–301

Paget-Gorman Sign System, 426
Paget-Gorman Systematic Sign
    linguistics of, 458-459
    tense formation in, 455
Paired associate training, 537
PAL System, 758
Parent counseling, in aural
        habilitation, 182-183
Parent involvement, in intervention
        strategy, 379
Parent training
    center-based, 699-701
    films in, 754
    group, 706-708
    home-based, 703-705
    incentives, 721-724
    media programs for, 763-764
    outcome of, 710-716
    participation in, by social level,
        717-719
    school-home, 701-703
    simulated home, 705-706
Parents (of developmentally
        disabled)
    attitude of, and progress of child,
        695
    roles and responsibilities of,
        694-696
    as teachers, 695, 696-698
Parsons Language Sample, 83
Patterning
    encoding and transmission in,
        15-19, 25
    linguistic
        phonemic, 16-17
        syntactic, 17-18
        vocal, 16
    nonverbal
        fingerspelling and signing, 18
        gestures, 19
        movement or posture, 19
        pointing, 18
        writing, 18
    reception and decoding of, 23-28
Peabody Rebus Reading Program,
        586-589
Perseveration, described, 23
Phenylketonuria, 128

Phoneme contrast development,
        theoretical models of,
        335-336
Phonemes, defined, 331
Phonemic patterning, 16-17
Phonetically balanced words, 157
Phonologic goals, for severely
        handicapped, 338-341
Phonotypy, 569-570
Piaget, theory of cognitive
        development, 7
Piagetian theory, 374
Pictographs, 554, 583
Pidgin language, defined, 426-427
Pointing, 18
Positive reinforcement, 234
Postnatal infections, and hearing
        impairment, 57-58
Posture, as communication, 19
Prelinguistic behavior, 374-375
"Premackese," 594
Prematurity
    factors associated with, 57
    and hearing impairment, 56-57
Prerequisite behavior, 256
Prevalence, defined, 36
Progressive Matrices, 209
Project LIFE, 674, 758
Pronouns
    case of, 103
    determiner-nominal distinction
        of, 104
    gender of, 104
    number distinctions of, 103-104
Psychodiagnostics
    with hearing-impaired, general
        principles of, 204-206
    in schools, 220-221
Psycholinguistic Color System,
        562-563
Psychologic examination, of
        mentally retarded and
        multiply handicapped
        hearing-impaired, 202-220
Punishment, defined, 234
Pure tone audiometer, in determin-
        ing hearing loss, 48

Randall's Island Performance
Tests, 210
Ratio schedules, 240–241
READ Project, 676, 708–710, 711,
712, 717
Reading
aided by television, 746
functional analysis of, 280–284
Rebus, 583–591
Rebus principle, 554, 579
The Rebus Reading Series,
584–585
Rebus systems, 583–591
Receptive language training, 250
Recruitment, defined, 154
Reference thresholds, developed by
ASA, ANSI, and ISO,
48–49
Reinforcement, 234–235
Reinforcement contingencies,
239–242
conditional reinforcer, 240
intermittent reinforcement, 240
interval schedules, 240–241
ratio schedules, 240–241
Respondent behavior, 233
Response class, 242, 243–245
Response development (phones),
344
procedures in, 349–356
Response proclivity, 5–6
Reverberation, 313–314
Rh factor, and hearing impairment,
56
Rochester method, 465, 467
Role-taking, 115–116
Rorschach Ink Blot Test, 214
Rotter Incomplete Sentences
Blank, 215
Rubella
and hearing impairment, 54–55
and lowered intelligence, 55
and mental retardation, 55

Sarah, 12, 287, 289, 525–527, 594
Scanning, 615–619
Scarlet fever, and hearing impair-
ment, 58

SEE, *see* Signing Exact English
Seeing Essential English, 426
Seizures, febrile, 41
Sensory capability, 5, 6
Siblings (of developmentally
disabled), programs for,
719–720
SIG, 441, 444
Siglish, 426
Sign language, teaching method for,
513–514
Sign space, 435–436
Signed English, 426, 594–597
linguistics of, 463–465
tense formation in, 455
in total communication program,
513, 514
Signing, 18
Signing Exact English, 426
linguistics of, 459–462
tense formation in, 455
Signs, two-handed, 442–443
Simultaneous communication, 504
Sound targets, 351–355
Sound treatment, of rooms,
314–315
Special Experience Room, 768
Specific learning disabilities, 38
Speech, as adaptive behavior, 17
Speech aids, 355
Speech audiometry, 155–159
Speech discrimination, in assessing
communicative abilities,
157–158
Speech disorders, and mental
retardation, 59–60
Speech perception, 6
Speech sample, as phonologic test,
361-362
Speech signals, 304
Speechreading, 181–182, 213
*Standards for Residential Facilities
for the Mentally Retarded,*
511
Stimulus
defined, 10
role of, in communication, 10–11
Stimulus class, 242, 245–250

Stimulus control, 235–239
Stimulus equivalence, 245
Stimulus fading, 237–238
Stimulus pattern equivalency,
    11–14
Stimulus shaping, 237–238
Supportive personnel
  acceptance by professionals,
      667–668
  attendants
    attitudes of, 663–665
    and innovative programming,
        664
  attitude changes, through media,
      748–749
  background characteristics of,
      661–663
  benefits of
    to handicapped, 668–671
    to professionals, 668
    to selves, 668
  coordination of, 658–660
  direct-care staff (attendants),
      655–656
  with hearing-impaired retarded
    in communication program-
        ming, 671–672
    in hearing aid care and use,
        671
    in using sign language, 672
  motivating, 680–681
  "new careers" concept and,
      656–657
  organization of
    medical model, 660
    team model, 660–661
  supervising, 679–681
  teacher aides, 656
  training of, 674-679
    media programs for, 763–764
  volunteers
    citizen advocate, 658
    Domestic Volunteer Service
        Act, 657
    Foster Grandparent program,
        657
    SWEAT program, 657

Syllabary
  Cherokee, 579, 580
  Gleitman and Rozin, 579–580,
      582
  Japanese, 579, 581
  nonpictographic, 552
  pictographic, 552
Syllabic systems, 579–580
Symbol Accentuation, 564–566
Syntactic patterning, 17–18
Syntax, 79–80
  assessment of, 95–104
  model of, 99–100
  as redundancy, 97–98
  as rules, 96–97
  as semantic relationships, 98
Syphilis, congenital, and hearing
      impairment, 58

TAB, 441, 444
"Talking" typewriter, 761
Target behaviors, 256–258
Task analysis
  in complex performances,
      252–258
  defined, 253
Ten-Vowel Alphabet, *see*
      Alphabets
Test of Auditory Comprehension
      of Language (TACL),
      99–103
Test for Preschool Deaf Children
      (Dr. Alathena Smith's), 211
Tests (psychologic)
  achievement, 213
  aptitude, 217–218
  for brain damage, 212
  of communication skills,
      213–217
  of intelligence, 206–207
  personality, 207–212
Thematic Apperception Test, 214
Therapy, speech and language, 176
T. O., *see* Traditional Orthography
Total communication
  defined, 503
  importance of, 504–505

24-hour approach to, 505–518
administrative considerations,
506–507
clients for, 508–509
living area in, 511–514
sample schedule for, 515
staff selection, 509–510
staff training, 510–511
Touchette procedure, 238
Traditional orthography, 551, 552,
557–566, 633–634
controlled, 552, 557–562
elaborated, 552, 562–566
Transfer
in learning, 279–280
of response mode, in language
acquisition, 286–287
Transmission, in patterning, 15–19
Tympanometry, 167–169
Type-token ratio, in speech, 229

UNIFON, *see* Alphabets

Video Articulator, 756–757
Vineland Social Maturity Scale,
211
Visible Speech Translator, 756
VISTA, 657
Visual/auditory reception, and
comprehension, 316–317

Visual defects, among hearing-
impaired, 201
Vocabulary, development of,
105–107
Vocabulary skills
assessment of, 109–113
specific, assessment of, 111–113
Peabody Picture Vocabulary
Test, 109, 110, 111–113
standardized, 109
Vocal patterning, 16
Vocalization, development of,
329–331
Vowels, acoustics of, 304

Weschler Performance Scale, 216
Weschler Performance Scale for
Adults, evaluation of, 208
Weschler Performance Scale for
Children, evaluation of, 208
Weschler Preschool and Primary
Scale of Intelligence
Performance Subtests, 208
Whooping cough, and hearing
impairment, 58
Wisconsin General Test Apparatus,
674
Words in Color, 563
Writing, 18

Y cord arrangement (of hearing
aids), 307